CARDIOLOGY
— IN AIDS —

Edited by
Steven E. Lipshultz, M.D.

Professor of Pediatrics
University of Rochester School of Medicine and Dentistry

Chief, Division of Pediatric Cardiology
Children's Hospital at Strong and University of Rochester Medical Center
Rochester, NY

Associate in Cardiology
Children's Hospital
Boston, MA

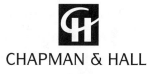

CHAPMAN & HALL

I(T)P® International Thomson Publishing
Thomson Science

New York • Albany • Bonn • Boston • Cincinnati • Detroit • London • Madrid • Melbourne
Mexico City • Pacific Grove • Paris • San Francisco • Singapore • Tokyo • Toronto • Washington

JOIN US ON THE INTERNET
WWW: http://www.thomson.com
EMAIL: findit@kiosk.thomson.com

Point your browser to: **http://www.chaphall.com** or
http://www.thomson.com/chaphall/med.html for Medicine

A service of **I** (**T**) **P**®

Cover Design: Andrea Meyer, Emdash, Inc.

Copyright © 1998
Chapman & Hall

Printed in the United States of America

For more information, contact:

Chapman & Hall
115 Fifth Avenue
New York, NY 10003

Chapman & Hall
2-6 Boundary Row
London SE1 8HN
England

Thomas Nelson Australia
102 Dodds Street
South Melbourne, 3205
Victoria, Australia

Chapman & Hall GmbH
Postfach 100 263
D-69442 Weinheim
Germany

International Thomson Editores
Campos Eliseos 385, Piso 7
Col. Polanco
11560 Mexico D.F.
Mexico

International Thomson Publishing-Japan
Hirakawacho-cho Kyowa Building, 3F
1-2-1 Hirakawacho-cho
Chiyoda-ku, 102 Tokyo
Japan

International Thomson Publishing Asia
221 Henderson Road #05-10
Henderson Building
Singapore 0315

1 2 3 4 5 6 7 8 9 10 XXX 01 00 99 98

Library of Congress Cataloging-in-Publication Data

Cardiology in AIDS / edited by Steven E. Lipshultz.
     p.   cm.
Includes bibliographical references and index.
ISBN 0-412-08861-4
1. Cardiovascular system—Diseases. 2. AIDS (Disease)—Complications. I. Lipshultz, Steven E.,
1954-   . [DNLM: 1. Acquired Immunodeficiency Syndrome—complications. 2. HIV Infections—complications. 3. Cardiovascular Diseases—etiology. 4. Cardiovascular Diseases—virology.
WC 503.5 C267 1998]   RC669 C274   1998
616.1—dc21
DNLM/DLC
for Library of Congress   97-42609
                                      CIP

British Library Cataloguing in Publication Data available

To order this or any other Chapman & Hall book, please contact **International Thomson Publishing, 7625 Empire Drive, Florence, KY 41042.** Phone: (606) 525-6600 or 1-800-842-3636. Fax: (606) 525-7778, e-mail: order@chaphall.com.

For a complete listing of Chapman & Hall's titles, send your requests to **Chapman & Hall, Dept. BC, 115 Fifth Avenue, New York, NY 10003.**

Contents

Part 3   Pathogenesis

Preface

HIV infection has had a global impact on the health of people and on our understanding of basic concepts of disease. HIV infection has major consequences for the cardiovascular system and has become one of the leading causes of acquired heart disease. *Cardiology in AIDS* was written to inform the cardiology community about HIV cardiovascular-related complications and to provide primary care providers and infectious and immunologic colleagues with information about the cardiologic aspects of HIV infection. This is an area where with proper testing, early cardiac abnormalities can be detected and treatments are often effective. It is also an area where a substantial amount of clinically occult disease occurs that is easily attributed to other organ systems. The overall goals of this book are to improve the care of HIV-infected patients and their families and to stimulate additional investigations into the causes and treatments of HIV-associated cardiovascular disease. This book is dedicated to the many patients and families affected by this infection as well as to their care providers.

Having been privileged to be a care provider in this field, I have witnessed this epidemic and have watched this infection go from a rapidly fatal illness to a chronic illness. I hope to witness it become an eradicated illness. Along those lines, this book is also dedicated to Dr. Constance Weinstein of the National Heart, Lung, and Blood Institute (NHLBI) of the National Institutes of Health (NIH). Dr. Weinstein was among the leaders within the NIH to champion the cause of pushing for further investigations on cardiovascular disease in children and adults with HIV infection. In fact, most of the chapters in this book were completed with the support of NIH funds that specifically arose out of programs Dr. Weinstein was instrumental in bringing to the investigative arena. On the occasion of Dr. Weinstein's retirement, this book is also dedicated to her deep convictions and strong leadership in this field.

For the past nine years I have been privileged to have been a member of the P^2C^2 study group. This NHLBI multicenter study of heart and lung complications in children of HIV-infected mothers has demonstrated how NIH-sponsored research can not only lead to major scientific advances in understanding disease, but can also significantly improve patient health and functioning as illustrated by Chapter 30. On this the 50th anniversary of the NHLBI, this study represents how both research and patient care objectives can be met jointly. I would like to thank the many dedicated care providers, staff, and patients involved with this study, all of whom have been both my collaborators and teachers. On Kenneth McIntosh, Chief of Infectious

Diseases at Boston Children's Hospital, and the Children's Hospital AIDS program deserve special thanks.

I would like to acknowledge a number of other people who have helped make this book possible. I am grateful to the contributing authors of the various chapters for providing outstanding and current information concerning this complex field. I am also grateful to Rachel Rossetti for her dedication and hard work in coordinating this book's production and to Christine Messere and Drs. Nandini Moorthy and Elizabeth Bancroft, all of whom helped coordinate production of this book. Special thanks go to Mr. Jonathan Harrington for providing medical editing and Emily Flynn Macintosh for providing some of the graphics and illustrations seen throughout this book. I would also like to acknowledge Chapman and Hall, in particular, Lauren Enck and Catherine Felgar for their support and encouragement. Finally, the patience and support from my family in this project has been invaluable.

It is my hope that this book will enable clinicians and scientists to better understand this field and that it will ultimately lead to improved care of infected patients and their families.

Steven E. Lipshultz, M.D.

Contributors

Inas Al-Attar, M.D.
Former Fellow in Pediatric Infectious Diseases
Children's Hospital
Boston, MA
Chairperson of the Department of Pediatrics
Princeton Community Hospital
Infectious Diseases Consultant
Princeton, WV

Roxellen Auletto, R.N.
Department of Cardiology
Children's Hospital
Boston, MA

Anne-Marie Boller, M.A.
Department of Cardiology
Children's Hospital
Boston, MA

Nicholas A. Boon, M.D., F.R.C.P.
Consultant Cardiologist
Department of Cardiology
Royal Infirmary
Edinburgh, Scotland
United Kingdom

J. Timothy Bricker, M.D.
Professor and Chief
The Lillie Frank Abercrombie Section of
    Cardiology
Department of Pediatrics
Baylor College of Medicine
Chief of Cardiology
Texas Children's Hospital
Chief of Pediatric Cardiology
Texas Heart Institute
Houston, TX

Stephen Chanock, M.D.
Senior Staff Fellow
Pediatric Oncology Branch
National Cancer Institute
Bethesda, MD

Melvin D. Cheitlin, M.D.
Emeritus Professor of Medicine
University of California, San Francisco
Former Chief of Cardiology at San Francisco
    General Hospital
San Francisco, CA

Steven D. Colan, M.D.
Associate Professor of Pediatrics
Harvard Medical School
Senior Associate in Cardiology
Director, Cardiac Noninvasive Lab
Children's Hospital
Boston, MA

Peter F. Currie, M.B., Ch.B., M.R.C.P. (UK)
British Heart Foundation
Junior Research Fellow
Department of Cardiology
Royal Infirmary
Edinburgh, Scotland
United Kingdom

Rachel Diness, M.S.W., L.C.S.W.
Social Worker
Heart/Lung Study
Department of Cardiology, AIDS Program
Children's Hospital
Boston, MA

Quentin Eichbaum, Ph.D.
Fellow in the Department of Infectious Diseases
Children's Hospital
Boston, MA

Judith Epstein, M.D.
Fellow, Division of Infectious Diseases
Children's Hospital
Boston, MA

Vernat Exil, M.D., F.A.A.P.
Fellow of Pediatric Cardiology
Washington University School of Medicine
Robert Wood Johnson Scholar
St. Louis Children's Hospital
St. Louis, MO

Roy Freeman, M.D.
Director, Autonomic and Peripheral Nerve
   Laboratory
Department of Neurology
Beth Israel Deaconness Medical Center
Boston, MA

Alistair I. Fyfe, M.D., Ph.D.
Assistant Professor of Medicine in Cardiology
UCLA
Los Angeles, CA

Amy L. Giantris
Department of Cardiology
Children's Hospital
Boston, MA

Nina Greenbaum, M.P.H., C.H.E.S
Department of Cardiology
Children's Hospital
Boston, MA

Michelle A. Grenier, M.D.
Assistant Professor of Pediatric Cardiology
University of Rochester School of Medicine and
   Dentistry
Rochester, NY

Lisa K. Hornberger, M.D.
Assistant Professor of Pediatrics
Director, Fetal Cardiac Program
University of Toronto
The Hospital for Sick Children
Toronto, Ontario

Judith Hsia, M.D.
Associate Professor of Medicine
Division of Cardiology
George Washington University Medical Center
Washington, D.C.

Janice M. Hunter, R.N., M.S.
Division of Respiratory Diseases
Children's Hospital
Boston, MA

Hal B. Jenson, M.D.
Professor, Departments of Pediatrics and of
   Microbiology
Chief, Pediatric Infectious Diseases
University of Texas Health Science Center
San Antonio, TX

Vijay V. Joshi, M.D.
Director of Pediatric Pathology
Department of Pathology and Laboratory
  Medicine
Connecticut Children's Medical Center and
  Hartford Hospital
Hartford, CT

Samuel Kaplan, M.D.
Professor of Pediatric Cardiology
Kurlin Heart Center
Department of Pediatric Cardiology
UCLA Medical Center
Los Angeles, CA

Nancy Karthas, R.N., M.S., P.N.P.
Clinical HIV Coordinator
Children's Hospital
Boston, MA

Carol Kasten-Sportès, M.D.
Fellow, Division of Pediatric Genetics
University of Michigan Medical Center
Ann Arbor, MI

Wyman Lai, M.D., M.P.H.
Assistant Professor of Pediatrics
Division of Pediatric Cardiology
Mount Sinai Medical Center
New York, NY

Robert J. Lederman, M.D.
Fellow in Cardiology
University of California, San Francisco
San Francisco, CA

Karen Lewis, R.N., M.P.H.
Pediatric Pulmonary Division
Department of Pediatrics
Boston Medical Center
Boston, MA

William Lewis, M.D.
Professor and Director of Cardiovascular
  Pathology
Department of Pathology and Laboratory
  Medicine
University of Cincinnati College of Medicine
Cincinnati, OH

Steven E. Lipshultz, M.D.
Professor of Pediatrics
University of Rochester School of Medicine
  and Dentistry
Chief, Division of Pediatric Cardiology
Children's Hospital at Strong and
  University of Rochester Medical Center
Rochester, NY
Associate in Cardiology
Children's Hospital
Boston, MA

Daniel R. Lucey, M.D., M.P.H.
Medical Officer
Office of Vaccines Research and Review
Food and Drug Administration
Rockville, MD

Jonathan M. Mann, M.D., M.P.H.
Francois-Xavier Bagnoud Professor of Health
  and Human Rights
Professor of Epidemiology and International
  Health
Harvard School of Public Health
Boston, MA

Tracie L. Miller, M.D.
Associate Professor of Pediatrics
Division of Pediatric Gastroenterology and
  Nutrition
University of Rochester Medical Center
Rochester, NY

L. Nandini Moorthy, M.B.B.S., M.D.
Pediatric Resident
Department of Pediatrics
UNC Hospital
Chapel Hill, NC

Edward O'Rourke, M.D.
Medical Director of Infection Control
Children's Hospital
Assistant Professor of Pediatrics
Harvard Medical School
Boston, MA

E. John Orav, Ph.D.
Associate Professor of Medicine (Biostatistics)
Harvard Medical School
Section of Clinical Epidemiology
Division of General Internal Medicine
Brigham and Women's Hospital
Boston, MA

Brad H. Pollock, M.P.H., Ph.D.
Associate Professor and Director, Division of
    Epidemiology
Department of Health Policy and Epidemiology
University of Florida College of Medicine
Gainesville, FL

Sheryl Ross, R.N.
Pediatric Pulmonary Division
Department of Pediatrics
Boston Medical Center
Boston, MA

Arwa Saidi, M.B., B.Ch.
Fellow in Pediatric Cardiology
Texas Children's Hospital
Houston, TX

J. Philip Saul, M.D.
Associate Professor
Department of Pediatrics
Division of Health Sciences and Technology
Children's Hospital
Harvard Medical School
Boston, MA

Richard P. Shannon, M.D.
Claude R. Joyner Professor of Medicine
Chairman, Department of Medicine
Allegheny General Hospital
Pittsburgh, PA

Thomas J. Starc, M.D.
Associate Clinical Professor of Pediatrics
Babies & Children's Hospital
Columbia Presbyterian Medical Center
New York, NY

Suzanne Steinbach, M.D.
Assistant Professor in Pediatrics
Boston University School of Medicine
Boston, MA

Daniel Tarantola, M.D.
Director, International AIDS Program
Francois-Xavier Bagnoud Center for Health and
    Human Rights
Lecturer in Population and International Health
Harvard School of Public Health
Boston, MA

Jeffrey A. Towbin, M.D.
Associate Professor of Pediatrics (Cardiology)
    and Molecular and Human Genetics
Baylor College of Medicine
Director, Phoebe Willingham Muzzy Pediatric
    Molecular Cardiology Laboratory
Baylor College of Medicine, Texas Children's
    Hospital
Texas Children's Hospital Foundation
Chair of Pediatric Cardiac Research
Houston, TX

Constance Weinstein, Ph.D.
Leader, Congenital and Infectious Research
    Group
Division of Heart and Vascular Diseases
National Heart, Lung, and Blood Institute
National Institutes of Health
Bethesda, MD

Ms. Barrie Wing
Fall River, MA

Julia C. L. Wong, M.B.B.S., M.Med.
Senior Lecturer
Department of Pediatrics
National University of Singapore
Pediatric Cardiologist and Senior Registrar
National University Hospital
Republic of Singapore

Introduction

To my knowledge, this is the first book to be written on HIV infection and AIDS that focuses on vascular and cardiac complications. It is a rich compendium of clinical experience and information that have been reported in a wide diversity of professional journals. In an effort to be as up-to-date as possible, the editor included some data that had not yet been published when the book went to press. Most of the authors have treated AIDS patients or have conducted HIV-related research on disorders of the cardiovascular system and have given much thought to the complex questions of etiology and pathology. The conviction that physicians should be aware of the possibility that some of a patient's symptoms may relate to cardiovascular abnormalities has been the impetus for the production of this book. Physicians who treat AIDS patients are overwhelmingly busy, and it is a tribute to their dedication that these authors took precious personal time to prepare their contributions.

In the early years of the AIDS epidemic periodic reports appeared in the literature on cardiovascular involvement in the syndrome, but the possibility of AIDS patients needing cardiac care seemed remote because death occurred too soon from other causes. However, improvements in therapy allowed patients to live longer, and the potential for cardiovascular complications became greater. The National Heart, Lung, and Blood Institute, recognizing this potential, established a study of AIDS-associated heart disease in adults in 1987 and a study of the pediatric and pulmonary complications of AIDS in 1988. These studies confirmed the early reports of cardiac complications of AIDS and provided physicians treating HIV-infected patients with a clear rationale to monitor cardiac status.

Thus, heart and vascular system are added to the long list of organs and systems affected by HIV infection. In this context, the information on epidemiology creates an alarming picture of the number of persons who will be infected with HIV by the year 2000. These numbers will affect patient volume in a variety of specialties, including cardiology, and they foretell a burden of clinical care that health systems around the world may be inadequate to bear. The information in Chapters 3 to 9 and 29 seems to indicate that the impact in terms of cardiovascular disease will fall most heavily on pediatric cardiologists unless the rate of vertical transmission of HIV can be dramatically reduced.

As the reader will appreciate, the etiology of cardiovascular complications in HIV-infected patients is poorly understood because, in addition to lifestyle factors, there are many potential mechanisms that could result in dysfunction and disease of the cardiovascular system. The reader should pay close attention to Chapter 1 because it provides the background for nearly every chapter that follows. The life cycle of the virus, its subtypes, and the pathogenesis of HIV disease, must be understood in order to develop hypotheses concerning dysfunction and disease of the cardiovascular system in HIV-infected patients. With each succeeding chapter, it becomes increasingly clear that vascular and cardiac complications may derive from dysfunction and disease of other organs and systems and from intercurrent illnesses. For example, Chapter 11 not only describes a diverse array of lung disorders and diseases but also includes an important discussion on the impact of lung impairment on cardiac function, especially how respiratory symptoms may obscure cardiac symptoms. Chapter 12 describes a variety of vascular lesions that may cause damage to other organs, including the heart. The existence of these lesions may go unrecognized until autopsy.

Since myocarditis and cardiomyopathy are the most common cardiac diseases associated with HIV infection, it is appropriate that a chapter be devoted to the defining features of these diseases in HIV-negative as well as HIV-positive patients. In both sets of patients, it is a common observation that myocarditis and/or dilated cardiomyopathy do not develop in all individuals infected with cardiotropic viruses. This raises the question of genetic susceptibility and, in the case of HIV infection, the relation of the clade to cardiovascular susceptibility as well as the role of opportunistic infections.

The diagnosis and appropriate treatment of cardiovascular complications are mentioned in several chapters. For the physician, Chapters 24 and 25 provide comprehensive overviews of treatment strategies and clinical experience, while Chapter 5 provides a carefully considered discussion of the role of exercise in the regimen of treatment for HIV-infected patients both with and without cardiac complications. However, clinical care does not reside solely with the physician. Nurses, social workers, psychologists, and other professionals are involved. Complicating factors include the varying socioeconomic status of patients, their lifestyles, and the wide age range from infancy to old age, as well as the trauma suffered by families of many of the patients. Chapter 27 describes in practical detail the issues that can be approached most sensitively by a multidisciplinary team approach.

Chapter 30 tells the poignant story of a mother with an HIV-infected infant. Not only does it encompass the pain and suffering of the patient, but it also illustrates the consequences within the family. Furthermore, as the story progresses, one is amazed at the large number of physicians and nurses involved in optimal care of a single patient's illness. Some of the health-care workers treated the patient before her HIV status was known. Thus, Chapter 28 is extremely important, elaborating as it does on the need for infection control and careful adherence to recommended precautions on the part of health-care workers.

In summary, this book contains much knowledge gathered in one place for the first time and from that point of view should greatly facilitate the search for information by those who treat patients and those who are actively involved in research or are planning a research program on the cardiovascular complications of AIDS.

Constance Weinstein, Ph.D.

Part 1
Overview

1

HIV Infection and AIDS

Daniel R. Lucey, M.D., M.P.H., and Stephen Chanock, M.D.

From 1981 to 1996 more than 500,000 people in the United States were diagnosed with the acquired immunodeficiency syndrome (AIDS). This chapter addresses the current understanding of the classification of human immunodeficiency virus (HIV) as well as recent trends in the epidemiology of the HIV infection, particularly as they relate to the virology and transmission of the virus. The human immunodeficiency viruses type 1 and type 2 (HIV-1 and HIV-2) that cause AIDS can be distinguished from other known and putative human retroviruses by clinical assays and by more sophisticated sequence analysis. We discuss the viral life cycle of HIV and the evolution of both nomenclature and the recent global subtyping into an increasing number of "clades," as defined by molecular analysis of specific viral isolates. The current case definitions of AIDS from the Centers for Disease Control and Prevention (CDC) for adults and adolescents (1993 definition) and for infants and children (1994 definition) are reviewed in detail.

Basic issues in the pathogenesis of HIV/AIDS are briefly addressed. Among the recent findings discussed are the potential contribution of cytotoxic T lymphocytes, production of noncytotoxic antiretroviral soluble factors by CD8+ T lymphocytes, type 1/type 2 cytokine dysregulation, and extracellular trapping of HIV by follicular dendritic cells

within lymph nodes. These alterations contribute to the profound immunosuppression, marked by loss of both number and function of CD4+ T lymphocytes, that is, induced by HIV infection. In addition, recent evidence has shown that the burden of virus may be higher than previously predicted, even during the asymptomatic stage of HIV disease. This observation underscores the complexity of interaction between virus and host immune response.

Clinical manifestations of HIV-1 disease are briefly presented, with an emphasis on the classification system for adults and children alike. Newer antiretroviral regimens, including HIV protease inhibitors and combinations of anti-HIV drugs, are discussed. The 1995 recommendations for the prophylaxis and treatment of 17 of the more common opportunistic infections associated with HIV are reviewed, as well as the putative novel human herpesvirus recently reported to be the cause of Kaposi's sarcoma. New virologic tests are presented, including the HIV RNA plasma assays and an HIV p24 antigen detection assay licensed in 1996 for routine testing of the American blood supply. Last, we discuss the current status of preventive and therapeutic vaccines against HIV-1. In this context, we emphasize the concept of an HIV/AIDS "Apollo Program" to coordinate an international collaboration that will pool global resources to develop effective preventive strategies, including vaccines, and effective therapies for HIV-infected patients.

Introduction to Human Retroviruses 1971–1996: Evolution of the Nomenclature

The two viruses that can cause the acquired immunodeficiency syndrome (AIDS) are named the "human immunodeficiency virus type 1" (HIV-1) and the "human immunodeficiency virus type 2" (HIV-2). Both are RNA viruses within the genus *Lentivirus* of the family Retroviridae. A distinguishing feature of this family of viruses is the presence of an enzyme termed *reverse transcriptase,* which transcribes their viral nucleic acid in a "reverse" direction, namely, from RNA to DNA.[1,2]

HIV-1 and HIV-2 were not the first human retroviruses to be isolated or, for that matter, to be implicated in human disease (Table 1-1).[3–5] In 1971, a retrovirus called "human foamy virus" or *Spumavirus* was reported and presumably linked to one or more human diseases. However, follow-up studies have failed to confirm these initial reports.[6,7] On the other hand, animal spumaviruses are found in a variety of nonhuman primates. Theoretically, these agents may be of concern in humans undergoing xenotransplantation (transfer of nonhuman bone marrow, such as baboon marrow or solid organs, into humans).

In 1980, the first report of a retrovirus subsequently proven to cause disease in humans was published.[8] The "human T-lymphotropic virus type I" (HTLV-I) was implicated in a rare type of adult T-lymphocytic leukemia/lymphoma. Since this report, others have linked HTLV-I infection to a devastating neurologic disorder affecting the spinal cord, termed "tropical spastic paraparesis," or "HTLV-I-associated myelopathy."[9,10] Recent seroepidemiologic studies indicate that in populations with a high incidence of HTLV-I infection, a minority of individuals develop either oncologic or neurologic manifestations of infection. In 1982, "human T-lymphotropic virus type II" (HTLV-II) was reported to be associated with a variant of hairy cell leukemia. Subsequent studies have determined that HTLV-II is causally related to this type of leukemia in only a small number of patients, if at all.[11,12] Similiar to HTLV-I, infection with HTLV-II may be associated with a spastic myelopathy syndrome, although this is still an area of active investigation. Neither of these two viruses, HTLV-I or HTLV-II, causes AIDS.

In 1983 and 1984, three independent laboratories reported identification of a retrovirus from persons with AIDS.[13–15] Initially, each of these three laboratories gave the same virus different names: "lymphadenopathy virus," "human T-lymphotropic virus type III" (HTLV-III), or "AIDS-associated retrovirus." In 1986, a subcommittee of the International Committee on the Taxonomy of Viruses resolved the confusion over nomenclature by assigning the virus a new name, "human immunodeficiency virus" (HIV, or HIV-1).[16] Subsequent analysis has confirmed that each of these laboratories identified the same agent.

Table 1-1. Original Terminology, Date Named, and Current Terminology for Human Retroviruses Reported Since 1980

Abbrev.	Original Terminology	Date Named	Current Terminology Abbrev.
HTLV-1	Human T-lymphotropic virus I	1980	HTLV-I
HTLV-II	Human T-lymphotropic virus II	1982	HTLV-II
LAV-I	Lymphadenopathy virus I	1983	HIV-1
HTLV-III	Human T-lymphotropic virus III	1984	HIV-1
ARV	AIDS-associated retrovirus	1984	HIV-1
HTLV-IV	Human T-lymphotropic virus IV	1985	(None)
HIV-1	Human immunodeficiency virus I	1986	HIV-2
LAV-2	Lymphadenopathy virus 2	1986	HIV-2
HIV-2	Human immunodeficiency virus 2	1986	HIV-2
HTLV-V	Human T-lymphotropic virus V	1987	HTLV-V

In 1986, another human immunodeficiency virus (HIV-2) was reported from people with AIDS in West Africa.[17] People with HIV-2 infection have been reported from Europe, North America, South America, and Asia. In the United States, HIV-2 has been reported in only 62 people as of June 1995.[18] Of these 62 people, 24 were identified in New York, 10 in Massachusetts, and 9 in Maryland (Figure 1-1). HIV-2 appears to cause progression to symptomatic disease and AIDS more slowly than HIV-1, suggesting its pathogenicity may be lower than that of HIV-1.[19] It is also notable that HIV-2 may be less efficiently transmitted vertically from mother to fetus.[20] One group of investigators has proposed that infection with HIV-2 confers partial protection against infection with HIV-1. Nearly all people with clinically significant HIV or AIDS in the United States are infected with HIV-1.

There have been reports of two other putative human retroviruses, termed "human T-lymphotropic virus type IV" (HTLV-IV) and "human T-lymphotropic virus type V" (HTLV-V). In 1985 HTLV-IV was reported, but this virus was eventually shown to be a nonhuman primate retrovirus that was later determined to be a laboratory contaminant.[21-23] In 1987, there were reports of a new retrovirus, called HTLV-V, which was isolated from a small cohort of patients with cutaneous T-lymphocyte leukemia/lymphoma, but the clinical significance of this report has yet to be confirmed by other investigators.[24]

In 1992, several groups reported a putative retroviruslike agent in a small number of patients with low CD4+ T-lymphocyte counts.[25,26] This agent was presumed to be the cause of an immunodeficient state that resembled HIV in an emerging group of rare patients. This new entity was called "idiopathic CD4+ lymphocytopenia (ICL)" and was defined on the basis of a clinical history compatible with a significant immune deficiency (e.g., AIDS-like opportunistic infections) and no evidence of HIV infection. In fact, HIV infection must be excluded to make the diagnosis of idiopathic CD4+ lymphocytopenia. Subsequent work by several laboratories failed to identify a retroviral cause, and the syndrome remains an enigma.[27-30]

CDC Revised Classification System for HIV Infection and AIDS

The most recent CDC classification system for HIV infection in adults and adolescents was published in January 1993.[31] Several additions to the previous AIDS surveillance case definition were made. In persons with established HIV infection, these

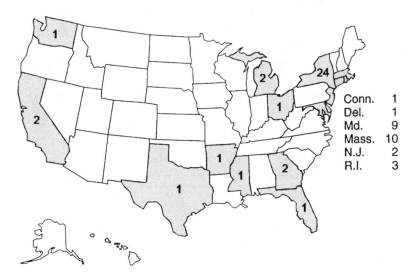

Figure 1-1. Number of persons reported with HIV-2 infection, by state—USA, December 1987–June 1995. (From Ref. 18, with permission.)

Table 1-2. Conditions Included in the 1993 AIDS Surveillance Case Definition

Candidiasis of bronchi, trachea, or lungs	Lymphoma, immunoblastic (or equivalent term)
Candidiasis, esophageal	Lymphoma, primary, of brain
Cervical cancer, invasive*	*Mycobacterium avium-intracellulare* complex of *M. kansasii*,
Coccidioidomycosis, disseminated or extrapulmonary	disseminated or extrapulmonary
Cryptococcosis, extrapulmonary	*Mycobacterium tuberculosis*, any site (pulmonary* or extra-
Cryptosporidiosis, chronic intestinal (>1 month duration)	pulmonary)
Cytomegalovirus disease (other than liver, spleen, or nodes)	*Mycobacterium,* other species or unidentified species, dissem-
Cytomegalovirus retinitis (with loss of vision)	inated or extrapulmonary
Encephalopathy, HIV-related	*Pneumocystis carinii* pneumonia
Herpes simplex: chronic ulcer(s) (>1 month duration); or	Pneumonia, recurrent*
bronchitis, pneumonitis, or esophagitis	Progressive multifocal leukoencephalopathy
Histoplasmosis, disseminated or extrapulmonary	*Salmonella* septicemia, recurrent
Isosporiasis, chronic intestinal (>1 month duration)	Toxoplasmosis of brain
Kaposi's sarcoma	Wasting syndrome due to HIV
Lymphoma, Burkitt's (or equivalent term)	

*Added in the 1993 expansion of the AIDS surveillance case definition.

From Ref. 32, with permission.

changes included CD4+ T-lymphocyte counts < 200 cells/μl, or a CD4+ T-lymphocyte percentage <14%, even in asymptomatic persons, as well as pulmonary tuberculosis, recurrent pneumonia, or invasive cervical cancer at any CD4+ T-lymphocyte level. In addition, the AIDS-defining clinical conditions used in the previous (1987) CDC AIDS surveillance case definition were retained (Table 1-2).

A matrix of three CD4+ T-lymphocyte categories ("1, 2, or 3") and three clinical categories ("A, B, or C") were created in this new classification system (Table 1-3). Category 1 includes CD4+ T-lymphocyte counts > 500 cells/μl, category 2 counts of 200–499 cells/μl, and category 3 counts of <200 cells/μl. Category 3 alone is AIDS-defining, regard-

less of clinical status. Thus, in the presence of HIV infection, AIDS can now be diagnosed solely on immunologic grounds (CD4+ T-lymphocyte count < 200 cells/μl), even in the absence of clinical signs or symptoms.

Clinical category A includes asymptomatic persons as well as those with acute HIV infection or with progressive lymphadenopathy. Category B includes patients who are symptomatic but without AIDS-defining conditions. Specifically, category B conditions include bacillary angiomatosis (due to *Bartonella henselae* or *B. quintana*), oral candidiasis, vulvovaginal candidiasis (persistent, frequent, or poorly responsive to therapy), cervical dysplasia (moderate or severe) or cervical carcinoma in situ,

Table 1-3. 1993 Revised Classification System for HIV Infection and Expanded AIDS Surveillance Case Definition for Adolescents and Adults*

CD4+ T Lymphocyte Categories	Clinical Categories		
	A: Asymptomatic, Acute (Primary) HIV Infection or PGL	B: Symptomatic, Not A or C Conditions§	C: AIDS-Indicator Conditions
1: ≥500 cells/μl	A1	B1	C1
2: 200–499 cells/μl	A2	B2	C2
3: <200 cells/μl	A3	B3	C3

From Ref. 32, with permission.

PGL, persistent generalized lymphadenopathy.

*Table 1-2. See text for discussion.

Persons with AIDS-indicator conditions (category C) as well as those with CD4+ T-lymphocyte counts <200/μl (categories A3 or B3) are reportable as AIDS cases in the United States and territories, effective January 1, 1993.

Table 1-4. Immunologic Categories Based on Age-Specific CD4+ T-Lymphocyte Counts and Percentage of Total Lymphocytes

| Immunologic Category | Age of Child (years) | | | | | |
| | <1 | | 1–5 | | 6–12 | |
	µl	(%)	µl	(%)	µl	(%)
1 No evidence of suppression	≥1500	(≥25)	≥1000	(≥25)	≥500	(≥25)
2 Evidence of moderate suppression	750–1499	(15–24)	500–999	(15–24)	200–499	(15–24)
3 Severe suppression	<750	(<15)	<500	(<15)	<200	(<15)

From Ref. 31, with permission.

fever (>38.4°C) or diarrhea for >1 month, oral hairy leukoplakia, herpes zoster involving two separate episodes or more than one dermatome, idiopathic thrombocytopenic purpura, listeriosis, pelvic inflammatory disease—especially if complicated by tuboovarian abscess, and peripheral neuropathy. Category C includes 25 conditions, including opportunistic infections, tumors, central nervous system abnormalities, wasting syndrome, pulmonary tuberculosis, invasive cervical cancer, and recurrent pneumonia (Table 1-2).

The updated classification for children under 13 years of age was published in September 1994[32] and is notable for the incorporation of CD4+ T-lymphocyte counts and CD4+ T-lymphocyte percentages into a matrix of clinical categories. The age-adjusted CD4+ T-lymphocyte counts and CD4+ percentages are summarized for children in three groupings: <1 year, 1 to 5 years, and 6 to 12 years of age (Table 1-4). The three immunologic categories, which are a rough estimation of risk for disease progression, are category 1 with no evidence of immunosuppression, category 2 with evidence of moderate suppression, and category 3 with severe suppression. As in adults, laboratory measurements of alterations in immune function provide a crude estimate of risk for infectious complications. Age-adjusted CD4+ T-lymphocyte values for severe suppression included: <1 year of age: CD4+ T-lymphocyte count <750 cells/µl or <15%; 1–5 years of age: CD4+ T-lymphocyte count <500 cells/µl or <15 %; 6–12 years of age: <200 cells/µl or <15 %). The clinical categories in the 1994 pediatric HIV classification scheme were devised to further delineate the progression of HIV disease (Table 1-5). These include N, no signs or symptoms; A, mild signs or symptoms; B, moderate signs or symptoms; and, C, severe signs or symptoms. The specific conditions for category A include lymphadenopathy (>0.5 cm at two sites),

Table 1-5. Pediatric HIV Classification by Clinical and Immunologic Categories

| Immunologic Categories* | Clinical Categories | | | |
	N: No Signs/ Symptoms	A: Mild Signs/ Symptoms	B:† Moderate Signs/ Symptoms	C:† Severe Signs/ Symptoms
1: No evidence of suppression	N1	A1	B1	C1
2: Evidence of moderate suppression	N2	A2	B2	C2
3: Severe suppression	N3	A3	B3	C3

Freom Ref. 31, with permission.

*Children whose HIV infection status is not confirmed are classified by using the above grid with a letter E (for perinatally exposed) placed before the appropriate classification code (e.g., EN2).

†Both category C and lymphoid interstitial pneumonitis in category B are reportable to state and local health departments as AIDS.

hepatomegaly, splenomegaly, dermatitis, parotitis, and recurrent or persistent upper respiratory tract infection, sinusitis, or otitis media. Categories B and C have longer lists of specific clinical conditions (Table 1-6). Category C includes AIDS-de- fining conditions listed in the 1987 surveillance case definition. Lymphoid interstitial pneumonitis is now listed under category B (moderately symptomatic), although it continues to be reportable as an AIDS-defining condition (Table 1-7).

Table 1-6. Clinical Categories (Mild, Moderate, and Severe) for Children with HIV Infection

Category N: Not Symptomatic

Children who have no signs or symptoms considered to be the result of HIV infection or who have only one of the conditions listed in category A.

Category A: Mildly Symptomatic

Children with two or more of the conditions listed below but none of the conditions listed in categories B and C.

- Lymphoadenopathy (≥0.5 cm at more than two sites; bilateral = one site)
- Hepatomegaly
- Splenomegaly
- Dermatitis
- Parotitis
- Recurrent or persistent upper respiratory infection, sinusitis, or otitis media

Category B: Moderately Symptomatic

Children who have symptomatic conditions other than those listed for category A or C that are attributed to HIV infection. Examples of conditions in clinical category B include, but are not limited to, the following:

- Anemia (<8 g/dl), neutropenia (<1,000/mm³), or thrombocytopenia (<100,000/mm³) persisting ≤30 days
- Bacterial meningitis, pneumonia, or sepsis (single episode)
- Candidiasis, oropharyngeal (thrush), persisting (>2 months) in children >6 months of age
- Cardiomyopathy
- Cytomegalovirus infection, with onset before 1 month of age
- Diarrhea, recurrent or chronic
- Hepatitis
- Herpes simplex virus stomatitis, recurrent (more than two episodes within 1 year)
- Herpes simplex virus bronchitis, pneumonitis, or esophagitis with onset before 1 month of age
- Herpes zoster (shingles) involving at least two distinct episodes or more than one dermatome
- Leiomyosarcoma
- Lymphoid interstitial pneumonia or pulmonary lymphoid hyperplasia complex
- Nephropathy
- Nocardiosis
- Persistent fever (lasting >1 month)
- Toxoplasmosis, onset before 1 month of age
- Varicella, disseminated (complicated chickenpox)

Category C: Severely Symptomatic

Children who have any condition listed in the 1987 surveillance case of definition for AIDS, with the exception of lymphoid interstitial pneumonia (see Table 1-7).

From Ref. 31, with permission.

Table 1-7. Conditions Included in Clinical Category C for Children Infected With HIV

Category C: Severely Symptomatic*

- Serious bacterial infections, multiple or recurrent (i.e., any combination of at least two culture-confirmed infections within a 2-year period), of the following types: septicemia, pneumonia, meningitis, bone or joint infection, or abscess of an internal organ or body cavity (excluding otitis media, superficial skin or mucosal abscesses, and indwelling catheter-related infections)
- Candidiasis, esophageal or pulmonary (bronchi, trachea, lungs)
- Coccidioidomycosis, disseminated (at site other than or in addition to lungs or cervical or hilar lymph nodes)
- Cryptococcosis, extrapulmonary
- Cryptosporidiosis or isosporiasis with diarrhea persisting >1 month
- Cytomegalovirus disease with onset of symptoms at age >1 month (at a site other than liver, spleen, or lymph nodes
- Encephalopathy (at least one of the following progressive finds present for at least 2 months in the absence of a concurrent illness other than HIV infection that could explain the findings):
  - —Failure to attain or loss of developmental milestones or loss of intellectual ability, verified by standard developmental scale or neuropsychological tests;
  - —Impaired brain growth or acquired microcephaly demonstrated by head circumference measurements or brain atrophy demonstrated by computed tomography or magnetic resonance imaging (serial imaging is required for children <2 years of age);
  - —Acquired symmetric motor deficit manifested by two or more of the following: paresis, pathologic reflexes, ataxia, or gait disturbance
- Herpes simplex virus infection causing a mucocutaneous ulcer that persists for >1 month; or bronchitis, pneumonitis, or esophagitis for any duration affecting a child >1 month of age
- Histoplasmosis, disseminated (at a site other than or in addition to lungs or cervical or hilar lymph nodes)
- Kaposi's sarcoma
- Lymphoma, primary, in brain
- Lymphoma, small, noncleaved cell (Burkitt's), or immunoblastic or large cell lymphoma of B-lymphocyte or unknown immuno-logic phenotype
- *Mycobacterium tuberculosis*, disseminated or extrapulmonary
- *Mycobacterium,* other species or unidentified species, disseminated (at a site other than or in addition to lungs, skin, or cervical or hilar lymph nodes)
- *Mycobacterium avium-intercellulare* complex or *M. kansasii*, disseminated (at site other than or in addition to lungs, skin, or cervical or hilar lymph nodes)
- *Pneumocystis carinii* pneumonia
- Progressive multifocal leukoencephalopathy
- *Salmonella* (nontyphoid) septicemia, recurrent
- Toxoplasmosis of the brain with onset at >1 month of age
- Wasting syndrome in the absence of a concurrent illness other than HIV-infection that could explain the following findings:
  - —Persistent weight loss >10% of baseline *or*
  - —Downward crossing of at least two of the following percentile lines on the weight-for-age chart (e.g., 95th, 75th, 50th, 25th, 5th) in a child ≥1 year of age *or*
  - —>5th percentile on weight-for-height chart on two consecutive measurements, ≥30 days apart *plus*
  - —Chronic diarrhea (i.e., at least two loose stools per day for ≥30 days) *or*
  - —Documented fever (for ≥30 days, intermittent or constant)

From Ref. 31, with permission.

*See the 1987 AIDS surveillance case definition for diagnosis criteria.

The 1994 revised pediatric classification system also provided an updated definition for HIV infection, which can be problematic to define in children born to infected mothers (less than one-third are actually infected) (Table 1-8). The diagnosis of HIV infection can be established in a child <18 months of age known to be seropositive or born to an HIV-infected mother, or in a patient who has an AIDS-defining clinical condition, if positive viral testing on two separate determinations (not including cord blood) from one or more of the following three HIV tests is confirmed: HIV culture, HIV polymerase chain reaction, HIV antigen (p24 core). Defini-

tions for perinatally HIV-exposed and for HIV sero-reverters were also provided (Table 1-8).

Epidemiology of the HIV-1/AIDS Epidemic: The Global Pandemic and HIV-1 Subtypes (Clades)

Globally, the World Health Organization (WHO) estimated that 1.5 million children and 18 million adults had been infected with HIV-1, resulting in at least 4.5 million people with AIDS, as of 1995.[33–35]

Table 1-8. 1994 Revised Pediatric HIV Classification System with Definitions for HIV Infection, Perinatally HIV-Exposed, and HIV Seroreverters

Diagnosis: HIV Infected

1. A child <18 months of age who is known to be HIV-seropositive or born to an HIV-infected mother and
   - has positive results on two separate determinations (excluding cord blood) from one or more of the following HIV detection tests:
     —HIV culture,
     —HIV polymerase chain reaction,
     —HIV antigen (p24),
                                                    or
   - meets criteria for AIDS diagnosis based on the 1987 AIDS surveillance case definition.
2. A child ≥18 months of age born to an HIV-infected mother or any child infected by blood, blood products, or other known modes of transmission (e.g., sexual contact) who
   - is HIV antibody-positive by repeatedly reactive EIA and confirmatory test (e.g., Western blot or IFA).
                                                    or
   - meets any of the criteria in example 1 above.

Diagnosis: Perinatally Exposed (Prefix E)

A child who does not meet the criteria above who
   - is HIV-seropositive by EIA and confirmatory test (e.g., Western blot or IFA) and is <18 months of age at the time of test;
                                                    or
   - has unknown antibody status, but was born to a mother known to be infected with HIV.

Diagnosis: Seroreverter (SR)

A child who is born to an HIV-infected mother and who
   - has been documented as HIV antibody-negative (i.e., two or more negative EIA tests performed at 6–18 months of age or one negative EIA test after 18 months of age);
                                                    and
   - has had no other laboratory evidence of infection (has not had two positive viral detection tests, if performed);
                                                    and
   - has not had an AIDS-defining condition.

This definition of HIV infection replaces the definition published in the 1987 AIDS surveillance case-definition.

From Ref. 31, with permission.
EIA, enzyme immunoassay; IFA, immunofluorescence assay.

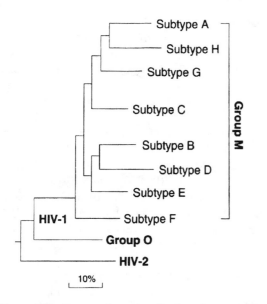

Figure 1-2. Degree of genetic relatedness between different subtypes or "clades" or subtypes of HIV-1 and HIV-2. Group M refers to "majority" of HIV-1 subtypes. Group O refers to "outlier" subtype. (From Ref. 36, with permission.)

Molecular analysis of the RNA sequence of viruses isolated from patients in different parts of the world has provided a scientific basis for identifying different HIV-1 subtypes, or *clades*. HIV-1 clades are classified on the basis of sequence variation in the envelope and core (*gag*) genes and have been divided into two groups: group M (majority) and group O (outlier). Group M consists of at least nine clades: A, B, C, D, E, F, G, H, I. Group O consists only of the outlier clade O recently reported from West Africa and Europe[36–38] (Figures 1-2 and 1-3). Evidence of recombination between two clades or dual infection with viruses of different clades (e.g., clades E and B in Thailand, and clades B and F in Brazil) has recently been reported.[39,40] In January 1996, the CDC published a global map illustrating the known distribution of different HIV-1 clades[36] (Figure 1-3). Additional clades are likely to be found throughout the world as more systematically obtained samples are studied. Moreover, expanding international travel will certainly lead to the global spread of HIV-1 clades and possibly new "emerging" HIV epidemics.

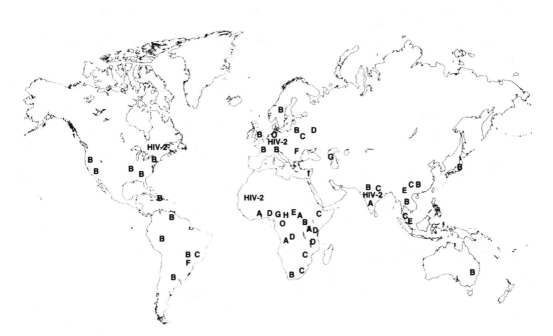

Figure 1-3. Global distribution of HIV-1 clades and HIV-2 as of 1995. (From Ref. 36, with permission.)

Clade A has been found primarily in Africa; clade B in North and South America, Europe, Africa, Asia, and Australia; clade C in Africa, Asia, and South America; clade D in Africa; clade E in Asia and Africa; clade F in Europe; clade G in Africa and Russia; clade H in Africa; clade I in Cyprus; and, clade O in Africa and Europe.[36] It is a matter of concern that clade O is so divergent from other HIV-1 subtypes that some HIV-1 antibody tests do not detect it.[41,42] It has also been proposed that HIV-2 be subtyped into different clades.[36,43]

One implication of finding multiple HIV-1 clades is that vaccine development may be further impeded if HIV-1 clade-specific immunity predominates. HIV vaccines may need to include components of multiple HIV clades to confer protection in populations where more than one clade is endemic.[44] Another implication has been raised by Essex and colleagues. In 1996, they suggested that HIV-1 clade E, which is endemic in Thailand, is more readily transmitted heterosexually than is clade B, which is endemic in the United States, much of Europe, and Australia. This theory is based on the finding that clade E virus replicates better than clade B virus in Langerhans cells, which may be especially important in the sexual transmission of HIV-1. They propose that the rate of heterosexual transmission of HIV will increase in the West if clade E virus is introduced there.[45]

Epidemiology of the HIV-1 Epidemic in the United States

A total of 501,310 persons with AIDS were reported in the United States between 1981 and October 31, 1995.[34] The gender, age, race or ethnicity, HIV-exposure category, and geographic location of these half-million Americans have been summarized by the CDC (Table 1-9). Some of the changes in these demographic characteristics in the United States are important to emphasize, in part because efforts and resources expended through public health education to prevent the spread of infection must take these factors into account. For example, women comprised 8% of AIDS patients from 1981 to 1987,

but between 1993 and 1995, the percentage rose to 17.5%. At the same time, the percentage of cases acquired by heterosexual transmission increased from 2.5% to 10.1%. Another trend of great concern is the increasing proportion of cases among injection drug users, which jumped from 17.2% to 27.3% during this same time. An evaluation of the incidence of AIDS in different racial or ethnic groups was reported for 1994. Overall, the AIDS case rates per 100,000 population were higher for African-Americans (101/100,000) and Hispanics (51/100,000) than for whites (17/100,000), indicating an overrepresentation in minority populations. HIV infection among adolescents has increased significantly and represents another major public health challenge.

In October 1995, the cumulative number of AIDS cases due to perinatal HIV transmission was 6,124, accounting for the majority of children with AIDS. During this same time, AIDS was diagnosed in 4,258 hemophiliacs, but the number of new cases (in particular, newly acquired HIV infection) has dropped sharply in hemophiliacs because of the availability of recombinant antihemophilia factor and changes in blood banking techniques. Among nonhemophiliac transfusion recipients, a total of 7,700 have been reported with AIDS. As noted previously, very few cases (<100) of AIDS due to HIV-2 have been reported in the United States.[18]

Nearly all HIV-positive U.S. citizens living in this country are thought to have clade B infection, although this awaits confirmation in large surveys.[46] In 1995, however, the U.S. military reported five personnel infected with either clade A, D, or E after returning from overseas assignments where these clades are endemic (e.g., Thailand, Uganda, Kenya).[47] Similiarly, clade E infections occurring among South American military personnel while stationed in Southeast Asia have also been reported as the probable source for introduction of clade E into South America.[36] One of the five U.S. military personnel who had clade E infection has recently been reported to have been involved through sexual contact in the first recognized case of HIV-1 clade E transmission within the United States.[48] No cases of HIV-1 clade O have been detected in this country, although retrospective serologic searches have been performed.[42] HIV-1 clade O infections should

Table 1-9. Number and Percentage of Persons with AIDS, by Demographics and Other Characteristics, in the United States From October 1981–October 1995.

Characteristic	1981–1987 No.	1981–1987 (%)	1988–1992 No.	1988–1992 (%)	1993–Oct 1995 No.	1993–Oct 1995 (%)	Cumulative No.	Cumulative (%)
Sex								
Male	46,317	92.0	177,807	87.5	204,356	82.5	428,480	85.5
Female	4,035	8.0	25,410	12.5	43,383	17.5	72,828	14.5
Age group (yr)								
0–4	653	1.3	2,766	1.4	2,013	0.8	5,432	1.1
5–12	100	0.2	669	0.3	616	0.2	1,385	1.1
13–19	100	0.4	758	0.4	1,343	0.5	2,300	0.5
20–29	10,531	20.9	38,662	19.0	41,861	16.9	91,054	18.2
30–39	23,269	46.2	92,493	45.5	111,992	45.3	227,754	45.4
40–49	10,491	20.8	47,088	23.1	64,990	26.2	122,569	24.4
50–59	3,690	7.3	14,537	7.2	18,413	7.5	36,640	7.3
≥60	1,419	2.8	6,244	3.1	6,513	2.6	14,176	2.8
Race/ethnicity								
White, non-Hispanic	30,104	59.8	102,551	50.5	105,516	42.6	238,171	47.5
Black, non-Hispanic	12,794	25.4	63,319	31.2	94,158	38.0	170,271	34.0
Hispanic*	7,039	14.0	35,213	17.3	45,135	18.2	87,387	17.4
Asian/Pacific Islander	309	0.6	1,339	0.7	1,809	0.7	3,457	0.7
American Indian/ Alaskan Native	67	0.1	433	0.2	783	0.3	1,283	0.3
HIV-exposure category								
Men who have sex with men	32,246	64.0	110,934	54.6	111,257	44.9	254,437	50.8
Injection drug use	8,639	17.2	49,093	24.2	67,708	27.3	125,440	25.0
Men who have sex with men and inject drugs	4,193	8.3	14,252	7.0	13,984	5.6	32,429	6.5
Hemophilia	505	1.0	1,744	0.9	2,009	0.8	4,258	0.8
Heterosexual contact	1,248	2.5	12,335	6.1	24,958	10.1	38,541	7.7
Transfusion recipients	1,285	2.6	3,894	1.9	2,521	1.0	7,700	1.6
Perinatal transmission	608	1.2	3,084	1.5	2,432	1.0	6,124	1.2
No risk reported	1,628	3.2	7,881	3.9	22,872	9.2	32,381	6.4
Region†								
Northeast	19,544	38.8	62,282	30.6	74,769	30.2	156,595	31.2
Midwest	3,770	7.5	20,352	10.0	24,914	10.1	49,036	9.8
South	12,960	25.7	65,926	32.4	86,462	34.9	165,348	33.0
West	13,550	26.9	46,675	23.0	53,729	21.7	113,954	22.7
U.S. Territories	516	1.0	7,889	3.9	7,566	3.1	15,971	3.2
Vital status								
Living	2,779	5.5	32,144	15.8	155,006	62.6	189,929	37.9
Decreased	47,573	94.5	171,073	84.2	92,735	37.4	311,381	62.1
Total‡	50,352	100	203,217	100	247,741	100	501,310	100

From Ref. 34, with permission.

*Persons of Hispanic origin may be of any race.

†Northeast = Connecticut, Maine, Massachusetts, New Hampshire, New Jersey, New York, Pennsylvania, Rhode Island, and Vermont; Midwest = Illinois, Indiana, Iowa, Kansas, Michigan, Minnesota, Missouri, Nebraska, North Dakota, Ohio, South Dakota, and Wisconsin; South = Alabama, Arkansas, Delaware, District of Columbia, Florida, Georgia, Kentucky, Louisiana, Maryland, Mississippi, North Carolina, Oklahoma, South Carolina, Tennessee, Texas, Virginia, and West Virginia; West = Alaska, Arizona, California, Colorado, Hawaii, Idaho, Montana, Nevada, New Mexico, Oregon, Utah, Washington, and Wyoming.

‡Includes persons for whom sex, race/ethnicity, or region are missing.

be expected in the United States, however, since they have now been found in Europe and West Africa.[36]

Historically, the earliest reported patient with HIV or AIDS in the United States was a 15-year-old sexually active male who presented in 1968 to a St. Louis hospital with lymphedema and *Chlamydia* infection[49] and later developed Kaposi's sarcoma. Autopsy specimens were preserved and subsequently serum and autopsy tissue were reported by Garry et al. to be positive for HIV-1 virus.[49] An initial report[50,51] that an English sailor died of HIV disease in 1959 has not been corroborated by another laboratory, nor could it be confirmed by the original investigators.[52,53] Finally, during the Ebola virus outbreak in Zaire in 1976, sera from several hundred people in the area of the outbreak were stored at the CDC and later were reported to show only <0.9% seroprevalence for HIV-1.[54] The virus could be grown from the serum of only one of these Zairean donors.[55,56] Coincidentally, this HIV isolate (clade A, "HZ321 strain") was later used as the viral stock for development of the gp120-depleted, inactivated, HIV therapeutic vaccine (see the section HIV Vaccines below).

Transmission

Since the replication cycle of HIV occurs exclusively within infected cells, transmission is believed to be strongly correlated with exposure to infected cells. Although the virus can be found extracellularly, HIV preferentially infects CD4+ lymphocytes and monocytes, and thus body fluids rich in lymphocytes and monocytes are the major vehicles for transmission. Acellular sources of HIV, such as plasma, serum, and factor VIII concentrate, are also well recognized to be able to transmit the virus.

The most important body fluids for HIV transmission are blood and semen. Other body fluids, such as vaginal and cervical secretions, amniotic fluid, breast milk, alveolar fluid, saliva, tears, throat swabs and cerebrospinal fluid, may be contaminated with infected lymphocytes or monocytes, but the efficiency of transmission by these body fluids is thought to be less than that through blood or semen.[57–70] Accordingly, transmission is highly cor-

related with high-risk activities involving direct exposure to, and inoculation with, blood or semen. HIV infection is acquired when infected material is introduced into the blood directly or through the skin or mucous membranes.[71] Infection is not acquired by casual contact, such as touching, hugging, and kissing. Several factors may contribute to the risk of transmission. These include the volume of contaminated material (usually contaminated with blood), the titer of HIV in the inoculum, possibly the clade (or the strain within a clade) of HIV, the route of exposure, and any antiretroviral therapy received by the source person.[57]

HIV infection can also be transmitted on the job by a single percutaneous exposure to HIV-infected blood, such as by a needle-stick injury, or by a mucosal exposure. The calculated risk associated with a single needle-stick has been estimated to be <0.2% (95% confidence interval: 0.1–0.5%).[72–75] There is no evidence for transmission by aerosols or insect bites. The efficacy of administering antiretroviral therapy following an exposure has recently been suggested by a multinational (United States, France, Britain) case-control study of healthcare workers.[76] Thus, many experts recommend offering intervention with an antiretroviral drug (zidovudine), while serial follow-up testing is performed over several months. The issue of HIV isolates that are resistant to zidovudine and possibly to other anti-HIV drugs has complicated the choice of postexposure chemoprophylaxis, and no clear national guidelines currently exist.

The risk of HIV transmission varies according to the route of exposure. Sexual transmission through anal or vaginal intercourse has been responsible for most of the AIDS cases in the United States. The risk from a single exposure has been difficult to quantify, but repeated exposure through unprotected sexual contact results in a higher risk of transmission. Recent trends indicate that the sharing of needles for drug injection has emerged as a significant risk factor. Transmission from contaminated blood transfusions was an important risk factor, but with improvements in blood banking, specifically screening techniques for donors and collected blood, transfusion-acquired HIV is a very rare event in 1996.

The blood supply in the United States is currently tested for antibody to HIV-1, HIV-2, and HTLV-I as well as other bloodborne pathogens (cytomegalovirus, hepatitis B, hepatitis C). In August 1995 the Food and Drug Administration (FDA) recommended routine testing of donated blood and plasma for HIV-1 p24 core antigen. In March 1996 the FDA licensed a test for p24 antigen specifically for use in screening the U.S. blood supply. The use of this test by blood banks will become mandatory by June 1996.[77] With a prescreening questionnaire and serologic testing for HIV, the risk of acquiring HIV-1 through a blood transfusion has dropped significantly. Rare cases arise at an estimated rate of 1 in 450,000 to 660,000 donations per year (18–27 donations per year in the United States) and are thought to occur when a donor is in the "window period," that is, within weeks of recent infection but before antibodies are detectable by commercial screening tests.[77] Very rarely, an HIV-positive person does not develop detectable antibodies. One such example was reported in March 1996, in a patient who was a frequent plasma donor.[78] No cases of HIV transmission are known to have resulted from this donor because plasma is routinely heat-inactivated or treated by a solvent and detergent method that inactivates enveloped viruses such as HIV. This very rare patient had a typical clade B virus, was not hypogammaglobulinemic, and had measurable levels of antibodies against other viruses, such as cytomegalovirus and Epstein-Barr virus. Thus, the reason for the absence of antibody to HIV in this patient is unknown and is currently under intense investigation. Use of the new HIV p24 antigen test might have identified this patient at the time of some of his plasma donations.

The risk factors for children with HIV infection have shifted dramatically during the last decade. Initially, a substantial proportion of these children, usually hemophiliacs or neonates, were recipients of contaminated blood products. At the same time that transfusion-acquired infection was decreasing, HIV infection began to increase in women of child-bearing age,[34,35,79] who can transmit the virus to their offspring perinatally. The term "perinatal" has been chosen because evidence suggests that infection can take place in utero, intrapartum, and postpartum. The specific factors that influence the timing of infection and perhaps the long-term clinical course

are still not well defined. The results of a large randomized study (ACTG 076), in which pregnant women were given zidovudine or a placebo, demonstrated a significant reduction in HIV transmission: 8.3% with zidovudine versus 25% with placebo.[80]

Breast-feeding may be an additional risk factor for transmission.[81–87] In the United States, HIV-infected women are recommended not to breast-feed, whereas in less-developed countries this recommendation is more controversial because of other concerns, such as the risk of transmission of waterborne pathogens associated with formula preparation.[80–87] Serologic testing of young children is difficult because of interference from passively acquired maternal antibodies. Culture techniques, HIV antigen detection, and molecular diagnostics (e.g., polymerase chain reaction) have contributed greatly to the early detection of children who are actually infected.

Knowledge of the risk factors for HIV transmission has led to recommendations for the prevention of infection. Abstention from high-risk activities has been advocated as the cornerstone of prevention. Barrier protection with condoms has been advocated for prevention of sexual transmission. The practice of universal precautions by health-care workers,[87,88] in and out of the hospital environment, includes the use of safe practices and barrier precautions when contact with potentially infected material is anticipated. Health-care workers should handle sharp objects with techniques that minimize the risk of injuries (e.g., not recapping needles).

HIV-1 Life Cycle

The viral life cycle of HIV-1 has been summarized by Greene[89] (Figure 1-4). The HIV-1 envelope protein is a glycoprotein of 160 kDa consisting of two subunits, gp120 and gp41. The initial step in HIV-1 infection requires the binding of gp120 to the CD4 molecule on the surface of a CD4+ T lymphocyte, monocyte, or microglial cell. Other cell types may express low levels of CD4, but their importance for both intracellular replication and immunopathogenesis of HIV is less clear.[90–92] After gp120 binds to CD4 on the cell surface, the virus fuses with the

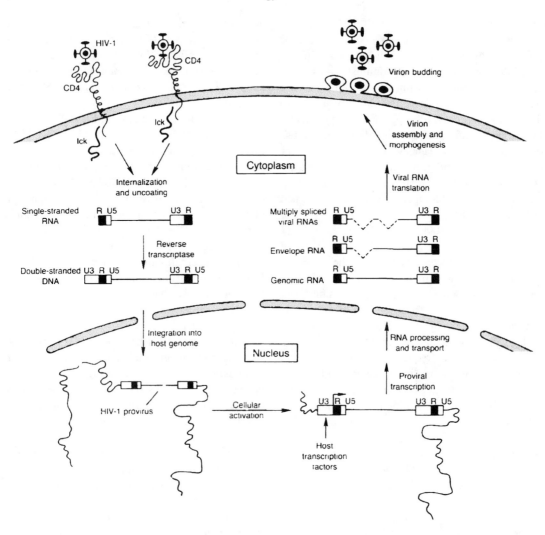

Figure 1-4.   HIV-1 life cycle. (From Ref. 89, with permission.)

cell membrane, presumably by binding to a second, unidentified receptor that binds gp41. Several other coreceptors for the HIV-1 envelope protein have been suggested, including galactosyl ceramide and CD26, although both are putative ligands for gp120 and not gp41.[90,93,94] The substance P receptor, a seven-transmembrane G protein, has been hypothesized as the "fusion receptor" for gp41 based on similiarities between the fusion domains of retroviruses and paramyxoviruses such as respiratory syncytial virus and measles virus.[95] Other putative receptors for gp41 have also been proposed, and evidence for an unidentified protein of 44 to 46

kDa has been accumulating. What has emerged from recent studies is a complex set of interactions between viral proteins and several potential cellular receptors that are required for HIV infection.[96]

Once inside the cell, viral genomic RNA is reverse-transcribed into DNA, which then is integrated into the genome of the infected cell. During cell division, the HIV provirus is transcribed into both unspliced HIV mRNA and multiply spliced HIV mRNA. The unspliced HIV mRNA becomes genomic RNA for new virus particles and is translated into the three structural proteins of HIV-1 (gag, pol, and env). These three structural proteins comprise the core (gag), which includes the p24 and p17 proteins, the polymerase, which includes the reverse transcriptase enzyme and the HIV protease, and the envelope (gp41, gp120, and gp160). The gag proteins can bind to cellular proteins such as cyclophilin A and B, and the HIV matrix protein p17 has structural homology to the cytokine interferon gamma, properties that may contribute to HIV pathogenesis.[97-100] The spliced HIV mRNA is translated into HIV regulatory and accessory proteins, of which there are at least six: tat, nef, rev, vpr, vpu, and vif. These nonstructural proteins assist with the transport and assembly of new infectious virions, which eventually bud off the surface of infected T lymphocytes, carrying with them selected cellular proteins, with the potential to infect new cells and repeat this cycle.

Some of the proteins on the surface of the HIV-1 virion include class I (ß2-microglobulin) and class II major histocompatibility complex (MHC) molecules (HLA-DR), actin, ubiquitin, cyclophilin A, and lymphocyte adhesion and signaling molecules. To emphasize this point, Arthur and colleagues[101] have calculated that on the surface of each HIV virion, there are more molecules (roughly 375 to 600) of β2-microglobulin and HLA-DR than HIV gp120 (216 molecules). The 1995 Los Alamos HIV database lists 14 exterior proteins on the HIV virion and 5 internal proteins.[37]

Pathogenesis of HIV-1 Disease

Laboratory and clinical findings over the past several years have expanded and modified our understanding of the pathogenesis of HIV disease.[102-111] After HIV enters the body, it is distributed throughout and appears to concentrate in lymphoid tissues. Viral replication is not stopped, and it is apparent that the inability to shut down viral replication may be a critical factor in HIV pathogenesis. Recently, two separate laboratories have demonstrated that the half-life of an individual HIV-1 virus in the peripheral blood of patients is only 2 days[112,113] and that an estimated 1 billion viruses are turned over during this time. Accordingly, an incessant battle,[114] or "virological mayhem,"[115] between the virus and the immune system appears to be occurring during the later stages of infection and possibly during earlier stages as well. Since approximately 50% of HIV-positive adults in the United States progress to AIDS within 10 years,[116] it is remarkable that the immune system can defend itself against such large quantities of virus for so long.

This intense interaction between the virus and the immune system also appears to occur during the earlier, clinically quiescent stage of HIV disease. The mechanism(s) responsible for the short half-life of the virus have not yet been defined, although lysis of CD8+ cytotoxic T lymphocytes and programmed death (apoptosis) of infected cells are leading possibilities. Both lysis by cytotoxic T lymphocytes and programmed cell death have also been implicated in the death of CD4+ T lymphocytes that are not infected with the virus.

Viremia during acute HIV infection (e.g., within 2 to 6 weeks after initial infection) increases to high levels but begins to decline as CD8+ cytotoxic T lymphocytes appear and before neutralizing antibody is detectable by standard assays.[117-120] One of the central aspects of HIV pathogenesis is the predilection of the virus for CD4+ lymphocytes. These cells are critical to the coordination of many immune responses, including those directed at controlling or eliminating HIV infection. Over time, the number of circulating CD4+ lymphocytes decreases, indicating that the ability to repopulate these cells may be defective. In light of the tropism of HIV for hematopoietic cells (CD34+ lymphocytes as well as CD4+ lymphocytes), it is not surprising to observe the high frequency of neutropenia, anemia, and thrombocytopenia.

Although HIV can infect CD4+ T lymphocytes and monocytes or macrophages[121-133] in the peripheral blood, reservoirs of the virus and its CD4+ target cells also exist in lymphoid tissue.[124-127] Integral to the pathogenesis of HIV in lymph nodes is the interaction of the virus with follicular dendritic cells. These cells are critical for antigen presentation. The role of follicular dendritic cells in HIV pathogenesis continues to be actively investigated. Whether lymph node follicular dendritic cells are actually infected with HIV or not is still controversial. However, HIV is known to be trapped extracellularly by lymph node follicular dendritic cells via complement and antibody bound to circulating

HIV. Fixed to the extracellular receptors for either complement or antibodies (Fc receptors), viral particles may contact and subsequently infect other T lymphocytes and macrophages. Over time, it is also postulated that the failure to clear HIV from follicular dendritic cells may partially account for changes in lymph node architecture and function.[133] As a consequence of the binding of an antibody–virus complex to follicular dendritic cells, the neutralizing function of antibody may be lost, permitting the free virion to infect another cell.[126,127] If such a mechanism exists in vivo, it could partially explain the inability of neutralizing antibody against HIV to prevent chronic, progressive disease, resulting in AIDS. Moreover, the loss of activity by neutralizing antibody after binding to follicular dendritic cells within lymph nodes could lead to an increase in susceptibility to infection in recipients of HIV-preventive vaccines. No evidence to support this prediction, however, has emerged from HIV vaccine studies involving HIV-negative volunteers.[134]

The balance between cellular and humoral immunity is disrupted by HIV infection. Specifically, this is evident in the dysregulation of selected cytokines, which were classically divided into two groups known as TH1 and TH2, secreted by distinctive helper cells. In humans, we now know that cells other than CD4+ T lymphocytes produce these cytokines. Thus, the nomenclature of "TH1" and "TH2" has been changed to "type 1" and "type 2" cytokines. Type 1 cytokines primarily promote cellular immune responses and include interleukin-2 (IL-2), interferon gamma (IFN-γ), tumor necrosis factor-β (TNF-β), and IL-12. Type 2 cytokines primarily promote antibody production and include IL-4, IL-5, IL-6, IL-10, and IL-13. Some of these cytokines are cross-regulatory (Figure 1-5). For example, IFN-γ and IL-12 decrease levels of IL-4 and IL-10, and vice versa. This cytokine model was originally described in 1986 using murine helper cell (CD4+) clones.[135] This cytokine model has been applied to the study of a wide range of human infectious, neoplastic, and inflammatory diseases, including HIV/AIDS .[136]

Clerici and Shearer initially proposed that type 1 cytokines and cellular immunity can protect against HIV infection, as well as against HIV disease progression if infection does occur.[106–107,137–138] HIV disease progression has been linked to the loss of helper cell function, including loss of IL-2 production in response to soluble antigens and mitogens.[139–142] It has also been shown that CD4+ T lymphocytes that produce type 1 cytokines are less susceptible to HIV infection than CD4+ T lymphocytes that produce type 2 cytokines.[143] Clerici and Shearer further proposed that type 2 cytokines promote apoptosis of uninfected, type 1 cytokine-producing CD4+ T lymphocytes.[144] On the basis of cytokine model, it was postulated that immune-based HIV therapy with type 1 cytokines such as IL-2 or IL-12 would be beneficial, and giving IL-4, IL-10, or IL-13 would be detrimental. Preliminary

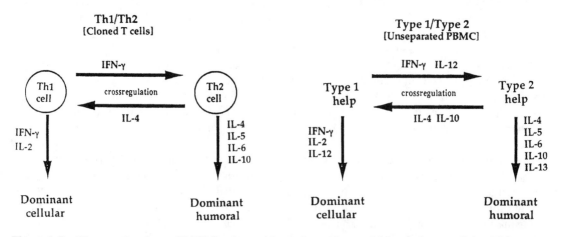

Figure 1-5. The cross-regulatory Th1/Th2 and type 1/ type 2 cytokine model in relation to cellular (Th1, or type 1) and humoral (Th2, or type 2) immune responses.

therapeutic trials with IL-2 and standard antiretroviral therapy have resulted in increases in CD4+ T-lymphocyte counts, but the results are still too preliminary to address the overall clinical benefit.[145,146] Cytokine-based therapy is not without risk. For example, late-stage patients receiving IL-2 were shown to have increased viral load. Moreover, patients at all stages of HIV disease experienced a range of toxicities.[145] Clinical studies are also under way to evaluate the potential clinical usefulness of one or more of the following cytokines: IL-4, IL-10, IL-12, and IL-15. Despite the fact that IL-12 was well tolerated in patients with HIV and cancer, the phase II study was marred by increased morbidity and at least one death attributed to the cytokine.[147] Phase I trials with IL-15, a cytokine functionally similiar to IL-2, are under consideration. IL-15 binds two of the three IL-2 receptor subunits, can enhance helper cell responses to HIV gp120 and lymphokine activated killer cell activity, and does not appear to induce any greater HIV replication than IL-2.[148–154]

On the basis of the type 1–type 2 cytokine model, it is not surprising that some people exposed to HIV have not generated a detectable antibody response. Instead, they have produced a T-lymphocyte response (e.g., CD8+ cytotoxic T lymphocyte or T-lymphocyte proliferation) that may have antiviral activity. Evidence for such antibody-negative, T lymphocyte-reactive, HIV-exposed persons has now been presented by many laboratories. Such people include those frequently exposed to sexual partners who are HIV-positive, health-care workers occupationally exposed to HIV, and infants born to HIV-positive mothers.[155–163] Recently, several investigators have reported a small number of infants born to infected mothers who eventually clear HIV infection.[164–172] Although the basis of this observation is poorly understood, the therapeutic implications are significant.

CD8+ T lymphocytes are recognized to have antiviral capability against a wide range of viruses by functioning as cytotoxic T lymphocytes. HIV may avoid lysis by cytotoxic T lymphocytes by mutation.[173] The role of CD8+ T lymphocytes in protecting against HIV infection and disease progression, however, may involve more than their ability to become cytotoxic T lymphocytes. Levy

and colleagues have argued that CD8+ T lymphocytes also elaborate soluble factors that have anti-HIV activity but are not cytolytic. These CD8+ cellular antiviral factors have not been definitely identified,[174,175] but their activity has recently been corroborated by several other laboratories. One group reported that these CD8+ T-lymphocyte antiviral factors may be a combination of three chemotactic cytokines or "chemokines": RANTES, Macrophage Inflammatory Protein-1 alpha and Macrophage Inflammatory Protein-1 beta.[176] Continued work on the pathogenesis of HIV is necessary to confirm or refute the recent major findings summarized above. An essential goal of such research is to establish the immune correlates of protection against HIV infection and disease in order to improve HIV therapies and rationally design better HIV vaccines.

Like the immunopathogenesis of HIV disease, the neuropathogenesis of HIV disease is complex and incompletely understood.[90,177–180] The importance of interactions between brain microglial cells (which can be infected by HIV), neurons (which appear not to be infected), and astrocytes (which may be infected without producing new virus) has been the focus of recent laboratory work.[178,181] The American Academy of Neurology AIDS Task Force recently updated its nomenclature and research case definitions for neurologic manifestations of human immunodeficiency virus disease.[182] As noted previously, HIV-associated neurologic disease is particularly common in infants and children. Neurologic abnormalities due to HIV in adults are well recognized by clinicians and supported by data from the Multicenter AIDS Cohort Study, which has followed patients for nearly a decade.[183] Many of the methodological tools being applied to studies of peripheral blood and lymph nodes are also being applied to studies of cerebrospinal fluid and brain tissue. For example, HIV RNA is now being quantified in the cerebrospinal fluid by the polymerase chain reaction,[184] and the sequences of HIV isolates from cerebrospinal fluid, brain, blood, and spleen are being compared.[185,186] In 1994, Power and colleagues[187] reported that relatively small changes in HIV envelope sequences from brain isolates distinguished patients with dementia from those without dementia.

Common immunologic assays have also been applied to the study of the nervous system in HIV disease. For example, antibody against the HIV V3 loop (the HIV principal neutralizing determinant) has been detected in the cerebrospinal fluid, although it appears not to neutralize autologous virus.[188,189] Nonspecific markers of immune activation, such as β2-microglobulin and neopterin, have also been found to increase slowly in asymptomatic patients.[190,191] At the time of neurologic symptoms, however, they are usually markedly increased, and may decrease with antiretroviral therapy.

Clinical Manifestations of HIV/AIDS and Newer Therapies

A current understanding of the clinical manifestations of HIV infection in children, adolescents, and adults has emerged over the first 15 years of the epidemic. It is evident that a great spectrum of clinical complications is observed in HIV-infected persons. Patients with HIV infection are plagued with chronic problems of persistent fevers, weight loss, diarrhea, and night sweats. Moreover, alterations in host defense by loss of T lymphocytes or of humoral antibody response render patients susceptible to a spectrum of opportunisitic infections. Recently, guidelines for the prophylaxis and prevention of opportunistic infections associated with HIV infection have been presented.[192] The management of these infections is essential because many patients die from complications of HIV infection. The increased susceptibility of HIV-positive patients to neoplastic processes, especially lymphomas and Kaposi's sarcoma, has generated great interest in the basic mechanisms of cancer. The clinical management of the HIV patient with cancer is further complicated by the increased susceptibility to opportunistic infections before the start of antineoplastic therapy (itself a major risk factor for infectious complications).[193]

HIV infection in children, in particular in children with perinatally acquired infection, manifests clinical features that are different from those in adults with HIV infection. Children with HIV infection are more prone to recurrent or serious bacterial infections, neurodevelopmental abnormalities, and lymphocytic interstitial pneumonitis with salivary gland enlargement. On the other hand, children are less likely to develop Kaposi's sarcoma, other cancers (e.g., lymphomas), and the opportunistic infections toxoplasmosis, cryptococcosis, and histoplasmosis, which are usually a consequence of reactivation in the adult population.[193] Factors that contribute to these differences between children and adults with HIV infection include infection during the normal development of immunity, blunted responses to standard pediatric vaccines, and immunosuppression secondary to coinfection with opportunistic pathogens. Older children who acquire infection after birth and adolescents frequently progress in a manner similar to adult patients.[194]

Because immunodeficient young children may have higher CD4+ T-lymphocyte counts than immunodeficient older children and adults, serious infections may develop when their CD4 T-lymphocyte counts are high compared with those in older children and adults.[195-198] In 1995, the CDC issued new recommendations for prophylaxis against *Pneumocystis carinii* pneumonia, the most important opportunistic pathogen in children with HIV infection.[198,199] All infants between 4 and 6 weeks of age who are at risk for HIV infection as well as those shown to be infected, or in whom the diagnosis of HIV is indeterminate, should begin prophylaxis and continue during their first year of life, regardless of their CD4+ lymphocyte counts. Continued prophylaxis may extend beyond the first year of life but will be guided by age-corrected changes in CD4+ cell levels and whether or not *P. carinii* pneumonia has occurred previously.

In 1995, national guidelines were published for the prevention of initial and recurrent disease for 17 opportunistic infections in HIV-positive children and adults.[200-202] Specific dosing regimens are given, as well as first choice and alternative choices of drugs, vaccines, and preventive behaviors. These recommendations are also graded according to the strength of the supportive data. The 17 infections are *P. carinii* pneumonia, toxoplasmic encephalitis, cryptosporidiosis, microsporidiosis, tuberculosis, disseminated *Mycobacterium avium* complex, bacterial respiratory infections, bacterial enteric infections, *Bartonella* infections, candidiasis, cryptococcosis, histoplasmosis, coccidioidomycosis, cytomegalovirus, herpes simplex virus, varicella-zoster virus, and human papillomavirus infection. The following changes from the previous guidelines were made:

1. For patients unable to tolerate sulfa drugs, the preferred prophylaxis for *P. carinii* is either dapsone or dapsone and pyrimethamine, rather than aerosolized pentamidine.

2. For patients with CD4+ T-lymphocytes <100/µl who are seropositive for toxoplasma, chemoprophylaxis against toxoplasmic encephalitis with trimethoprim–sulfamethoxazole—or for intolerant patients, with either dapsone or dapsone and pyrimethamine—is recommended.

3. The threshold for prophylaxis against disseminated *Mycobacterium avium* complex disease (with rifabutin or, alternatively, with clarithromycin or azithromycin) was decreased from a CD4+ T-lymphocyte count of 100 cells/µl to 75 cells/µl.

These guidelines represent an invaluable resource for the clinical care of the HIV-positive person. The success of prophylaxis for *P. carinii* pneumonia has resulted in a smaller proportion of patients presenting with *P. carinii* pneumonia as their initial AIDS-defining opportunistic infection.[201] Although all opportunistic infections pose serious problems for patients, the spread of tuberculosis, an increasing proportion of which is multidrug-resistant, is especially worrisome. The incidence of tuberculosis has increased nationally and globally during the HIV/AIDS epidemic. This increase is in part due to the enhanced susceptibility to tuberculosis infection in immunocompromised patients, such as those with HIV, who have profound defects in cell-mediated immunity. In addition, the burden of mycobacteria may be greater in HIV-positive patients, which probably translates into an increase in the likelihood of transmission to others. Strategies to control multiply-resistant tuberculosis have been proposed. These include use of a rapid diagnostic method for evaluation of sputum,[202] strict isolation procedures for infected persons, and directly observed therapy (DOT) by health-care workers to ensure compliance and optimize the likelihood of cure. Ultimately, rapid iden-

tification of resistant strains will improve control measures and permit the selection of an effective antimycobacterial regimen sooner. Standard care currently requires initial therapy for tuberculosis to include four drugs (isoniazid, rifampin, pyrazinamide, and ethambutol or streptomycin) until the in vitro susceptibilities of the patient's isolate are known.

Another recent clinical development has been the discovery of a novel human herpesvirus agent (HHV-8) that may be the cause of Kaposi's sarcoma-associated virus.[203] The initial finding by Chang and colleagues has been corroborated in both HIV-positive and HIV-negative persons with Kaposi's sarcoma.[204,205] This herpesvirus has now been seen by electron microscopy and grown in culture. More recently, this virus has also been reported in other conditions, including brain and body cavity lymphomas, angiosarcomas, and Castleman's disease,[206,207] but it appears to be most closely linked to Kaposi's sarcoma. Whether antiherpesvirus drugs are active against this virus or will prove useful in treating Kaposi's sarcoma are questions under active investigation.

A clinical cohort of patients termed "long-term nonprogressors" have been extensively studied over the past few years.[208–213] These patients represent a small percent (<10%, depending on the precise definition and patient population) of patients who have been infected for 8 to 10 years yet appear to be clinically asymptomatic, with normal levels of CD4+ T lymphocytes. Frequently, these patients have low levels of circulating virus and their lymph node architecture is generally preserved, suggesting adequate control of HIV replication. In the patients studied to date, a brisk cellular (by cytotoxic T lymphocytes) and humoral (neutralizing antibody titers) immune response to HIV has been preserved over time. However, a central issue is determining whether these patients are truly nonprogressors or simply slow progressors. In either case, intense interest in these patients is driven by the implications of understanding their response to viral infection. Identifying a specific immune correlate of protection in these patients would have clear implications for developing better therapies and vaccines. This group may be a heterogeneous collection of individuals, in some of whom host factors may predominate, while in others viral factors, such as mutations in selected genes (e.g., *nef*), may be important. One such patient from the United States and several Australian patients who received blood tranfusions from an HIV-positive donor whose virus had an altered *nef* gene have been reported.[212,213]

Over the past decade, many important insights into the life cycle and immunopathogensis of HIV infection have formed the foundation for strategies to control the virus. The most intense effort has been devoted to developing antiretroviral agents. The first agents licensed for treatment of HIV infection were inhibitors of reverse transcriptase. These drugs can prevent the spread of new infection but do not block replication of integrated virus.[214–216] The first two drugs approved for general use, zidovudine (AZT) and didanosine (ddI), delay clinical progression and improve surrogate markers. However, the emergence of resistant strains that develop on therapy with the potential of spreading throughout a community has undermined the efficacy of these agents. Furthermore, they may have minimal impact on long-term survival when used during early-stage HIV disease. Other reverse transcriptase blockers, such as zalcitabine (ddC), lamivudine (3TC), stavudine (d4T), and nevaripine, have been added and are frequently used in combination. Zidovudine monotherapy is no longer considered standard care for adults with HIV disease.

In late 1995 the first protease inhibitor, saquinivir, was approved for use in combination therapy. In early 1996, two other protease inhibitors, ritonavir and indinavir, were approved. With the advent of these new drugs, the era of HIV monotherapy will likely end. It will be important to develop guidelines for the choice of combination therapy based upon current information, in a manner similar to recommendations following the publication of the Concorde zidovudine trial in 1993.[215–219] The introduction of these new antiretroviral agents and a better understanding of the immunopathogenesis of HIV now permit the use of combination therapy in a manner similiar to antineoplastic chemotherapy. The clear advantage lies in selecting the most effective combination of drugs while minimizing the pressure to develop resistance. On the other hand, significant side effects, interactions with other drugs, expense, and possible cross-resistance are important factors for consideration in the selection of these medications.

Use of the HIV protease inhibitors and combination anti-HIV drug regimens has been closely tied to the development of new assays to measure HIV viral load (HIV RNA) in plasma. At least three such assays are well into development, two of which are based on the polymerase chain reaction and one is based on the branched-chain DNA assay.[220,221] These highly sensitive assays can detect HIV RNA in plasma at all stages of HIV infection. The highest levels have been measured in the weeks immediately following initial infection and during the late stages of advanced AIDS.[222] The utility of these assays in patient care remains to be determined. However, they may be able to measure clinically relevant changes in viral load in response to therapeutic interventions. Another potential use of these assays may be to predict long-term clinical outcome based on plasma HIV RNA levels soon after initial infection[224] as well as during later stages of the disease. Similarly, measuring HIV mRNA in peripheral blood mononuclear cells has been used to predict disease progression soon after HIV seroconversion and during later stages of disease.[224–226] An additional potential application of plasma HIV RNA assays is in the determination of the risk of perinatal HIV transmission from mother to infant.[223] Because of the finding that HIV is present and replicating even during the clinically asymptomatic stage, an increasing number of clinicians and investigators favor treating HIV "early and hard."[227]

HIV Vaccines

More than 25 candidate HIV vaccines have entered clinical trials since 1987.[228–230] However, not one has been licensed for widespread use. Many research groups have studied vaccines made of recombinant forms of the envelope protein gp160 or one of its subunits, gp 120. At the same time, HIV vaccine development has progressed along two pathways, one of which has focused on preventing infection in HIV-negative persons, a true "preventive" vaccine, while the other one has concentrated on developing "therapeutic" strategies for those already infected.[231] The latter is intended to boost or enhance immunity against preexisting infection.

No preventive HIV vaccines have entered phase III clinical efficacy trials in the United States. Two gp120 vaccines were considered for phase III trials in this country, but in June 1994 it was decided that such trials did not warrant the support of the National Institutes of Health (NIH).[232,233] Recently, these candidate vaccines have entered phase I studies in Thailand. The evaluators were concerned that these vaccines failed to induce sufficient neutralizing antibody against HIV strains isolated from patients, although they were successful against laboratory strains adapted to grow in neoplastic cell lines.[234] Subsequently, the NIH has published a detailed agenda for HIV vaccine development presenting the criteria for advancement from small phases I and II trials to large phase III efficacy trials.[235]

The basic virology of HIV underscores many problems inherent in vaccine development. Differences in HIV clades could undermine effective immunity. It may be necessary to develop regional strategies, directed at specific clades. It is not clear whether a vaccine derived from one clade will confer protection against infection with HIV of another clade, or even against a divergent strain within the same clade (subtype). If cross-clade, or at least cross-strain, protection does not exist, the choice of vaccine strains will be critical to the success of a vaccine study. For example, Thailand has both clade B and clade E viruses. Most of the clade B strains in Thailand (termed B-) are somewhat divergent in their principal neutralizing determinant (V3 loop, or third hypervariable region) from the clade B virus used in the two gp120 vaccine products recently tested there in small studies.[236–239] Such amino acid sequence divergence in the V3 loop might account for differences in immunologic responses, including induction of specific neutralizing antibodies. At the same time, data from such clinical trials can provide crucial information for a better understanding of HIV immunopathogenesis and the design of optimal HIV vaccines. For example, the breakthrough infections documented in the HIV preventive vaccine trials in the United States

should permit a better understanding of the role of vaccine-induced humoral and cell-mediated immunity against HIV.[134,240,241]

In 1996, the first phase III study in the United States for therapeutic immunization of HIV-infected persons was begun. The product being tested is an inactivated HIV virion clade A, "HZ321 strain" isolated from the serum of a Zairean woman in which the gp120 envelope is depleted but not completely removed. This approach was initially proposed by Jonas Salk in 1987.[231] Other HIV therapeutic vaccines have taken a different approach and used exclusively the envelope portions of the virus (gp160, or gp120). In 1996, a 608-person United States trial of a gp160 therapeutic vaccine and a similiar 278-person Canadian study failed to show any evidence of efficacy.[242] An earlier phase 1 study of this product by the U.S. Army reported no reduction in HIV viral burden.[243] At least two other intermediate-size trials of other HIV therapeutic vaccines have also recently ended without demonstrating efficacy.[244]

Looking toward the future development of HIV vaccines, several novel candidates have been proposed. These include use of canarypox vectors in an attempt to enhance anti-HIV cellular as well as humoral immune responses.[245] Unlike vaccinia, canarypox virus does not replicate in mammalian cells and is therefore considered safer than vaccinia. Other novel approaches, which have undergone preclinical tests, include nucleic acid vaccines.[246,247] These so-called DNA, or naked DNA vaccines are entering small clinical trials. It is anticipated that other novel strategies will be studied in the near future. A better understanding of the basic biology of HIV infection and its immunopathogenesis will form the rational basis for new preventive approaches. At the same time, complex ethical and social issues are inseparably linked with the scientific development of HIV vaccines in both developed and less developed countries.[248–251]

Conclusion

Investigation into the biologic and clinical problems of HIV infection has yielded many new insights, some of which already have had important implications for therapeutic and preventive strategies. The development of several classes of antiretroviral agents forms the cornerstone for the next generation of therapeutic interventions, which will employ combinations of agents. At the same time, the classification of HIV infection continues to be updated on the basis of recognition of clinical patterns. It is also anticipated that advances in the detection of viral load and other surrogate markers of disease will be introduced into clinical practice, primarily to predict or identify stages of disease. In turn, these findings will influence choices of antiretroviral therapy and prevention of opportunistic infections. Since the prevention and treatment of opportunistic infections has resulted in significant improvements in outcome, another challenge will be to refine further therapeutic and prophylactic strategies based on identification of clinical risk factors for opportunistic infections. This will be all the more daunting in the age of restricted economic opportunities for health care.

Over the past 15 years, preventive measures against acquisition of HIV have resulted in changes in the epidemiology of HIV infection. For example, transfusion-associated infection is now very rare. The use of zidovudine in pregnant women with HIV infection has reduced the rate of transmission to offspring. Refinements of this approach with new agents or interventions may further reduce the number of children infected with HIV. Public health measures designed to reduce high-risk activities have been partially successful, but complex societal and economic reasons may have militated against a more successful outcome. The challenge of the future will be to integrate new scientific findings with clinical therapeutics and preventive measures, including not only vaccine development but essential behavioral changes to avoid HIV exposure and transmission.

HIV vaccine development has not progressed as rapidly as some had predicted in the mid-1980s. This is not surprising in light of the complex behavior of the HIV virus. The call for more basic science in HIV research is appropriate and should not be ignored.[111] In this regard, resources are provided to the reader for continually evolving, state-of-the-art information on HIV clinical trials, recommendations on new therapeutic drug combinations, use of viral load measurements, and HIV basic science (see Table 1-10). With a better understanding of the pathogenesis and virology of HIV, we may develop better vaccines and make optimal use of antiretroviral therapies. To accomplish these goals, however, even greater collaborative efforts will be necessary between persons and institutions involved in the epidemic. We propose an "HIV/AIDS Apollo Program" as a unifying image for international collaborative research on HIV. The increasingly recognized number of HIV subtypes, the lack of access to affordable anti-HIV drugs for the majority of infected persons worldwide, and the need

Table 1-10. References for State-of-the-Art Information on HIV Clinical Trials, HIV-1 Immunologic and Virology Information

1. CDC National AIDS Clearinghouse: tel: (301)458-5231

2. American Foundation for AIDS Research (AMFAR): tel: (301)468-1287.

3. HIV Clinical Trial information: tel: 1-800-TRIALS-A

4. Los Alamos HIV Virology and Immunology Databases: tel: (505)665-0480.

5. NIH reference guide to major clinical trials in patients infected with HIV: Spooner KM, Lane HC, Masur H. *Clinical Infectious Diseases* 1996;23:15–27.

6. Grady C. The search for an AIDS vaccine: ethical issues in the development and testing of a preventive HIV vaccine. Bloomington, IN: Indiana University Press, 1995.

7. Carpenter CC, Fischl MA, Hammer SM, et al. Antiretroviral therapy for HIV infection in 1996. recommendations of an international panel. *JAMA* 1996;276:146–154.

8. CDC. Initial therapy for tuberculosis in the era of multidrug resistance. *MMWR* 1993;42(RR-7):1–8.

9. CDC. Update: Provisional Public Health Service Recommendations for chemoprophylaxis after occupational exposure to HIV. *JAMA* 1996;276:90–92.

for effective HIV preventive measures combine to require an unprecedented international collaborative research effort. The original Apollo Space Program resulted in the successful landing of a man on the moon. The result of a successful "HIV/AIDS Apollo Program" would be to accelerate development of HIV vaccines and behavioral interventions that are effective internationally to prevent HIV infection, and to provide global access to effective therapies for persons living with HIV/AIDS.

In 1996, six papers were published reporting identification of several HIV-1 coreceptors for the post-CD4 binding "fusion" step of HIV entry into a cell.[252–257] One of these coreceptors has been termed *fusion*. It appears to be used preferentially by syncytia-inducing strains of HIV-1 that infect T-lymphocyte lines and that occur during advanced HIV disease. Another coreceptor is a β-chemokine receptor termed *chemokine receptor 5*. It appears to be used preferentially by nonsyncytia-inducing strains of HIV-1 that infect macrophages and T lymphocytes and that occur during earlier stages of HIV disease. Both coreceptors have seven transmembrane domains and are G proteins. Other "fusion" coreceptors may soon be reported. Other recent developments include the first report of a patient in the United States with the HIV-1 "outlier" clade O, FDA approval of the first plasma HIV RNA viral load test, and licensure of the ninth anti-HIV drug (nevirapine). Finally, new recommendations for the use of anti-HIV combination drugs, including protease inhibitors, and for postexposure prophylaxis for health-care workers have been published.[258]

References

1. Temin HM, Mitzutani S. RNA-dependent polymerase in virions of Rous sarcoma virus. *Nature* 1970;211–213.

2. Baltimore D. Viral RNA-dependent DNA polymerase. *Nature* 1970;226:1209–1211.

3. Coffin JM. In: Fields (ed). *Retroviridae and Their Replication in Virology*. New York: Lippincott-Raven, 1990:1437–1500.

4. Broder S. Pathogenic human retroviruses. *N Engl J Med* 1988;318:243–245.

5. Lucey DR. The first decade of human retroviruses: a nomenclature for the clinician. *Milit Med* 1991; 156:155–157.

6. Achong BG, Mansel PWA, Epstein MA, et al. An unusual virus in cultures from a human nasopharyngeal carcinoma. *J Natl Cancer Inst* 1971;46: 299–302.

7. Flugel RM. Spumaviruses: a group of complex retroviruses. *J AIDS* 1991;4:739–750.

8. Poiesz BJ, Ruscetti FW, Gazdar AF, et al. Detection and isolation of type C retrovirus particles from fresh and cultured lymphocytes of a patient with cutaneous T-cell lymphoma. *Proc Natl Acad Sci USA* 1980;77:7415–7419.

9. Gessain A, Vernant JC, Maurs L, et al. Antibodies to human T-lymphotropic virus type-1 in patients with tropical spastic paraparesis. *Lancet* 1985;2: 407–409.

10. Osame M, Usuku K, Izumo S, et al. HTLV-I associated myelopathy, a new entity. *Lancet* 1986;1: 1031–1032.

11. Kalyanaraman VS, Sarngadharan MG, Robert-Guroff M, et al. A new subtype of human T-cell leukemia virus (HTLV-II) associated with a T-cell variant of hairy-cell leukemia. *Science* 1982;218: 571–573.

12. Lion T, Razvi N, Golomb HM, et al. B-lymphocytic hairy cells contain no HTLV-II DNA sequences. *Blood* 1988;72:1428.

13. Barre-Sinousi F, Chermann JC, Fey F, et al. Isolation of T-cell lymphotropic retrovirus from a patient at risk for AIDS. *Science* 1983;220:868–871.

14. Popovic M, Sarnagadharan MG, Read E, et al. Detection, isolation, and continuous production of cytopathic retroviruses (HTLV-III) from patients with AIDS and pre-AIDS. *Science* 1984;224: 487–500.

15. Levy JA, Hoffman AD, Kramer SM, et al. Isolation of lymphocytopathic retroviruses from San Franciscan patients with AIDS. *Science* 1985; 225:840–842.

16. Coffin J, Haase A, Levy JA, et al. What to call the AIDS virus. *Nature* 1986;321:10.

17. Clavel F, Guetard D, Brun-Vezzinet F, et al. Isolation of a new human retrovirus from West African patients with AIDS. *Science* 1986;233:343–346.

18. Centers for Disease Control and Prevention. Update: HIV-2 infection among blood and plasma donors—United States, June 1992–June 1995. *MMWR* 1995;44:603–606.

19. Marlink R, Kanki P, Thior I, et al. Reduced rate of disease development after HIV-2 infection as compared to HIV-1. *Science* 1994;265:1587–1590.

20. Adjorlolo-Johnson G, De Cock KM, Ekpini E, et al. Prospective comparison of mother-to-child transmission of HIV-1 and HIV-2 in Abidjan, Ivory Coast. *JAMA* 1994;272:462–466.

21. Kanki PJ, Barin F, M'Boup, et al. New human T-lymphotropic retrovirus related to simian T-lymphotropic virus type III (STLV-III AGM). *Science* 1986;232:238–242.

22. Kestler HW, Li Y, Yathirajulu MN, et al. Comparison of simian immunodeficiency virus isolates. *Nature* 1988;331:619–622.

23. Mulder C. A case of mistaken non-identity. *Nature* 1988;331:562–563.

24. Manzari V, Gismondi A, Barillari G, et al. HTLV-V: a new human retrovirus isolated in a tac-negative T-cell lymphoma/leukemia. *Science* 1987;238:1581–1583.

25. Centers for Disease Control and Prevention. Unexplained CD4+ T-lymphocyte depletion in persons without evident HIV infection-United States. *MMWR* 1992;41:541–545.

26. Smith DK, Neal JJ, Holmberg SD, et al. Unexplained opportunistic infections and CD4+ T-lymphocytopenia without HIV infection: an investigation of cases in the United States. *N Engl J Med* 1993;328:373–380.

27. Ho DD, Cao Y, Zhu T, et al. Idiopathic CD4+ T-lymphocytopenia: immunodeficiency without evidence of HIV infection. *N Engl J Med* 1993;328:380–385.

28. Spira TJ, Jones BM, Nicholson JKA, et al. Idiopathic CD4+ T-lymphocytopenia: an analysis of five patients with unexplained opportunistic infections. *N Engl J Med* 1993;328:386–392.

29. Duncan RA, Von Reyn CF, Alliegro GM, et al. Idiopathic CD4+ T-lymphocytopenia: four patients with opportunistic infections and no evidence of HIV infection. *N Engl J Med* 1993;328:393–398.

30. Fauci AS. CD4+ T-lmphocytopenia without HIV infection: no lights, no camera, just facts. *N Engl J Med* 1993;328:429–431.

31. Centers for Disease Control and Prevention. 1994 revised classification system for human immunodeficiency virus infection in children less than 13 years of age. *MMWR* 1994;43(RR-12):1–19.

32. Centers for Disease Control and Prevention. 1993 revised classification scheme for HIV infection and expanded surveillance case definition for AIDS among adolescents and adults. *MMWR* 1992;41:RR-17.

33. WHO. *The Current Global Situation of the HIV/AIDS Pandemic.* Geneva: World Health Organization, 1995.

34. Centers for Disease Control and Prevention. First 500,000 AIDS cases—United States, 1995. *MMWR* 1995;44(46):849–852.

35. Rosenberg PS. Scope of the AIDS epidemic in the United States. *Science* 1995;270:1372–1375.

36. Hu DJ, Dondero TJ, Rayfield MA, et al. The emerging genetic diversity of HIV. *JAMA* 1996;275:210–216.

37. Myers G, Korber B, Hahn BH, et al. *Human Retroviruses and AIDS 1995 (Virology Database).* Los Alamos, NM: Los Alamos National Laboratory, 1995.

38. Korber BT, Brander C, Walker BD, et al. *HIV Molecular Immunology Database.* Los Alamos, NM: Los Alamos National Laboratory, 1995.

39. Sabino EC, Shaper EG, Morgado MG, et al. Identification of HIV type 1 envelope genes recombinant between subtypes B and F in two epidemiologically linked individuals from Brazil. *J Virol* 1994;68:6340–6346.

40. Artenstein A, Van Cott TC, Mascola JR, et al. Dual infection with HIV-1 subtypes in Thailand. *J Infect Dis* 1995;171:805–810.

41. Loussert-Ajaka I, Ly TD, Chaix ML, et al. HIV-1/HIV-2 seronegativity in HIV-1 subtype O infected patients. *Lancet* 1994;343:1393–1394.

42. Schable C, Zekeng L, Pau CP, et al. Sensitivity of US HIV antibody tests for detection of HIV-1 group O infections. *Lancet* 1994;344:1333–1334.

43. Gao F, Yue L, Robertson DL, et al. Genetic diversity of HIV-2: evidence for distinct sequence subtypes with differences in virus biology. *J Virol* 1994;68:7433–7447.

44. Rowe PN. HIV subtypes raise vaccine anxieties. *Lancet* 1996;347:603.

45. Soto-Ramirez LE, Renjifo B, McLane MF, et al. HIV-1 Langerhans' cell tropism associated with heterosexual transmission of HIV. *Science* 1996;271:1291–1293.

46. Brodine SK, Mascola JR, Weiss PJ, et al. Detection of diverse HIV-1 genetic subtypes in the USA. *Lancet* 1995;346:1198–1199.

47. Artenstein AW, Coppola J, Brown AE, et al. Multiple introductions of HIV-1 subtype E into the western hemisphere. *Lancet* 1995;346:1197–1198.

48. Artenstein AW, Ohl CA, Van Cott TC, et al. Transmission of HIV-1 subtype E in the United States. *JAMA* 1996;276:99–100..

49. Garry RF, Witte MN, Gottlieg A, et al. Documentation of an AIDS virus infection in the United States in 1968. *JAMA* 1988;260:2085–2087.

50. Corbitt G, Bailey AS, Williams G. HIV infection in Manchester, 1959. *Lancet* 1990;336:51.

51. Williams G, Stretton TB, Leonard JC. Cytomegalic inclusion disease and *Pneumocystis carinii* infection in an adult. *Lancet* 1960;2:951–955.

52. Zhu T, Ho D. Was HIV present in 1959? [Letter]. *Nature* 1995;374:503–505.

53. Bailey AS, Corbitt G. Was HIV present in 1959? [Lette]. *Lancet* 1996;347:189.

54. Nzilambi N, De Cock KM, Forthal DN, et al. The prevalence of infection with HIV over one ten year period in Zaire. *N Engl J Med* 1988;318:276–279.

55. Getchell JP, McCormick JB, Srinivasan A, et al. Isolation of an HIV virus from a serum sample collected in 1976 in central Africa. *J Infect Dis* 1987;156:833–837.

56. Srinivasan A, York D, Butler D, et al. Molecular characterization of HIV-1 isolated from a serum collected in 1976: nucleotide sequence comparison to recent isolates and generation of hybrid HIV. *AIDS Res Hum Retrov* 1989;5:121–129.

57. Simonds RJ , Chanock SJ. Medical issues related to caring for human immunodeficiency virus-infected children in and out of the home. *Pediatr Infect Dis J* 1993;12:845–852.

58. Ho DD, Schooley RE, Rota TR, et al. HTLV-III in the semen and blood of a healthy homosexual man. *Science* 1984;226:451–3.

59. Vogt MW, Witt DJ, Craven DZ, et al. Isolation patterns of the human immunodeficiency virus from cervical secretions during the menstrual cycles of women at risk for the acquired immunodeficiency syndrome. *Ann Intern Med* 1987;106:380–382.

60. Mundy DC, Schinazi RF, Gerber AR, et al. Human immunodeficiency virus isolated from amniotic fluid. *Lancet* 1987;2:459–460.

61. Thiry L, Sprecher-Goldberger S, Jonckheer T, et al. Isolation of AIDS virus from cell-free breast milk of three healthy virus carriers. *Lancet* 1985; 2:891–892.

62. Ziza J-M, Brun-Vezinet F, Venet A, et al. Lymphadenopathy-associated virus isolated from bronchoalveolar lavage fluid in AIDS-related complex with lymphoid interstitial pneumonitis. *N Engl J Med* 1985;313:183.

63. Ho DD, Byington RE, Schooley RT, et al. Infrequency of isolation of HTLV-III virus from saliva in AIDS. *N Engl J Med* 1985;313:1606.

64. Levy JA, Greenspan D. HIV in saliva. *Lancet* 1988;2:1248.

65. Groopman JE, Salahuddin SZ, Sarngadharan MG, et al. HTLV-III in saliva of people with AIDS-related complex and healthy homosexual men at risk for AIDS. *Science* 1984;226:447–449.

66. Fujikawa LS, Palestine AG, Nussenblatt RB, et al. Isolation of human T-lymphotropic virus type III from the tears of a patient with the acquired immunodeficiency syndrome. *Lancet* 1985;2:529–530.

67. Kawashima H, Bandyopadhyay S, Rutstein R, et al. Excretion of human immunodeficiency virus type 1 in the throat but not in urine by infected children. *J Pediatr* 1991;118:80–82.

68. Ho DD, Rota TR, Schooley RT, et al. Isolation of HTLV-III from cerebrospinal fluid and neural tissues of patients with neurologic syndromes related to the acquired immunodeficiency syndrome. *N Engl J Med* 1985;313:1493–1497.

69. Li JJ, Huang YQ, Poiesz BJ, Zaumetzger-Abbot L, et al. Detection of human immunodeficiency virus type 1 (HIV-1) in urine cell pellets from HIV-1-seropositive individuals. *J Clin Microbiol* 1992;30:1051–1055.

70. Michaelis BA, Levy JA. Recovery of human immunodeficiency virus from serum. *JAMA* 1987; 257:1327.

71. Donegan E, Stuart M, Niland JC, et al. Infection with human immunodeficiency virus type 1 (HIV-1) among recipients of antibody-positive blood donations. *Ann Intern Med* 1990;113:733–739.

72. Gerberding JL, Bryant-LeBlanc CE, Nelson K, et al. Risk of transmitting the human immunodeficiency virus, cytomegalovirus, and hepatitis B virus to health care workers exposed to patients with AIDS and AIDS-related conditions. *J Infect Dis* 1987;156:1–8.

73. Henderson DK, Fahey BJ, Willy M, et al. Risk for occupational transmission of human immunodeficiency virus type 1 (HIV-1) associated with clinical exposures. *Ann Intern Med* 1990;113:740–746.

74. Marcus R, CDC Cooperative Needlestick Study Group. Surveillance of health-care workers exposed to blood from patients infected with the human immunodeficiency virus. *N Engl J Med* 1988;319:1118–1123.

75. Gerberding, JL. Management of occupational exposures to blood-borne viruses. *N Engl J Med* 1995;332:444–451.

76. Centers for Disease Control and Prevention. Case-control study of HIV seroconversion in health-care workers after percutaneous exposure to HIV-infected blood—France, United Kingdom, and United States, January 1988–August 1994. *MMWR* 1995;44.

77. Centers for Disease Control and Prevention. U.S. Public Health Service guidelines for testing and counseling blood and plasma donors for human immunodeficiency virus type 1 antigen. *MMWR* 1996;45:1–9.

78. Centers for Disease Control and Prevention. Persistent lack of detectable HIV-1 antibody in a person with HIV infection—Utah, 1995. *MMWR* 1996;45/No. 9:181–185.

79. Hirschfeld S, Chanock SJ. Selected issues in human immunodeficiency virus infection in adolescents. *Curr Opin Pediatr* 1992;4:599–605.

80. Connor EM, Sperling RS, Gelber R, et al. Reduction of maternal-infant transmission of human immunodeficiency virus type 1 with zidovudine treatment. *N Engl J Med* 1994;331:1173–1180.

81. Peckham C, Gibb D. Mother-to-child transmission of the human immunodeficiency virus. *N Engl J Med* 1995;333:298–302.

82. Dunn DT, Newell ML, Mayaux MJ. Mode of delivery and vertical transmission of HIV-1: a review of prospective studies. *J AIDS* 1994;7:1064–1066.

83. Kliks SC, Wara DW, Landers DV, et al. Features of HIV-1 that could influence maternal-child transmission. *JAMA* 1994;272:467–474.

84. Dunn DT, Newell ML, Ades AE, et al. Risk of human immunodeficiency virus type 1 transmission through breast feeding. *Lancet* 1992;340:585–588.

85. *Consensus Statement from WHO/UNICEF Consultation of HIV Transmission and Breastfeeding.* Geneva: World Health Organization, 1992.

86. Centers for Disease Control and Prevention. Recommendations for assisting in the prevention of perinatal transmission of human T-lymphotrophic virus type III/lymphadenopathy-associated virus and acquired immunodeficiency syndrome. *MMWR* 1985;34:721–726.

87. Ruff AJ, Halsey NA, Coberly J , et al. Breast-feeding and maternal-infant HIV-1 transmission. *J Pediatr* 1992;121:325–329.

88. Centers for Disease Control and Prevention. Update: universal precautions for prevention of transmission of human immunodeficiency virus, hepatitis B virus, and other bloodborne pathogens in health-care settings. *MMWR* 1988;37:377–382, 387–388.

89. Greene W. The molecular biology of human immunodeficiency virus type 1 infection. *N Engl J Med* 1991;324:308–315.

90. Levy J. The pathogenesis of HIV. *Microbiol Rev* 1993;57:183–289.

91. McCune JM. HIV-1: the infective process in vivo. *Cell* 1991;64:351–364.

92. Lucey DR, Nicholson-Weller A, Weller PF. Mature human eosinophils have the capacity to express HLA-DR. *Proc Natl Acad Sci USA* 1989;86:1348–1351.

93. Cohen JC. HIV "cofactor" comes in for more heavy fire. *Science* 1993;262:1971.

94. Bhat S, Spitalnik SL, Gonzalez-Scarano F, et al. Galactosyl ceramide or a derivative is an essential component of the neural receptor for human immunodeficiency virus type 1 envelope glycoprotein gp120. *Proc Natl Acad Sci USA* 1991;88:7131–7134.

95. Lucey DR, Novak K, Poloni V, et al. Characterization of substance P binding to human monocytes/macrophages. *Clin Diagn Lab Immunol* 1994;1:330–335.

96. Qureshi NM, Coy DH, Garry RF, et al. Characterization of a putative cellular receptor for HIV-1 transmembrane glycoprotein using synthetic peptides. *AIDS* 1990;553–558.

97. Luban J, Bossolt KL, Franke EK, et al. Human immunodeficiency virus type 1 gag protein binds to cyclophilins A and B. *Cell* 1993;73:1067–1078.

98. Franke EK, Hui Yuan HE, Luban J. Specific incorporation of cyclophilin A into HIV-1 virions. *Nature* 1994;372:359.

99. Thali M, Bukovsky A, Kondo E, et al. Functional association of cyclophilin A with HIV-1 virions. *Nature* 1994;372:363.

100. Matthew S, Barlow P, Boyd J, et al. Structural similarity between the p17 matrix protein and interferon-gamma. *Nature* 1994;370:666–668.

101. Arthur LO, Bess JW, Sowder RC, et al. Cellular proteins bound to immunodeficiency vitruses: implications for pathogenesis and vaccines. *Science* 1992;258:1935–1938.

102. Weiss R. How does HIV cause AIDS? *Science* 1993;260:1273–1279.

103. Haynes BF, Pantaleo G, Fauci AS. Toward an understanding of the correlates of protective immunity to HIV infection. *Science* 1996;271: 324–328.

104. Clerici M, Shearer GM. The Th1-Th2 hypothesis of HIV infection: new insights. *Immunol Today* 1994;15:575–581.

105. Shearer GM, Clerici M. Protective immunity against HIV infection: has nature done the experiment for us? *Immunol Today* 1996;17:21–24.

106. Fauci AS, Pantaleo G, Stanley S, et al. Immunopathogenic mechanisms of HIV infection. *Ann Intern Med* 1996;124:654–663.

107. McCune MM. Viral latency in HIV disease. *Cell* 1995;82:183–188.

108. Schnittman SM, Greenhouse JJ, Lane HC, et al. Frequent detection of HIV-1-specific mRNAs in infected individuals suggests ongoing active viral expression in all stages of disease. *AIDS Res Hum Retrov* 1991;7:361–367.

109. Bonyhadi ML, Rabin L, Salimi S, et al. HIV induces thymus depletion in vivo. *Nature* 1993; 363:728–732.

110. Schnittman SM, Denning SM, Greenhouse JJ, et al. Evidence for susceptibility of intrathymic T-cell precursors and their progeny carrying T-cell antigen receptor phenotypes TCRαβ+ and TCR γδ+ to human immunodeficiency virus infection: a mechanism for CD4+ (T4+) lymphocyte depletion. *Proc Natl Acad Sci USA* 1990;87:7727–7731.

111. Fields BN. AIDS: time to turn to basic science. *Nature* 1994;369:95–96.

112. Wei X, Ghosh SK, Taylor ME, et al. Viral dynamics in human immunodeficiency virus type 1 infection. *Nature* 1995;373:117–122.

113. Ho DD, Neumann AU, Perelson AS, et al. Rapid turnover of plasma virions and CD4 lymphocytes in HIV-1 infection. *Nature* 1995;373:123–126.

114. Coffin JM. HIV population dynamics in vivo: implications for genetic variation, pathogenesis, and therapy. *Science* 1995;267:483–489.

115. Wain-Hobson S. Virological mayhem. *Nature* 1995;373:102.

116. Rutherford GH, Lifson AR, Hessol NA, et al. Course of HIV-1 infection in a cohort of homosexual and bisexual men: an 11-year followup study. *BMJ* 1990;301:1183–1188.

117. Koup RA, Safrit JT, Cao Y, et al. Temporal association of cellular immune responses with the initial control of viremia in primary human immunodeficiency virus type 1 syndrome. *J Virol* 1994;68: 4650–4655.

118. Koup RA, Ho DD. Shutting down HIV. *Nature* 1994;370:416.

119. Niu MT, Stein DS, Schnittman SM. Primary human immunodeficiency virus type 1 infection: review of pathogenesis and early treatment intervention in humans and animal retrovirus infections. *J Infect Dis* 1993;168:1490–1501.

120. Pantaleo G, Demarest JF, Soudeyns H, et al. Major expansion of CD8+ T cells with a predominant Vß usage during the primary immune response to HIV. *Nature* 1994;370:463–467.

121. Gartner S, Markovits P, Markovitz DM, et al. The role of mononuclear phagocytes in HTLV-III/LAV infection. *Science* 1986;233:215–219.

122. Yu X, McLane MF, Ratner L, et al. Killing of primary CD4+ T-cells by non-syncytium-inducing macrophage-tropic human immunodeficiency virus type 1. *Proc Natl Acad Sci USA* 1994;91: 10237–10241.

123. Lucey DR, Hensley RE, Ward WW, et al. CD4+ monocytes in HIV infection: an early increase is followed by a progressive decline. *J AIDS* 1991; 4:24–30.

124. Embretson J, Zupancic M, Ribas JL, et al. Massive covert infection of helper T lymphocytes and macrophages by HIV during the incubation period of AIDS. *Nature* 1993;362:359–362.

125. Pantaleo G, Graziosi C, Demarest JF, et al. HIV infection is active and progressive in lymphoid tissue during the clinically latent stage of disease. *Nature* 1993;362:355–358.

126. Heath SL, Tew JG, Szakal AK, et al. Follicular dendritic cells and human immunodeficiency virus infectivity. *Nature* 1995;377:740–744.

127. Schrager LK, Fauci AS. Trapped but still dangerous. *Nature* 1995;377:680–681.

128. Frankel SS, Wenig BM, Burke AP, et al. Replication of HIV-1 in dendritic cell-derived syncytia at the mucosal surface of the adenoid. *Science* 1996;272:115–117.

129. Donaldson YK, Bell JE, Ironside JW, et al. Redistribution of HIV outside the lymphoid system with onset of AIDS. *Lancet* 1994;343:383–385.

130. Degrassi A, De Maria A, Lisignoli G, et al. Transfer of HIV-1 to human tonsillar stromal cells following cocultivation with infected lymphocytes. *AIDS Res Hum Retrov* 1994;10:675–682.

131. Tamalet C, Lafeuillade A, Tourres C, et al. Inefficacy of neutralizing antibodies against lymph node HIV-1 isolates in patients with early stage HIV infection. *AIDS* 1994;8:388–389.

132. Ebnet K, Kaldjian EP, Anderson AO, et al. Orchestrated information transfer underlying leukocyte endothelial interactions. *Annu Rev Immunol* 1996;14:155–177.

133. Frost SD, McLean AR. Germinal centre destruction as a major pathway of HIV pathogenesis. *J AIDS* 1994;7:236–244.

134. Belshe RB, Bolognesi DP, Clements ML, et al. HIV infection in vaccinated volunteers. *JAMA* 1994;272:431.

135. Mosman TR, Cherwinski H, Bond MW, et al. Two types of murine helper T cell clones: definition according to profiles of lymphokine activities and secreted proteins. *J Immunol* 1986;136:2348–2357.

136. Lucey DR, Clerici M, Shearer GM. Type 1/type 2 cytokine dysregulation in human infectious, neoplastic, and inflammatory diseases. *Clin Microbiol Rev* 1996;9:532–562.

137. Salk J, Bretscher PA, Salk PL, et al. A strategy for prophylactic vaccination against HIV. *Science* 1993;260:1270–1274.

138. Shearer GM, Clerici M, Lucey DR. Cytokines and HIV infection. *Semin Virol* 1994;5:449–455.

139. Lucey DR, Melcher GP, Hendrix CW, et al. Human immunodeficiency virus infection in the U.S. Air Force: seroconversions, clinical staging, and assessment of a T helper cell functional assay to predict change in CD4+ T cell counts. *J Infect Dis* 1991;164:631–637.

140. Dolan MJ, Clerici M, Blatt, SP. *In vitro* T-cell function, delayed-type hypersensitivity skin testing, and CD4+ T-cell subset phenotyping independently predict survival time in patients infected with human immunodeficiency virus. *J Infect Dis* 1995;172:79–87.

141. Meyaard L, Otto SA, Hooibrink B, et al. Quantitative analysis of CD4+ T cell function in the course of human immunodeficiency virus infection. *J Clin Invest* 1994;94:1947–1952.

142. Miedema F, Petit AJC, Terpstra FG, et al. 1988. Immunological abnormalities in human immunodeficiency virus (HIV)-infected asymptomatic homosexual men: HIV affects the immune system before CD4+ T-helper cell depletion occurs. *J Clin Invest* 1988;82:1908–1914.

143. Romagnani S, Maggi E, Del Prete G. HIV can induce a Th1 to Th0 shift, and preferentially replicates in CD4+T-cell clones producing Th2-type cytokines. *Science* 1994;145:611–617.

144. Clerici M, Sarin A, Coffman RL, et al. Type 1/type 2 cytokine modulation of T-cell programmed cell death as a model for human immunodeficiency virus pathogenesis. *Proc Natl Acad Sci USA* 1994;91:11811–11815.

145. Kovacs JA, Baseller M, Dewar RJ, et al. Increases in CD4 T-lymphocytes with intermittent courses of interleukin–2 in patients with human immunodeficiency virus infection. *N Engl J Med* 1995;332:567–575.

146. Clark AG, Holodny M, Schwartz D, et al. Decrease in HIV provirus in peripheral blood mononuclear cells during zidovudine and human rIL-2 administration. *J AIDS* 1992;5:52.

147. Cohen J. IL-12 deaths: explanation and a puzzle. *Science* 1995;270:908.

148. Grabstein KH, Eisenman J, Shanebeck K, et al. Cloning of a T cell growth factor that interacts with the ß chain of the interleukin–2 receptor. *Science* 1994;264:965–968.

149. Bamford RN, Grant AJ, Burton JD, et al. The interleukin (IL) 2 receptor β chain is shared by IL-2 and a cytokine, provisionally designated IL-T, that stimulates T-cell proliferation and the induction of lymphokine-activated killer cells. *Proc Natl Acad Sci USA* 1994;91:4940–4944.

150. Burton JD, Bamford RN, Peters C, et al. A lymphokine, provisionally designated interleukin T and produced by a human adult-T-cell leukemia line, stimulates T-cell proliferation and the induction of lymphokine-activated killer cells. *Proc Natl Acad Sci USA* 1994;91:4935–4939.

151. Giri JG, Kumaki S, Ahdieh M, et al. Identification and cloning of a novel IL-15 binding protein that is structurally related to the alpha chain of the IL-2 receptor. *EMBO J* 1995;15:3654–3663.

152. Seder RA, Grabstein KH, Berzofsky JA, et al. Cytokine interactions in HIV-infected individuals:

roles of IL-2, IL-12, and IL-15. *J Exp Med* 1995; 182:1067–1073.

153. Mori AT, M. Suko M, Kaminuma O, et al. IL-15 promotes cytokine production of human T helper cells. *J Immunol* 1996;156:2400–2405.

154. Lucey DR, Pinto LA, Bethke FR, et al. Immunologic and virologic effects on peripheral blood mononuclear cells from HIV-1 infected patients. (Submitted for publication).

155. Langlade-Demoyen P, Ngo-Giang-Huong N, Ferchal F, et al. Human immunodeficiency virus (HIV) *nef*-specific cytotoxic T lymphocytes in noninfected heterosexual contact of HIV-infected patients. *J Clin Invest* 1994;93:1293–1297.

156. Clerici M, Giorgi JV, Chou CC, et al. Cell-mediated immune response to human immunodeficiency virus (HIV) type 1 in seronegative homosexual men with recent sexual exposure to HIV-1. *J Infect Dis* 1992;165:1012–1019.

157. Clerici M, Sison AV, Berzofsky JA, et al. Cellular immune factors associated with mother-to-infant transmission of HIV. *AIDS* 1993;7:1427–1433.

158. Ranki AM, Mattinen S, Yarchoan R, et al. T-cell response towards HIV in infected individuals with and without zidovudine therapy, and in HIV-exposed sexual partners. *AIDS* 1989;3:63–69.

159. Cheynier R, Langlade DP, Marescot MR, et al. Cytotoxic T lymphocyte responses in the peripheral blood of children born to human immunodeficiency virus-1-infected mothers. *Eur J Immunol* 1992;2:2211–2217.

160. Rowland-Jones SL, Nixon DF, Aldhous MC, et al. HIV-specific cytotoxic T-cell activity in an HIV-exposed but uninfected infant. *Lancet* 1993;341:860–861.

161. Rowland-Jones SL, Nixon DF, Aldhous MC, et al. HIV-specific cytotoxic T-cells in HIV-exposed but uninfected Gambian women. *Nature Med* 1995;1:59–64.

162. Pinto L, Sullivan J, Berzofsky JA, et al. ENV-specific cytotoxic T lymphocyte responses in HIV seronegative health care workers occupationally exposed to HIV-contaminated body fluids. *J Clin Invest* 1995;96:867–876.

163. Fowke K, Rutherford J, Ball B, et al. Cellular immune responses correlate with protection against HIV-1 among women resistant to infection. *Can J Infect Dis* 1995;6–8.

164. Baur A, Schwarz N, Ellinger S, et al. Continuous clearance of HIV in a vertically infected child. [Letter]. *Lancet* 1989;21:1045.

165. Bryson YJ, Pang S, Wei L, et al. Clearance of HIV infection in a vertically infected infant. *N Engl J Med* 1995;332:833–838.

166. European Collaborative Study. Mother-to-child transmission of HIV infection. *Lancet* 1988;2: 1039–1042.

167. Bryson YJ, Chen ISY. Clearance of 2 HIV in an infant: reply. *N Engl J Med* 1995;333:319–320.

168. Roques PA, Gras G, Parnet-Mathieu F, et al. Clearance of HIV infection in 12 perinatally infected children: clinical, virological and immunological data. *AIDS* 1995;9:F19–26.

169. Bryson YJ. HIV clearance in infants-a continuing saga. *AIDS* 1995;9:1373–1375.

170. McKintosh K, Burchett SK. Clearance of HIV-lessons from newborns. *N Engl J Med* 1995;332: 883–884.

171. Bakshi SS, Tetali S, Abrams EJ, et al. Repeatedly positive human immunodeficiency virus type 1 DNA polymerase chain reaction in human immunodeficiency virus-exposed seroreverting infants. *Pediatr Infect Dis J* 1995;14:658–662.

172. Newell ML, Dunn D, De Maria A, et al. Detection of virus in vertically exposed HIV-antibody-negative children. *Lancet* 1996;347:213–215.

173. Meier U-C, Klenerman P, Griffin P, et al. Cytotoxic T lymphocyte lysis inhibited by viable HIV mutants. *Science* 1995;270:1360–1362.

174. Walker CM, Moody DJ, Stites DP, et al. CD8+ lymphocytes can control HIV infection *in vitro* by suppressing virus replication. *Science* 1986; 234:1563.

175. Mackewicz CE, Blackbourn DJ, Levy JA. CD8+ T-cells suppress human immunodeficiency virus replication by inhibiting viral transcription. *Proc Natl Acad Sci USA* 1995;92:2308–2312.

176. Cocchi F, DeVico AL, Garzino-Demo A, et al. Identification of RANTES, MIP-1 alpha and MIP-1 beta as the major HIV-suppressive factors produced by CD8+ T-cells. *Science* 1995;270:1811–1815.

177. Hollander H, Levy JA. Neurologic abnormalities and recovery of human immunodeficiency virus from cerebrospinal fluid. *Ann Intern Med* 1987; 106:692–695.

178. Nottet HSLM, Gendelman HE. Unraveling the neuroimmune mechanisms for the HIV-1 associated cognitive/motor complex. *Immunol Today* 1995;16:441–448.

179. Resnick L, Berger JR, Shapshak P, et al. Early penetration of the blood-brain barrier by HIV. *Neurology* 1988;38:9–14.

180. Wesselingh SL, Griffin DE. Local cytokine responses during acute and chronic viral infections of the central nervous system. *Semin Virol* 1994; 5:457–463.

181. Epstein LG, Gendelman HE. Human immunodeficiency virus type 1 infection of the nervous system: pathogenetic mechanisms. *Ann Neurol* 1993; 33:429–436.

182. American Academy of Neurology AIDS Task Force. Nomenclature and research case definitions for neurologic manifestations of human immunodeficiency virus-type 1 infection. *Neurology* 1991; 41:778–785.

183. Bacellar H, Munoz A, Miller EN, et al. Temporal trends in the incidence of HIV-1 related neurologic diseases: Multicenter AIDS Cohort Study, 1985–1992. *Neurology* 1994;44:1892–1900.

184. Conrad AJ, Schmid P, Syndulko K, et al. Quantifying HIV-1 RNA using the polymerase chain reaction on cerebrospinal fluid and serum of seropositive individuals with and without neurologic abnormalities. *J AIDS* 1995;10:425–435.

185. Epstein LG, Kuiken C, Blumberg BM, et al. HIV-1 V3 domain variation in brain and spleen of children with AIDS: tissue-specific evolution within host-determined quasispecies. *Virology* 1991; 180:583–590.

186. Korber BTM, Kunstman KJ, Patterson BK, et al. Genetic differences between blood and brain-derived viral sequences from human immunodeficiency virus type 1-infected patients: evidence of conserved elements in the V3 region of the envelope protein of brain-derived sequences. *J Virol* 1994;68:7467–7481.

187. Power C, McArthur JC, Johnson RT, et al. Demented and nondemented patients with AIDS differ in brain-derived human immunodeficiency virus type 1 envelope sequences. *J Virol* 1994; 68:4643–4649.

188. Von Gegerfelt A, Chiodi F, Keys B, et al. Lack of autologous neutralizing antibodies in the cerebrospinal fluid of HIV-1 infected individuals. *AIDS Res Hum Retrov* 1992;8:1133–1138.

189. Lucey DR, Van Cott TC, Loomis LD, et al. Measurement of cerebrospinal fluid antibody to the HIV-1 principal neutralizing determinant (V3 loop). *J AIDS* 1993;6:994–1001.

190. Lucey DR, McGuire SA, Abbadessa S, et al. Cerebrospinal fluid neopterin levels in 159 neurologically asymptomatic persons infected with the human immunodeficiency virus (HIV-1): relationship to immune status. *Viral Immunol* 1993;6: 267–271.

191. Lucey DR, McGuire SA, Clerici M, et al. Comparison of spinal fluid β2-microglobulin levels with CD4+ T-cells, *in vitro* T helper cell function, and spinal fluid IgG parameters in 163 neurologically normal adults infected with the human immunodeficiency virus type 1. *J Infect Dis* 1991;163: 971–975.

192. Centers for Disease Control and Prevention. USPHS/IDSA guidelines for the prevention of opportunistic infections in persons infected with human immunodeficiency virus: a summary. *MMWR* 1995;44:1–34.

193. Chanock SJ, Pizzo PA. Infection prevention strategies for children with cancer and AIDS: contrasting dilemmas. *J Hosp Infect* 1995;30(Suppl): 197–208.

194. Gayle HD, D'Angelo LJ. Epidemiology of acquired immunodeficiency syndrome and human immunodeficiency virus infection in adolescents. *Pediatr Infect Dis J* 1991;10:322–328.

195. McKinney RE, Wilfert, CM. Lymphocyte subsets in children younger than 2 years old: normal values in a population at risk for human immunodeficiency virus infection and diagnostic and prognostic application to infected children. *Pediatr Infect Dis J* 1992;11:639–644

196. Erkeller-Yuksel FM, Deneys V, Hannet I, et al. Age-related changes in human blood lymphocyte subpopulations. *J Pediatr* 1992;120:216–220.

197. Landay A, Ohlsson-Wilhelm B, Giorgi JV. Application of flow cytometry to the study of HIV infection. *AIDS* 1990;4:479–497.

198. Centers for Disease Control and Prevention. 1995 revised guidelines for prophylaxis against *Pneumocystis carinii* pneumonia for children infected with or perinatally exposed to human immunodeficiency virus. *MMWR* 1995;44.

199. Grubman S, Simonds RJ. New PCP prophylaxis guidelines. *Pediatr Infect Dis J* 1996;15:165–168.

200. Powderly WG. Prophylaxis for HIV-related infections: a work in progress. *Ann Intern Med* 1996; 124:342–344.

201. Hoover DR, Saah AJ, Bacellar H, et al. Clinical manifestations of AIDS in the era of *Pneumocystis*

prophylaxis: Multicenter AIDS Cohort Study. *N Engl J Med* 1993;329:1922–1926.

202. Frankel DH. FDA approves rapid test for smear-positive tuberculosis. *Lancet* 1996;347:48.

203. Chang Y, Cesarman E, Pessin MS, et al. Identification of herpesvirus-like DNA sequences in AIDS-associated Kaposi's sarcoma. *Science* 1994; 266:1865–1869.

204. Moore PS, Chang Y. Detection of herpesvirus-like DNA sequences in Kaposi's sarcoma in patients with and without HIV infection. *N Engl J Med* 1995;332:1181–1185.

205. Chuck S, Grant RM, Katongole-Mbidde E, et al. Frequent presence of a novel herpesvirus genome in lesions of human immunodeficiency virus-infected Kaposi's sarcoma. *J Infect Dis* 1996;173: 248–251.

206. Gyulai R, Kemeny L, Kiss M, et al. Herpesvirus-like DNA in angiosarcoma in a patient without HIV infection. *N Engl J Med* 1996;334:540–541.

207. Soulier H, Grollet L, Oksenbhandler E, et al. Kaposi's sarcoma-associated herpesvirus-like DNA sequences in multicentric Castleman's disease. *Blood* 1995;86:1276–1280.

208. Cao Y, Qin L, Zhang L, et al. Virologic and immunologic characterization of long-term survivors of human immunodeficiency virus type 1 infection. *N Engl J Med* 1995;332:201–208.

209. Pantaleo G, Menzo S, Vaccarezza M, et al. Studies in subjects with long-term nonprogressive human immunodeficiency virus infection. *N Engl J Med* 1995;332:209–216.

210. Baltimore D. Lessons from people with nonprogressive HIV infection. *N Engl J Med* 1995;332: 259–260.

211. Zuger A. The long goodbye. *NY Times Mag.* 1993; July 25:23.

212. Deacon NJ, Tsykin A, Solomon A, et al. Genomic structure of an attenuated quasispecies of HIV-1 from a blood transfusion donor and recipients. *Science* 1995;270:988–991.

213. Kirchhoff F, Greenough TC, Brettler DB, et al. Brief report: absence of intact *nef* sequences in a long-term nonprogressive HIV-1 infection. *N Engl J Med* 1995;332:228–232.

214. Hirsch MS, D'Aquila RT. Therapy for human immunodeficiency virus infection. *N Engl J Med* 1993;328:1686–1695.

215. Volberding PA, Lagakos SW, Koch MA, et al. Zidovudine in asymptomatic human immunode-ficiency virus infection. *N Engl J Med* 1990;322: 941–949.

216. Sande MA, Carpenter CJ, Cobbs CG, et al. Antiretroviral therapy for adult HIV-infected patients. *JAMA* 1993;270:2583–2589.

217. Aboulker JR, Swart AM. Preliminary analysis of the Concorde trial. *Lancet* 1993;341:889–890.

218. Eron JJ, Benoit SL, Jemsek J, et al. Treatment with lamivudine, zidovudine, or both in HIV-positive patients with 200 to 500 CD4+ cells per cubic millimeter. *N Engl J Med* 1995;333:1662–1669.

219. Markowitz M, Saag M, Powderly WG, et al. A preliminary study of ritonavir, an inhibitor of HIV-1 protease to treat HIV-1 infection. *N Engl J Med* 1996;333:1534–1539.

220. Mascolini M. An FDA-OK'd viral load test? The wait may be nearly over. *J Int Assoc Phys AIDS Care* 1996:Jan:6–9.

221. Volberding PA. HIV quantification: clinical applications. *Lancet* 1996;347:71–73.

222. Piatek M, Saag MS, Yang LC, et al. High levels of HIV-1 in plasma during all stages of infection determined by competitive PCR. *Science* 1993; 259:1749–1754.

223. Dickover RE, Garratty EM, Herman SA, et al. Identification of levels of maternal HIV-1 RNA associated with risk of perinatal transmission. *JAMA* 1996;275:599–605.

224. Mellors JW, Kingsley LA, Rinaldo CR, et al. Quantitation of HIV-1 RNA in plasma predicts outcome after seroconversion. *Ann Intern Med* 1995;122:573–579.

225. Saksela K, Stevens C, Rubinstein R, Baltimore D. Human immunodeficiency virus type 1 mRNA expression in peripheral blood cells as an early marker of risk for progression to AIDS. *Ann Intern Med* 1995;123:641–648.

226. Greene WC. Predicting progression to AIDS. *Ann Intern Med* 1995;123:726–727.

227. Ho DD. Time to hit HIV, early and hard. *N Engl J Med* 1995;333:450–451.

228. Walker MC, Fast PE. Clinical trials of candidate AIDS vaccines. *AIDS* 1994;8:S213–S236.

229. Vermund SH, Schultz AM, Hoff R. Prevention of HIV/AIDS with vaccines. *Curr Opin Infect Dis* 1994;7:82–94.

230. Hilleman R. Whether and when an AIDS vaccine? *Nature Med* 1995;1:1126–1129.

231. Salk J. Prospects for the control of AIDS by immunizing seropositive individuals. *Nature* 1987;327: 473–476.

232. Cohen J. U.S. panel votes to delay real-world vaccine trials. *Science* 1994;264:1839.

233. Rowe PM. AIDS vaccines not ready for phase III trials. *Lancet* 1994;343:1626.

234. Mascola JR, Snyder SW, Weislow OS, et al. Immunization with envelope subunit vaccine products elicits neutralizing antibodies against laboratory-adapted but not primary isolates of human immunodeficiency virus type 1. *J Infect Dis* 1996; 173:340–348.

235. National Institutes of Allergy and Infectious Diseases. *HIV/AIDS Research Agenda*. Bethesda, MD: National Institutes of Health, December 1995.

236. Moore J, Anderson R. The WHO and why of HIV vaccine trials. *Nature* 1994;372:313–314.

237. Cohen J. Thailand weighs AIDS vaccine tests. *Science* 1995;270:904–907.

238. Berman PW, Nurthy KK, Wrin T, et al. Protection of MN-rgp120-immunized chimpanzees from heterologous infection with a primary isolate of HIV type 1. *J Infect Dis* 1996;13:52–59.

239. Kalish ML, Baldwin A, Raktham S, et al. The evolving molecular epidemiology of HIV-1 envelope subtypes in injecting drug users in Bangkok, Thailand: implications for HIV vaccine trials. *AIDS* 1995;9:851–857.

240. Kahn JO, Steimer KS, Baenziger J, et al. Clinical, immunologic and virologic observations related to HIV-1 infection in a volunteer in an HIV-1 vaccine clinical trial. *J Infect Dis* 1995;171:1343–1347.

241. O'Toole C, Muller S, Nara P, et al. Immunologic mechanism for human immunodeficiency virus type 1 gp120 vaccine failure. *J Infect Dis* 1996; 173:512–513.

242. Kaiser J. AIDS vaccine trial disappointing. *Science* 1996;272:341.

243. Vahey M, Birx DL, Michael NL, et al. Assessment of *gag* DNA and genomic RNA in peripheral blood mononuclear cells in HIV-infected patients receiving intervention with a recombinant gp160 subunit vaccine in phase I study. *AIDS Res Hum Retrov* 1994;10:649–655.

244. Holden C. AIDS vaccine therapy trial launched. *Science* 1996;271:501.

245. Egan MA, Pavlat WA, Tartaglia J, et al. Induction of HIV-1 specific cytolytic T-lymphocyte response in seronegative adults by a nonreplicating, host-range-restricted canary-pox vector (ALVAC) carrying the HIV-1 MN gene. *J Infect Dis* 1995; 171:1623–1627.

246. Robinson HL, Lu S, Feltquate DM, et al. DNA vaccines. *AIDS Res Hum Retrov* 1996;12:455–457.

247. McDonnell WM, Askaria FK. DNA vaccines. *N Engl J Med* 1996;334:42–45.

248. Haynes BF. Scientific and social issues of HIV vaccine development. *Science* 1993;260:1279–1286.

249. Lurie P, Bishaw M, Chesney MA, et al. Ethical, behavioral, and social aspects of HIV vaccine trials in developing countries. *JAMA* 1994;271: 295–301.

250. Grady C. The search for an AIDS vaccine: ethical issues in the development and testing of a preventive HIV vaccine. Bloomington, IN: Indiana University Press, 1995.

251. Anonymous. Coming clean about needle exchange. *Lancet* 1995;346:1377.

252. Feng Y, Broder CC, Kennedy PE, Berger EA. HIV-1 entry cofactor: functional cDNA cloning of a seven-transmembrane, G protein-coupled receptor. *Science* 1996;272:872–877.

253. Choe H, Farzan M, Sun Y, et al. The beta-chemokine receptors CCR3 and CCR5 facilitate infection by primary HIV-1 isolates. *Cell* 1996;85:1135–1148.

254. Doranz BJ, Rucker J, Yi Y, et al. A dual-tropic primary HIV-1 isolate that uses fusin and the beta-chemokine receptors CKR-5, CKR-3, and CKR-2b as fusion cofactors. *Cell* 1996;85:1149–1158.

255. Deng H, Liu R, Ellmeier W, et al. Identification of a major co-receptor for primary isolates of HIV-1. *Nature* 1996;381:661–666.

256. Dragic T, Litwin V, Allaway GP, et al. HIV-1 entry into CD4+ cells is mediated by the chemokine receptor CC-CKR-5. *Nature* 1996;381:667–673.

257. Alhkatib G, Combadiere C, Broder CC, et al. CC CKR5: a RANTES, MIP-1alpha, MIP-1 beta receptor as a fusion cofactor for macrophage-tropic HIV-1. *Science* 1996;272:1955–1958.

258. Anonymous. From the Centers for Disease Control and Prevention. Update: provisional public health service recommendations for chemoprophylaxis after occupational exposure to HIV. *JAMA* 1996; 272:90–92.

2

Global Overview of the HIV/AIDS Pandemic

Daniel Tarantola, M.D., and Jonathan M. Mann, M.D., M.P.H.

The pandemic of human immunodeficiency virus (HIV) infection and acquired immunodeficiency syndrome (AIDS) continues to expand, and its impact on individuals and society is increasingly felt. Since more than two-thirds of new HIV infections worldwide are estimated to be due to heterosexual transmission, and an increasing proportion of these are in women, the number of infected children is growing rapidly.[1a]

By January 1996, about 3 million children had acquired HIV infection through mother-to-child transmission. Because of the rapid evolution of pediatric HIV infection to the onset of AIDS and the short survival once pediatric AIDS has set in, most of these children have died. About one-quarter of all AIDS-related deaths have occurred in children infected perinatally. More than 85% of children infected perinatally were in sub-Saharan Africa. During 1995, approximately 500,000 children were born with HIV infection (about 1,400 per day), and of these children 67% were in sub-Saharan Africa, 30% in Southeast Asia, 2% in Latin America, and 1% in the rest of the world. By January 1996, about one million children were living with HIV/AIDS, of whom 65% were in sub-Saharan Africa. HIV incidence among children in sub-Saharan Africa, Southeast Asia, and the Caribbean was higher than the incidence among adults in all other regions in the world. The prevalence of HIV infection or AIDS among children was almost 35 times higher in the developing world than in the industrialized world.

The pandemic of HIV infection and AIDS also affects children through the premature death of their parents. Since the beginning of the pandemic, more than 9 million children under 15 years of age have lost their mothers to AIDS. Of these maternal orphans, 90% were in sub-Saharan Africa, and in this region, as well as in the rest of the world, one in every three children orphaned was under 5 years of age.

This chapter provides estimates of the prevalence and incidence of HIV infection and AIDS in adults (15–49 years old) and children infected perinatally for 10 geographic areas of affinity (GAAs) and for the world.[2] It attempts to project a panoramic view of the HIV infection and AIDS pandemic, which, over time, has become increasingly fragmented, complex, and powerful.

Data Used in Estimating the Status, Trends, and Impact of HIV Infection and AIDS

Notifications of HIV infection obtained through mandatory testing schemes, as imposed in a number of countries, are not reliable sources of information for surveillance purposes or for estimating the status, trends, or impact of the pandemic. A survey conducted in 1993–1994 indicated that 36 countries imposed involuntary HIV testing on individuals assumed to belong to "high-risk" groups.[3] The most frequent targets of involuntary HIV testing were military recruits, patients with tuberculosis, prisoners, foreign laborers applying for work permits, applicants for residence permits, and pregnant women. The selectivity and mandatory nature of such testing diminishes considerably the epidemiologic value of the data obtained. Furthermore, the quality of such information varies considerably from one population to the next due to differences in public awareness, commitment to voluntary testing, access to diagnostic services, protection of confidentiality, and actions taken in the event of a positive result.

Voluntary HIV testing may provide useful information when the rate of acceptance of a proposed test, combined with counseling, both before and after the test, is high. For example, in Sweden almost all pregnant women attend antenatal clinics where they are offered voluntary HIV testing; the acceptance rate has exceeded 97%.[4] In addition, an estimated 87% of patients attending sexually transmitted disease clinics in Sweden agreed to be tested. By 1992, one-quarter of the men and one-third of the women in Sweden had been tested for HIV at least once.[5] People more likely to have been tested lived in large urban areas and had higher educational levels.

In the United States, 25 of the 50 states have laws or regulations requiring confidential named reporting of HIV infection, but this reporting is considered to be less complete than the reporting of AIDS cases.[6] In a large number of countries, voluntary testing is at least theoretically offered to adults in the sexually active age group. However, access to testing schemes is limited by many factors, including the lack of diagnostic facilities and reagents. The persisting gap in both industrialized and developing countries between the capacity to test for HIV infection and the availability of counseling further limits the coverage of testing schemes and biases the samples of persons who request an HIV test.

An increasing number of countries have established *sentinel surveillance systems* along guidelines from the World Health Organization (WHO) Global Programme on AIDS. These systems, based on anonymous HIV testing performed on residual blood samples initially collected for other purposes than HIV diagnosis, help monitor epidemic trends and guide policy development and management decisions. The estimates that follow are derived from published and unpublished cross-sectional studies of HIV prevalence in individuals deemed to represent as closely as possible the sexually active adult population in countries around the world (women attending antenatal clinics, in particular) and from sentinel surveillance schemes.[7] The methods used to estimate HIV infections, AIDS cases, and AIDS-related deaths were detailed in the first volume of *AIDS in the World*.[8]

As HIV prevalence surveys in children are too scarce to provide a global picture, the estimates of HIV prevalence in this population are limited to infants who have acquired HIV infection perinatally from their mothers. These estimates are based on a model that takes into account age-specific HIV prevalence in women in the reproductive age group (15–49 years old); age-specific fertility rates in various world regions, and rates of transmission from HIV-infected pregnant women to their offspring.[9]

Geographic Distribution of HIV-1 and HIV-2

Two strains of HIV are currently involved in the global HIV pandemic: HIV-1 and HIV-2. Found in almost every country around the world since its discovery in 1983, HIV-1 has been extensively researched, and several subtypes of this virus—also called *clades*—have now been recognized. They differ genetically, biologically, and serologically.[10,11] Some regions of the world have only one clade, while other regions have two or more coexisting clades.[12,13]

In contrast to the wide spread HIV-1, HIV-2 is found mostly in West Africa and in countries that are linked to this region through patterns of population mobility (France, southern Africa, Latin America, and the Caribbean). In addition to structural, serologic, and pathogenic differences between HIV-1 and HIV-2, epidemiologic studies have shown that the former is transmitted more efficiently than the latter.[14–16] In areas where HIV-2 was involved in most of the infections when it was initially recognized in 1986, the prevalence of this virus is being overtaken by that of HIV-1. Regardless of differences in pathogenesis and transmission patterns, prevention strategies remain identical for both types of HIV. Since HIV-2 accounts for less than 1% of all HIV infections worldwide, the estimates presented below for HIV-1 may be considered also to include HIV-2.

Cumulative Incidence of HIV Infection

From the beginning of the pandemic until January 1, 1996, an estimated 30.1 million people worldwide had been infected with HIV. Of these, 27.4 million were adults (15.8 million men and 11.7 million women) and 2.7 million were children. The largest numbers of HIV-infected people were in sub-Saharan Africa (18.9 million; 63% of global total) and Southeast Asia (6.8 million; 23%) (Table 2-1). Since the beginning of the pandemic, the most of the HIV infections (over 27 million; 92%) have occurred in the developing world. The number of HIV-infected people in Southeast Asia is now more than three times the total number of infected people in the entire industrialized world (Figure 2-1).

The global cumulative number of HIV infections among adults has tripled since the beginning of the decade, from nearly 10 million in 1990 to over 30 million in 1996.

Reported and Estimated AIDS Cases

In every country, national health authorities have the responsibility of collecting and reporting health information to WHO. Since 1986, WHO has monitored the reporting of AIDS by countries. Official reporting of AIDS provides a broad indication of the evolution of the pandemic. The official reporting of AIDS is constrained by several factors. First, national health authorities differ widely in their capability, interest, and willingness to collect or report information about AIDS. Second, even when intentions are ideal, reporting is based on AIDS case definitions that may vary widely among countries or from one reporting period to another. Finally, reporting is often delayed or incomplete, and seldom includes pediatric AIDS cases, partly because of the shortcomings of the pediatric AIDS case definition. The global reporting of AIDS to WHO by countries does not include pediatric cases. Thus, official AIDS reports may help define general trends, particularly where HIV epidemics have matured, but inadequately reflect HIV spread and, therefore, are poor indicators of the current status or impact of the epidemic.

Table 2-1. Cumulative HIV Infections as of January 1, 1996, by Geographic Area of Affinity*

GAA	Adults	Men	Women	Children†	Total
North America	1,269,000	1,087,000	181,000	16,000	1,285,000
Western Europe	829,000	691,000	138,000	8,000	836,000
Oceania	31,000	28,000	3,000	<1,000	32,000
Latin America	1,477,000	1,182,000	295,000	70,000	1,547,000
Sub-Saharan Africa	16,550,000	7,881,000	8,670,000	2,327,000	18,877,000
Caribbean	467,000	280,000	187,000	31,000	498,000
Eastern Europe	37,000	34,000	3,000	<1,000	38,000
Southeast Mediterranean	76,000	63,000	13,000	<1,000	77,000
Northeast Asia	179,000	149,000	30,000	1,000	180,000
Southeast Asia	6,535,000	4,356,000	2,178,000	228,000	6,762,000
Total world	27,449,000	15,751,000	11,699,000	2,682,000	30,131,000

From Ref. 1, with permission.

*Columns and rows may fail to sum due to rounding off to the nearest 1,000.

†HIV infection acquired before or at birth.

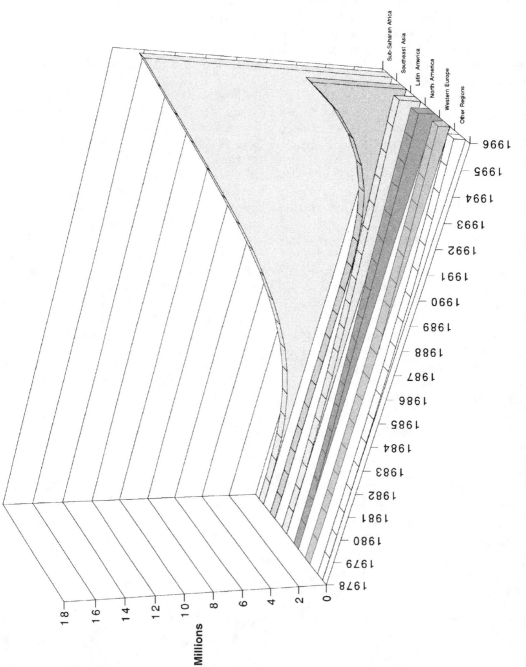

Figure 2-1. Cumulative number of HIV-infected adults, by GAA and by the year, 1978–1996 (as of January 1 of each year).

Table 2-2. Cumulative AIDS Cases as of January 1, 1996, by Geographic Area of Affinity*

GAA	Adults	Men	Women	Children†	Total
North America‡	443,000	380,000	63,000	7,000	449,000
Western Europe	193,000	161,000	32,000	3,000	195,000
Oceania	9,000	8,000	0,000	<1,000	9,000
Latin America	518,000	414,000	104,000	62,000	579,000
Sub-Saharan Africa	6,367,000	3,032,000	3,335,000	2,046,000	8,413,000
Caribbean	133,000	80,000	53,000	27,000	160,000
Eastern Europe	7,000	7,000	<1,000	<1,000	7,000
Southeast Mediterranean	12,000	10,000	2,000	<1,000	12,000
Northeast Asia	12,000	10,000	2,000	<1,000	12,000
Southeast Asia	332,000	221,000	111,000	206,000	537,000
Total world	8,024,000	4,321,000	3,703,000	2,351,000	10,375,000

From Ref. 1, with permission.

*Columns and rows may fail to sum due to rounding off to the nearest 1,000.

†HIV infection acquired before or at birth.

‡AIDS cases in North America have been estimated on the basis of the 1987 revised CDC AIDS Surveillance Case definition.

By the end of 1995, over 1.4 million AIDS cases had been reported to WHO. Of the 190 countries and territories, 160 (86%) had reported at least one case.[17] However, by reconstructing and modeling HIV epidemic curves for each world region, we estimate that 10.4 million people developed AIDS from the beginning of the pandemic until January 1, 1996. Of these people, 8.4 million (81%) were in sub-Saharan Africa, 0.7 million were in Latin America and the Caribbean (7%), and 0.7 million were in North America, western Europe, and Oceania combined (6%) (Table 2-2). In Southeast Asia, where the pandemic gained intensity more recently, it is estimated that 0.5 million people have already developed AIDS. Of the 2.4 million children with AIDS, the large majority (2 million or 85%) were in sub-Saharan Africa.

AIDS-Related Deaths

The life expectancy of people with AIDS—both adults and children—who have access to early and sustained therapy has increased considerably in recent years, largely due to prevention and treatment of opportunistic infections. Detailed information on disease progression rates has been available from the industrialized world through cohort studies of homosexual men and people infected with HIV-1

through blood transfusions.[18,19] Relatively little is known about disease progression in developing countries. Studies in Africa, however, suggest that both incubation and symptomatic survival periods are shorter—perhaps far shorter—there than in the industrialized world.[20] Accordingly, the estimates of deaths presented in this chapter are based on survival rates applied to adults and children that differ in the developing and in the industrialized world.[9]

By January 1, 1996, 9.2 million people are estimated to have died from AIDS worldwide, or 89% of all people with AIDS. The total number of people having died from AIDS includes about 7.6 million people in sub-Saharan Africa (83%), 0.7 million in Latin America, 0.4 million in Southeast Asia, 358,000 in North America, 144,000 in western Europe, and 26,000 in the rest of the world.

New HIV Infections, AIDS, and AIDS-Related Deaths in 1995

New HIV infections, cases of AIDS, and AIDS-related deaths during a calendar year illustrate the current magnitude and global distribution of the epidemic. Worldwide during 1995, 4.7 million new HIV infections occurred (an average of 13,000 new infections each day). Of these, 2.4 million (an average of nearly 7,000 new infections per day) occur-red in Southeast Asia and 1.9 million infections (over 5,000 new infections per day) were in sub-Saharan Africa. The industrialized world accounted for about 170,000 new HIV infections (nearly 500 new infections per day; less than 4% of the global total). In 1995, 1.7 million women were newly HIV-infected (over 4,500 per day; 40% of all new adult infections). During 1995, approximately 500,000 children were born with HIV infection (about 1,400 per day); of these children, 67% were in sub-Saharan Africa, 30% in Southeast Asia, 2% in Latin America, and 1% in the Caribbean (Table 2-3).

Therefore, in all GAAs, from thousands to mil-lions of people are still becoming infected with HIV each year. The number of adults becoming infected each year seems to have reached a plateau in western Europe, the Caribbean, and sub-Saharan Africa. The annual number of new infections also appears to have decreased, at least temporarily, in North America, Oceania, and the Southeast Mediterra-nean. However, in recently affected areas, such as Southeast and Northeast Asia, HIV incidence (new infections per year) is rising steeply (Figure 2-2).

Analysis of HIV incidence in 1995 indicates the comparative rate of increase of the HIV pandemic in various populations. The worldwide incidence of (new) HIV infections in 1995 was estimated at 82.9 per 100,000 population: 145 per 100,000

adults (men and women, 15–49 years old) and 75.5 per 100,000 in children (under 5 years old). The highest HIV incidence for adults and children com-bined was in sub-Saharan Africa (318 per 100,000), followed by Southeast Asia (164 per 100,000), and the Caribbean (140 per 100,000). The incidence of HIV in other GAAs was at or below 50 per 100,000.

HIV incidence was higher in women than in men in sub-Saharan Africa. (607 vs 561 per 100,000). However, in all other GAAs, HIV incidence was higher among men. The incidence of HIV infection among children varied among GAAs, from less than 1 per 100,000 in eastern Europe, Southeast Mediterranean, and Northeast Asia, to 310 per 100,000 in sub-Saharan Africa. HIV incidence among children in sub-Saharan Africa, Southeast Asia, and the Caribbean was higher than HIV inci-dence among adults in all other regions of the world.

During 1995 an estimated 1.9 million people developed AIDS, including 1.5 million adults and 400,000 children (Table 2-4). Of people newly de-veloping AIDS, 74% were in sub-Saharan Africa and 13% were in Southeast Asia. Thus, in 1995, over twice as many people developed AIDS in Southeast Asia than in all the industrialized coun-tries of the world. Globally, the estimated incidence of AIDS in 1994 was 32.5 per 100,000 (Table 2-5). The highest incidence occurred among women in sub-Saharan Africa.

Table 2-3. New HIV Infections, January 1, 1995 Through December 31, 1995, by Geographic Area of Affinity*

GAA	Adults	Men	Women	Children†	Total
North America	70,000	60,000	10,000	2,000	72,000
Western Europe	88,000	73,000	15,000	1,000	89,000
Oceania	2,000	2,000	<1,000	<1,000	2,000
Latin America	110,000	88,000	22,000	9,000	119,000
Sub-Saharan Africa	1,547,000	737,000	810,000	345,000	1,892,000
Caribbean	45,000	27,000	18,000	5,000	50,000
Eastern Europe	5,000	4,000	<1,000	<1,000	5,000
Southeast Mediterranean	11,000	9,000	2,000	<1,000	11,000
Northeast Asia	47,000	39,000	8,000	<1,000	48,000
Southeast Asia	2,298,000	1,532,000	766,000	153,000	2,450,000
Total world	4,223,000	2,572,000	1,651,000	516,000	4,739,000

From Ref. 1, with permission.

*Columns and rows may fail to sum due to rounding off to the nearest 1,000.

†HIV infection acquired before or at birth.

Year	North America	Western Europe	Oceania	Latin America	Sub-Saharan Africa	Caribbean	Eastern Europe	Southeast Mediterranean	Northeast Asia	Southeast Asia	Total world
1978	0	0	0	0	0	0					0
1979	1,000	<1,000	0	0	<1,000	0					2,000
1980	18,000	1,000	<1,000	1,000	41,000	<1,000					62,000
1981	50,000	6,000	<1,000	18,000	152,000	1,000					227,000
1982	96,000	14,000	<1,000	49,000	373,000	5,000					537,000
1983	156,000	29,000	1,000	96,000	730,000	13,000	0				1,025,000
1984	228,000	50,000	2,000	160,000	1,243,000	25,000	<1,000				1,708,000
1985	310,000	78,000	4,000	238,000	1,921,000	42,000	1,000	0			2,593,000
1986	398,000	115,000	6,000	328,000	2,762,000	64,000	3,000	<1,000			3,676,000
1987	491,000	160,000	8,000	429,000	3,756,000	91,000	5,000	4,000	<1,000	<1,000	4,944,000
1988	586,000	212,000	10,000	539,000	4,890,000	123,000	7,000	8,000	1,000	7,000	6,384,000
1989	682,000	272,000	13,000	654,000	6,145,000	159,000	10,000	13,000	4,000	41,000	7,993,000
1990	777,000	339,000	16,000	773,000	7,498,000	198,000	13,000	20,000	10,000	138,000	9,782,000
1991	869,000	411,000	19,000	894,000	8,929,000	241,000	16,000	27,000	21,000	357,000	11,784,000
1992	958,000	488,000	21,000	1,015,000	10,414,000	285,000	20,000	36,000	38,000	774,000	14,048,000
1993	1,043,000	570,000	24,000	1,135,000	11,932,000	330,000	24,000	45,000	62,000	1,484,000	16,647,000
1994	1,123,000	654,000	27,000	1,252,000	13,463,000	376,000	28,000	55,000	93,000	2,597,000	19,668,000
1995	1,198,000	741,000	29,000	1,367,000	15,003,000	421,000	33,000	65,000	132,000	4,237,000	23,226,000
1996	1,269,000	829,000	31,000	1,477,000	16,550,000	467,000	37,000	76,000	179,000	6,535,000	27,449,000

Figure 2-2. Cumulative adult HIV infections as of January 1, 1996, by GAA. *Note:* Columns and rows may fail to sum due to rounding off to the nearest 1,000. (From Ref. 8, with permission.)

Table 2-4. New AIDS Cases, January 1, 1995 Through December 31, 1995, by Geographic Area of Affinity*

GAA	Adults	Men	Women	Children†	Total
North America‡	62,000	53,000	9,000	1,000	63,000
Western Europe	37,000	31,000	6,000	<1,000	38,000
Oceania	2,000	1,000	<1,000	<1,000	2,000
Latin America	85,000	68,000	17,000	8,000	93,000
Sub-Saharan Africa	1,074,000	511,000	562,000	301,000	1,375,000
Caribbean	26,000	16,000	10,000	4,000	30,000
Eastern Europe	2,000	1,000	<1,000	<1,000	2,000
Southeast Mediterranean	3,000	3,000	<1,000	<1,000	3,000
Northeast Asia	5,000	4,000	<1,000	<1,000	5,000
Southeast Asia	160,000	107,000	53,000	87,000	248,000
Total world	1,455,000	795,000	660,000	403,000	1,858,000

From Ref. 1, with permission.

*Columns and rows may fail to sum due to rounding off to the nearest 1,000.

†HIV infection acquired before or at birth.

‡AIDS cases in North America have been estimated on the basis of the 1987 revised CDC AIDS Surveillance Case definition.

People Living with HIV Infection and with AIDS in 1996

On January 1, 1996, an estimated 20.3 million people were living with HIV infection that had not yet evolved to AIDS, including 19.4 million adults (11.4 million men and 8 million women) along with about 850,000 children (Table 2-6). In addition, on January 1, 1996, an estimated 1.2 million people worldwide were living with AIDS, including 1.1 million adults (618,000 men and 472,000 women) and about 62,000 children (Table 2-7).

On January 1, 1996, there were 18 people living with HIV infection for each person living with AIDS. Depending upon the rate of new HIV infection and the duration of the epidemic, this ratio should gradually decline. The ratio is also influenced by the number of perinatally infected children, since progression from HIV infection to AIDS and the duration of life after the onset of AIDS are shorter in these children than among adults.

Table 2-5. Incidence of AIDS Cases, January 1 Through December 31, 1995, Rates per 100,000 by Geographic Area of Affinity

GAA	Adults	Men	Women	Children*	Total
North America†	39.9	68.3	11.4	5.1	21.5
Western Europe	19.2	31.7	6.5	2.2	9.8
Oceania	10.2	17.9	2.3	0.8	5.4
Latin America	36.9	59.1	14.8	14.0	20.9
Sub-Saharan Africa	405.4	389.4	421.1	270.5	230.7
Caribbean	138.1	166.4	110.1	105.7	84.6
Eastern Europe	0.8	1.4	0.1	<0.1	0.4
Southeast Mediterranean	1.4	2.2	0.5	<0.1	0.6
Northeast Asia	0.6	0.9	0.2	0.1	0.3
Southeast Asia	21.5	27.8	14.7	43.3	16.6
Total world	49.9	53.5	46.3	59.0	32.5

From Ref. 1, with permission.

*HIV infection acquired before or at birth.

†AIDS cases in North America have been estimated on the basis of the 1987 revised CDC AIDS Surveillance Case definition.

Table 2-6.   Persons Living With HIV (Not Yet Progressed to AIDS) on January 1, 1996, by Geographic Area of Affinity*

GAA	Adults	Men	Women	Children†	Total
North America	826,000	708,000	118,000	11,000	837,000
Western Europe	636,000	530,000	106,000	6,000	642,000
Oceania	23,000	20,000	3,000	<1,000	23,000
Latin America	959,000	767,000	192,000	17,000	976,000
Sub-Saharan Africa	10,183,000	4,849,000	5,334,000	626,000	10,809,000
Caribbean	334,000	200,000	134,000	9,000	343,000
Eastern Europe	30,000	27,000	3,000	<1,000	30,000
Southeast Mediterranean	64,000	54,000	11,000	<1,000	65,000
Northeast Asia	167,000	139,000	28,000	2,000	169,000
Southeast Asia	6,203,000	4,135,000	2,068,000	175,000	6,378,000
Total world	19,425,000	11,430,000	7,995,000	847,000	20,272,000

From Ref. 1, with permission.

*Columns and rows may fail to sum due to rounding off to the nearest 1,000.

†HIV infection acquired before or at birth.

Therefore, on January 1, 1996, an estimated 21.4 million people worldwide were living with HIV infection or AIDS (Table 2-8). Of these, 11.6 million (54%) were in sub-Saharan Africa, about 6.4 million (30%) were in Southeast Asia, 1 million (5%) were in Latin America, 928,000 (4%) were in North America, 694,000 (3%) were in western Europe, and 583,000 (3%) were in the rest of the world. About 41% of all adults living with HIV infection or AIDS were women, and 4% of all people living with HIV infection or AIDS were children. The majority of people living with HIV infection or AIDS were in the developing world (including 92% of all adults, 97% of all women, and 98% of all children).

Finally, the point prevalence of HIV infection and AIDS was derived by dividing the number of people living with HIV infection or AIDS at the beginning of 1996 by the total population. Prevalence provides another perspective on the challenges posed by the pandemic, as it indicates the proportion of the population directly affected by HIV infection or AIDS. On January 1, 1996, the prevalence of HIV infection in the world—not

Table 2-7.   Persons Living With AIDS on January 1, 1996, by Geographic Area of Affinity*

GAA	Adults	Men	Women	Children†	Total
North America‡	91,000	78,000	13,000	<1,000	91,000
Western Europe	52,000	43,000	9,000	<1,000	52,000
Oceania	2,000	2,000	<1,000	<1,000	2,000
Latin America	60,000	48,000	12,000	1,000	61,000
Sub-Saharan Africa	756,000	360,000	396,000	47,000	803,000
Caribbean	18,000	11,000	7,000	<1,000	19,000
Eastern Europe	2,000	2,000	<1,000	<1,000	2,000
Southeast Mediterranean	4,000	4,000	<1,000	<1,000	4,000
Northeast Asia	6,000	5,000	0,000	<1,000	6,000
Southeast Asia	100,000	67,000	33,000	12,000	112,000
Total world	1,090,000	618,000	472,000	62,000	1,152,000

From Ref. 1, with permission.

*Columns and rows may fail to sum due to rounding off to the nearest 1,000.

†HIV infection acquired before or at birth.

‡AIDS cases in North America have been estimated on the basis of the 1987 revised CDC AIDS Surveillance Case definition.

Table 2-8. Persons Living With HIV or AIDS on January 1, 1996, by Geographic Area of Affinity*

GAA	Adults	Men	Women	Children†	Total
North America	916,000	785,000	131,000	12,000	928,000
Western Europe	688,000	573,000	115,000	6,000	694,000
Oceania	25,000	22,000	3,000	<1,000	25,000
Latin America	1,019,000	815,000	204,000	19,000	1,038,000
Sub-Saharan Africa	10,939,000	5,209,000	5,730,000	673,000	11,612,000
Caribbean	352,000	211,000	141,000	10,000	362,000
Eastern Europe	32,000	29,000	3,000	<1,000	32,000
Southeast Mediterranean	69,000	57,000	11,000	<1,000	69,000
Northeast Asia	173,000	144,000	29,000	2,000	174,000
Southeast Asia	6,303,000	4,202,000	2,101,000	186,000	6,490,000
Total world	20,516,000	12,048,000	8,467,000	909,000	21,424,000

From Ref. 1, with permission.

*Columns and rows may fail to sum due to rounding off to the nearest 1,000.

†HIV infection acquired before or at birth.

counting people living with AIDS—was estimated at 355 per 100,000. The highest prevalence was in sub-Saharan Africa (1,814 per 100,000), and the lowest was in eastern Europe (7 per 100,000).

The global prevalence of AIDS on January 1, 1996, was 20 per 100,000. AIDS prevalence in sub-Saharan Africa was about 4 times higher than in North America, more than twice as high as in the Caribbean, and 18 times higher than in Southeast Asia (where a major increase in the prevalence of AIDS is expected by the end of the decade). Therefore, the combined global prevalence of HIV infection and AIDS on January 1, 1996 was 375 per 100,000. The prevalence of HIV infection and AIDS was 12 times higher in the developing world than in the industrialized world. Compared with the industrialized world, the prevalence of HIV infection and AIDS in the developing world was almost 9 times higher among men, 37 times higher among women, and 35 times higher among children.

AIDS Orphans

For the purpose of this summary, orphans are defined as noninfected children younger than 15 whose biologic mother died of AIDS. No estimates can be made of the number of children who lost their biologic father or their stepfather to AIDS or can of the number of children who lost both parents to the pandemic.

In 1995 alone, 1.6 million children younger than 15 have their mothers to AIDS, including 1.4 million (87.5%) in sub-Saharan Africa. Two-thirds of these children were younger than 10; one-third were younger than 5 (Table 2-9). Since the beginning of the pandemic, 8.7 million children have lost their mothers to AIDS, 95% of whom were in sub-Saharan Africa (Table 2-10). The emotional, physical, and social stress created by the rapidly growing number of AIDS orphans on families, communities, and nations requires measures that go well beyond the limited coping capacity of extended, traditional social support systems.

Regional Trends

The epicenter of the global pandemic of HIV infection and AIDS is now shifting gradually from sub-Saharan Africa to Southeast Asia. The great diversity and complexity of social and cultural networks in Southeast Asia are severe constraints to the accurate forecasting of the course of the pandemic in this heavily and densely populated region.[21] While data suitable for estimating the status and trends of the pandemic are abundant in several countries, in particular in Thailand, they remain fragmentary in other countries in the region, such as India, which accounts for over 70% of the adult population in the GAA.[22–25]

In sub-Saharan Africa, where the present esti-

Table 2-9. Annual Maternal AIDS Orphans,* January 1 Through December 31, 1995 (Newly Orphaned), by Geographic Area of Affinity†

GAA	<5 years old	<10 years old	<15 years old
North America	2,500	5,500	8,000
Western Europe	1,500	3,000	5,000
Oceania	<500	<500	<500
Latin America	9,000	20,000	31,000
Sub-Saharan Africa	394,500	911,500	1,431,500
Caribbean	4,500	10,000	17,000
Eastern Europe	<500	<500	<500
Southeast Mediterranean	<500	500	500
Northeast Asia	500	1000	1000
Southeast Asia	49,000	100,000	108,000
Total world	461,000	1,000,000	1,600,500

From Ref. 2, with permission.

*Maternal AIDS orphans are defined as the surviving non-HIV-infected children of a mother who died of AIDS.

†Columns and rows may fail to sum due to rounding to the nearest 500.

mates assume that HIV incidence peaked in the early 1990s, the incidence may decline further if prevention efforts, targeting young people and women in particular, are considerably enhanced. In December 1995, an expert panel meeting held in Kampala, Uganda, concluded that there were clear signs that the rate of new infection among young adults seemed to have reached a plateau or even to have declined in some areas that had been hard hit by the epidemic in the mid-1980s.[26] In most parts of sub-Saharan Africa, however, HIV was still spreading with sustained intensity in both urban and rural populations. Between 1990 and 1993, HIV prevalence rates in pregnant women increased from 10% to 30% in Francistown, Botswana, reaching or passing levels that had been documented in pregnant women in several East African cities in the early 1990s. By contrast, rates in similar populations in Nigeria, which has more than one-third of the sub-Saharan population, remained below 5%.

In western Europe HIV incidence trends vary considerably: increasing markedly in Italy and Spain, remaining steady in Belgium; and even decreasing in the Netherlands.[27] Noticeably, the num-

Table 2-10. Cumulative Maternal AIDS Orphans* as of January 1, 1996, by Geographic Area of Affinity*

GAA	<5 years old	<10 years old	<15 years old
North America	18,900	39,000	52,000
Western Europe	8,000	17,000	24,000
Oceania	500	1000	1000
Latin America	56,500	125,000	177,000
Sub-Saharan Africa	2,420,000	5,545,000	8,106,500
Caribbean	23,500	55,000	81,000
Eastern Europe	<500	500	1000
Southeast Mediterranean	1000	1,500	1,500
Northeast Asia	1000	2,000	2,000
Southeast Asia	102,000	198,500	207,000
Total world	2,603,500	5,983,500	8,653,000

From Ref. 2, with permission.

*Maternal AIDS orphans are defined as the surviving non-HIV-infected children of a mother who died of AIDS.

†Columns and rows may fail to sum due to rounding to the nearest 500.

ber of AIDS cases attributed to heterosexual transmission in western and eastern Europe combined increased from 2,215 in 1991 to 4,301 in 1994—a 94% increase—while the number of AIDS cases due to injection-drug use and to homosexual or bisexual contact increased by 52% and 13%, respectively, during the same period.

In the United States through June 1995, men who have sex with men continued to account for the largest population of persons with AIDS-defining opportunistic illnesses, but the rate of growth in this risk category has slowed.[28] By contrast, persons infected through injection-drug use and their heterosexual partners accounted for an increasing proportion of persons with AIDS-defining opportunistic infections. Several shifts are being noted through the analysis of AIDS surveillance data: emerging trends among women, blacks, and Hispanics, persons in moderate and small-sized metropolitan areas and in the rural South, persons infected through heterosexual contacts, minority homosexual/bisexual men, and young men who have sex with men. While, overall, these data suggest that the AIDS epidemic is reaching a plateau, at least temporarily, its future course will be determined by the strength of prevention programs specifically designed to respond to the specific needs of people who are marginalized on the basis of gender, race, behaviors, or cultural, social, and economic grounds.

Current trends observed in Latin America show that significant shifts are occurring in risk factors associated with reported AIDS cases in this region. Transmission through homosexual/bisexual contacts continue to account for most AIDS cases in South America, but throughout the continent, the absolute number and the proportion of newly diagnosed AIDS cases attributed to heterosexual transmission are increasing steeply. In Central America and the Caribbean, 80% of all HIV transmissions are due to heterosexual contact.[29]

The Pandemic of HIV Infection and AIDS at the Doorstep of the Twenty-First Century

In 1992 the Global AIDS Policy Coalition projected that by the end of the year 2000, a cumulative total of between 38 and 110 million adults would have been infected with HIV since the beginning of the pandemic.[1b] This broad range took into account major uncertainties prevailing at that time about the future course of the pandemic in Asia, Latin America, and eastern Europe, and about the magnitude, quality, and sustainability of the global response.

If current epidemic trends persist through the end of the century, it is most likely that about 60 to 70 million adults will have been infected with HIV by the end of the year 2000. Of these adults, about 33 million (51%) will be in Southeast Asia and 24 million (38%) in sub-Saharan Africa.[30] Probably by the turn of the century more HIV infections will have occurred in adults in Southeast Asia than in any other world region. Because most HIV infections in this region occur through heterosexual contact, one must foresee and prepare for a further rise in the number of children born with HIV infection and thus requiring extensive care and support.

References

1. (a) Mann J, Tarantola D, Netter T. *AIDS in the World.* Cambridge, MA: Harvard University Press, 1992:33. (b) *Ibid.* pp. 885–892.

2. Mann J, Tarantola D. The state of the pandemic and its impact. In: *AIDS in the World, Vol. II: The Global AIDS Policy Coalition.* New York: Oxford University Press, 1996:5–40.

3. Gruskin S, Hendriks A, Tomasevski K, et al. Worldwide trends in the laws and practices in the context of HIV/AIDS: a survey of government national AIDS program managers. Poster presented at the Eighteenth International Conference on HIV/AIDS, Yokohama, August 1994.

4. Larsson G, Spangberg L, Lindgren S, Bohlin AB. Screening for HIV in pregnant women: a study of maternal opinion. *AIDS Care* 1990;2:223–228.

5. Blaxhult A, Anagrius C, Arneborn C, et al. Evaluation of HIV testing in Sweden, 1985–1991. *AIDS* 1993;7:1625–1631.

6. Centers for Disease Control and Prevention. *HIV/AIDS Surveill Rep* 1994.

7. HIV/AIDS Surveillance Database; HIV/AIDS Literature Review. International Programs Center, Population Division; U.S. Bureau of the Census, July 1995.

8. Mann J, Tarantola D, Netter T. *AIDS in the World: Methods for the Estimation of the Number of HIV Infections, AIDS Cases, and Deaths in the World, January 1, 1992, and Projections to 1995 and the Year 2000.* Cambridge, MA: Harvard University Press, 1992:871–891.

9. Mann J, Tarantola D. Estimating the status and trends of the HIV/AIDS pandemic, 1996. In: *AIDS in the World, Vol. II.* New York: Oxford University Press, 1996:487–490.

10. Evans LA, McHugh TM, Stites DP, Levy JA. Differential ability of human immunodeficiency virus isolates to productively infect human cells. *J Immunol* 1987;138:3415–3418.

11. Levy JA. Pathogenesis of human immunodeficiency virus infection. *Microbiol Rev* 1993;57:183–289.

12. McCutchan FE. The global distribution of HIV-1 genotypes. In: Mann J, Tarantola D (eds). *AIDS in the World, Vol. II.* New York: Oxford University Press, 1996:180–183.

13. Weniger BG, Takebe Y, Ou C-Y, et al. The molecular epidemiology of HIV in Asia. *AIDS* 1994;8: S13–S28.

14. De Cock KM, Brun-Vezinet F. Epidemiology of HIV-2 infection. *AIDS* 1989;3:S89–S95.

15. Kanki PJ, De Cock KM. Epidemiology and natural history of HIV-2. *AIDS* 1994;8:S85–S93.

16. Adjorlolo-Johnson G, De Cock KM, Ekpini E, et al. Prospective comparison of mother-to-child transmission of HIV-1 and HIV-2 in Abidjan, Côte d'Ivoire. *JAMA* 1994;272:462–466.

17. World Health Organization. *Wkly Epidemiol Rec* 1995;70(50):355–357.

18. Goedert JJ, Kessler CM, Aledort L, et al. Prospective study of human immunodeficiency virus type 1 infection and the development of AIDS in subjects with haemophilia. *N Engl J Med* 1989;321:1141–1148.

19. Whitmore-Overton SE, Tillett HE, Evans BG, Allardice GM. Improved survival from diagnosis of AIDS in adult cases in the United Kingdom and bias due to reporting delays. *AIDS* 1993;7:415–420.

20. Mulder DW, Nunn AJ, Kamali A, et al. Two-year HIV-1 associated mortality in a Ugandan rural population. *Lancet* 1994;343:989–990.

21. Chin J. Scenario for the AIDS epidemic in Asia: Asia-Pacific population. *Res Abstr (Honolulu)* 1995;Feb.

22. Brown T, Sittitrai W. Estimates of recent HIV infection levels in Thailand. *Research Report No. 9.* Bangkok: Program on AIDS, Thai Red Cross Society, 1993.

23. Brown T, Xenos P. *AIDS in Asia: The Gathering Storm: Analysis.* Honolulu: East-West Center No. 16, August 1994.

24. Kaldor J, Effler P, Sarda R, et al. HIV and AIDS in Asia and the Pacific: an epidemiological overview. *AIDS* 1994;8:S165–S172.

25. Jain M, Jacob JT, Keusch G. Epidemiology of HIV and AIDS in India. *AIDS* 1994;8:S61–S75.

26. AIDSCAP and the Harvard School of Public Health's François-Xavier Bagnoud Center for Health and Human Rights. *Report on the Workshop on the Status and Trends of the HIV/AIDS Epidemic in Africa, Kampala, December 8–9, 1995.*

27. European Centre for the Epidemiological Monitoring of AIDS (Saint Maurice, France). Q Rep 1995(2):5–10.

28. Centers for Disease Control and Prevention. *HIV/AIDS Surveill Rep* 1995;7:1.

29. AIDS surveillance in the Americas. *Pan Am Health Organ Reg* Program AIDS/STD, Q Rep 1995; Sep.

30. *Pan Am Health Organ Reg Program AIDS/STD. Q Rep* 1995;Mar.

3

Prospective Studies of HIV-Associated Heart Disease in Adults in the United States

Judith Hsia, M.D.

The initial cases of immunodeficiency in previously healthy young men were reported on the East and West Coasts of the United States in the summer of 1981.[1,2] Autopsy evidence that this new illness, the acquired immunodeficiency syndrome (AIDS), affected the heart followed in 1983[3]; however, clinical heart disease was not reported until 1986.[4] Subsequent data on the prevalence, variety of manifestations, and pathophysiology of heart disease in human immunodeficiency virus (HIV) infection have been derived from autopsy series and case reports, as well as both retrospective and prospective clinical studies. No randomized treatment trials have been carried out with HIV-associated heart disease as an endpoint.

This chapter examines prospective studies of HIV-associated heart disease in adults in the United States (Table 3-1). In evaluating these reports, the observations may be affected by the characteristics of the population studied, for example, the stage of infection during which the persons were studied. During the early years of the AIDS pandemic, the etiologic agent had not yet been identified, and no serologic test for HIV was available. Consequently, the diagnosis was made on the basis of clinical criteria, which included the presence of an AIDS-defining illness, usually atypical pneumonia or Kaposi's sarcoma. By the time the first group of patients were prospectively evaluated for HIV-associated heart disease, serologic tests had been developed, and the Centers for Disease Control and Prevention (CDC) had released a classification system for HIV infection,[5] which included categories for asymptomatic patients, those with lymphadenopathy, and those with AIDS-defining illnesses. The classification system was revised in 1993[6] to rely more heavily on circulating CD4-lymphocyte counts, a change that has affected some of the more recent prospective studies.

In addition to the stage of disease, a review of these studies should include data on the presence or absence of acute illness, the demographic characteristics of the population studied (age, sex, and risk factors for HIV), and geographic locations, as well as current and past treatment.

New Jersey, 1988

The first prospective study of heart disease was carried out the same year that clinical cardiomyopathy in HIV infection was reported. Between October and December 1986, 15 consecutive patients with serologically confirmed HIV infection who met the CDC criteria for AIDS were screened at Raritan Bay Medical Center in Perth Amboy, New

Table 3-1. Prospective Adult Studies of HIV-Associated Heart Disease in U.S. Adults

Study	No. of Subjects	Population	Data Collected
New Jersey, 1988	12	AIDS	ECG, echocardiography, radionuclide ventriculography
New York City, 1989	27	HIV and AIDS	Echocardiography
Washington, DC, 1989	60	HIV and AIDS	ECG, echocardiography, Holter monitoring
San Francisco, 1989	70	HIV and AIDS, in- and outpatients	Echocardiography, clinical status
San Diego, 1991	70	HIV and AIDS, in- and outpatients	Echocardiography
Baltimore, 1993	108	HIV and AIDS, in- and outpatients	Echocardiography, clinical status, endomyocardial biopsy
Washington, DC, 1993	439	HIV and AIDS, in- and outpatients	Echocardiography, signal-averaged ECG, clinical status, endomyocardial biopsy

Jersey, for a prospective study of cardiac function[7]: 10 men and 2 women agreed to participate (Table 3-2); 8 were intravenous drug users, 3 were homosexual, 2 had both risk factors, and 1 was the spouse of a drug user. None had a history of ischemic or alcoholic heart disease or evidence of cardiovascular disease on the basis of the history or physical examination.

Abnormal 12-lead electrocardiograms (ECGs) were present in 9 of the 12 patients (75%); 7 had nonspecific ST-T wave changes, 1 had right bundle branch block, and 1 had a low-voltage QRS complex. Radionuclide ventriculography identified two subjects with left ventricular ejection fraction and those with right ventricular ejection fraction more than 1 SD below the value normal. Echocardiograms were obtained in 9 of the 12 participants. One patient with a normal ECG and radionuclide ventriculogram had a pericardial effusion. Thus, 6 of the 12 subjects had either abnormal ventricular function or pericardial effusion.

The presence of right ventricular dysfunction might have been attributable to pulmonary disease associated with HIV infection, rather than to an effect of HIV on the heart, particularly since five of the patients had previously been treated for pneumonitis. The relationship between reduced right ventricular ejection fraction and past pulmonary infection was not specified. Nonetheless, two patients had unsuspected left ventricular dysfunction, and one had a previously unidentified pericardial effusion. This study design did not include follow-up; however, five of the participants were known to have died subsequently from noncardiac causes. There was no relation between the presence of heart abnormalities and survival.

Before this report, autopsy series and retrospective analyses had suggested that cardiac lesions occurred in 25% to 75% of patients with AIDS, despite the apparently low prevalence of clinical heart disease. The results of this prospective, albeit small, study supported the view that heart disease

Table 3-2. Demographic Characteristics of Study Populations

Study	Age Range (Mean)	No. Male (%)	Asymptomatic/ARC/AIDS	Risk Group: Homosexual/IDU/Other
New Jersey, 1988	26–57 (NA)	10/12 (83)	0/0/12	3/8/1
New York City, 1989	29–53 (37)	27/27 (100)	0/0/27	27/0/0
Washington, DC, 1989	NA (36)	59/60 (98)	25 asymptomatic or ARC/35 AIDS	NA
San Francisco, 1989	23–54 (37)	67/70 (96)	6/13/51	65/3/2
San Diego, 1991	24–64 (38)	69/70 (99)	20/6/44	No IVDU
Baltimore, 1993	NA	57/69 (83)	48 asymptomatic or ARC/21 AIDS	25 IVDU
Washington, DC, 1993	18–64 (38)	389/429 (91)	298 asymptomatic or ARC/131 AIDS	355/44/30

ARC, AIDS-related complex; IDU, intravenous drug user; NA, not available.

could be identified in most patients with AIDS by means of noninvasive imaging.

New York City, 1989

The second prospective study was also carried out in the Northeast. The Beth Israel Medical Center and Mount Sinai School of Medicine recruited 27 homosexual men with AIDS for an echocardiographic study.[8] Characteristics of the study population are summarized in Table 3-2. As in the New Jersey study, none of the men had evidence of heart disease on the basis of the history or physical examination. The most common AIDS-defining illness was *Pneumocystis carinii* pneumonia, which had been diagnosed in 26 of the 27 participants. Other opportunistic infections included *Mycobacterium avium-intracellulare* infection in 4 patients and cytomegalovirus infection in 2. In addition, 7 patients had Kaposi's sarcoma, and 1 had lymphoma. This study included, for comparison, a group of 21 asymptomatic homosexual men, 12 of whom were HIV-seropositive.

The left atrial dimension, left ventricular wall thickness and left ventricular cavity size, adjusted for body surface area, were no different in the group with AIDS than in the asymptomatic subjects. By contrast, the shortening fraction was abnormally reduced in 8 of the 27 patients with AIDS (30%) but in only 1 of the 21 asymptomatic subjects (5%, $P < .05$). Small pericardial effusions were observed in 7 of the patients with AIDS (26%), 2 of whom also had reduced shortening fraction, but in only 1 of the asymptomatic participants (5% $P = .05$). Neither the interval since the development of AIDS nor the type of AIDS-defining illness was associated with the presence of cardiac abnormalities. Overall, echocardiographic abnormalities were present in 13 of the 27 AIDS patients (48%), none of whom had clinical evidence of heart disease. This prevalence is similar to that in the preceding study.

Although 12 subjects in the asymptomatic control group were HIV-seropositive, the authors do not state whether the two subjects in that group with echocardiographic abnormalities were HIV-seropositive. The prevalence of heart disease at earlier stages of HIV infection remained unknown

at the time of this study. The evaluation of HIV-infected patients before the development of AIDS was carried out in the following study.

Washington, D.C., 1989

A third East Coast, urban population was studied in the District of Columbia[9]. 60 consecutive HIV-infected subjects were recruited at the George Washington University Medical Center (Table 3-2); 25 had not yet developed AIDS-defining illnesses, 24 had AIDS and active opportunistic infections, and 11 had AIDS without opportunistic infections at the time of study. Of the subjects who had not yet developed AIDS, 48% were hospitalized, and of those with full-blown AIDS, 94% were hospitalized. Risk factors for the acquisition of HIV infection were not stated.

Electrocardiographic abnormalities (repolarization abnormalities in 13 patients, bundle branch block in 4, and pathologic Q waves in 4) were identified in 22 of 50 participants (44%). Echocardiographic abnormalities (pericardial effusion in 9 patients, left ventricular dilatation in 9, and wall motion abnormalities in 9) were identified in 21 of 60 participants (35%). The prevalence of electrocardiographic or echocardiographic abnormalities did not differ according to the presence or absence of AIDS or active opportunistic infection.

CD4+ lymphocyte counts were available for 36 patients. The range was 0 to 832/mm³ (mean: 145). Echocardiographic abnormalities were significantly more frequent in subjects with CD4+ lymphocyte counts <100/mm³ (12 of 22, 55%) than in those with CD4+ lymphocyte counts >100/mm³ (1 of 14, 7%; $P < .01$). This was the first prospective study in the United States that reported the relative prevalence of cardiac abnormalities in relation to the CD4+ lymphocyte count in HIV infection.

As in previous studies, pericardial disease and dilated cardiomyopathy were the predominant cardiac abnormalities reported. This study also considered arrhythmia as a manifestation of HIV infection for the first time. Holter monitoring was performed on 43 subjects, 2 of whom had unsustained ventricular tachycardia and 1 of whom had 472 premature ventricular contractions per hour. These 3 subjects also had abnormal EKGs and echocardiograms. Although none had symptomatic arrhythmia, this study raised the possibility that arrhythmias may have been overlooked as a manifestation of HIV-associated heart disease.

San Francisco, 1989

The initial West Coast experience with heart disease in HIV infection was also reported in 1989.[10] In San Francisco, 82 consecutive patients from the University of California, San Francisco, AIDS clinic were asked to participate in an echocardiographic study. The characteristics of the 70 patients who agreed to participate are summarized in Table 3-2. HIV infection was thought to have been acquired through homosexual contact in 65 (93%), blood transfusion in 3 (4%), intravenous drug use in 3 (4%), and heterosexual contact in 2 (3%). Of the 70 participants, 45 (64%) were hospitalized and 25 (36%) were ambulatory. The mean CD4+ count was significantly lower in the hospitalized patients (131 ± 186 vs 333 ± 217/mm³, $P < .05$). At the time of study, 25 patients (36%) were receiving zidovudine.

Significant echocardiographic abnormalities were identified only in the hospitalized patients. Eight patients had dilated cardiomyopathy, and seven had pericardial effusions; other abnormalities identified by echocardiography included a mediastinal mass in one patient and pleural effusions in four. All the participants with cardiac abnormalities had AIDS except one, who had cardiomyopathy and AIDS-related complex. These observations supported the view that heart disease was predominantly a late manifestation of HIV infection. The prevalence of heart disease was 21% (15 of 70 patients), which was somewhat lower than in earlier reports.

None of the eight patients with cardiomyopathy had other apparent causes of left ventricular dysfunction, such as coronary disease, hypertension, excessive alcohol consumption, or prior treatment with anthracycline derivatives. Four of the eight had symptoms of congestive heart failure, which were successfully treated by conventional means, that is, the administration of digoxin and diuretics

and afterload reduction. Within 6 months after echocardiography, four of the subjects with dilated cardiomyopathy had died: two as a consequence of heart failure and two from opportunistic infections. Treatment with zidovudine did not appear to provide protection against the development of cardiomyopathy, since half the patients with cardiomyopathy had received this treatment.

Of the seven patients with pericardial effusions, one had a large effusion with tamponade, and the remaining six had small effusions. Pericardial fluid was not available for analysis from any of the patients. The cause of the cardiomyopathy and pericardial effusions in the patients in this study could not be confirmed in the absence of tissue or pericardial fluid samples and remains a topic of considerable interest and speculation.

San Diego, 1991

The first prospective study in the United States that used serial echocardiography was reported from San Diego (Table 3-2).[11] Between 1987 and 1989, initial echocardiograms were performed in 70 ambulatory study participants, with a second study performed in 52 patients after a mean interval of 9 ± 3 months (range: 6–16) A third echocardiogram was obtained in 29 of the patients within an average of 15 ± 3 months (range: 12–21) after the initial study.

Of the 70 study subjects, 50 had symptomatic infection, and 20 were asymptomatic. Despite the predominance of patients with AIDS, the prevalence of cardiac abnormalities in this entirely ambulatory population differed considerably from that reported in previous studies, which included a large proportion of hospitalized participants. The most common abnormality was right heart dilatation, which was present on the baseline echocardiogram in 7 of the 50 subjects with symptomatic HIV infection (11%) and in 1 of the 20 asymptomatic participants (5%). On the first follow-up echocardiogram, right heart enlargement had resolved in 5 of the 8 patients, persisted in 3, and was newly observed in 7 patients (Figure 3-1). Of those with right heart enlargement on their first follow-up echocardiogram, abnormality had resolved in 3 patients on

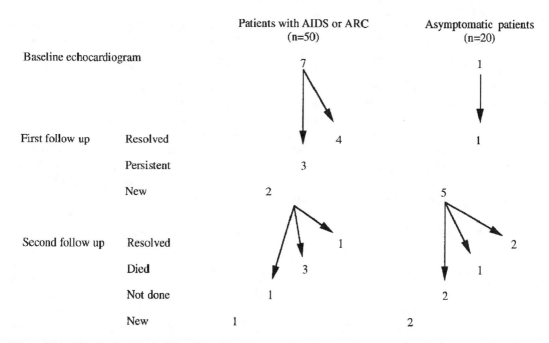

Figure 3-1. Echocardiographic follow-up of patients with right heart enlargement. Echocardiographic right heart enlargement was present in 8 of 70 patients with HIV infection at baseline. A second echocardiogram was obtained in 52 of the subjects after a mean of 9 ± 3 months, and a third was obtained in 29 subjects 15 ± 3 months after the baseline study. (From Ref. 13, with permission.)

subsequent study. The cause of right heart enlargement was not apparent in the majority of the subjects; recent *P. carinii* pneumonia was diagnosed in only 4 of the patients with right heart enlargement observed on one or more echocardiogram.

The most prevalent cardiac abnormalities in earlier echocardiographic studies were cardiomyopathy and pericardial effusion, which were found predominantly or, in some cases, exclusively, in hospitalized patients. In the San Diego study of ambulatory patients, reduced left ventricular ejection fraction was observed on the baseline echocardiogram for 6 of the 52 subjects who had serial studies (12%). The ejection fraction reverted to the normal range in 3 of the 6 patients on follow-up study. The 3 patients with persistently abnormal ejection fractions all died within 1 year after the baseline study. Reduced ejection fraction was newly observed on the follow-up study of a single patient. Of the 7 patients with left ventricular dysfunction, all either had AIDS or AIDS-related complex, but none had symptoms of congestive heart failure or required pharmacologic treatment for heart failure. In contrast to the Washington, D.C., study, CD4+ lymphocyte counts did not differ significantly in patients with and without left ventricular dysfunction (198 ± 82 and 249 ± 255/mm^3).

Pericardial effusions were observed on the baseline echocardiograms in nine subjects, none of whom had either clinical or echocardiographic evidence of hemodynamic compromise. Three of these patients had no symptoms associated with HIV infection; the remaining six had either AIDS or AIDS-related complex. During follow-up, the effusions resolved in seven of the nine patients. Among subjects without effusions on baseline echocardiography, new effusions developed in seven patients during follow-up, including two with impending cardiac tamponade. No pericardial fluid analyses were reported among the patients with AIDS or AIDS-related complex; however, CD4+ lymphocyte counts were significantly lower in those with effusions than in those without effusions (68 ± 74/ mm^3 vs 290 ± 248/mm^3, $P < .001$).

The most striking observation in this study was the transience of cardiac abnormalities associated with HIV infection. The resolution of left ventricular dysfunction, right heart enlargement, and pericardial effusion might have been unexpected in view of the inexorable nature of HIV infection itself. Nonetheless, persistent left ventricular dysfunction appeared to be associated with a poor prognosis, since the three patients with persistently reduced left ventricular ejection fractions all died within 1 year after their baseline study. Similarly, four of the seven subjects with new effusions identified on their first follow-up echocardiogram died before their second follow-up study.

Baltimore, 1993

Most patients infected with HIV are thought to have been infected either through homosexual contact or through intravenous drug use. Nearly all the participants in the prospective studies discussed thus far were homosexual. A report from the Johns Hopkins Medical Institutions in 1993, however, included a substantial number of patients thought to have acquired HIV infection through intravenous drug use.[12] Thus, for the first time, investigators were in a position to describe differences or similarities in manifestations of heart disease between the two risk groups.

The study population consisted of 69 patients from the Johns Hopkins HIV Clinic (Table 3-2), 61 of whom were ambulatory at the time of enrollment and 25 (36%) of whom were intravenous drug users. Echocardiographic evidence of global left ventricular dysfunction was observed at baseline in 10 of the 69 subjects (14%). During follow-up (mean: 12 months) of the 59 patients with initially normal echocardiograms, another 11 patients developed left ventricular dysfunction, an incidence of 18% per year. Of the 21 patients with cardiomyopathy on either the baseline or the follow-up echocardiogram, only one had symptoms of congestive heart failure. The likelihood of left ventricular dysfunction was not affected by sex, race, risk group, or the presence or absence of a history of AIDS-defining illness. As in the Washington, D.C., study, CD4+ lymphocyte count <100/mm³ was more com-

mon among patients with left ventricular dysfunction than among those without this abnormality (62% vs 35%, $P = .04$).

The pathophysiology of cardiomyopathy and other forms of HIV-associated heart disease was the topic of considerable speculation at the time of this study. Endomyocardial biopsies were performed in the study participants with left ventricular dysfunction, as well as in HIV-seropositive patients referred for evaluation of cardiomyopathy. The results of the biopsies are discussed later in this book.

Washington, D.C., 1993

The largest of the prospective studies of heart disease in HIV infection was carried out at George Washington University.[13] The study population included 389 men and 40 women (Table 3-2). This was the first study to include more than a handful of women. Of the men, 355 were homosexual and 33 were past or current intravenous drug users. Of the women, 11 (28%) were intravenous drug users, and the remainder were thought to have contracted HIV through heterosexual contact.

The mean duration of follow-up was 24 ± 17 months, during which a marked progression of disease took place. A total of 130 patients (30%) died from the sequelae of HIV infection, and AIDS developed in 45 patients (10%). The CD4+ lymphocyte counts fell from 325 ± 244 to 247 ± 235/mm³ ($P < .001$), and calculated body surface area fell from 1.91 ± 0.18 m² to 1.89 ± 0.18 m² ($P < .001$).

For the group as a whole, the left ventricular dimension (5.18 ± 0.6 cm) was normal at baseline, but the left ventricular mass index was reduced, as compared with the normal value (86 ± 16 g/m², $P < .001$). Serial echocardiograms were obtained at 4-month intervals, with an average of six studies per participant. During follow-up, the left ventricular end-diastolic dimension increased ($P < .01$), but there was no significant change in the left ventricular mass index.

Among the 256 subjects with initially normal echocardiograms, new abnormalities, summarized in Table 3-3, developed in 53 (21%). The interval since known seroconversion, age, initial CD4+ lym-

Table 3-3. New Abnormalities Among 256 Patients With Normal Baseline Echocardiograms

Abnormality	No. of Patients
Left ventricular dilatation	22
Dilated, hypokinetic left ventricle with or without pericardial effusion	8
Isolated pericardial effusion	8
Diastolic dysfunction	9
Right heart dilatation	1
Left ventricular hypertrophy	3
Intracardiac mass	2

phocyte count, race, sex, disease stage, and history of zidovudine treatment did not differ in these subjects as compared with echocardiograms that remained normal. The duration of follow-up was longer, 23 ± 15 months vs 29 ± 15 months, in the group of patients with new abnormalities detected during follow-up ($P > .01$). Symptomatic heart failure requiring anticongestive treatment occurred in eight patients, half of whom had cardiomyopathy at baseline.

In an effort to shed light on the cause of HIV-associated cardiomyopathy, endomyocardial biopsies were performed in a subgroup of study participants with normal and abnormal ventricular contractility.[14] HIV gene sequences were identifiable in individually microdissected cardiocytes and dendritic cells from all the patients. Efforts to identify cytomegalovirus or picornaviruses by in situ hybridization were unfruitful. Multivariate analysis failed to identify any potentially cardiotoxic drugs that were consistently associated with echocardiographic evidence of left ventricular dysfunction. These observations were thought to increase the likelihood that HIV was responsible for the cardiomyopathy. The reason some patients develop heart disease and others do not, when all appear to harbor the virus in their cardiocytes, remains unexplained.

Pericardial effusions were observed on at least 1 echocardiogram in 71 of the men (18%) and in none of the women.[15] Age, race, and interval since known seroconversion did not affect the likelihood of pericardial effusion. The disease stage was more advanced in the patients with effusions, and a larger proportion of these patients met the clinical criteria for AIDS (78% vs 26%, $P < .0001$). The patients with effusions also had a lower CD4+ lymphocyte count ($119 \pm 180/mm^3$ vs $333 \pm 265/mm^3$, $P < .001$, and smaller body surface area (1.79 ± 0.14 vs 1.90 ± 0.19, $P < .001$) than the patients without effusions. Pericardial effusions were large in 13 subjects, moderate in 10, and small in 48.

Follow-up echocardiograms were obtained in 33 of the subjects with pericardial effusions; in 9 subjects the effusions had resolved spontaneously, in 3 they had increased in size and in 15 they were unchanged, including 4 of the 10 patients with moderate effusions and 3 of the 13 with large effusions. Despite the potential for spontaneous resolution, the presence of a pericardial effusion was a significant predictor of death; among the subjects with known vital status at the end of the study, 53 of 60 subjects with effusions were dead, as compared with 165 of the 279 subjects without effusions ($P < .0001$). In a multivariate logistic regression analysis that included CD4+ lymphocyte count, body surface area, presence of AIDS, and treatment with zidovudine or didanosine as variables, the relationship between pericardial effusion and death persisted.

Pericardial effusion was thought to have an infectious cause in 38 of the 71 patients (54%) and was attributed to congestive heart failure in 16 patients (23%) with concurrent severe global hypokinesia. Malignant effusion was suspected in 1 patient with an intracardiac mass. Pericardial fluid was analyzed in 14 of the 71 patients (20%), 4 of whom had cardiomyopathy. Lymphoma was diagnosed on the basis of cytologic studies in 2 patients, and *Staphylococcus aureus* infection, *Mycobacterium avium-intracellulare* infection, and hyphae characteristic of fungal infection in one patient each. Concurrent malignancy and multiple infections were frequent, but the discordance between the results of pericardial fluid studies and those of other organ systems was complete. This observation underscored the diagnostic value of pericardiocentesis. Although the yield was relatively low, none of the identified causes would have been predicted from other diagnostic studies.

These observations differ from those of earlier studies in two respects: the incidence of left ventricular dysfunction was lower than in the Baltimore study and the prevalence of right heart dilatation was lower than in the San Diego study. On the other hand, the observation that cardiomyopathy and pericardial effusion were the most common cardiac abnormalities and were often reversible was consistent with the findings in the previous studies.

In the Baltimore study, the incidence of new left ventricular dysfunction was 18% per year. In the Washington, D.C., study, new left ventricular dysfunction was identified in 8 of 256 subjects over 2 years, an incidence of 1.6% per year. If left ventricular dilatation is considered an early manifestation of cardiomyopathy, the incidence is 6%, which is still quite a bit lower than in Baltimore.

The San Diego and New Jersey studies reported a predominance of right-sided cardiac abnormalities; no clear relationship between pulmonary disease and right heart dilatation was observed. In the Washington, D.C., study, *P. carinii* pneumonia was reported in 62 patients, pneumonia due to other pathogens in 17, and infiltrating lymphocytic pneumonitis in 2. Overall, 26% of the study participants had pulmonary disease, yet symptomatic right heart failure without left ventricular systolic dysfunction was rare. One patient with a right atrial mass obstructing tricuspid outflow had symptomatic right heart failure, and another patient had asymptomatic right heart dilatation. By contrast, 14 of 50 subjects in the San Diego study had right heart dilatation.

The 1989 Washington, D.C., study raised the possibility that ventricular arrhythmias are a manifestation of HIV-associated heart disease. Consequently, signal-averaged electrocardiography, a noninvasive technique for assessing the risk of arrhythmia,[16] was performed in 225 participants in the 1993 Washington, D.C., study.[17] At baseline, 9 subjects (4%) had a QRS duration > 144 ms, 55 (24%) had low root-mean-square voltage (<20 μV), and 43 (19%) had prolonged low-amplitude signal duration (>39 ms). The test showed that 22 patients had a single abnormal variable, 29 patients had two abnormal variables, and 9 patients had all 3 abnormal variables. Overall, 60 patients (27%) had at least one abnormal variable. By contrast, all signal-averaged EKG values were normal in a group of 12 seronegative, age-matched men ($P = .03$, as compared with the HIV-seropositive group). Age, race, HIV risk group, CD4+ lymphocyte count, interval since seroconversion, history of AIDS-defining illness, past or current zidovudine treat-

ment, and ventricular function were similar in study patients with and those without late potentials.

Clinically important ventricular arrhythmias occurred in only 4 of the 429 subjects during follow-up: 2 with aborted sudden death and 2 with unsustained but symptomatic ventricular tachycardia.[18] Three of these patients had severe, dilated cardiomyopathy, and one had normal ventricular function. None was receiving pentamidine, which has been implicated as a proarrhythmic agent,[19] and none had abnormal findings on signal-averaged electrocardiography. One patient had biopsy-confirmed myocarditis at the time and was treated with corticosteroids; the myocarditis and ventricular tachycardia resolved. In a second patient, ventricular tachycardia could not be induced during electrophysiologic testing. This individual was treated with procainamide because of persistent presyncope; his symptoms resolved. A third patient underwent endomyocardial biopsy, which showed interstitial hemorrhage but no infiltrate. He was treated for congestive heart failure but without antiarrhythmic agents. The fourth patient was resuscitated successfully following cardiac arrest. She had normal ventricular function, and declined further evaluation. Thus, ventricular arrhythmias are uncommon but potentially life-threatening manifestations of HIV-associated heart disease, particularly in patients with cardiomyopathy. Signal-averaged electrocardiography was not helpful in identifying persons at risk.

Conclusions

Although the observations in these prospective studies of adults in the United States are not wholly consistent, a number of conclusions can be drawn.

1. Left ventricular dilatation and dysfunction and pericardial effusion were the most common cardiac abnormalities, tended to occur late in the course of HIV infection, and were often unsuspected.

2. Left ventricular dysfunction and pericardial effusion resolved spontaneously in a substantial proportion of patients.

3. Clinical signs of cardiomyopathy were less common than echocardiographic evidence of left ventricular dysfunction.

4. Pericardiocentesis had a low diagnostic yield, but the information obtained was valuable because of the complete lack of concordance between infections or malignancies in the pericardium and those in other organ systems.

5. Life-threatening arrhythmia was infrequent and was usually associated with cardiomyopathy.

References

1. Masur H, Michelis MA, Greene JB, et al. An outbreak of community-acquired *Pneumocystis carinii* pneumonia: manifestations of cellular immune dysfunction. *N Engl J Med* 1981;305:1431–1438.

2. Gottlieb MS, Schroff R, Schanker HM, et al. *Pneumocystis carinii* pneumonia and mucosal candidiasis in previously healthy homosexual men: evidence of a new acquired cellular immunodeficiency. *N Engl J Med* 1981;305:1425–1431.

3. Reichert CM, OíLeary TJ, Levens DL, et al. Autopsy pathology in the acquired immune deficiency syndrome. *Am J Pathol* 1983;112:357–382.

4. Cohen IS, Anderson DW, Virmani R, et al. Congestive cardiomyopathy in association with the acquired immune deficiency syndrome. *N Engl J Med* 1986;315:628–630.

5. Centers for Disease Control, Department of Health and Human Services. Revision of the case definition of acquired immunodeficiency syndrome for national reporting—United States. *Ann Intern Med* 1985;103:402–403.

6. CDC. 1993 revised classification system for HIV infection and expanded surveillance case definition for AIDS among adolescents and adults. *MMWR* 1992;41:1–19.

7. Raffanti SP, Chiaramida AJ, Sen P, et al. Assessment of cardiac function in patients with the acquired immunodeficiency syndrome. *Chest* 1988; 93:592–594.

8. Hecht S, Berger M, Van Tosh A, Croxson S. Unsuspected cardiac abnormalities in the acquired immune deficiency syndrome: an echocardiographic study. *Chest* 1989;96:805–808.

9. Levy WS, Simon GL, Rios JC, Ross AM. Prevalence of cardiac abnormalities in human immunodeficiency virus infection. *Am J Cardiol* 1989;63: 86–89.

10. Himelman RB, Chung WS, Chernoff DN, et al. Cardiac manifestations of human immunodeficiency virus infection: a two-dimensional echocardiographic study. *J Am Coll Cardiol* 1989;13:1030–1036.

11. Blanchard DG, Hagenhoff C, Chow LC, et al. Reversibility of cardiac abnormalities in human immunodeficiency virus (HIV)- infected individuals: a serial echocardiographic study. *J Am Coll Cardiol* 1991;17:1270–1276.

12. Herskowitz A, Vlahov D, Willoughby S, et al. Prevalence and incidence of left ventricular dysfunction in patients with human immunodeficiency virus infection. *Am J Cardiol* 1993;71:955–958.

13. Hsia J, McQuinn LB. AIDS Cardiomyopathy. *Resident Staff Physician* 1993;39:21–24.

14. Rodriguez ER, Nasim S, Hsia J, et al. Cardiac myocytes and dendritic cells harbor human immunodeficiency virus in infected patients with and without cardiac dysfunction: detection by multiplex, nested, polymerase chain reaction in individually microdissected cells from right ventricular endomyocardial biopsy tissue. *Am J Cardiol* 1991;68:1511–1520.

15. Hsia J, Ross AM. Pericardial effusion and pericardiocentesis in human immunodeficiency virus infection. *Am J Cardiol* 1994;74:94–96.

16. Coto H, Maldonado C, Palakurthy P, Flowers NC. Late potentials in normal subjects and in patients with ventricular tachycardia unrelated to myocardial infarction. *Am J Cardiol* 1985;55:384–390.

17. Hsia J, Colan SD, Adams S, Ross AM. Late potentials and their relation to ventricular function in human immunodeficiency virus infection. *Am J Cardiol* 1991;68:1216–1220.

18. Mohanty N, Adams S, Hsia J. Cardiac problems in persons with AIDS. *Choices Cardiol* 1992;6:1–3.

19. Eisenhauer MD, Eliasson AH, Taylor AJ, et al. Incidence of cardiac arrhythmias during intravenous pentamidine therapy in HIV-infected patients. *Chest* 1994;105:389–394.

4

Prospective Adult Cardiovascular Morbidity and Mortality Studies: The World

Peter F. Currie, M.B., M.R.C.P., and Nicholas A. Boon, M.D., F.R.C.P.

Epidemiology of AIDS outside the United States

According to estimates by the World Health Organization (WHO), as many as 18 million adults and 1.5 million children may have been infected with the human immunodeficiency virus (HIV).[1] The virus can be transmitted by penetrative sexual intercourse, injection of drugs with contaminated needles and syringes, administration of infected blood products, and vertically from mother to child.[2]

Homosexual males still constitute the largest group of HIV-positive patients in the United States, while HIV infection is particularly common among injection-drug users in Europe. This situation contrasts with that in WHO-defined "pattern II" African countries and Asia, where HIV is transmitted mainly by heterosexual contact.[3] In developed countries, modification of risk behavior by homosexuals and injection-drug users has resulted in a reduction of viral spread in these groups.[4] Unfortunately, heterosexual risk behavior has been affected to a much lesser extent in the United Kingdom, and in certain populations in the United States the rate of growth of heterosexually acquired HIV infection is higher than that of HIV acquired by other routes.[5,6]

In Europe over 128,000 cases of acquired immunodeficiency syndrome (AIDS) have been reported to date,[1] with the highest incidence, 14 cases per 100,000 people, in Spain.[1] In the United Kingdom, 9,865 AIDS cases had been reported by the end of 1994.[1] The majority of these were in the major cities, particularly Edinburgh, where it is estimated that approximately 1 in 150 people aged between 15 and 35 is infected with the virus.[7]

Retrospective analysis of stored sera has shown that HIV was spreading rapidly among drug users in the United States as early as 1979[8] and had already appeared in Italy.[9] It seems likely that drug users at U.S. Air Force bases were important vectors for HIV infection[10] and that contact among the highly mobile population of drug users across Europe helped spread the virus farther afield.

Increasing numbers of people in the Third World are at risk from HIV infection, and AIDS is now endemic in many parts of Africa and Asia. The incidence of AIDS in Zambia was 239.3 per 100,000 people by the end of 1994,[1] and case rates of over 30 per 100,000 are not uncommon in many African nations.[1] Thailand is experiencing an explosive rise in the numbers of AIDS patients, with 13,246 cases reported at the end of 1994.[1] This probably reflects the silent increase in the number of HIV-positive people in Southeast Asia as a whole.

59

HIV is similar to, and may be a variant of, the simian immunodeficiency virus, a relatively innocuous retrovirus that infects chimpanzees. In some African societies it is a customary sexual practice to paint the genital area with monkey blood and it has been suggested that HIV may have crossed the species boundary in this way.[11] This may explain the importance of heterosexual contact in the spread of HIV infection and the extremely high incidence of AIDS in many African countries. It seems likely that sociosexual practices in Southeast Asia are also important in the dissemination of the virus. For example, HIV seropositivity in female Thai prostitutes rose from 3.5% in June 1989 to 29.5% by the end of 1993.[12]

Cardiac Involvement in HIV Infection

The cardiovascular manifestations of HIV infection are now well recognized as a significant cause of morbidity and mortality throughout the world, but it seems likely that their prevalence has been underestimated in the Third World, where diagnostic and autopsy facilities are often inadequate. Heart muscle disease is well recognized in Europe and the United States. Pericardial disease, on the other hand, appears to be particularly important in Africa.

There are also a few reports of endocarditis and cardiac cancer from other countries.

Nonbacterial Thrombotic Endocarditis

Nonbacterial thrombotic endocarditis (NBTE) is a condition of unknown etiology in which friable clumps of platelets and red blood cells adhere to the cardiac valves. This was one of the commonest cardiac abnormalities described in early autopsies of U.S. patients with AIDS, being reported in approximately 10% of autopsies before 1989 (Table 4-1). Although it has been suggested that particulate matter from injection drug use may predispose to the development of thrombotic vegetations,[13] NBTE has never been a feature of HIV infection outside the United States despite the high proportion of drug users in Europe.

We have performed autopsies on 118 HIV-positive adults, 42 of whom died before AIDS developed and 76 of whom had an AIDS-defining illness. Of those with AIDS, the risk factors for HIV infection were intravenous drug use in 41 patients, homosexual contact in 28, heterosexual contact in 4 (including 1 African), and receiving contaminated blood products in 3 others. NBTE vegetations were discovered on the mitral valve of a male homosexual with no history of drug abuse. This is the only case of NBTE in our series, which suggests that

Table 4-1. Prevalence of Nonbacterial Thrombotic Endocarditis in Early HIV Postmortem Series

Author (Ref.)	Year	No. of Cases	No. of Autopsies (%)	Valves Involved	Symptoms
Garcia et al. (104)	1983		Case report	Mitral + aortic	Systemic emboli
Snider et al. (105)	1983	2	50 (4)	NA	Systemic emboli
Fink et al. (84)	1984	1	4 (25)	Tricuspid + pulmonary	Nil
Guarda et al. (106)	1984	2	13 (15)	Tricuspid + mitral	DIC
				Aortic, tricuspid + mitral	Systemic emboli
Cammarosano and Lewis (107)	1985	3	41 (7)	Tricuspid	Systemic emboli
				Mitral	Systemic emboli
				All	
Roldan et al. (59)	1987	4	54 (7)	Tricuspid + mitral	Nil
				Tricuspid + mitral	
				Tricuspid + mitral	
				NA	
Klatt et al. (35)	1988	7	187 (4)	NA	NA

DIC, disseminated intravascular coagulation; NA, not available.

in the United Kingdom the prevalence is less than 1%.[14]

There is no apparent explanation for the low prevalence of NBTE in the United Kingdom, although it has been suggested recently that the incidence of NBTE in patients with AIDS is falling in the United States.[15] This is surprising, given the growing interest in the cardiac manifestations of AIDS, and raises the possibility that the prevalence of the condition was overestimated in the past.

Infective Endocarditis

Injection-drug use is a major risk factor for both HIV infection and infective endocarditis, yet there are relatively few reports of this condition in drug users with AIDS. Since the immunologic abnormalities associated with HIV infection render patients susceptible to bacterial infections,[16] it is also surprising that infective endocarditis is rarely found in HIV-positive patients from other risk groups.[17]

The relation between immunosuppression and the development of infective endocarditis is not clear. Animal studies have shown that granulocytopenia can adversely affect the ability of rabbits to sterilize bacterial vegetations[18,19] and may increase susceptibility to experimental endocarditis.[20,21] Although these models suggest that abnormal white blood cell function may be a predisposing factor, the pathogenesis of endocarditis in humans is probably very complex.

It is possible that the natural history of some forms of infective endocarditis is modified by the specific immunodeficiency associated with early HIV infection. For example, a minor change in the inflammatory reaction at an early stage of the infection could impair vegetation formation and limit valvular damage. *Salmonella* endocarditis, for example, is often associated with devastating cardiac complications in HIV-negative patients,[22] but it appears to be responsive to antibiotic treatment and may even have a reasonable prognosis in patients with AIDS.[23,24] It has also been suggested that bacterial endocarditis may be less common in HIV-positive than in HIV-negative injection-drug users.[25]

We examined the prevalence of infective endocarditis in a 4-year, prospective, echocardiographic survey of 296 HIV-positive adults.[14] The majority (68.6%, 203/296) were current or previous injection-drug users, but homosexual (17.6%, 52/296), heterosexual (9.5%, 28/296), and bisexual males (2.4%, 7/296), blood product recipients (1.0%, 3/296), and patients with multiple risk factors (1.0%, 3/296) were also included. Only six cases of infective endocarditis, including one confirmed at autopsy, were identified by echocardiography, all involving injection-drug users. At the same time, the incidence of clinically diagnosed infective endocarditis in all HIV-positive patients attending our regional specialist HIV unit has decreased with the decline in injection-drug use—and despite the increased number of HIV-positive patients (Figure 4-1).

In a large-scale survey, Miro and colleagues[26] examined 17,592 episodes of infection diagnosed in injection-drug users over a 14-year period in Spain. Infective endocarditis was diagnosed in 1,175 cases (7%), of which 80% involved the right heart. *Staphylococcus aureus* was the commonest bacterial organism, although there was a high proportion of *Streptococcus viridans* infection in those patients with left heart endocarditis.[27] The clinical presentation of bacterial endocarditis was the same for HIV-positive and HIV-negative drug users. AIDS was diagnosed in 2,889 of those studied.

In a similar study of 46 drug users in Chicago, Nahass and colleagues[28] confirmed that, if properly treated, infective endocarditis has a good outcome in asymptomatic HIV-positive patients with well-preserved immune function but runs a more fulminant course in the late stages of HIV infection when immunosuppression is more advanced. Rare cases of fungal endocarditis with species such as *Aspergillus fumigatus* and *Pseudalleschira boydii* also occur during the late stages of HIV infection both in drug users[29] and in patients with other risk factors.[30,31]

Our own experience suggests that the incidence of endocarditis in HIV-positive injection-drug users is falling or is at a constant low level,[32] while hospitalization for HIV infection and AIDS has increased dramatically.[26,33,34] This may reflect an unexpected benefit of needle-exchange schemes, oral opiate substitute prescription programs, and the continuing education of drug users in general.

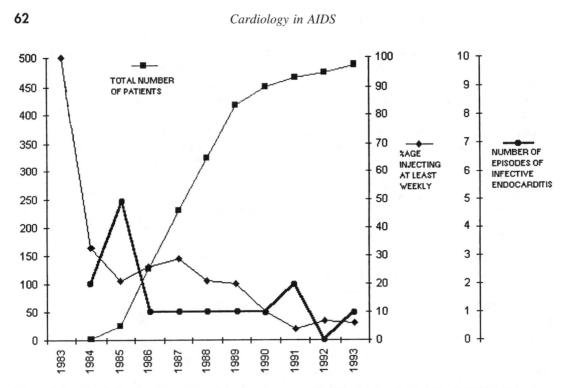

Figure 4-1. Graph showing the total number of patients attending the Edinburgh City Hospital HIV clinic along with the total number of episodes of infective endocarditis and percentage number of drug users injecting at least weekly by year.

Pericardial Disease

Pericardial disease is common in HIV infection[15] and can take many forms, ranging from a small pericardial effusion complicating generalized fluid retention or cardiac dysfunction to classical pericarditis or cardiac tamponade.[35,36] Clinically significant effusions are usually due to secondary viral or bacterial infection or malignant infiltration.

Pericardial effusion is a major problem in Africa,[37] where up to 72% of patients with serosanguineous effusions have been found to be HIV-positive.[38] There is a clear association between pericarditis and typical or atypical mycobacterial infection in Africa,[39] and pericardial effusion in itself is strongly suggestive of HIV infection in some African countries.[38,40] Tuberculous pericarditis has also been reported as the first manifestation of AIDS in continental Europe[41] but is uncommon in Edinburgh, possibly because most of the at-risk population received prophylactic Calmette-Guérin bacillus vaccination in childhood.

Surgical intervention is not always beneficial in patients with AIDS who have large pericardial effusions.[42] However, there are no data on the long-term outcome of such measures in patients at an earlier stage of HIV infection. We used pericardiocentesis and pericardiectomy to treat a pericardial tamponade due to *S. aureus* in an HIV-positive drug user who has remained well for more than 5 years.[43] Culture of pericardial biopsy or fluid from symptomatic effusions may also be useful in identifying treatable opportunistic infections or malignancy.[44]

Cardiac Malignancy

Kaposi's sarcoma is the commonest AIDS-related neoplasm, affecting up to 35% of patients,[45] particularly male homosexuals, who appear to be most at risk.[46] Cardiac Kaposi's sarcoma occurs most often as part of a disseminated process, although a single case of primary cardiac involvement was described in France as early as 1983.[47] The tumor is an endothelial cell neoplasm and was shown to have a predilection for the subpericardial fat around coronary arteries in two European autopsy cases.[48] It is unusual for Kaposi's sarcoma to be associated with symptoms of cardiac dysfunction, although a case of fatal hemorrhagic cardiac tamponade was described by Monsuez and co-workers.[49]

Primary cardiac lymphoma is extremely rare in HIV-negative persons, accounting for less than 10% of all primary malignant cardiac tumors.[50] B-lymphocyte and non-Hodgkin's lymphomas have been described widely in the United States in both autopsy and echocardiographic studies but are found only infrequently elsewhere.[49,51] In contrast to Kaposi's sarcoma, cardiac lymphoma commonly gives rise to clinical symptoms of tamponade, heart failure, and conduction abnormalities.

HIV-Related Heart Muscle Disease

Introduction

Cardiac failure due to dilated cardiomyopathy was described in three patients with AIDS in 1986.[52] Initially, the clinical significance of this new entity was not clear, but it has since become apparent from echocardiographic and autopsy studies that cardiac dysfunction is an important cause of morbidity and mortality in AIDS. Although the reported prevalence of left ventricular dysfunction in HIV infection varies from 2%[53] to over 40%,[54] it has become accepted that symptomatic heart failure will develop in approximately 5% of patients, most of whom will have end-stage AIDS.[55-57]

Autopsy and Histopathologic Data

The Dallas criteria for the histologic diagnosis of myocarditis require the presence of an inflammatory infiltrate of the myocardium with adjacent myocyte necrosis or degeneration that is not typical of ischemia. The term "borderline myocarditis" may be used in situations where an inflammatory infiltrate is found in isolation or myocardial necrosis occurs without an acute inflammatory response.[58]

Although the use of these strict definitions may be inappropriate in the context of the impaired immune response associated with HIV infection and AIDS, all three of these histologic patterns of myo-carditis have been described in patients at different stages of the disease: lymphocytic infiltration with myocyte necrosis fulfilling the Dallas criteria,[48,59-62] lymphocytic infiltration without inflammation,[15,63] and myocyte damage in the absence of inflammatory infiltration.[64-66] These differences, compounded by possible sampling errors, make the prevalence of myocarditis difficult to establish,[67] with estimates ranging from 12.5%[52] to 53%.[68]

Furthermore, significant numbers of infiltrating CD8+ and CD45+ lymphocytes have been found in association with increased HLA class I antigen expression on apparently histologically normal endomyocardial biopsy specimens from HIV-positive patients with cardiac failure.[69] These immunohistochemical findings are indistinguishable from those in other HIV-positive patients with heart failure who had histologic evidence of myocarditis, suggesting that simple histologic methods may be insufficient to rule out this diagnosis in patients with AIDS. This may also partly explain the apparent lack of correlation between myocarditis and left ventricular dysfunction noted in some surveys.

Baroldi and colleagues[48] described the autopsy findings in 26 patients with AIDS, including 8 who had undergone antemortem echocardiographic assessment. Abnormal left ventricular function had been documented before death in 6 of these patients, all of whom had evidence of lymphocytic infiltration of the myocardium. The Dallas criteria for the diagnosis of myocarditis were met in 4 of the 6 patients, and lymphocytic infiltration alone was found in the remaining 2 subjects. No pathologic irregularities were discovered in the 2 patients with normal echocardiograms. No macroscopic evidence of heart muscle disease was seen in 5 other patients with myocarditis.

In a similar study from the United States (Table 4-2), biventricular dilatation was found in 7 of 71 autopsies of patients with AIDS[60]: 4 of these patients died of heart failure and the other 3 died of sepsis. Evidence of myocarditis was found in all these patients and in 30 other patients, 9 of whom had evidence of myocardial infection by specific opportunistic pathogens.

A subsequent retrospective study of 26 of these patients with myocarditis found cardiac abnormalities in 15 of them, including cardiac failure, pericar-

Table 4-2. Comparison of the Major Autopsy Studies from the United States and Europe

Author (Ref.)	Cases	Risk Factor For HIV	Main Cardiac Findings	Cardiac Symptoms
Anderson et al. (60)	71	Homosexual male (75%) Injection drug user (7%) Heterosexual contact (4%) Haitian (1%) Risk factors denied (13%)	Myocarditis (52%) Biventricular dilatation (10%) Right ventricular dilatation (17%) Specific opportunistic pathogens (13%)* Acid-fast bacilli (2) Cytomegalovirus (2) *Toxoplasma gondii* (2) *Histoplasma capsulatum* (1) *Candida* sp. (1)	Heart failure (6%)
Baroldi et al. (48)	26	Injection drug user (77%) Homosexual male (12%) Blood product (4%) African travel (4%) Multiple (4%)	Lymphocytic myocarditis (35%) Lymphocytic infiltrate (27%) Epicardial lymphocytic infiltrate (15%) Kaposi's sarcoma (8%) Specific opportunistic pathogens (11%) *Toxoplasma* (1) *Sarcosporidium* (1) *Cryptococcus* (1)	None reported

*Discovered in patients with evidence of disseminated infection

ditis, and ventricular tachycardia, or a left ventricular ejection fraction of <44% when radionuclide ventriculography was used.[70] Serious cardiac abnormalities were more common in patients with myocarditis than in those with normal histologic findings.

The nature of the lymphocytic infiltrates found in 34 autopsy samples from Italian patients with AIDS, was studied further by using immunohistochemical methods.[71] The Dallas criteria were met in only 26% of the cases, with borderline myocarditis in a further 32%. The inflammatory cells were found to be CD8+ lymphocytes and were similar in appearance in patients with or without myocyte necrosis. These cells resembled the lymphocytes found in HIV-negative "idiopathic" myocarditis and suggest a common pathogenic mechanism. Cytomegalovirus antigens were also found in five samples with well-defined myocarditis, although there was evidence of disseminated infection in these patients.

There were clear differences between the European and American patients in these studies, reflecting the variation in risk factors for HIV infection in the respective populations. However, it is clear that risk behavior and geographic location

are not important factors in the pathogenesis of myocarditis in AIDS patients.

Myocarditis can be diagnosed clinically in HIV-positive patients on the basis of symptoms and physical findings. Nonspecific conduction defects or repolarization abnormalities may be present on the EKG, and the chest radiograph may reveal cardiac enlargement or pulmonary congestion. Echocardiography is usually nondiagnostic, but wall thickness was found to lie at the lower end of normal in HIV-positive adults with histologically proven myocarditis.[48] Similarly, left ventricular dyskinesia may itself represent a nonspecific marker of myocarditis in patients with AIDS.[48,63,72,73]

Echocardiographic Studies

Echocardiography has become an important tool both in the assessment of individual HIV-positive patients and in cross-sectional population surveys, and has helped to reinforce the clinical importance of all the cardiac complications of AIDS (Table 4-3).

Cardiac abnormalities were a common finding in an early study of 102 consecutive Italian patients with AIDS. Although none of them had cardiac symptoms, left ventricular functional abnormalities

Table 4-3. Major Cross-Sectional Echocardiographic Studies Outside the United States

Author (Ref.)	Country	Cases	Major Risk Factor for HIV	Major Echocardiographic Abnormalities
Corallo et al. (54)	Italy	102	Injection drugs (71%) Homosexual male (26%)	Left ventricular dysfunction (54%) Significant pericardial effusion (30%)
Monsuez et al. (49)	France U.S.	86	Homosexual male (40%) Injection drugs (34%)	Significant pericardial effusion (15%) Dilated cardiomyopathy (6%) Left ventricular dysfunction (9%)
Lindvig et al. (81)	Denmark	24	Homosexual male (92%)	Right ventricular dilatation (38%) Left ventricular dilatation (4%) Pericardial effusion (21%)
Jacob et al. (74)	UK	173	Injection drugs (69%) Homosexual male (22%)	Dilated cardiomyopathy (7%) Left ventricular dilatation (3%) Right ventricular dilatation (4%)
De Castro et al. (86)	Italy	114	Injection drugs (74%) Homosexual male (21%)	Dilated cardiomyopathy (17%) Pericardial effusion (18%) Mitral valve prolapse (4%) Septal hypokinesis (14%)
Akhras et al. (75)	UK	124	Homosexual male (100%)	Pericardial effusion (37%) Mitral valve prolapse (27%) Dilated cardiomyopathy (13%) Left ventricular dysfunction (3%) Right ventricular dilatation (4%)
Coudray et al. (76)	France	51	Homosexual male (67%) Heterosexual (22%) Injection drugs (10%)	Evidence of diastolic dysfunction in symptomatic and asymptomatic HIV patients
Hakim et al. (77)	Zimbabwe	157	Heterosexual contact (100%)	Dilated cardiomyopathy (9%) Left ventricular dysfunction (22%) Right ventricular dilatation (6%) Pericardial effusion (19%)

were found in 54% of patients, including moderate pericardial effusions in 30% and vegetations in 4 patients. Cardiac Kaposi's sarcoma was specifically diagnosed in 3 patients.[54]

Monsuez and colleagues[49] evaluated 46 patients with AIDS from Paris and 40 from Miami: 18 patients had symptoms of cardiac disease and a lower average CD4+ lymphocyte count than the asymptomatic group. Although there was a significant difference in the number of echocardiographic abnormalities between the symptomatic and the asymptomatic patients, they consisted mostly of pericardial effusion with or without features of tamponade.

A group of 173 HIV-positive patients from all the major risk groups in Edinburgh included 13 patients with dilated cardiomyopathy and 6 with left ventricular dysfunction abnormalities.[74] This study confirmed that myocardial dysfunction was associated with advanced disease, as shown by low CD4+ lymphocyte counts, but serologic tests found no evidence of more frequent opportunistic infections with either cytomegalovirus or *Toxoplasma* in these patients than in patients with normal echocardiograms. Most patients with cardiac dysfunction had been exposed to zidovudine, but the proportion of patients treated and the mean total dose were similar in patients with or without myocardial dysfunction, and the drug therefore did not appear to be implicated in the pathogenesis of heart muscle disease.

A much higher proportion of patients with symptomatic heart failure was found in a study of 124 HIV-positive homosexual men in London. Of the 101 of these men with AIDS, 16 had cardiomyopathy and 4 had isolated left ventricular dysfunction.[75] No such abnormalities were found in the 23 HIV-positive patients without AIDS. In contrast to the patients in the Edinburgh study, who were mostly injection-drug users, cardiac dysfunction was commonly associated with opportunistic *Pneumocystis carinii*, cytomegalovirus, *Toxoplasma*, and *Mycobacterium avium-intracellulare* complex infections. However, the higher prevalence of opportunistic infections in the London patients could have been due to their more advanced disease.

A subsequent echocardiographic study of 51 HIV-positive patients, including 23 with AIDS, showed evidence of left ventricular diastolic dysfunction at an early stage of HIV infection.[76] Increased isovolumetric relaxation time and decreased early mitral peak flow velocity were noted, as were abnormalities in Doppler-derived indices of diastolic dysfunction. These abnormalities were equally frequent in asymptomatic HIV-positive patients and those with AIDS but were more uncommon in HIV-negative controls. Diastolic dysfunction appeared to be independent of systolic impairment, which was also identified in 11 patients. These findings suggest that some form of cardiac dysfunction may occur at an early stage of HIV infection, but their clinical significance remains unclear.

There was little information on the prevalence of functional cardiac abnormalities in HIV-positive patients in Africa until a recent cross-sectional echocardiographic survey of seropositive, heterosexual subjects in Zimbabwe. The diagnostic criteria were similar to those used in European studies. Patients with preexisting cardiovascular disease were excluded, there were no hemophiliacs, and all denied any history of injection-drug use. *P. carinii* or pulmonary tuberculosis had been diagnosed in 32 patients (20%), and 37 (24%) had symptoms of congestive heart failure. Dilated cardiomyopathy was found in 14 patients (9%), left ventricular dysfunction in 33 (22%), and isolated right ventricular dilatation in 30 (19%); these results were similar to the results from developed countries. As expected, pericardial disease was also common, with pericardial effusion demonstrated in 28 patients, 3 of whom had evidence of tamponade.[77]

It seems clear, therefore, that significant left ventricular dysfunction can occur in any patient with HIV infection, regardless of risk behavior and geographic location.

Right Ventricular Involvement in HIV Infection

Right ventricular hypertrophy is one of the most common cardiac abnormalities found at autopsy in HIV-positive patients,[53] and functional abnormalities of the right ventricle have been reported frequently in both echocardiographic studies[74,78,79] and blood pool nucleotide studies.[80] In most cases, right ventricular dilatation occurs in isolation,[56,74,81] although some cases are clearly part of the global process that leads to biventricular dysfunction and four-chamber dilatation.[52,65,82]

Isolated right ventricular dysfunction is probably secondary to changes in the pulmonary circulation rather than a result of primary myocardial disease,[56,74,75] and some cases have been associated with elevated pulmonary vascular resistance and pulmonary artery pressures[79] or HIV-induced pulmonary arteritis.[83] Pulmonary hypertension could result from multiple microvascular pulmonary emboli following drug injection or from the recurrent bronchopulmonary infections that are a hallmark of HIV infection.[79] Tricuspid incompetence may also result in volume overload and was the cause of right ventricular dysfunction in a patient with AIDS and with nonbacterial thrombotic endocarditis.[84]

Right ventricular hypertrophy may be evident on the EKG, but echocardiography remains the most useful method of assessing right ventricular function (Figure 4-2). Doppler ultrasound studies are also useful in determining right ventricular systolic pressure.[79]

Natural History Studies

Despite the continued interest in HIV-related heart muscle disease, there has been little information about the natural history of cardiac dysfunction in patients with AIDS. Some anecdotal reports had suggested that dilated cardiomyopathy and clinically overt heart failure in particular were associated with a poor prognosis,[49,52,53,57] but others suggested that reduced ejection fraction[80] or right ventricular dilatation[74,81] had no effect on mortality. The need for long-term prospective clinical studies was clear.

In 1994, we reported on the outcome of 296 HIV-positive patients who had been assessed by serial echocardiography over a 4-year period.[56] All

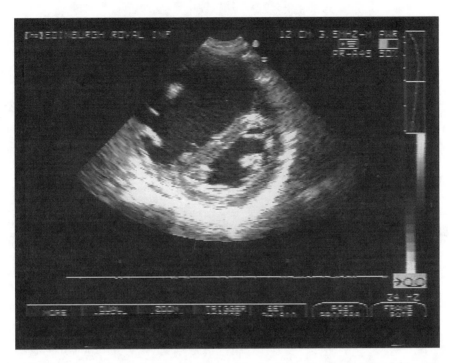

Figure 4-2. Parasternal short axis view of right ventricular dysfunction in an HIV-positive drug user.

the major risk groups for HIV infection in the United Kingdom were represented (203 injection drug users, 52 homosexual men, 28 who had contracted the virus through heterosexual contact, 7 bisexual men, 3 blood-product recipients, and 3 with multiple risk factors).

The mean CD4+ lymphocyte count was 153×10^6 cells per liter (range: 0 to 1,178; normal range: $500–1400 \times 10^6$ cells per liter), but over 90% of the cohort showed evidence of immunosuppression, with a CD4+ lymphocyte count $<400 \times 10^6$ cells per liter, including 146 patients who had a count $<100 \times 10^6$ cells per liter. According to criteria from the Centers for Disease Control, 100 patients had AIDS and 89 had advanced HIV infection without AIDS.

In our group of 296 patients, 44 (15%) had cardiac dysfunction: 13 (4%) had dilated cardiomyopathy, 12 (4%) had isolated right ventricular dilatation, and 19 (6%) had borderline left ventricular dysfunction; 9 of the 13 patients with dilated cardiomyopathy and 7 of the 19 with borderline left ventricular dysfunction had signs and symptoms of heart failure; 6 of the 12 patients with right ventricular dilatation had breathlessness, but this was more frequently attributable to pulmonary causes. The patients with dilated cardiomyopathy, but not those with isolated right ventricular dilatation or borderline left ventricular dysfunction, had lower CD4+ lymphocyte counts than the patients with structurally normal hearts.

The survival of patients with dilated cardiomyopathy was poor and was significantly worse than for patients with structurally normal hearts or other forms of heart muscle disease. The outcome was independent of many factors, including CD4+ lymphocyte count, age, sex, and risk group for HIV infection (Figure 4-3).

The excess mortality in patients with cardiomyopathy remained significant even when compared to that of subjects with CD4+ lymphocyte counts less than 20×10^6 cells per liter, the highest count in our cardiomyopathy group (Figure 4-3). The median survival to AIDS-related death was 101 days in those with cardiomyopathy, compared with 472 days in 59 patients with normal hearts at a similar stage of HIV infection. Patients with isolated right and borderline left ventricular dysfunction did not

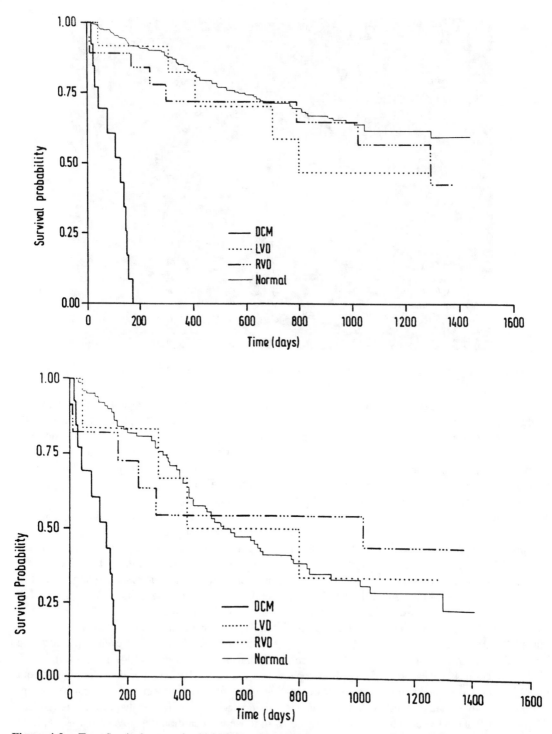

Figure 4-3. **Top:** Survival curves for 296 HIV-positive patients with structurally normal hearts or with evidence of cardiac dysfunction. **Bottom:** Time to death related to AIDS in 81 patients with CD4+ cell counts less than 20 × 10[6] cells per liter (From Ref. 56, with permission.)

differ significantly from patients without evidence of cardiac involvement.

Also in 1994, De Castro and colleagues[85] reported on the effects of acute-onset left ventricular dysfunction in a population of 136 HIV-positive Italian patients who had been studied previously over a 4-year period[86]: 60% were injection-drug users, 22% were homosexual men, and 18% partners at risk; 68% had AIDS, 19% had advanced HIV infection, and 12.5% had asymptomatic HIV infection. All had structurally normal hearts at the time of enrollment.

In seven patients (5%), with a mean CD4+ lymphocyte count of 56×10^6 cells per liter, acute left ventricular dysfunction developed during a mean follow-up time of 415 days. This diagnosis was based on clinical, radiologic, or echocardiographic findings, which included global hypokinesis and decreased ejection fraction (<45% by Simpson's rule) or shortening fraction (<28%). Left ventricular dilatation per se was not required as a diagnostic criterion, as five of these patients had normal left ventricular dimensions and only two had features of dilated cardiomyopathy.

Cardiac failure was the cause of death in six of the seven patients and occurred at a mean time of 41 days from the diagnosis of cardiac dysfunction. Autopsy examination later revealed lymphocytic myocarditis in three cases and cryptococcal myocarditis in another.

In another five patients with AIDS, dilated cardiomyopathy developed, with progressive biventricular dilatation and decreased ejection fraction. One died from noncardiac causes, but the others survived to the end of the study despite symptoms of cardiac failure. Twelve patients with an established diagnosis of dilated cardiomyopathy were not included, as their cardiac abnormalities had been present at enrollment.

Both of these natural history studies clearly demonstrate that some forms of HIV-related heart muscle disease are associated with a poor prognosis. We have shown that HIV-positive patients with dilated cardiomyopathy are at risk of an early death from an AIDS-related condition, independent of their CD4+ lymphocyte count. The Italian study suggests that those cases of symptomatic acute left ventricular dysfunction that are associated with a

lymphocytic myocarditis have a similarly grave outlook.

There are differences in the terminology and criteria for left ventricular dysfunction used in these reports, which may explain some of the apparent variance in the outcome of patients with isolated left ventricular dysfunction. Nevertheless, it seems likely that some immunocompromised patients can develop a self-limiting myocarditis that does not progress to overt left ventricular failure, while others may present with an aggressive lymphocytic myocarditis that carries a particularly poor prognosis.

We believe that the outlook for patients with isolated right ventricular dilatation is much less gloomy, probably because this is often due to transient pulmonary hypertension associated with bronchopulmonary infection rather than primary myocardial disease.[79]

Observations on the Pathogenesis of HIV-Related Heart Muscle Disease

The etiology of HIV-related heart muscle disease has yet to be clearly established. Nevertheless, cases may appear to be related to the idiopathic lymphocytic myocarditis that is a frequent postmortem finding in patients with ventricular dysfunction.[48,70] This may be due to a direct or an indirect effect of HIV or, more rarely, cytomegalovirus infection,[69] but other potential pathogenic factors, including nutritional deficiencies, opportunistic infections, and cardiotoxic effects of antiretroviral drugs, require further investigation.

Although it is clear that HIV can infect interstitial cells within the myocardium,[30] there is only scanty evidence to suggest the virus can enter the cardiac myocyte. The results of cell culture studies and polymerase chain reaction work can be difficult to interpret because of the possibility of contamination with the patient's own infected blood.[87] Immunohistochemical studies on HIV-positive patients in Edinburgh have shown no evidence of gp120 or p24 antigen expression in the heart, suggesting that intracellular replication of HIV does not occur.[88]

Abnormally elevated circulating immune complexes and autoantibodies are frequently found in patients with AIDS; autoimmune processes are well recognized in HIV infection.[89–94] It seems plausible therefore that myocyte damage could occur indirectly through some autoimmune mechanism. IgA and IgG obtained from HIV-positive hemophiliacs have been shown to have a negative inotropic effect on isolated rat atria, possibly through modulation of cholinergic receptors,[95] similar to findings in patients with Chagas' cardiomyopathy.[96]

We assessed the frequency of circulating cardiac and disease-specific autoantibodies in a series of 74 HIV-positive patients by immunofluorescence and enzyme-linked immunosorbent assay (ELISA); 28 (38%) of these patients had dilated cardiomyopathy or isolated left ventricular dysfunction, and 9 (12%) had isolated right ventricular dysfunction. Antiheart antibodies detected by immunofluorescence were commoner in the HIV-positive patients with heart muscle disease than in HIV-negative controls. Abnormal anti-α myosin autoantibody levels were also found more frequently in the HIV-positive patients with heart muscle disease than in those with structurally normal hearts or in HIV-negative controls. This would support a role for cardiac autoimmunity in the pathogenesis of HIV-related heart muscle disease.[97]

Similarly, opportunistic infection, nutritional deficiencies, or drugs may induce a toxic myocarditis. However, although a variety of organisms have been identified in the myocardium of AIDS patients, the majority of these have been found on a background of disseminated infection and are infrequently associated with localized myocarditis.[48,60] Isolated infection with adjacent myocarditis has rarely been described,[49,98,99] and a clear etiologic link between opportunistic infection and AIDS myocarditis has yet to be established.

Treatment of HIV-Related Heart Muscle Disease

Despite their poor outlook, HIV-positive patients with dilated cardiomyopathy should be offered appropriate palliative therapy. Common agents such as diuretics and digoxin are often useful, but angiotensin-converting enzyme inhibitors may be poorly tolerated because many patients already have a low systemic vascular resistance (P.F. Currie and A.J. Jacob, unpublished observations).

Clinical trials evaluating the efficacy of conventional heart failure treatment would be worthwhile.

Zidovudine (azidothymidine) may be involved in the development of some cases of HIV-related heart muscle disease, although this remains controversial.[74,100,101] In addition to competitively inhibiting HIV RNA-dependent DNA polymerase (reverse transcriptase), it causes a specific, dose-dependent, reversible skeletal myopathy by inhibiting mitochondrial γ DNA polymerase.[102,103] The drug did not appear to cause cardiac dysfunction in our studies.[74] However, improvements in left ventricular function have been reported in cardiomyopathy patients who have stopped the treatment.[100] It seems reasonable, therefore, to discontinue zidovudine therapy for a month in those patients who develop cardiac dysfunction while receiving the drug. This should be followed by reassessment and possible reintroduction of the drug if there is no improvement in cardiac function.

Pyrimethamine and clindamycin were used to treat a patient with heart failure and dilated cardiomyopathy in whom *Toxoplasma* myocarditis was suspected on the basis of clinical findings and a positive bronchoalveolar lavage result.[73] Although a myocardial biopsy did not find *Toxoplasma*, his general condition improved, with a complete recovery of ventricular function. Similarly, immunosuppressive therapy has been used to treat two patients with myocarditis presumed to be secondary to HIV itself.[63]

The improvement in cardiac function noted in these cases may be due to specific treatment, although the condition may also be self-limiting. However, the fact that some forms of myocarditis associated with HIV may be curable suggests that right ventricular endomyocardial biopsy may be useful in selected patients. Right ventricular dysfunction secondary to pulmonary infection may also respond to treatment and is potentially reversible with antibiotic therapy.[49,78]

Conclusion

Despite the differences among the groups of patients affected by HIV throughout the world, it is clear that cardiac involvement is common and occurs in all patient groups. HIV-related heart failure seems destined to become more frequent in Africa and Asia where HIV infection is now endemic. Similarly, improvements in clinical surveillance and the treatment of previously fatal opportunistic infections in Western countries will allow more patients to survive to a later stage of disease, only to succumb to organ failure such as heart muscle disease. Even if only 5% of HIV-positive patients survive to develop symptomatic ventricular dysfunction, this will have serious social and economic implications throughout the world.

The pathogenesis of cardiac dysfunction in AIDS is at present poorly understood, although it is similar to idiopathic dilated cardiomyopathy in HIV-negative patients. Current prospective studies on well-defined HIV-positive populations in many countries may ultimately yield insight into the causes of this and other forms of heart muscle disease.

Acknowledgments

We thank Mrs. Jean Cunningham for her expert secretarial assistance. Dr. Peter Currie is funded by the British Heart Foundation.

References

1. World Health Organization Global Statistics, December 1994. *AIDS* 1995;9:409–410.

2. Rogers DE, Gellin BG. The bright spot about AIDS: it is very tough to catch. *AIDS* 1990;4: 695–696.

3. Potts M, Anderson R, Boily M-C. Slowing the spread of human immunodeficiency virus in developing countries. *Lancet* 1991;338:608–613.

4. Taylor A, Frischer M, Green ST, et al. Low and stable prevalence of HIV among drug injectors in Glasgow. *Int J STD AIDS* 1994;5:105–107.

5. Communicable Disease (Scotland) Unit. AIDS News Supplement. *CDS Weekly Rep* 1992;43.

6. Lifson AR. Preventing HIV: have we lost our way? *Lancet* 1994;343:1306–1307.

7. Brettle RP. Implications of the Edinburgh AIDS epidemic for the United Kingdom. *J Infect* 1990; 20:215–217.

8. Des Jarlais DC, Friedman SR, Novick M, et al. HIV-1 infection among intravenous drug users in Manhattan, New York City, from 1977 through 1987. *JAMA* 1989;261:1008–1012.

9. Lazzarin A, Crocchiolo P, Galli M, et al. Milan as a possible starting point of LAV/HTLV-III epidemic among Italian drug addicts. *Boll Ist Sieroter Milan* 1986;66:9–13.

10. Francheschi S, Tirelli U, Vaccher T, et al. Increased prevalence of HTLV-III antibody among drug users from Italian provinces with US military base. *Lancet* 1986;i:804.

11. Karpas A. Origin and spread of AIDS. *Nature* 1990;348:578.

12. Hanenberg RS, Rojanapithayakorn W, Kunasoll P, et al. Impact of Thailand's HIV-control programme as indicated by the decline of sexually transmitted diseases. *Lancet* 1994;344:243–245.

13. Livornese LL, Korzeniowski OM. Pathogenesis of endocarditis. In: Kaye D (ed). *Infective Endocarditis,* 2nd Ed. New York: Lippincott-Raven, 1992.

14. Currie PF, Sutherland GR, Bell JE, et al. Is human immunodeficiency virus a risk factor for endocarditis? [Abstract P294]. *Eur Heart J* 1995;16:33.

15. Lewis W, Grody WN. AIDS and the heart: review and consideration of pathogenic mechanisms. *Cardiovasc Pathol* 1992;1:53–64.

16. Wit DJ, Craven DE, McCabe WR. Bacterial infection in adult patients with the acquired immunodeficiency syndrome (AIDS) and AIDS-related complex. *Am J Med* 1987;82:900–906.

17. Currie PF, Sutherland GR, Jacob AJ, et al. A review of endocarditis in acquired immunodeficiency syndrome and human immunodeficiency virus infection. *Eur Heart J* 1995;16:15–18.

18. Yersin BR, Glauser MP, Freedman LR. Effect of nitrogen mustard on the natural history of right sided streptococcal endocarditis in rabbits: role for cellular host defences. *Infect Immun* 1982;35: 320–325.

19. Meddens MJM, Thompson J, Eulderink F, et al. Role of granulocytes in experimental *Streptococcus sanguis* endocarditis. *Infect Immun* 1982;36: 325–332.

20. Meddens MJM, Thompson J, Bauer WC, et al. Role of granulocytes and monocytes in experimental *Staphylococcus epidermidis* endocarditis. *Infect Immun* 1983;41:145–153.

21. Meddens MJM, Thompson J, Bauer WC, Van Furth R. Role of granulocytes and monocytes in experimental *Escherichia coli* endocarditis. *Infect Immun* 1984;43:491–496.

22. Tunkel AR, Mandell GL. Infecting micro-organisms. In: Kaye D (ed). *Infective Endocarditis,* 2nd Ed. New York: Lippincott-Raven, 1992.

23. Kinney EL, Monsuez JJ, Kitzis M, Vittecoq D. Treatment of AIDS-associated heart disease. *Angiology* 1989;40:970–976.

24. Bestetti RB, Figueiredo JF, De C, Da Costa JC. Salmonella tricuspid endocarditis in an intravenous drug abuser with human immunodeficiency virus infection. *Int J Cardiol* 1991;30:361–362.

25. Roberts J, Navarro C, Johnson A, et al. Cardiac involvement in intravenous drug abusers with and without acquired immunodeficiency syndrome. [Abstract]. *Circulation* 1989;80(Suppl II):1285.

26. Grupo de Trabajo para el Estudio de Infecciones en Drogadictos. Estudio multicentrico de las complicaciones infecciosas en adictos a drogas por via parenteral en Espana: analisis final de 17,592 casos (1977–1991). *Enferm Infecc Microbiol Clin* 1996; 13:532–539.

27. Miro JM, Gatell JM. Estudio multicentrico de las complicaciones infecciosas en adictos a drogas por via parenteral en Espana: analisis de 11,645 casos (1977–1988). *Enferm Infecc Microbiol Clin* 1990;9:514–519.

28. Nahass RG, Weinstein MP, Bartels J, Gocke DJ. Infective endocarditis in intravenous drug users: a comparison of human immunodeficiency virus type 1-negative and -positive patients. *J Infect Dis* 1990;162:967–970.

29. Henochowicz S, Mustafa M, Lawrinson WE, et al. Cardiac aspergillosis in acquired immune deficiency syndrome. *Am J Cardiol* 1985;55:1239–1240.

30. Raffanti SP, Fyfe B, Carreiro S, et al. Native valve endocarditis due to *Pseudalleschira boydii* in a patient with AIDS: case report and review. *Rev Infect Dis* 1990;12:993–996.

31. Cox JN, di Dio F, Pizzolato GP, et al. *Aspergillus* endocarditis and myocarditis in a patient with the acquired immunodeficiency syndrome (AIDS). *Virchows Arch Pathol Anat* 1990;417:255–259.

32. Currie PF, Sutherland GR, Jacob J, et al. Endocarditis and human immunodeficiency virus infection. *Br Heart J* 1994;71:13.

33. Weisse AB, Heller DR, Schimenti RJ, et al. The febrile parenteral drug user: a prospective study in 121 patients. *Am J Med* 1993;94:274–280.

34. Sande MA, Lee BL, Mills J, Chambers HF. Endocarditis in intravenous drug users. In: Kay D (ed). *Infective Endocarditis,* 2nd Ed. New York: Lippincott-Raven, 1992:345–359.

35. Klatt EC, Meyer PR. Pathology of the heart in acquired immunodeficiency syndrome (AIDS). [Letter]. *Arch Pathol* 1988;112:114.

36. Eisenberg MJ, Gordon AS, Schiller NB. HIV-associated pericardial effusions. *Chest* 1992;102: 956–958.

37. Malu K, Longo-Mbenza B, Luhrhuma Z, et al. Pericardite et syndrome d'immunodeficience acquise. *Arch Mal Coeur* 1988;81:207–211.

38. Taelman G, Kagame A, Batungwanayo J, et al. Pericardial effusion and HIV infection. [Letter]. *Lancet* 1990;335:924.

39. Elliot AM, Halwiindi B, Hayes RJ, et al. The impact of human immunodeficiency virus on presentation and diagnosis of tuberculosis in a cohort study in Zambia. *J Trop Med Hyg* 1993;96:1–11.

40. Cegielski JP, Ramaiya K, Lallinger GJ, et al. Pericardial disease and human immunodeficiency virus in Dar es Salaam, Tanzania. *Lancet* 1990; 335:209–212.

41. Dalli E, Quesada A, Juan G, et al. Tuberculous pericarditis as the first manifestation of acquired immunodeficiency syndrome. *Am Heart J* 1987; 114:905–906.

42. Flum DR, McGinn JT, Tyras DH. The role of the pericardial window in AIDS. *Chest* 1995; 107:1522–1525.

43. Currie PF, Wright RA, Campanella C, et al. Long-term survival following pericardiectomy for *Staphylococcus aureus* pericarditis in an HIV-positive drug user. *Eur Heart J* 1997;18:526–527.

44. Andress JD, Polish LB, Clark DM, Hossack KF. Transvenous biopsy diagnosis of cardiac lymphoma in an AIDS patient. *Am Heart J* 1989;118: 421–423.

45. Moskowitz L, Hensley GT, Chan JC, et al. Immediate causes of death in acquired immunodeficiency syndrome. *Arch Pathol* 1985;109:735–738.

46. Ambrose RA, Eun-Young L, Sharer LR, et al. The acquired immunodeficiency syndrome in intravenous drug abusers and patients with a sexual risk. *Hum Pathol* 1987;18:1109–1114.

47. Autran BR, Gorin I, Leibowitch M, et al. AIDS in a Haitian woman with cardiac Kaposi's sarcoma and Whipple's disease. *Lancet* 1983;i:767–768.

48. Baroldi G, Corallo S, Moroni M, et al. Focal lymphocytic myocarditis in acquired immunodeficiency syndrome (AIDS): a correlative morphologic and clinical study in 26 consecutive fatal cases. *J Am Coll Cardiol* 1988;12:463–469.

49. Monsuez J, Kinney EL, Vittecoq D, et al. Comparison among acquired immune deficiency syndrome patients with and without clinical evidence of cardiac disease. *Am J Cardiol* 1988;62:1311–1313.

50. McAllister HA, Fenoglio JJ Jr. Tumors of the cardiovascular system. In: McAllister HA, Fenoglio JJ (eds). *Atlas of Tumor Pathology*. Washington, DC: Armed Forces Institute of Pathology, 1978:111–119.

51. Pousset F, Le Heuzey J-Y, Pialoux G, et al. Cardiac lymphoma presenting as atrial flutter in an AIDS patient. *Eur Heart J* 1994;15:862–864.

52. Cohen IS, Anderson DW, Virmani R, et al. Congestive cardiomyopathy in association with the acquired immunodeficiency syndrome. *N Engl J Med* 1986;315:628–630.

53. Lewis W. AIDS: cardiac findings from 115 autopsies. *Prog Cardiovasc Dis* 1989;32:207–215.

54. Corallo S, Mutinelli MR, Moroni M, et al. Echocardiography detects myocardial damage in AIDS: prospective study in 102 patients. *Eur Heart J* 1988;9:887–892.

55. Herskowitz A, Vlahov D, Willoughby S, et al. Prevalence and incidence of left ventricular dysfunction in patients with human immunodeficiency virus infection. *Am J Cardiol* 1993;71:955–958.

56. Currie PF, Jacob AH, Foreman AR, et al. HIV related heart muscle disease: prognostic implications. *BMJ* 1994;309:1605–1607.

57. Himelman B, Chung WS, Chernoff DN, et al. Cardiac manifestations of human immunodeficiency virus infection: a two-dimensional echocardiographic study. *J Am Coll Cardiol* 1989;13:1030–1036.

58. Aretz TH, Billingham ME, Edwards WD, et al. Myocarditis: a histopathologic definition and classification. *Am J Cardiovasc Pathol* 1987;1:3–14.

59. Roldan EO, Moskowitz L, Hensley GT. Pathology of the heart in acquired immunodeficiency syndrome. *Arch Pathol* 1987;111:943–946.

60. Anderson DW, Virmani R, Reilly JM, et al. Prevalent myocarditis at necropsy in the acquired immunodeficiency syndrome. *J Am Coll Cardiol* 1988;11:792–799.

61. Beschorner WE, Baughman K, Turnicky RP, et al. HIV associated myocarditis: pathology and immunopathology. *Am J Pathol* 1990;137:1365–1371.

62. Wu T-C, Pizzorno MC, Hayward GS, et al. In situ detection of human cytomegalovirus immediate-early gene transcripts within cardiac monocytes of patients with HIV-associated cardiomyopathy. *AIDS* 1992;6:777–785.

63. Levy WS, Varghese PJ, Anderson DW, et al. Myocarditis diagnosed by endomyocardial biopsy in human immunodeficiency virus infection with cardiac dysfunction. *Am J Cardiol* 1988;62:658–659.

64. Welch K, Finkbeiner W, Alpers CE, et al. Autopsy findings in the acquired immune deficiency syndrome. *JAMA* 1984;252:1152–1159.

65. Corboy JR, Fink L, Miller WT. Congestive cardiomyopathy in association with AIDS. *Radiology* 1987;165:139–141.

66. Kaminski HJ, Katzman M, Wiest PM, et al. Cardiomyopathy associated with the acquired immune deficiency syndrome. *AIDS* 1988;1:105–110.

67. Jacob AJ, Boon NA. HIV cardiomyopathy: a dark cloud with a silver lining? *Br Heart J* 1991;66:1–2.

68. Levy WS, Simon GL, Riso JC, Ross AM. Prevalence of cardiac abnormalities in human immunodeficiency virus infection. *Am J Cardiol* 1989;63:86–89.

69. Herskowitz A, Wu TC, Willoughby S, et al. Myocarditis and cardiotropic viral infection associated with severe left ventricular dysfunction in late stage infection with human immunodeficiency virus. *J Am Coll Cardiol* 1994;24:1025–1032.

70. Reilly JM, Cunnion RE, Anderson DW, et al. Frequency of myocarditis, left ventricular dysfunction and ventricular tachycardia in the acquired immune deficiency syndrome. *Am J Cardiol* 1988;62:789–793.

71. Parravicini C, Baroldi G, Gaiera G, Lazzarin A. Phenotype of intramyocardial leukocytic infiltrates in acquired immunodeficiency syndrome (AIDS): a postmortem immunohistochemical study in 34 consecutive cases. *Mod Pathol* 1991;4:559–565.

72. Lafont A, Wolff M, Marche C, et al. Overwhelming myocarditis due to *Cryptococcus neoformans*

in an AIDS patient. [Letter]. *Lancet* 1987;ii:1145–1146.

73. Grange F, Kinney EL, Monsuez J, et al. Successful therapy for *Toxoplasma gondii* myocarditis in acquired immunodeficiency syndrome. *Am Heart J* 1990;120:443–444.

74. Jacob AJ, Sutherland GR, Bird AG, et al. Myocardial dysfunction in patients infected with HIV: prevalence and risk factors. *Br Heart J* 1992;68:549–555.

75. Akhras F, Dubrey S, Gazzard B, Noble MIM. Emerging patterns of heart disease in HIV infected homosexual subjects with and without opportunistic infections: a prospective colour flow echocardiographic study. *Eur Heart J* 1994;15:68–75.

76. Coudray N, De Zuttere D, Force G, et al. Left ventricular diastolic dysfunction in asymptomatic and symptomatic human immunodeficiency virus carriers: an echocardiographic study. *Eur Heart J* 1995;16:61–76.

77. Hakim JG, Matenga JA, Siziya S. Myocardial dysfunction in human immunodeficiency virus infection: an echocardiographic study of 157 hospitalised patients in Zimbabwe. *Heart* 1996;76:161–165.

78. Blanchard DG, Hagenhoff C, Chow LC, et al. Reversibility of cardiac abnormalities in human immunodeficiency virus (HIV)-infected individuals: a serial echocardiographic study. *J Am Coll Cardiol* 1991;17:1270–1276.

79. Himelman RB, Dohrmann M, Goodman P, et al. Severe pulmonary hypertension and cor pulmonale in the acquired immunodeficiency syndrome. *Am J Cardiol* 1989;64:1396–1399.

80. Raffanti SR, Chiaramida AJ, Sen P, et al. Assessment of cardiac function in patients with the acquired immunodeficiency syndrome. *Chest* 1988;93:592–594.

81. Lindvig K, Nielsen TL, Videbœk R, Pedersen C. Echocardiographic screening in 24 consecutive AIDS patients. *Dan Med Bull* 1990;37:449–451.

82. Stewart JM, Kaul A, Gromische DS, et al. Symptomatic cardiac dysfunction in children with human immunodeficiency virus infection. *Am Heart J* 1989;117:140–144.

83. Coplan NL, Shimony RY, Ioachim HL, et al. Primary pulmonary hypertension associated with human immunodeficiency viral infection. *Am J Med* 1990;89:906–909.

84. Fink L, Reichek N, St John Sutton MG. Cardiac abnormalities in acquired immune deficiency syndrome. *Am J Cardiol* 1984;54:1161–1163.

85. De Castro S, D'Amati G, Gallo P, et al. Frequency of development of acute global left ventricular dysfunction in human immunodeficiency virus infection. *J Am Coll Cardiol* 1994;24:1018–1024.

86. De Castro S, Migliau G, Silvestri A, et al. Heart involvement in AIDS: a prospective study during various stages of the disease. *Eur Heart J* 1992;13:1452–1459.

87. Dittrich H, Chow L, Denaro F, Spector S. Human immunodeficiency virus, coxsackie virus, and cardiomyopathy. [Letter]. *Ann Intern Med* 1988;108:308.

88. Jacob AJ, Rebus S, Bird AG, et al. Can HIV infect the heart? [Abstract]. *Eur Heart J* 1992;13:370.

89. Sloand EM, Klein HG, Banks SM, et al. Epidemiology of thrombocytopenia in HIV infection. *Eur J Haematol* 1992;48:168–172.

90. Bettaieb A, Fromont P, Louache F, et al. Presence of cross-reactive antibody between human immunodeficiency virus (HIV) and platelet glycoproteins in HIV-related immune thrombocytopenic purpura. *Blood* 1992;80:162–169.

91. Procaccia S, Blasio R, Villa P, et al. Rheumatoid factors and circulating immune complexes in HIV-infected individuals. *AIDS* 1991;5:1441–1446.

92. Chou K, Kauh YC, Jacoby RA, Webster GF. Autoimmune bullous disease in a patient with HIV infection. *J Am Acad Dermatol* 1992;24:1022–1023.

93. Golding H, Robey FA, Gates FT, et al. Identification of homologous regions in human immunodeficiency virus I gp 41 and human MHC class II beta 1 domain. I. Monoclonal antibodies against the gp 41-derived peptide and patients' sera react with native HLA class II antigens, suggesting a role for autoimmunity in the pathogenesis of acquired immune deficiency syndrome. *J Exp Med* 1988;167:914–923.

94. Klaassen RJLK, Vlekke ABJ, von dem Borne AEGK. Neutrophil-bound immunoglobulin in HIV infection is of autoantibody nature. *Br J Haematol* 1991;77:403–409.

95. de Bracco MME, Borda E, Galassi N, et al. Autoantibodies in HIV-infected patients that modulate the cholinergic activity of the heart and gut tissue. *Autoimmunity* 1993; 14:307–314.

96. Gorelik G, Genaro AM, Sterin-Borda L, et al. Autoantibodies bind and activate adrenergic and

cholinergic lymphocyte receptors in Chagas' disease. *Clin Immunol Immunopathol* 1990;55:221–236.

97. Currie PF, Goldman JH, Wright RA, et al. Immune mechanisms in patients with human immunodeficiency virus related heart muscle disease. [Abstract P1717]. *Eur Heart J* 1995;16:301.

98. Tschirhart D, Klatt EC. Disseminated toxoplasmosis in acquired immunodeficiency syndrome. *Arch Pathol* 1988;112:1237–1241.

99. Adair OV, Randive N, Krasnow N. Isolated toxoplasma myocarditis in acquired immune deficiency syndrome. *Am Heart J* 1989;118:856–857.

100. Herskowitz A, Willoughby S, Baughman, et al. Cardiomyopathy associated with antiretroviral therapy in patients with HIV infection: a report of six cases. *Ann Intern Med* 1992;116:311–313.

101. Lipshultz SE, Orav EJ, Sanders SP, et al. Cardiac structure and function in children with human immunodeficiency virus infection treated with zidovudine. *N Engl J Med* 1992;327:1260–1265.

102. Simpson MV, Chin CD, Keilbaugh SA, et al. Studies on inhibition of mitochondrial DNA replication of 3′-azido–3′-dioxythymidine and other dideoxynucleoside analogues which inhibit HIV-1 replication. *Biochem Pharmacol* 1989;38:1033–1036.

103. Peters BS, Winer J, Landon DN, et al. Mitochondrial myopathy associated with chronic zidovudine therapy in AIDS. *Q J Med* 1993;86:5–15.

104. Garcia I, Fainstein V, Rios A, et al. Nonbacterial thrombotic endocarditis in a male homosexual with Kaposi's sarcoma. *Arch Intern Med* 1983;143:1243–1244.

105. Snider WD, Simpson DM, Neilsen S, et al. Neurological complications of acquired immune deficiency syndrome: analysis of 50 patients. *Ann Neurol* 1983;14:403–418.

106. Guarda LA, Luna MA, Smith JL, et al. Acquired immune deficiency syndrome: post mortem findings. *Am J Clin Pathol* 1984;81:549–557.

107. Cammarosano C, Lewis W. Cardiac lesions in acquired immune deficiency syndrome (AIDS). *J Am Coll Cardiol* 1985;5:703–706.

5

Cardiovascular Morbidity and Mortality in Pediatric HIV Infection

Anne-Marie Boller, M.A., Inas Al-Attar, M.D., E. John Orav, Ph.D., and Steven E. Lipshultz, M.D.

Clinically significant cardiac problems are important to children with human immunodeficiency virus (HIV) infection. We are beginning to understand the types of cardiac disease that affect these children and the risk factors associated with them. Unfortunately, cardiovascular disease in HIV-infected children is often clinically occult or is erroneously attributed to other organ systems. Cardiac involvement may occur at any stage of HIV disease progression and in any region of the heart—pericardium, epicardium, myocardium, and endocardium. Recent advances in the treatment of HIV disease have led to increased survival among children; along with an increase in cardiac morbidity and mortality.

This chapter reviews cardiovascular abnormalities in children with HIV infection. We start by discussing the different patterns of survival in HIV-infected children. Clinically significant cardiac abnormalities in infected children are described, including the signs and symptoms associated with these abnormalities. We review the rates of occurrence of these cardiac abnormalities in HIV-infected children and describe noncardiac predictors of cardiac morbidity, cardiac-associated mortality, and overall mortality in these children.

Patterns of Survival

Currently, HIV is the leading cause of death in people between the ages of 24 and 45, and it was the seventh leading cause of death in children between 1 and 4 years old in 1992.[1,2] By the year 2000, it is estimated that as many as 120 million people worldwide may be infected with the virus, including 10 million children.[3] Since the incidence of heart failure in HIV-infected children is 10%, by the year 2000, the worldwide incidence of pediatric heart failure could exceed the incidence of adult heart failure in the United States.

Survival following HIV infection typically follows a bimodal curve, with rapid progressors and long-term survivors.[4-11] On the basis of mathematical modeling, Auger and coworkers[12] determined that the median incubation period to the development of acquired immunodeficiency syndrome (AIDS) for perinatally infected children was 4.8 years, with AIDS developing in 20% of the children in the first year of life and developing in the remainder at a constant rate of 8% per year.

The first mode of the pediatric HIV survival curve is characterized by short-term survival. Rapid progressors experience a severe disease course,

77

Table 5-1. Mean and Median Times Spent in Each Stage of Pediatric HIV Disease

Stage	Mean Time		Median Time	
	Mo (yr)	95% CI: mo	Mo (yr)	95% CI: mo
N	10 (0.8)	9–11	7 (0.6)	6–7
A	4 (0.3)	3–4	3 (0.2)	2–3
B	65 (5.4)	60–70	45 (3.8)	42–48
C	34 (2.8)	31–37	24 (2.0)	21–26

Modified from Ref. 9.

N, asymptomatic HIV infection; A, mild signs or symptoms of HIV disease; B, moderate signs or symptoms of HIV disease; C, severe signs and symptoms of HIV disease; CI, confidence interval.

usually occurring within the first year of life and characterized by encephalopathy and *Pneumocystis carinii* pneumonia.[4,8,11,13–15] Children in whom AIDS is diagnosed within the first year of life have the shortest survival time following diagnosis.[4,6,16] In the European Collaborative Study, HIV-infected infants had a 15% mortality rate in their first year.[17] A complementary study demonstrated that 10% to 25% of infected children had a fulminant course characterized by encephalopathy, *P. carinii* pneumonia, and death.[18] *P. carinii* pneumonia tends to develop between 3 and 6 months of age and is associated with high mortality, while neurologic manifestations often appear during the second half of the first year.[17]

The second mode of the pediatric HIV survival curve occurs in children who have long-term survival. Up to 50% of infected children will survive 2 years after their AIDS diagnosis.[5] Progression to AIDS slows after the first year of life to an annual rate of 6% to 8%, with mortality rates that decrease

at the same rate.[7,17] A recent update from the Pediatric Spectrum of Disease Project revealed an estimated mean survival time of 9.4 years from birth in a cohort of 2,148 perinatally infected, HIV-positive children.[9] Using the 1994 revised classification system for pediatric HIV disease, this study determined the estimated mean time spent in each stage of the disease, the estimated survival time for each stage, and the estimated mean time to the development of AIDS [1994 Centers for Disease Control (CDC) pediatric HIV classification, Category C] (Tables 5-1, 5-2, and 5-3). Barnhart and colleagues[9] showed that, on the average, children progress to moderate symptoms (1994 CDC pediatric HIV classification, Category B) by the second year of life and tend to remain in this category without significant progression for more than half their expected lives. Many previous studies have noted a significant percentage of their pediatric HIV population surviving longer than 5 years.[5,7–10,14] In another study, approximately 75% to 90% of the infected children were long-term

Table 5-2. Estimated Mean and Median Times to Severe Symptomatic HIV Disease from Milder Disease Stages

From Stage	Mean Time to C		Median Time to C: mo (yr)	Proportion of C Within 5 Years (95% CI)
	mo (yr)	95% CI: mo		
N	79 (6.6)	5.7–7.5	60 (5.0)	0.50 (0.40–0.60)
A	69 (5.7)	4.9–6.6	49 (4.1)	0.58 (0.47–0.69)
B	65 (5.4)	5.1–5.8	45 (3.8)	0.60 (0.49–0.71)

Modified from Ref. 9.

N, asymptomatic HIV infection; A, mild signs or symptoms of HIV disease; B, moderate signs or symptoms of HIV disease; C, severe signs and symptoms of HIV disease; CI, confidence interval.

Table 5-3. Estimated Mean and Median Survival Times from the Beginning of Each Stage to Death

From Stage	Mean Survival Time		Median Survival Time, mo (yr)	Proportion Surviving at Least 5 Years (95% CI)
	mo (yr)	95% CI: mo		
N	113 (9.4)	8.1–10.7	96 (8.0)	0.75 (0.68–0.82)
A	103 (8.6)	7.2–9.9	85 (7.1)	0.67 (0.61–0.74)
B	99 (8.2)	6.9–9.6	81 (6.8)	0.65 (0.56–0.73)
C	34 (2.8)	2.6–3.1	23 (1.9)	0.17 (0.10–0.24)

Modified from Ref. 9.

N, asymptomatic HIV infection; A, mild signs or symptoms of HIV disease; B, moderate signs or symptoms of HIV disease; C, severe signs and symptoms of HIV disease. CI, confidence interval.

survivors, with 50% surviving to age 9.[14] Long-term survival has been associated with lymphocytic interstitial pneumonitis and increased endogenous serum immunoglobulin levels.[7,13,19,20]

Although CD4+ lymphocyte counts decrease in conjunction with the degradation of the immune system in both adults and children, the diagnostic value of the CD4+ lymphocyte count is significantly different in these two populations. Recent articles discourage the use of isolated CD4+ lymphocyte counts as surrogate markers of the clinical effects of pediatric HIV disease progression.[10,21–23] In another study, de Martino et al.[24] suggested that immunologic abnormalities and clinical condition were together predictive of clinical outcome and should be considered in conjunction with one another. These conclusions complement the revised 1994 CDC pediatric HIV classification system, which conveys a child's infection status as the combination of immunologic status and clinical stage of disease.[25] The revised 1994 CDC classification system is described in Chapter 1 of this book. Table 5-4 lists the 1987 CDC pediatric classification system, as all of the recent studies cited in this chapter used this system.

The revised 1994 CDC classification system lists cardiomyopathy as a sign of moderately symptomatic HIV infection (Category B). Barnhart and colleagues[9] established that most infected children spend the greater part of their lives (an estimated mean of 65 months) in Category B. Although a lengthened period of moderately symptomatic disease is likely to be associated with the trend toward increasing survival rates among children, it may also contribute to the occurrence of cardiovascular morbidity and mortality in long-term survivors.

Clinical Manifestations of Cardiovascular Morbidity

Cardiovascular disease in HIV-infected children is often subclinical or is erroneously attributed to other organ systems. This section discusses the symptomatic forms of cardiovascular disease in HIV-infected children and highlights the signs of disease that may be observed by the experienced clinician. The echocardiogram remains the single most useful noninvasive diagnostic test to determine cardiac status in HIV-infected children, although the clinician should remain attentive to the development of any of the following signs and symptoms, which may indicate HIV-associated cardiovascular disease.[26]

Congestive Heart Failure

Congestive heart failure is characterized by the failure of the heart, as a pump, to maintain the circulation of blood, resulting in the development of congestion and edema in the tissues. Diagnostically, congestive heart failure may be defined by depressed left ventricular systolic function on echocardiography (fractional shortening < 25%), with accompanying signs and symptoms associated with heart failure. When these conditions persist and require anticongestive therapy for more than 30

Table 5-4. 1987 CDC Classification of HIV Infection in Children Under 13 Years of Age

Class P0. Indeterminate infection
Class P1. Asymptomatic infection
  Subclass A. Normal immune function
  Subclass B. Abnormal immune function
  Subclass C. Immune function not tested
Class P2. Symptomatic infection
  Subclass A. Nonspecific findings
  Subclass B. Progressive neurologic disease
  Subclass C. Lymphoid interstitial pneumonitis
  Subclass D. Secondary infectious diseases
    Category D1. Specified secondary infectious diseases listed in the CDC surveillance definition for AIDS: *Pneumocystis carinii* pneumonia; chronic cryptosporidiosis; disseminated toxoplasmosis with onset after 1 month of age; extraintestinal strongylidiasis; chronic isosporiasis; candidiasis (esophageal, bronchial, or pulmonary); extrapulmonary cryptococcosis; disseminated histoplasmosis; noncutaneous, extrapulmonary, or disseminated mycobacterial infection (any species other than *Mycobacterium leprae*); cytomegalovirus infection with onset after 1 month of age; chronic mucocutaneous or disseminated herpes simplex virus infection with onset after 1 month of age; extrapulmonary or disseminated coccidioidomycosis; nocardiosis; and progressive multifocal leukoencephalopathy
    Category D2. Recurrent serious bacterial infections, including patients with unexplained, recurrent, serious bacterial infections (two or more within a 2-year period), such as sepsis, meningitis, pneumonia, abscess of an internal organ, and bone/joint infections
    Category D3. Other specified secondary infectious diseases, such as oral candidiasis persisting for two months or more, 2 or more episodes of herpes stomatitis within a year, or multidermatomal or disseminated herpes zoster infection
  Subclass E. Secondary cancers
    Category E1. Specified secondary cancers listed in the CDC surveillance definition for AIDS, including patients with the diagnosis of one or more kinds of cancer known to be associated with HIV infection as listed in the surveillance definition of AIDS and indicative of a defect in cell-mediated immunity: Kaposi's sarcoma, B-cell non-Hodgkin's lymphoma, or primary lymphoma of the brain
    Category E2. Other cancers possibly secondary to HIV infection
  Subclass F. Other diseases possibly due to HIV infection, such as hepatitis, cardiopathy, nephropathy, hematologic disorders (anemia, thrombocytopenia), and dermatologic diseases

From Ref. 56, with permission.

days, the condition is usually referred to as chronic congestive heart failure.[27]

The younger HIV-infected child with congestive heart failure may present with a poor suck, diaphoresis, or a weak cry, though the latter may be attributable to the presence of oral candidiasis. Parents may report a change in the infant's or child's feeding patterns, which may include tiring while feeding, shortness of breath, or consumption of an inappropriate amount of formula. Signs of hypoxia may also be observed. The hypoxic infant may be uncharacteristically irritable or anxious, or exhibit a high level of fatigue and lethargy of unknown origin. Decreased urine output may be a sign of congestive heart failure.

The signs and symptoms associated with clinical congestive heart failure in infants and children are numerous. Clinical examination may reveal mottled extremities, decreased peripheral pulses and perfusion, edema, hepatosplenomegaly, and growth failure. Blood pressure and heart rate abnormalities may include tachycardia, decreased blood pressure, or a prolonged QTc interval on the electrocardiogram. Respiratory distress relating to congestive heart failure may manifest as tachypnea, dyspnea, nasal flaring, grunting, and costal retractions.

Dysrhythmias

Dysrhythmias are characterized by abnormalities of rate or rhythm, or an abnormal sequence of cardiac activation.

Infants and children experiencing dysrhythmias may present with a weak cry, poor suck, and inappropriate irritability and lethargy. Infants may fail to make eye contact or be unable to track objects within their view. The parents may report a change in the infant's or child's feeding patterns, which may include tiring while feeding, shortness of breath, or consumption of an inappropriate amount of formula. Parents may report periodic blue spells, diaphoresis, or seizures, and the clinician may note syncope upon examination. Hypoxic infants may appear irritable or anxious, with inappropriate fatigue and lethargy.

Certain dysrhythmias may result in symptomatic impaired cerebral perfusion. Respiratory distress may be noted, with signs of tachypnea, dyspnea, nasal flaring, grunting, and costal retractions. Clinical examination may reveal poor peripheral perfusion, edema, growth failure, tachycardia, or hepatosplenomegaly.

Abnormalities of Heart Rate and Blood Pressure

HIV-infected infants and children may experience a wide range of heart rate and blood pressure abnormalities, including resting sinus tachycardia, sinus bradycardia, hypotension, and hypertension.

Pericardial Disease, Pericardial Effusion With Tamponade, and Pericardial Inflammation

Pericardial disease may involve pericardial effusion of inflammatory or noninflammatory origin. The increased fluid in the pericardium may compress the heart, resulting in clinical symptoms (cardiac tamponade) or causing cardiac abnormalities.

The HIV-infected child with pericardial disease may report acute precordial pain or left shoulder pain. Numerous signs of congestive heart failure may also indicate pericardial disease, including hepatomegaly, peripheral edema, ascites, and the appearance of distended neck veins. The patient may present with or report a hacking cough, diaphoresis, or fever.

Heart rate and blood pressure abnormalities may include tachycardia or hypotension. Clinical examination may reveal paradoxical pulses, distant heart sounds, or a friction rub. The clinician should look

for signs of pericarditis and decreased cardiac output, leading to cerebral and renal hypoperfusion.

Pulmonary Hypertension

An elevated blood pressure in the pulmonary arterial bed may be primary or secondary to pulmonary disease or cardiac disease (e.g., fibrosis of the lung or mitral stenosis). Pulmonary hypertension may induce cardiac abnormalities, usually associated with the right ventricle.

HIV-infected infants with pulmonary hypertension may present with dyspnea, chest pain, dry cough, and a history of vomiting and blue spells. Infants and children may become fatigued easily.

A narrow second heart sound with a loud P2 component may be heard on physical examination. Patients with right ventricular failure due to pulmonary hypertension may present with hepatomegaly and ascites. Right ventricular hypertrophy may be found on electrocardiographic or echocardiographic examinations in the patient with pulmonary hypertension.

Description and Incidence of Cardiovascular Morbidity and Mortality

Cardiovascular Morbidity

Luginbuhl and associates[27] described the incidence of abnormal cardiac manifestations in pediatric HIV disease. Between January 1984 and February 1991, 81 HIV-infected patients followed at Children's Hospital, Boston, who had one or more cardiac evaluations, were included in the cohort and studied retrospectively. Cardiac morbidity endpoints were abnormalities in blood pressure and heart rate, cardiac arrest, and congestive heart failure.

Hemodynamic Abnormalities

Abnormal blood pressure was categorized as hypertension or hypotension. Hypertension was defined as blood pressure beyond the normal range for age (>95th percentile). Hypotension was defined as systolic blood pressure 65 mmHg or less in infants up to 1 year old and 70 mmHg or less in children older than 1 year. Blood pressure abnormalities were noted at echocardiography or in the medical record on at least two successive measurements or three measurements within a 24-hour period. Episodes of hypotension or hypertension occurring more than 7 days apart in the same patient were considered separate events.

In the Luginbuhl cohort, there were 21 noted episodes of hypertension (19%).[27] Hypertension was associated with various other conditions at diagnosis. Seven children had concurrent infections, four of which were *P. carinii* pneumonia. Two patients had documented renal failure during their hypertensive episode, while two others had congestive heart failure. One patient had hypertension while taking ceftriaxone sodium and another while taking amphotericin B.

In the same study, 19 episodes of hypotension were noted in 16 children (20%). Ten patients had infections during the hypotensive episode; 3 of these patients were undergoing treatment for *P. carinii* pneumonia. One child was hypotensive in conjunction with a respiratory arrest. One child had hypotension concurrently with pericardial effusion due to congestive heart failure, and one child had hypotension with nonketotic hyperglycemia coma. One patient was hypotensive following a cardiac arrest. Four patients had hypotension concurrently with medications, including amphotericin B, mezlocillin sodium, and trimethoprim–sulfamethoxazole. One patient had no known associations with the hypotensive episode.

Abnormal heart rates were categorized as tachycardia, bradycardia, or dysrhythmias. A dysrhythmia is any abnormality in the rate or regularity of the heartbeat or in the sequence of cardiac activation. Medical records, echocardiograms, electrocardiograms, and Holter monitor reports were analyzed for abnormal heart rate values, which were defined as values beyond the normal range for age (<2nd percentile and >98th percentile, for bradycardia and tachycardia, respectively) in a relaxed afebrile state during continuous monitoring for at least 1 minute, or as noted in the medical record on at least two successive measurements or on a minimum of three recordings within a 24-hour period.

Marked sinus dysrhythmia was defined as a heart rate that varied by more than 50 beats per minute.

The most common cardiac abnormality in this cohort was resting sinus tachycardia, noted in 52 patients (64%). For these 52 patients, the mean hematocrit at the time of tachycardia was 0.31; 10 patients had congestive heart failure either before or after their episode of tachycardia, and 9 patients (11%) had bradycardia.

Various types of dysrhythmias occurred in 35% of our patients, including atrial ectopy in 20 patients (25%), premature junctional beats in 3 patients (4%), premature ventricular beats in 12 patients (15%), ventricular tachycardia in 2 patients (2%), and ventricular fibrillation in 1 patient (1%); 14 children (17%) had marked sinus dysrhythmia.

Cardiac Arrest

Cardiac arrest was defined as the sudden onset of hemodynamic abnormalities severe enough to require chest compression in addition to pharmacologic intervention. Arrests were documented and confirmed through medical record abstraction. Seven (9%) of the patients studied by Luginbuhl and colleagues[27] had a total of eight cardiac arrests during the study. One arrest was temporally associated with flushing of a central line, three with medications (two with cardiac inotropic agents and one with trimethoprim–sulfamethoxazole), one with respiratory infection, one with sepsis, and one with both pericarditis and myocarditis. One arrest had no known associations. Six of the seven patients were successfully resuscitated. The one fatal arrest occurred in a patient with pericarditis, myocarditis, and inflammation of the conduction system, as noted at autopsy.

Chronic Congestive Heart Failure

The signs and symptoms of congestive heart failure are discussed above and should be considered during the examination of an HIV-infected child. Other HIV-associated illnesses may mimic the signs and symptoms of congestive heart failure, so that echocardiographic evaluation is useful in making the correct diagnosis.

Eight (10%) of the patients studied by Luginbuhl's group had chronic congestive heart failure upon evaluation, and another eight had transient heart failure.[27,28] The latter patients had depressed left ventricular fractional shortening (≤25%) but did not meet the definition of chronic congestive heart failure. Our results corroborate numerous other studies that document an approximately 10% rate of congestive heart failure in the pediatric HIV population.[27,29,30] These studies are reviewed in Chapter 24 of this book.

Cardiovascular Mortality

Luginbuhl and colleagues[27] also described the incidence of cardiac mortality in pediatric HIV disease. The endpoints were death with and without cardiac dysfunction, and overall mortality.

Overall Mortality

During the study period, 30 patients (37%) died; 10 of them (12%) had cardiac dysfunction.

Death With Cardiac Dysfunction

Death with cardiac dysfunction was defined as sudden death presumed secondary to a dysrhythmia, or death associated with significant left ventricular dysfunction. Left ventricular dysfunction was defined echocardiographically as markedly low contractility (stress velocity index more than two standard deviations below the mean) and depressed systolic function (fractional shortening ≤25%), both measured within 6 months before death.

Of the 10 patients who died with significant cardiac complications, 9 had significant ventricular dysfunction.

Al-Attar and coworkers[31,32] studied 68 HIV-infected children identified at the time of AIDS diagnosis between January 1984 and June 1994 and followed prospectively. During the study period, 43 patients (63%) died, 15 of them (22%) with cardiac dysfunction. Of the 15 patients who died with cardiac dysfunction, 14 were male. The definition of death with cardiac dysfunction was identical to that of Luginbuhl and colleagues.[27]

Death Without Cardiac Dysfunction

In the study of Luginbuhl and colleagues[27] 20 patients (25%) died with no evidence of cardiac dysfunction.

Predictors of Cardiovascular Morbidity

The study of Luginbuhl and collaborators[27] established significant clinical associations and predictors of cardiac morbidity in HIV-infected children who received one or more cardiac evaluations (Tables 5-5 and 5-6).

Al-Attar and coworkers[31,32] analyzed HIV disease progression and noncardiac predictors of cardiac morbidity in HIV-infected children. A retrospective review of medical records, echocardiograms, electrocardiograms, and Holter monitor reports was performed on 68 patients with a 1987 CDC-defined diagnosis of AIDS, who were followed from January 1984 through June 1994. Clinical and demographic characteristics were obtained at the time of the first AIDS-defining condition.

Both of these studies used Cox proportional hazards regression models to analyze noncardiac factors as potential predictors of serious cardiac events (congestive heart failure, significant dysrhythmias, tamponade, stroke with hemodynamic instability, and cardiac arrest) and hemodynamic abnormalities (hypertension, hypotension, tachycardia, and bradycardia). Significant associations and predictors of cardiac morbidity are portrayed in Figures 5-1 and 5-2.

Cardiovascular Morbidity

HIV Status

Both of the above studies relied on the 1987 CDC classification system for pediatric HIV disease (Table 5-4). Asymptomatic status was not a significant predictor of an adverse cardiac outcome.

Children with mildly symptomatic HIV disease who did not meet CDC diagnostic criteria for AIDS were designated as having AIDS-related complex, which is included in the 1987 pediatric CDC classification categories P2A, P2D3, and P2F. These children had the greatest risk of marked sinus dysrhythmia ($P < .001$) and tachycardia ($P < .001$) in comparison with children in other CDC pediatric categories of classification. By multivariate analysis, these two clinical associations remained significant, suggesting that tachycardia and marked sinus dysrhythmia are early findings in HIV disease.

Table 5-5. Univariate Analysis of CDC Pediatric Classification as a Correlate of Adverse Cardiac Outcomes

Cardiac Outcome	Relative Risk for 1987 CDC Pediatric HIV Classification			
	ARC (P2A, P2D3, P2F)* [n = 38]	LIP (P2C)* [n = 16]	Nonneurologic AIDS (P2D1, P2D2)* [n = 39]	Encephalopathy (P2B)* [n = 25]
Tachycardia	3.8	1.7	8.6	4.2
(*n* = 52)	(1.9–7.6)	(0.6–4.5)	(3.9–19.1)	(1.7–10.7)
Bradycardia	2.5	NS	8.9	12.4
(*n* = 9)	(0.4–16.6)		(1.5–52.5)	(2.0–75.9)
Hypertension	NS	2.8	27.1	13
(*n* = 15)		(0.5–14.2)	(7.6–96.5)	(3.6–46.5)
Hypotension	0.3	1.2	12.7	19.9
(*n* = 16)	(0.03–2.4)	(0.14–11.0)	(3.6–44.7)	(5.9–66.7)
Marked sinus	21.1	4.1	NS	6
dysrhythmia	(6.2–71.5)	(0.8–21.3)		(1.4–26.6)
(*n* = 14)				
Cardiac arrest	1.5	7	3.6	16.6
(*n* = 7)	(0.1–16.3)	(0.96–50.9)	(0.4–28.8)	(2.6–106.7)
Chronic congestive	1.1	2.9	2.7	6.2
heart failure	(0.2–6.4)	(0.3–32.8)	(0.4–16.4)	(1.2–31.8)
(*n* = 8)				
Death with cardiac	NS	3.7	66.7	34.5
dysfunction		(0.6–25.0)	(7.7–578.2)	(5.4–221.4)
(*n* = 10)				
Noncardiac death	NS	1.6	40	19.5
(*n* = 20)		(0.4–7.0)	(10.2–159.2)	(6.3–60.9)
Total deaths	NS	2.1	47	22.2
(*n* = 30)		(0.7–6.6)	(14.9–148.4)	(8.6–56.8)

From Ref. 27, with permission.
ARC, AIDS-related complex; LIP, lymphocytic interstitial pneumonitis; NS, not significant.
*P2 CDC classifications are described in Table 5-4.

AIDS-related complex was associated with cardiac arrest by multivariate analysis (*P* = .07). AIDS-related complex symptoms were not prognostic of other cardiac events, such as blood pressure abnormalities or congestive heart failure.[27]

Lymphocytic Interstitial Pneumonitis

By multivariate analysis, lymphocytic interstitial pneumonitis was related to cardiac abnormalities associated with the early course of HIV disease: tachycardia (*P* < .001), marked sinus dysrhythmia (*P* < .001), and cardiac arrest (*P* = .04). These findings may relate to autonomic imbalance and neuropathy, which are common in the early course of HIV infection and tend to worsen with disease progression.[33–39] Focal lymphocytic infiltration of the heart, analogous to lymphocytic interstitial pneumonitis in the lungs of HIV-infected children, may be associated with heart-rate abnormalities and dysrhythmias.[28] Lymphocytic interstitial pneumonitis was not associated with any cardiac abnormalities when the analysis was adjusted for other CDC pediatric classifications, nor was it related to severe cardiac abnormalities such as bradycardia, blood pressure abnormalities, or congestive heart failure.[27]

Nonneurologic, Non-Lymphocytic Interstitial Pneumonitis AIDS

Nonneurologic AIDS was defined as HIV infection together with opportunistic infection and/or severe bacterial infection, as defined in the 1987 pediatric CDC classification categories P2D1 and P2D2. Children with nonneurologic AIDS were at high risk for many severe cardiac outcomes by both univariate and multivariate analysis. Significant associations were found with tachycardia (*P* < .001),

Table 5-6   Multivariate Analysis of CDC Pediatric Classification as a Correlate of Adverse Cardiac Outcomes

Cardiac Outcome	Relative Risk for 1987 CDC Pediatric HIV Classification			
	ARC (P2A, P2D3, P2F)* [n = 38]	LIP (P2C)* [n = 16]	Nonneurologic AIDS (P2D1, P2D2)* [n = 39]	Encephalopathy (P2B)* [n = 25]
Tachycardia (n = 52)	14.1 (6.2–32.1)	6.3 (2.3–16.9)	16.4 (6.9–39.3)	3 (1.1–7.8)
Bradycardia (n = 9)	12.2 (1.1–131.6)	NS	10.3 (1.6–66.7)	16 (2.4–107.8)
Hypertension (n = 15)	NS	NS	27.1 (7.6–96.5)	NS
Hypotension (n = 16)	NS	NS	3.5 (0.9–13.9)	11.4 (2.8–45.6)
Marked sinus dysrhythmia (n = 14)	119 (17–829)	31 (3–279)	NS	57 (7–503)
Cardiac arrest (n = 7)	12.4 (0.8–184.9)	11.1 (1.1–112.2)	NS	32.8 (3.7–292.9)
Chronic congestive heart failure (n = 8)	NS	NS	NS	6.2 (1.2–31.8)
Death with cardiac dysfunction (n = 10)	NS	NS	21.6 (1.9–244.7)	10.3 (0.9–124.0)
Noncardiac death (n = 20)	NS	NS	12.6 (2.9–54.6)	7 (1.8–27.1)
Total death (n = 30)	NS	NS	14.9 (4.2–51.9)	7.5 (2.3–24.0)

From Ref. 27, with permission.

ARC, AIDS-related complex; LIP, lymphocytic interstitial pneumonitis; NS, not significant.

*P2 CDC classifications are described in Table 5-4.

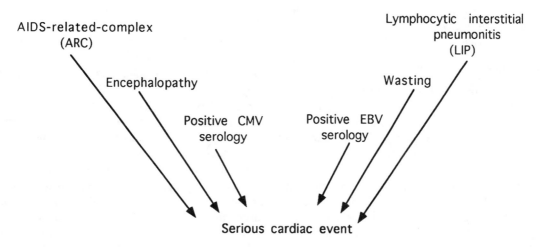

Figure 5-1.   Summary of noncardiac predictors of serious cardiac events, defined as congestive heart failure, cardiac arrest, dysrhythmias, and tamponade. (Based on Refs. 27, 31, and 32; see the sections Cytomegalovirus *and* Epstein-Barr Virus in this chapter for further details.)

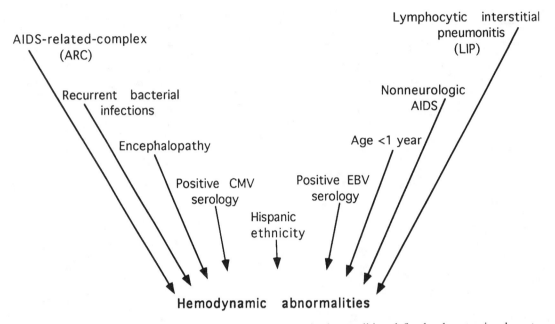

Figure 5-2.   Summary of noncardiac predictors of hemodynamic abnormalities, defined as hypotension, hypertension, tachycardia, and bradycardia. (Based on Refs. 27, 31, and 32; see the sections Cytomegalovirus *and* Epstein-Barr Virus in this chapter for further details.)

bradycardia $(P = .014)$, hypertension $(P < .001)$, and hypotension $(P = .08).$[27]

Al-Attar and colleagues[31,32] found that an age of less than 1 year at AIDS diagnosis, Hispanic ethnicity, a positive cytomegalovirus status, and recurrent serious bacterial infections predicted hemodynamic abnormalities, including hypertension, hypotension, tachycardia, and bradycardia (RR = 3.4, 2.5, 2.1, and 1.4, respectively; $P < .04$).

Encephalopathy

Encephalopathy was strongly associated with cardiac abnormalities found in the early and late stages of HIV disease progression. After adjustment for CDC classification, encephalopathy alone had the strongest correlation with cardiac arrest $(P < .002)$. Marked sinus dysrhythmia $(P < .001)$, bradycardia $(P = .004)$, tachycardia $(P = .03)$, and hypotension $(P < .001)$ were significantly associated with HIV infection children with encephalopathy.[27] Encephalopathy was the only risk factor prognostic of chronic congestive heart failure (P = .03). Encephalopathy may indicate autonomic nervous sys-

tem dysfunction. The results of the study of Luginbuhl and associates complement other reports that establish an association between autonomic neuropathy and HIV-associated peripheral and central nervous system disease.[34]

Cytomegalovirus

Of the 81 patients in the study of Luginbuhl and colleagues,[27] 75 had serologic testing for cytomegalovirus that was sufficient for analysis in this study. Of those tested, 33 children had positive cytomegalovirus serologic results. When analyses were controlled for zidovudine and intravenous immunoglobulin, cytomegalovirus was significantly associated with tachycardia, marked sinus dysrhythmia, and hypotension. Although previous studies have established an association between cytomegalovirus and myocarditis in HIV-infected patients, the analysis of Luginbuhl and colleagues did not reveal any cardiac abnormalities associated with cytomegalovirus infection after adjustment for CDC classification.[40-43]

Al-Attar and associates[31,32] found wasting, a history of prior cardiovascular abnormalities, and a positive cytomegalovirus status predictive of serious cardiac events, including congestive heart failure, significant dysrhythmias, tamponade, stroke with hemodynamic instability, and cardiac arrest (RR = 6.3, 4.1, and 2.6, respectively; $P < .05$).

A positive cytomegalovirus status, Hispanic ethnicity, recurrent bacterial infections, and an age of less than 1 year at AIDS diagnosis predicted hemodynamic abnormalities, including hypertension, hypotension, tachycardia, and bradycardia (RR = 3.4, 2.5, 2.1, and 1.4, respectively; $P = .04$).[31,32]

Epstein-Barr Virus

In the study of Luginbuhl and colleagues,[27] 66 children had serologic testing that allowed for longitudinal follow-up and analysis. In this group, 36 children had positive Epstein-Barr virus serologic results. In the reduced data set, all seven episodes of chronic congestive heart failure occurred in children with Epstein-Barr virus infection. After adjustment for zidovudine and intravenous immunoglobulin therapy, Epstein-Barr virus infection was significantly associated with tachycardia, bradycardia, hypertension, hypotension, and congestive heart failure. By multivariate analysis, controlling for CDC classification, Epstein-Barr virus was associated with an increased risk of bradycardia ($P = .04$). After adjustment for disease classification, Epstein-Barr virus had the strongest correlation with chronic congestive heart failure ($P < .001$).[27] This may be due to direct infection of the heart with Epstein-Barr virus.

Wasting

According to Al-Attar and coworkers,[31,32] wasting, a history of any prior cardiovascular abnormalities, and a positive cytomegalovirus status predicted serious cardiac events, including congestive heart failure, significant dysrhythmias, tamponade, stroke with hemodynamic instability, and cardiac arrest (RR = 6.3, 4.1, and 2.6, respectively; $P < .05$). The estimated median time to a serious cardiac event was 8 months for children with both wasting and a history of prior cardiac abnormalities, in con-

trast to more than 64 months for children with neither of these risk factors.

Predictors of Cardiovascular Mortality

Luginbuhl and associates[27] established significant clinical associations and predictors of cardiac mortality in HIV-infected children who received one or more cardiac evaluations (Tables 5-5 and 5-6).

Al-Attar and associates[31,32] analyzed HIV disease progression and noncardiac predictors of cardiac mortality in HIV-infected children. Clinical and demographic characteristics were obtained at the time of the first AIDS-defining condition.

Both studies used Cox proportional hazards regression models to analyze noncardiac factors as potential predictors of total deaths, deaths with cardiac dysfunction (i.e., death with significant left ventricular dysfunction [fractional shortening ≤25%] or sudden death, presumably related to a dysrhythmia), and deaths without cardiac dysfunction. Significant associations and predictors of cardiac and noncardiac mortality are portrayed in Figures 5-3, 5-4, and 5-5.

Cardiovascular Mortality

HIV Status

Luginbuhl and colleagues[27] found no association between AIDS-related complex symptoms and death with cardiac dysfunction.

Lymphocytic Interstitial Pneumonitis

Lymphocytic interstitial pneumonitis was not associated with any cardiac abnormalities when the analysis was adjusted for other CDC pediatric classifications, nor was it related to death with cardiac dysfunction.[27]

Nonneurologic, Non-Lymphocytic Interstitial Pneumonitis AIDS

Children with nonneurologic AIDS were at high risk by both univariate and multivariate analysis for many severe cardiac outcomes, including death with cardiac dysfunction ($P = .01$).[27]

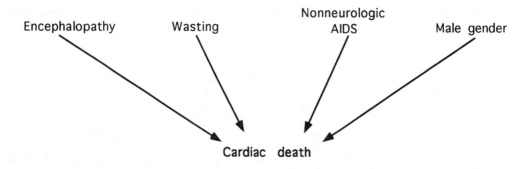

Figure 5-3. Summary of noncardiac predictors of cardiac mortality, defined as death with significant left ventricular dysfunction (fractional shortening ≤25%) or sudden death presumably related to a dysrhythmia. Nonneurologic AIDS, encephalopathy, wasting, and male gender are from models incorporating CD4+ lymphocyte count.[27,31,32] A decreased IgM level was predictive of cardiac mortality if CD4+ lymphocyte count was not incorporated into the model.[31,32] (Based on Refs. 27, 31, and 32; see text for further details.)

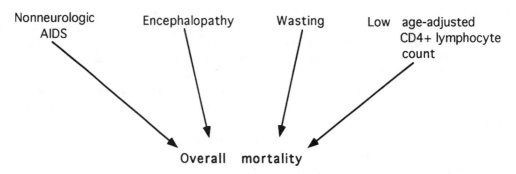

Figure 5-4. Summary of noncardiac predictors of overall mortality. Nonneurologic AIDS, encephalopathy, wasting, and low age-adjusted CD4+ lymphocyte count are from models incorporating CD4+ lymphocyte count.[27,31,32] Decreased IgG and a positive Epstein-Barr virus serologic result were predictive of overall mortality if CD4+ lymphocyte count was not incorporated into the model.[31,32] (Based on Refs. 31 and 32; see text for further details.)

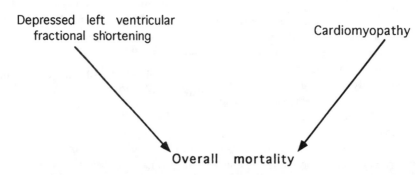

Figure 5-5. Summary of cardiac predictors of overall mortality. Based on Refs. 10, 13, 14, 44, and 46–49; see text for further details.)

Encephalopathy

Encephalopathy was strongly associated with cardiac abnormalities found in the early and late stages of HIV disease progression. There was a mild association between encephalopathy and death with cardiac dysfunction ($P = .01$).[27]

Al-Attar and colleagues[31,32] found encephalopathy to be a specific clinical correlate associated with cardiac death. Encephalopathy (RR = 37.7), wasting (RR = 327.3), and male gender (RR not computable) predicted cardiac death ($P < .03$). If CD4+ lymphocyte count (whose inclusion restricted sample size) was not incorporated in the model, a low IgM z score became a significant predictor of cardiac death (RR = 0.5; $P < .03$).

Cytomegalovirus

Of the 81 enrolled patients in the study of Luginbuhl and coworkers[27] 75 had serologic testing for cytomegalovirus that was sufficient for analysis in this study; 33 children had positive cytomegalovirus serologic results. When analyses were controlled for zidovudine and intravenous immunoglobulin, cytomegalovirus was significantly associated with death with cardiac dysfunction. However, after controlling for CDC classification by multivariate analysis, cytomegalovirus did not correlate with death with cardiac dysfunction.

Epstein-Barr Virus

In this study, 66 children had serologic testing that allowed for longitudinal follow-up and analysis, and 36 children were positive for Epstein-Barr virus. In the reduced dataset, there were 14 deaths,13 of which occurred in children with Epstein-Barr virus infection. After adjustment for zidovudine and intravenous immunoglobulin therapy, Epstein-Barr virus infection was significantly associated with death with cardiac dysfunction.[27]

Wasting

Wasting was found to be a specific clinical correlate associated with cardiac abnormalities and cardiac death.[31,32] Encephalopathy (RR = 37.7), wasting (RR = 327.3), and male gender (RR not computable) predicted cardiac death ($P < .03$).[31,32] If CD4+ lymphocyte count was not incorporated in the model (whose inclusion restricted sample

size), a low IgM z score became a significant predictor of cardiac death (RR = 0.5; $P < .03$).

Overall Mortality

HIV Status

Luginbuhl and colleagues[27] found no association between AIDS-related complex symptoms and overall mortality.

Lymphocytic Interstitial Pneumonitis

Lymphocytic interstitial pneumonitis was not associated with any cardiac abnormalities when the analysis was adjusted for other CDC pediatric classifications, nor was it related to overall mortality.[27]

Nonneurologic, Non-Lymphocytic Interstitial Pneumonitis AIDS

Children with nonneurologic AIDS were at high risk by both univariate and multivariate analysis for many severe cardiac outcomes, including death without cardiac dysfunction and overall mortality ($P < .001$).[27]

Encephalopathy

Encephalopathy was strongly associated with cardiac abnormalities found in the late stages of HIV disease progression. Noncardiac deaths ($P < .001$) and total deaths ($P < .001$) were significantly associated with HIV infection in children with encephalopathy.[27]

Al-Attar and colleagues[31,32] found by multivariate analysis that encephalopathy, wasting, and a low age-adjusted CD4+ lymphocyte count were significant predictors of overall mortality (RR = 7.1, 6.7, and 2.4, respectively; $P < .001$). The estimated median time to death for a child with encephalopathy, wasting, and a CD4+ lymphocyte z score three standard deviations below normal was 3 months; this was in contrast to a median time to death of more than 64 months if none of these risk factors was present.

Cytomegalovirus

In the cohort studied by Luginbuhl and colleagues,[27] 33 children tested positive for cytomegalovirus. When the analyses were controlled for zidovudine and intravenous immunoglobulin, cytomegalovirus was significantly associated with death without cardiac dysfunction. By multivariate analysis, cytomegalovirus was not associated with total deaths.

Epstein-Barr Virus

In this study, 36 children tested positive for Epstein-Barr virus. In the reduced dataset there were 14 deaths, 13 of which occurred in children with Epstein-Barr virus infection. After adjustment for zidovudine and intravenous immunoglobulin therapy, Epstein-Barr virus infection was significantly associated with noncardiac death.[27] Epstein-Barr virus was mildly associated with total deaths ($P = .06$).[27]

Al-Attar and colleagues[31,32] found a low IgG z score and a positive Epstein-Barr virus status to be significant predictors of mortality when CD4+ lymphocyte count (whose inclusion restricted sample size) was not incorporated in the model.

Wasting

Al-Attar and colleagues[31,32] found that wasting was significantly associated with overall mortality. By multivariate analysis, encephalopathy, wasting, and a low age-adjusted CD4+ lymphocyte count were significant predictors of overall mortality (RR = 7.1, 6.7, and 2.4, respectively; $P < .001$). The estimated median time to death for a child with encephalopathy, wasting, and a CD4+ lymphocyte z score three standard deviations below normal was 3 months; this was in contrast to a median time to death of more than 64 months if none of these risk factors was present.

Cardiac Predictors of Overall Mortality

Recent studies have documented cardiac abnormalities that are significantly associated with overall mortality, such as cardiomyopathy and decreased fractional shortening. These results are summarized in Figure 5-5. Of the HIV-infected children who died at one center, 25% died either of cardiomyopathy or suddenly of unexplained causes. Cardiac disease was the primary cause of death in these patients and a secondary cause of death in the majority (six of eight, 75%) of the remaining cases.[44] This study suggested a relation between cardiac disease and HIV symptoms, as each deceased patient had symptomatic P2 HIV disease.[45] At the same center, 83% of the children who died

had premorbid dysrhythmias or cardiomyopathy.[46] In a study by Stewart and associates,[47] six of eight children diagnosed with heart failure died within 2 months. A report from the P^2C^2 study[48] revealed that 7 of 9 (78%) HIV-positive newborns with severe left ventricular dysfunction (left ventricular fractional shortening <19%) and 12 of 42 (29%) of HIV-positive newborns with milder left ventricular dysfunction (left ventricular fractional shortening between 20% and 24%) died in 1 year.[48] This should be compared to the 8% cumulative incidence of death in HIV-positive newborns in 1 year and the 0% cumulative incidence of death in HIV-negative newborns (born to HIV-positive mothers) in 1 year.[48]

The multicenter Italian national study of 1,887 children born to HIV-infected mothers found cardiomyopathy to be associated with significantly shorter survival.[14] In the 6.5% of HIV-infected children with clinically relevant cardiomyopathy, the relative risk of death was 2.76 (1.94–3.93 confidence intervals, $P < .0001$). In another publication from this registry, cardiomyopathy was found in 7% of long-term survivors versus 21% of short-term survivors ($P = .002$).[10] HIV-infected children with cardiomyopathy were significantly less likely to have long-term survival beyond 5 years of age, although the presence of cardiomyopathy did not necessarily prevent long-term survival.[10] In a 1993 study of HIV-infected children in New York City, patients with cardiomyopathy, cardiomegaly, cor pulmonale, myocarditis, dysrhythmias, or congestive heart failure were classified in the most severe category of HIV disease progression (group 3). Although the study did not generate cardiac-specific statistics, group 3 was shown to have significantly shorter survival, a lower age at AIDS diagnosis, and the highest percentage of children dying within 3 months of diagnosis.[13]

A recent report from the P^2C^2 study examined left ventricular abnormalities in 197 HIV-infected children to determine if they independently predicted mortality. At enrollment, two patients had heart failure and significantly reduced left ventricular fractional shortening ($P < .001$), and 60 patients (30%) had a fractional shortening more than two standard deviations below normal. An increased risk of death was univariately related to depressed fractional shortening, increased left ventricular afterload, left ventricular mass and wall thickness at enrollment. After age, height, CD4+ lymphocyte *z* score, and progressive neurologic disease were controlled, fractional shortening proved a significant predictor of mortality.[49]

Conclusion

Cardiovascular morbidity and mortality occur in a significant percentage of pediatric patients with symptomatic HIV infection.[27,31,32] Serious cardiac events and death involving cardiac dysfunction are more likely in children with more advanced HIV disease and in older children. Advances in the treatment of HIV disease and the management of opportunistic infections have been successful in increasing survival in the pediatric population. According to multivariate analysis, a cohort of 68 children with AIDS, in recent years at an institution practicing

regular cardiac monitoring, had increased survival time and decreased risk of a serious cardiac event or cardiac death compared with children with AIDS in earlier years when cardiac monitoring did not occur.[31] This finding perhaps reflects improved follow-up and advances in the overall care of these patients. However, recent projections suggest an increase in cardiac morbidity and mortality with the advent of better treatment and prophylaxis of pulmonary and infectious diseases.[41,50–52]

Therapies that hinder HIV disease progression and the development of coinfections will, it is hoped, further increase survival time in this population. Maintenance of good nutrition and continued investigation of experimental treatments may also prove useful in reducing cardiac morbidity and mortality associated with advanced pediatric HIV disease. A recent study at our institution revealed the advantageous effects of intravenous immunoglobulin therapy in a pediatric HIV-infected population.[19]

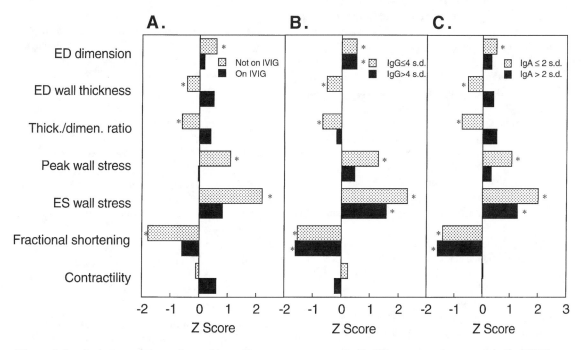

Figure 5-6. **A:** Average echocardiographic cardiac measurements on and off intravenous immunoglobulin (IVIG). **B:** Low and high endogenous IgG. **C:** Low and high endogenous IgA. All cardiac measurements are presented as age- or body surface area-adjusted *z* scores, so that an average of 0 represents a normal value, +1 represents a value one standard deviation above normal, and so on. *Average measurements that were significantly different from normal at $P \leq .05$ by analyses accounting for correlated measurements within children. ED, end-diastolic; ES, end-systolic.[49] (From Ref. 19, with permission.)

Higher endogenous serum IgG levels and intravenous immunoglobulin treatment were associated with significantly greater wall thickness and lower peak wall stress. Additionally, left ventricular contractility, fractional shortening, end-systolic wall stress, and thickness:dimension ratio all tended toward more normal values in association with intravenous immunoglobulin therapy and increased endogenous immunoglobulin levels (Figure 5-6). Serum endogenous IgA levels were significantly related to more normal left ventricular wall thickness and left ventricular thickness:dimension ratios. The improvement of cardiac functional parameters with immunomodulatory agents suggests that intravenous immunoglobulin therapy may have beneficial effects on the heart and help prevent heart disease.

Preliminary data suggest that serial monitoring of left ventricular function and early cardiac interventions reduce subsequent cardiac morbidity and related mortality in HIV-infected children.[31] The pediatric HIV population should, therefore, undergo routine monitoring of left ventricular function for the following reasons:

1. The prevalence of congestive heart failure is high in HIV-infected children and is likely to increase dramatically.[27,50,51]
2. Symptomatic left ventricular dysfunction is underreported, unless ventricular function is monitored by echocardiography, because clinical signs of congestive heart failure are often incorrectly attributed to pulmonary or infectious causes.[28]
3. Most HIV-infected children respond well to anticongestive therapy, especially if treatment is initiated early.[28,47]
4. Because HIV-infected children are at risk for hemodynamic abnormalities with therapeutic interventions, we should try to avoid inappropriate treatment.[27,28,30,33,53–55]

We hope that the monitoring program described in Chapter 24 of this book will cause a significant reduction in the development of symptomatic cardiac dysfunction in this population.

The prevention of heart failure is likely to be associated with reduced morbidity, better quality of life, and lower economic costs. Close monitoring as well as certain immunomodulatory therapies may be beneficial in lowering cardiac morbidity and mortality in the pediatric HIV-infected population.

References

1. Centers for Disease Control and Prevention. *HIV/ AIDS Surveillance Report.* 1995;6:1–33.
2. Kochanek KD, Hudson BL. Advance report of final mortality statistics, 1992. *Mon Vital Stat Rep* 1994; 43:1–76.
3. Mann J. AIDS in the world 1992: a global epidemic out of control? *Global AIDS Policy Coalition News* 1992;June:4.
4. Scott GB, Hutto C, Makuch RW, et al. Survival in children with perinatally acquired human immunodeficiency virus type 1 infection. *N Engl J Med* 1989;321:1791–1796.
5. European Collaborative Study. Natural history of vertically acquired human immunodeficiency virus-1 infection. *Pediatrics* 1994;94:815–819.
6. Rogers MF, Thomas PA, Starcher ET, et al. Acquired immunodeficiency syndrome in children: report of the Centers for Disease Contral National Surveillance, 1982–1985. *Pediatrics* 1987;79: 1008–1014.
7. Lepage P, van de Perre P, Van Vilet G, et al. Clinical and endocrinologic manifestations in perinatally human immunodeficiency virus type 1-infected children aged 5 years or older. *Am J Dis Child* 1991;145:1248–1251.
8. Blanche S, Tardieu M, Duliege AM, et al. Longitudinal study of 94 symptomatic infants with perinatally acquired human immunodeficiency virus infection. *Am J Dis Child* 1990;144:1210–1215.
9. Barnhart HX, Caldwell MB, Thomas P, et al. Natural history of human immunodeficiency virus disease in perinatally infected children: an analysis from the pediatric spectrum of disease project. *Pediatrics* 1996;97:710–716.
10. Italian Register for HIV Infection in Children. Features of children perinatally infected with HIV-1 surviving longer than 5 years. *Lancet* 1994;343: 191–195.
11. Krasinski K, Borkowsky W, Holzman RS. Prognosis of human immunodeficiency virus infection in children and adolescents. *Pediatr Infect Dis J* 1989; 8:216–220.

12. Auger I, Thomas P, De Gruttola V, et al. Incubation periods for paediatric AIDS patients. *Nature* 1988; 336:575–577.

13. Turner BJ, Denison M, Eppes SC, et al. Survival experience of 789 children with the acquired immunodeficiency syndrome. *Pediatr Infect Dis J* 1993; 12:310–320.

14. Tovo PA, de Martino M, Gabiano C, et al. Prognostic factors and survival in children with perinatal HIV-1 infection. *Lancet* 1992;339:1249–1253.

15. Lobato MN, Caldwell B, Ng P, Oxtoby MJ. Encephalopathy in children with perinatally acquired human immunodeficiency virus infection. *J Pediatr* 1995;126:710–715.

16. Blanche S, Rouzioux C, Moscato MLG, et al. A prospective study of infants born to women seropositive for human immunodeficiency virus type 1. *N Engl J Med* 1989;320:1643–1648.

17. Peckham C, Gibb D. Mother-to-child transmission of the human immunodeficiency virus. *N Engl J Med* 1995;333:298–302.

18. Wilfert CM, Wilson C, Luzuriaga K, Epstein L. Pathogenesis of pediatric human immunodeficiency virus type 1 infection. *J Infect Dis* 1994;170: 286–292.

19. Lipshultz SE, Orav EJ, Sanders SP, Colan SD. Immunoglobulins and left ventricular structure and function in pediatric HIV-infection. *Circulation* 1995;92:2220–2225.

20. Thomas P, Tejinder S, Williams R, Blum S. Trends in survival for children reported with maternally transmitted acquired immunodeficiency syndrome in New York City, 1982–1989. *Pediatr Infect Dis J* 1992;11:34–39.

21. Scientific Advisory Committee on Surrogate Markers of HIV. Consensus statement. *J AIDS Hum Retrov* 1995;10(Suppl 2):S114–S116.

22. Choi S, Lagakos SW, Schooley RT, Volberding PA. CD4+ lymphocytes are an incomplete surrogate marker for clinical progression in persons with asymptomatic HIV infection taking zidovudine. *Ann Intern Med* 1993;118:674–680.

23. Concorde Coordinating Committee. Concorde: MRC/ANRS randomized double-blind controlled trial of immediate and deferred zidovudine in symptom-free HIV infection. *Lancet* 1994;343:871–881.

24. deMartino M, Tovo PA, Galli L, et al. Prognostic significance of immunologic changes in 675 infants perinatally exposed to human immunodeficiency virus. *J Pediatr* 1991;119:702–709.

25. Centers for Disease Control and Prevention. 1994 revised classification system for human immunodeficiency virus infection in children less than 13 years of age. *MMWR* 1994;43:1–10.

26. Lane-McAuliffe E, Lipshultz SE. Cardiovascular complications in pediatric HIV infection. *Nurs Clin North Am* 1995;30:291–316.

27. Luginbuhl LM, Orav EJ, McIntosh K, Lipshultz SE. Cardiac morbidity and related mortality in children with HIV infection. *JAMA* 1993;269:2869–2875.

28. Lipshultz SE, Chanock S, Sanders SP, et al. Cardiovascular manifestations of human immunodeficiency virus infection in infants and children. *Am J Cardiol* 1989;63:1489–1497.

29. Lipshultz SE, Luginbuhl LM, McIntosh K, Orav EJ. Cardiac morbidity and mortality in children with symptomatic HIV infection. [Abstract]. *Circulation* 1992;86:I–362.

30. Lipshultz SE, Luginbuhl LM, Saul P, McIntosh K. Dysrhythmias, unexpected arrest and sudden death in pediatric HIV infection. [Abstract]. *Circulation* 1991;84:II–660.

31. Al-Attar I, Orav EJ, Exil V, Lipshultz SE. Predictors of cardiac morbidity and related mortality in children with the acquired immunodeficiency syndrome. [Abstract]. *Pediatr Res* 1995;37:169A.

32. Al-Attar I, Orav EJ, Exil V, et al. Survival patterns of pediatric patients with the acquired immunodeficiency syndrome. [Abstract]. *Pediatr Res* 1995; 37:169A.

33. Craddock C, Bull R, Pasvol G, et al. Cardiorespiratory arrest and autonomic neuropathy in AIDS. *Lancet* 1987;2:16–18.

34. Freeman R, Roberts MS, Friedman LS, Broadbridge C. Autonomic function and human immunodeficiency virus infection. *Neurology* 1990;40: 575–580.

35. Ruttimann S, Hilti P, Spinas GA, Dubach UC. High frequency of human immunodeficiency virus-associated autonomic neuropathy and more severe involvement in advanced stages of human immunodeficiency virus disease. *Arch Intern Med* 1991; 151:2441–2443.

36. Villa A, Foresti V, Confalonieri F. Autonomic nervous system dysfunction associated with HIV infection in intravenous heroin users. *AIDS* 1992;6: 85–89.

37. Scott G, Piaggesi A, Ewing DJ. Sequential autonomic function tests in HIV infection. *AIDS* 1990;4: 1279–1281.

38. Cohen J, Laudenslager M. Autonomic nervous system involvement in patients with human immunodeficiency virus infection. *Neurology* 1989;8: 111–112.

39. Villa A, Cruccu V, Foresti V, et al. HIV-related functional involvement of autonomic nervous system. *Acta Neurol* 1990;12:14–18.

40. Anderson DW, Virmani R. Emerging patterns of heart disease in human immunodeficiency virus infection. *Hum Pathol* 1990;21:253–259.

41. Kaul S, Fishbein MC, Siegel RJ. Cardiac manifestations of acquired immune deficiency syndrome: a 1991 update. *Am Heart J* 1991;122:535–544.

42. Acierno LJ. Cardiac complications in acquired immunodeficiency syndrome (AIDS): a review. *J Am Coll Cardiol* 1989;13:1144–1154.

43. Wu TC, Pizzorno MC, Hayward GS, et al. In situ detection of human cytomegalovirus immediate-early gene transcripts within cardiac myocytes of patients with HIV-associated cardiomyopathy. *AIDS* 1992;6:777–785.

44. Grenier MA, Karr SS, Rakusan TA, Martin GR. Cardiac disease in children with HIV: relationship of cardiac disease to HIV symptomatology. *Pediatr AIDS HIV Infect* 1994;5:174–179.

45. Rodriguez-Mahou M, Lopez-Long J, Lapointe N, et al. Autoimmune phenomena in children with human immunodeficiency virus infection and acquired immunodeficiency syndrome. *Acta Pediatr* 1994 (Suppl 400):31–34.

46. Grenier MA, Karr SS, Rakusan TA, Martin GR. Cardiac disease in children with HIV: relationship of cardic disease to HIV symptomatology. *Pediatr AIDS HIV Infect* 1994;5:174–178.

47. Stewart JM, Kaul A, Gromisch DS, et al. Symptomatic cardiac dysfunction in children with human immunodeficiency virus infection. *Am Heart J* 1989;117:140–144.

48. Starc TJ, Lipshultz S, Easley K, et al. Cardiac complications in HIV infected children: the NHLBI P^2C^2 study. [Abstract]. *Pediatr Res* 1995;37:189A.

49. Lipshultz SE, for the P^2C^2 Study Group. Cardiac dysfunction predicts mortality in children with HIV infection: the prospective NHLBI P^2C^2 HIV study. *Proc Natl Conf Retrov* 1996;65:415.

50. Lipshultz SE, Orav EJ, Sanders SP, et al. Cardiac structure and function in children with human immunodeficiency virus infection treated with zidovudine. *N Engl J Med* 1992;327:1260–1265.

51. Jacob AJ, Boon NA. HIV cardiomyopathy: a dark cloud with a silver lining. *Br Heart J* 1991;66:1–2.

52. Cotton P. AIDS giving rise to cardiac problems. *JAMA* 1990;263:2149.

53. Cohen AJ, Weiser B, Afzal Q, Fuhrer J. Ventricular tachycardia in two patients with AIDS receiving ganciclovir (DHPG). *AIDS* 1990;4:807–809.

54. Stein KM, Haronian H, Mensah GA, et al. Ventricular tachycardia and torsades de pointes complicating pentamidine therapy of *Pneumocystis carinii* pneumonia in the acquired immunodeficiency syndrome. *Am J Cardiol* 1990;66:888–890.

55. Wharton JM, Demopulos PA, Goldschlager N. Torsade de pointes during administration of pentamidine isethionate. *Am J Med* 1987;83:571–576.

56. Centers for Disease Control and Prevention. Classification system for human immunodeficiency virus (HIV) infection in children under 13 years of age. *MMWR* 1987;36:225–236.

Part 2
Specific Clinical Syndromes

6

Fetal Cardiovascular Changes

Lisa K. Hornberger, M.D.

An estimated 7,000 women infected with human immunodeficiency virus (HIV) give birth annually in the United States,[1] and 3.5 million women worldwide are thought to be infected with HIV, the majority of whom are of childbearing age.[2] Therefore, an ever-growing population of infants is at risk for vertically transmitted HIV infection. Infants of HIV-infected mothers are also at risk for other adverse effects developing in a chronically ill, HIV-infected mother.

Maternal HIV Infection and the Fetal Heart

Poor maternal heath, including that associated with HIV infection, can alter general fetal growth and development.[3–9] Maternal disease may also influence the development and function of the fetal cardiovascular system. For instance, transplacentally passed maternal autoantibodies associated with maternal connective tissue disorders may cause fetal heart block and cardiomyopathy.[10,11] Women with metabolic disorders, such as diabetes mellitus and phenylketonuria, are at increased risk for having an infant with structural heart disease.[12] Poor maternal

health during pregnancy may have adverse consequences for the cardiovascular system of the offspring even later in life. Inadequate maternal nutrition in pregnancy has been linked to an increased risk for coronary artery disease in adulthood.[5,13]

The fetal cardiovascular system may also be altered in the presence of maternal HIV infection, as suggested in the recent multicenter P^2C^2 HIV Study.[14] In this study, fetal echocardiography was performed in 174 fetuses of HIV-infected mothers (mean gestational age: 32.9 ± 3.7 weeks). Significant differences in cardiovascular structure and function were found between fetuses developing in HIV-infected mothers, irrespective of postnatal HIV infection status, and normal control fetuses (without maternal HIV infection or cardiovascular abnormalities). Fetuses of HIV-infected mothers had increased right and left ventricular wall thicknesses. They also had lower heart rates, increased peak mitral A (atrial systole) waves and mitral and tricuspid A/E (early ventricular diastole) wave ratios, increased right and left ventricular outflow velocities, and increased umbilical artery systolic: diastolic flow velocity ratios. Furthermore, tricuspid or mitral regurgitation, which is typically present in normal pregnancies, was found in several fetuses of HIV-infected mothers.

The cardiovascular changes identified in fetuses of HIV-infected mothers suggest a state of increased fetal myocardial growth, altered ventricular diastolic and systolic function, and increased placental vascular resistance. Increased circulating catecholamines or an elevated placental vascular resistance, as suggested by the increased umbilical systolic:diastolic blood flow velocities,[15–17] could increase myocardial growth in the fetus. The increase in myocardial growth may also be a secondary effect of altered maternal cytokines observed in HIV-infected patients.[18–20] Interleukin-1 (IL-1), for instance, which is elevated during HIV infection,[19] induces hypertrophy of neonatal cardiomyocytes in vitro.[21]

The increased ratio of peak late-to-early ventricular inflow velocities found in fetuses of HIV-infected mothers suggests the presence of abnormal biventricular diastolic function. This may be associated with increased ventricular wall thickness or may be secondary to increased afterload involving the systemic or placental circulations, as a similar ventricular inflow pattern in the presence of systemic hypertension has been demonstrated previously.[22,23] At lower heart rates, a reduced peak A wave velocity and decreased A:E wave ratio would be expected, in contrast to the observed increase in the A:E wave ratio.[24–26] Increased ventricular outflow velocities suggest the presence of altered systolic function. Increased force of contraction, for instance, perhaps associated with increased wall thickness or maternal factors that influence both ventricular contractility and mass, would result in higher peak ventricular outflow velocities.

Maternal HIV infection may also be associated with an increase in structural heart disease in the fetus and infant of an affected mother.[27,28] In the postnatal arm of the P^2C^2 HIV Study,[27] the prevalence of structural heart defects was 12.3% in 555 children of HIV-infected mothers. This prevalence is much greater than historical, population-based estimates of congenital cardiac abnormalities. In another study, Vogel and colleagues[28] found a 2.8% incidence of congenital heart disease in 175 children of HIV-infected mothers.

The etiology of the observed structural and functional cardiovascular abnormalities in the fetuses of HIV-infected mothers may be multifactorial. Maternal autoimmunity, abnormalities in cytokine production, malnutrition, viral coinfections, and drug and alcohol use, or a combination of these factors, may contribute. Anticardiovascular antibodies are commonly found in HIV-infected patients with cardiovascular impairment[29,30]; they can be transferred from mother to fetus through the placenta[31]; and, as alluded to earlier, they may induce fetal cardiovascular abnormalities.[32] Increased tumor necrosis factor-α (TNF-α) is commonly observed in HIV-infected patients.[33] Elevated TNF-α during pregnancy can cause placental injury and hemorrhage, premature onset of parturition, abortion, and impaired fetal growth.[34,35] Similar to TNF,[34,36,37] IL-1 and IL-6 are increased in pregnancy[36] and HIV infection,[38] and are known to have adverse cardiovascular effects, especially with HIV infection.[29,39]

HIV-infected patients are at considerable risk for micronutrient deficiencies, which may further influence fetal cardiovascular structure and function. Maternal vitamin A deficiency is associated with an increased risk of vertical HIV transmission[40] and fetal cardiovascular abnormalities.[41] Selenium deficiency, which is common with advanced HIV infection, is associated with cardiovascular abnormalities in HIV-infected patients[42] and poor postnatal outcome.[43] Maternal selenium levels at term are normally about 60% of the levels in nonpregnant adult women,[44] suggesting that if there is a threshold for cardiovascular effects, it may be lower with HIV infection.

Viral coinfections in HIV-infected pregnant women may also influence fetal cardiovascular structure and function. Maternal parvovirus B19 coinfection can result in fetal hydrops or stillbirth[45] and may be associated with cardiovascular abnormalities in HIV-infected patients.[46] Both Epstein-Barr virus and cytomegalovirus are associated with congestive heart failure in HIV-infected patients.[47] Many of the mothers in the fetal aspect of the P^2C^2 HIV Study had viral coinfections. Finally, maternal smoking and drug use, both legal and illegal, have been associated with cardiovascular abnormalities in newborns[48,49] and may be contributory.

Antenatal Cardiovascular Manifestations of Vertically Transmitted HIV Infection

Infants and children with vertically transmitted HIV infection frequently have abnormalities of cardiovascular structure and function. The cardiovascular abnormalities found in this population include lymphocytic pericarditis, myocarditis, endocarditis, vasculitis, abnormalities associated with malignancies, conduction disturbances, and dilated cardiomyopathy.[50–55] The etiology of these cardiovascular abnormalities and the timing of onset remain unclear. Data from the fetal aspect of the P^2C^2 HIV Study would suggest that vertically transmitted HIV infection is not typically associated with significant abnormalities of cardiac structure and function in the fetus.[14] In the P^2C^2 Study, when the findings from fetuses of HIV-infected mothers with postnatally confirmed HIV infection were compared with those from uninfected fetuses of HIV-infected mothers, the only difference was in the left ventricular diastolic dimension, which was smaller in the HIV-infected group. Other two-dimensional measurements and Doppler velocities did not differ for the two groups. This may be the result of the timing of HIV transmission. Although 10% to 30% of HIV-infected infants have symptoms of acquired immunodeficiency syndrome (AIDS) during the first few months of life, suggesting the effects of an intrauterine infection, the majority of infants and children do not develop AIDS until after the first year of life,[56,57] a finding consistent with transmission of HIV late in gestation or at the time of birth. Infants with vertically transmitted HIV infection also often have negative viral test results at birth, with peak viral production at 1 to 3 months of age.[57] Thus, abnormalities of cardiovascular function associated with perinatally acquired HIV infection might not be expected in the mid or even the early third trimester of affected infants.

Even in fetuses in which HIV is acquired in utero, structural and functional cardiovascular changes associated with HIV infection may be more subtle than are detectable by fetal echocardiography. The low vertical transmission rate in the fetal aspect of the P^2C^2 HIV Study[14] may also not have been sufficient to demonstrate more subtle changes or trends in Doppler blood flow patterns and velocities or cardiac dimensions. Furthermore, cardiovascular changes associated with vertically transmitted HIV infection may be primarily postnatal manifestations.

Two reports suggest that cardiovascular abnormalities may be associated with intrauterine transmission of HIV infection.[6,58] One 28-week fetus developing in a mother with clinical evidence of HIV infection was found to have a pericardial effusion. At birth, p24 antigen was identified in the pericardial fluid, and at autopsy there was evidence of vasculitis involving small vessels.[58] Another fetus with intrauterine demise at 32 weeks was found at fetopsy to have left heart obstructive lesions and placental infarcts with extensive HIV positivity in fetal tissues.[6] Cardiovascular abnormalities potentially related to vertically transmitted HIV infection are likely to be rare.

Uninfected infants of HIV-infected mothers are frequently lost to long-term follow-up because they have no obvious clinical abnormalities. The cardiovascular changes in the fetal aspect of the multicenter P^2C^2 HIV Study suggest that some infants have abnormalities related to development within an abnormal intrauterine environment. Shortly after birth, these infants have reduced left ventricular fractional shortening and depressed contractility, as well as increased left ventricular dimension and decreased wall thickness.[59] This may represent a response to normal perinatal changes in the systemic and pulmonary circulations, or perhaps a response to the absence of circulating maternal factors that had induced the antenatal abnormalities. Abnormal fetal growth[7,8] and an increase in fetal loss[6] have been observed with maternal HIV infection. In one study, fetal lung cells had arrested maturation when exposed to zidovudine,[60] suggesting the potential for abnormal organogenesis in fetuses of HIV-infected mothers treated with zidovudine. Furthermore, an earlier multicenter study[61] revealed an increased incidence of sudden death in children of HIV-infected mothers with or without postnatal HIV infection.

In summary, fetuses of HIV-infected mothers

can have abnormalities of cardiovascular structure and function. These abnormalities suggest altered myocardial growth, altered cardiovascular structure and function, and increased placental vascular resistance. They may be the direct or indirect consequences of maternal HIV infection or other maternal variables. Vertically transmitted HIV infection rarely may be associated with cardiovascular abnormalities in the fetus. Further investigation of the intrauterine environment during maternal HIV infection is needed to identify specific factors responsible for altering fetal cardiac growth and function.

References

1. Mofenson LM. Epidemiology and determinants of vertical HIV transmission. *Semin Pediatr Infect Dis* 1994;5:252–265.

2. United Nations Development Programme: Young women: silence, susceptibility, and the HIV epidemic. *Pediatr AIDS HIV Infect Fetus Adolesc* 1994;5:1–9.

3. Rosso P. Placental growth, development and function in relation to maternal nutrition. *Fed Proc* 1980;9:250.

4. Churchill JA, Moghissi KS, Evans TN, Frohman C. Relationships of maternal amino acid blood levels to fetal development. *Obstet Gynecol* 1969;33: 492–495.

5. Barker DJB, Gluckman PD, Godfrey KM, et al. Fetal nutrition and cardiovascular disease in adult life. *Lancet* 1993;341:938–941.

6. Langston C, Lewis DE, Hammill HA, et al. Excess intrauterine fetal demise associated with maternal human immunodeficiency virus infection. *J Infect Dis* 1995;172:1451–1460.

7. Braddick MR, Kreiss JK, Embree JE, et al. Impact of maternal HIV infection on obstetrical and early neonatal outcome. *AIDS* 1990;4:1001–1005.

8. Blanche S, Rouzioux C, Moscato M-L G, et al. and the HIV Infection in Newborns French Collaborative Study Group. A prospective study of infants born to women seropositive for human immunodeficiency virus type 1. *N Engl J Med* 1989;320: 1643–1648.

9. Marion RW, Wizma AA, Hutcheon RG, Rubinstein A. Human T cell lymphotrophic virus type III [HTLV-III] embryopathy: a new dysmorphic syndrome associated with intrauterine HTLV-III infection. *Am J Dis Child* 1986;140:638–640.

10. Scott JS, Maddison PJ, Taylor PV, et al. Connective tissue disease, antibodies to ribonucleoprotein, and congenital heart block. *N Engl J Med* 1983;309: 209–212.

11. Taylor PV, Scott JS, Gerlis LM, et al. Maternal autoantibodies against fetal cardiac antigens in congenital complete heart block. *N Engl J Med* 1986; 315:667–672.

12. Miller E, Hare JW, Cloherty JP, et al. Elevated maternal hemoglobin A1c in early pregnancy and major congenital anomalies in infants of diabetic mothers. *N Engl J Med* 1981;304:1331–1334.

13. Barker DJP, Osmond C, Simmonds SJ, Wield GA. The relation of head size and thinness at birth to death from cardiovascular disease in adult life. *BMJ* 1993;306:422–426.

14. Hornberger LK, Lipshultz SE, Easley KA, et al. Cardiac structure and function in fetuses of human immunodeficiency virus (HIV)-infected mothers: the prospective NHLBI P^{2}C^2 study. *J Am Coll Cardiol* 1995;25:30A.

15. Schulman H, Fleischer A, Stern W, et al. Umbilical velocity wave ratios in human pregnancy. *Am J Obstet Gynecol* 1984;148:985–990.

16. Giles WB, Trudinger BJ, Baird PJ. Fetal umbilical artery flow velocity waveforms and placental resistance: pathological correlations. *Br J Obstet Gynecol* 1985;92:31–38.

17. Trudinger BJ, Giles WB, Cook CM, et al. Fetal umbilical artery flow velocity waveforms and placental resistance: clinical significance. *Br J Obstet Gynecol* 1985;92:23–30.

18. Matsuyama T, Kobayashi N, Yamamoto N. Cytokines and HIV infection: is AIDS a tumor necrosis factor disease? *AIDS* 1991;5:1405–1417.

19. Sinicco A, Biglino A, Sciandra M, et al. Cytokine network and acute primary HIV-1 infection. *AIDS* 1993;7:1167–1172.

20. Clerici M, Hakim FT, Venzon DJ, et al. Changes in interleukin–2 and interleukin–4 production in asymptomatic human immunodeficiency virus-seropositive individuals. *J Clin Invest* 1993;91: 759–765.

21. Palmer JN, Hartogensis WE, Patten M, et al. Interleukin–1ß induced cardiac myocyte growth but inhibits cardiac fibroblast proliferation in culture. *J Clin Invest* 1995;95:2555–2564.

22. Gidding SS, Snider AR, Rochini AP, et al. Left ventricular diastolic filling in children with hypertrophic cardiomyopathy: assessment with pulsed Doppler echocardiography. *J Am Coll Cardiol* 1986;8:310–316.

23. Kitabatake A, Inoue M, Asao M, et al. Transmitral blood flow reflecting diastolic behavior of the left ventricle in health and disease: a study by pulsed Doppler technique. *Jpn Circ J* 1982;46:92–102.

24. Van der Mooren K, Barendregt LG, Wladimiroff JW. Fetal atrioventricular and outflow tract flow velocity waveforms during normal second half of pregnancy. *Am J Obstet Gynecol* 1991;165:668–674.

25. Voutilainen S, Kupari M, Hippelainen M, et al. Factors influencing Doppler indexes of left ventricular filling in healthy persons. *Am J Cardiol* 1991; 68:653–659.

26. Manca C, Aschieri D, Conti M, et al. Multivariate analysis of the variables affecting left ventricular filling in normal subjects. *Cardiology* 1992;80: 267–275.

27. Lai WW, Lipshultz S, Easley K, et al. for the P^{2}C^2 Study Group. Prevalence of congenital cardiovascular malformations (CCM) in children of HIV-infected mothers: the prospective P^{2}C^2 study. *Circulation* 1995;92:I–125.

28. Vogel RL, Alboliras ET, McSherry GD, et al. Congenital heart defects in children of human immunodeficiency virus positive mothers. *Circulation* 1988;78:II–17.

29. Herskowitz A, Willoughby S, Wu TC, et al. Immunopathogenesis of HIV-1 associated cardiomyopathy. *Clin Immunol Immunopathol* 1993;68: 234–241.

30. Kavanaugh-McHugh A, Rowe S, Ruff A, et al. Cardiac involvement in children with human immunodeficiency virus (HIV) infection: evidence for autoimmunity. *Proc Implic AIDS Mothers Child* 1989;1:85.C33.

31. Shearer WT, Duliege AM, Kline MW, et al. Transport of recombinant human CD4-immunoglobulin G across the human placenta: pharmacokinetics and safety in six mother-infant pairs in AIDS clinical trial group protocol 146. *Clin Diagn Labor Immunol* 1995;2:281–285.

32. Miyata K, Ono S, Tachikura T, et al. Cardiovascular malformations induced by anti-tissue sera and immunological cross-reaction. In: Clark EB, Takao A (eds). *Developmental Cardiology: Morphogenesis and Function.* Mount Kisco, NY: Futura Publishing, 1990:485–490.

33. Matsuyama T, Kobayashi N, Yamamoto N. Cytokines and HIV infection: is AIDS a tumor necrosis factor disease? *AIDS* 1991;5:1405–1417.

34. Heyborne KD, Witkin SS, McGregor JA. Tumor necrosis factor-α in midtrimester amniotic fluid is associated with impaired intrauterine fetal growth. *Am J Obstet Gynecol* 1992;167:920–925.

35. Bry K, Hallman M. Transforming growth factor-β opposes the stimulatory effects of interleukin-1 and tumor necrosis factor on amnion cell prostaglandin E$_2$ production: implication for preterm labor. *Am J Obstet Gynecol* 1992;167:222–226.

36. De M, Sanford TH, Wood GW. Detection of interleukin–1, interleukin–6, and tumor necrosis factor–α in the uterus during the second half of pregnancy in the mouse. *Endocrinology* 1992;131:14–20.

37. Odeh J. Tumor necrosis factor-α as a myocardial depressant substance. *Int J Cardiol* 1993;42: 231–238.

38. Gurram M, Chirmule N, Wang X-P, et al. Increased spontaneous secretion of interleukin 6 and tumor necrosis factor alpha by peripheral blood lymphocytes of human immunodeficiency virus-infected children. *Pediatr Infect Dis J* 1994;13:496–501.

39. Herskowitz A, Baughman KL. Effect of HIV infection on the heart. In: Braunwald E (ed). *Heart Disease Updates: Spring 1994.* Philadelphia: WB Saunders, 1994:1–10.

40. Semba RD, Miotti PG, Chiphangwi, et al. Maternal vitamin A deficiency and mother-to-child transmission of HIV-1. *Lancet* 1994;343:1593–1597.

41. Baird CD, Nelson MM, Monie IW, Evans HM. Congenital cardiovascular anomalies induced by pteroylglutamic acid deficiency during gestation in the rat. *Circ Res* 1954;2:544–554.

42. Kavanaugh-McHugh AL, Ruff A, Perlman E, et al. Selenium deficiency and cardiomyopathy in acquired immunodeficiency syndrome. *J Parenter Enter Nutr* 1991;15:347–349.

43. Sluis KB, Darlow BA, George PM, et al. Selenium and glutathione peroxidase levels in premature infants in a low selenium community (Christchurch, New Zealand). *Pediatr Res* 1992;32:189–194.

44. Dison PJ, Lockitch G, Halstead AC, et al. Influence of maternal factors on cord and neonatal plasma micronutrient levels. *Am J Perinatol* 1993;10: 30–35.

45. Brown T, Anand A, Ritchie L, et al. Intrauterine parvovirus infection associated with hydrops fetalis. *Lancet* 1984;2:1033–1034.

46. Nigro G, Pisano P, Krzysztofiak A. Recurrent Kawasaki disease associated with coinfection with parvovirus B19 and HIV-1. *AIDS* 1993;7:287–288.

47. Wu T-C, Pizzorno MC, Hayward GS, et al. In situ detection of human cytomegalovirus immediate-early gene transcripts within cardiac myocytes of patients with HIV-associated cardiomyopathy. *AIDS* 1992;6:777–785.

48. Lipshultz SE, Frassica JJ, Orav EJ. Cardiovascular abnormalities in infants prenatally exposed to cocaine. *J Pediatr* 1991;118:44–51.

49. Jacobson JL, Jacobson SW, Sokol RJ, et al. Effects of alcohol use, smoking, and illicit drug use on fetal growth in black infants. *J Pediatr* 1994; 124:757–764.

50. Lipshultz SE, Chanock S, Sanders SP, et al. Cardiovascular manifestations of human immunodeficiency virus infection in infants and children. *Am J Cardiol* 1989;63:1489–1497.

51. Luginbuhl LM, Orav EJ, McIntosh K, Lipshultz SE. Cardiac morbidity and related mortality in children with HIV infection. *JAMA* 1993;269:2869–2875.

52. Grenier MA, Karr SS, Rakusan TA, Martin GR. Cardiac disease in children with HIV: relationship of cardiac disease to HIV symptomatology. *Pediatr AIDS HIV Infect Fetus Adolesc* 1994;5:175–179.

53. Stewart JM, Kaul A, Gromisch DS, et al. Symptomatic cardiac dysfunction in children with human immunodeficiency virus infection. *Am Heart J* 1989;117:140–144.

54. Joshi VV, Gadol C, Connor E, et al. Dilated cardiomyopathy in children with acquired immunodeficiency syndrome: a pathologic study of five cases. *Hum Pathol* 1988;19:69–73.

55. Lipshultz SE, for the Pediatric Pulmonary and Cardiovascular Complications of Vertically Transmitted HIV Study. Cardiac dysfunction predicts mortality in HIV-infected children: the prospective NHLBI P2C2 Study [Abstract]. *Proc Conf Retrov Opportun Infect* 1996;130.

56. Peckham C, Gibb D. Mother-to-child transmission of the human immunodeficiency virus. *N Engl J Med* 1995;333:298–302.

57. Wilfert CM, Wilson C, Luzuriaga K, Epstein L. Pathogenesis of pediatric human immunodeficiency virus type 1 infection. *J Infect Dis* 1994;170: 286–292.

58. Rudin C, Meier D, Pavic N, et al. and the Swiss Study Group "HIV and Pregnancy." Intrauterine onset of symptomatic human immunodeficiency virus disease. *Pediatr Infect Dis J* 1993;12:411–414.

59. Lipshultz SE, Easley K, Kaplan S, et al. and the P^{2}C^2 Study Group. Abnormal left ventricular structure and function shortly after birth in infants of HIV-infected mothers: the prospective NHLBI P^{2}C^2 study. *Circulation* 1995;92:I–581.

60. DiMaio MF, Ting A, Hsu MT, et al. Effect of zidovudine on human fetal lung development. *Pediatr AIDS HIV Infect Fetus Adolesc* 1995;6:83–90.

61. Kind C, Brandle B, Wyler C-A, et al. and the Swiss Neonatal HIV Study Group. Epidemiology of vertically transmitted HIV-1 infection in Switzerland: results of a nationwide prospective study. *Eur J Pediatr* 1992;151:442–448.

7

Congenital Cardiovascular Malformations

Wyman W. Lai, M.D., M.P.H.

Vertical Transmission of Human Immunodeficiency Virus

The rate of vertical transmission of human immunodeficiency virus (HIV) is estimated at 20% to 30% in the United States and as high as 39% in Africa.[1] There is a significant association between high maternal viral load and mother–infant transmission.[2] Intervention with zidovudine during pregnancy may reduce the viral load and is associated with an approximately two-thirds reduction in mother–infant transmission.[3,4]

Because the critical period of normal fetal cardiac development is about from day 20 to day 50,[5] the timing of vertical transmission is important in the assessment of HIV as a potential cardiac teratogen. HIV has been detected in fetal tissue as early as the eighth week of gestation.[6] Controversy exists as to the rate of early maternal–fetal transmission. A comprehensive review of the rate and timing of maternal–fetal transmission is beyond the scope of this chapter but is available to the reader.[1,7]

The percentage of fetuses of HIV-positive mothers determined to be HIV-positive varies widely between studies, from a low of 0% to 2%[7,8] to a high of 60% to 80%.[9–11] The lack of uniform criteria for the diagnosis of fetal HIV infection has been a problem and accounts for some of the variation in the reported rates of early maternal–fetal transmission. In addition, there are significant methodological differences between studies, and sample sizes are frequently small.

Less controversy exists in postnatal studies, which indicate that in most vertically transmitted cases, infection occurs late in pregnancy or at delivery.[12,13] This postnatal experience does not exclude the possibility of early maternal–fetal transmission but suggests that it is rare.

Teratogenic Effect of HIV

HIV has been proposed as a teratogenic agent, but its effect on organogenesis is still under investigation. Earlier studies examining HIV-seropositive children suggested a malformation syndrome consisting of growth failure, microcephaly, and dysmorphic craniofacial features.[14–16] Later studies looking at the effect of perinatal HIV exposure on infected and uninfected children failed to identify craniofacial dysmorphism in these children when compared to normal groups controlled for age and race.[17,18] These studies, however, confirmed the existence of growth retardation and possibly microcephaly, but one group attributed these features to chronic postnatal illness and progressive central nervous system involvement in the HIV-infected patients.[18]

Some, but not all, studies of children born to HIV-infected mothers have found an increased incidence of low birthweight in the HIV-infected children.[19-23] Two groups have demonstrated that differences in birthweight between HIV-infected and HIV-uninfected children could be attributed to maternal drug use during pregnancy.[21,24]

Congenital Cardiovascular Malformations

Early Reports

Because of the importance of dilated cardiomyopathy in the clinical course of patients with HIV infection, few early reports focused on the prevalence of congenital cardiovascular malformations in this population. One exception is a series reported in an abstract by Vogel and colleagues[25] of 5 cases of congenital heart disease from a population of 175 children exposed to maternal HIV infection (2.8%): 1 atrial septal defect, 1 tricuspid atresia, 1 ventricular septal defect, 1 tetralogy of Fallot, and 1 ventricular septal defect with pulmonary stenosis. Three of the five children required catheterization and surgery. Another abstract reported that 4 of 133 HIV-infected children had congenital heart disease (3.0%).[26] Neither of the two studies was controlled for possible case selection bias and other potential confounders.

Prospective Studies

Two prospective multicenter studies have examined the prevalence of congenital cardiovascular malformations in children of HIV-infected mothers. The Italian Multicenter Study reported 5 cases from a population of 486 children born to HIV-infected mothers (1.1%). In this study, 4 of the cases occurred in the group of 165 HIV-infected children (2.4%): 1 patent foramen ovale and patent ductus arteriosus; 1 atrial septal defect and ventricular septal defect; 1 pulmonary artery stenosis; and 1 ventricular septal defect, left superior vena cava, patent ductus arteriosus, and peripheral pulmonary steno-

sis. The other case (pulmonary artery stenosis) occurred in the group of 92 HIV-uninfected children (1.1%). There were 229 children classified as HIV-indeterminate with no cases of congenital cardiovascular malformations noted.[20] The difference in the rate of congenital cardiovascular malformations in HIV-infected versus HIV-uninfected children was not statistically significant. Although study methodology pertaining to congenital cardiovascular malformation prevalence was not provided, a standard method of case ascertainment was presumably used, namely, the referral of suspected cases to a pediatric cardiology center for diagnosis. Children were routinely followed at 6-month intervals.

Preliminary and as yet unconfirmed data from the National Heart, Lung, and Blood Institute (NHLBI) P^{2}C^2 Study indicated a congenital cardiovascular malformation prevalence of 12.3% (95% CI: 9.5–15.0%) in 555 children of HIV–infected mothers. Most of the lesions were clinically inapparent and were detected by multiple early routine echocardiograms as part of the study protocol. There was no difference in the prevalence of congenital cardiovascular malformations between HIV-infected ($n = 84$) and HIV-uninfected children ($n = 414$), with rates of 13.1% and 11.6%, respectively. The proportion of children with congenital cardiovascular malformations diminished over time.[27]

The distribution of lesions in children of HIV-infected mothers is relatively unremarkable (see Table 7-1). As noted by the authors of the NHLBI P^{2}C^2 Study, certain echocardiographic diagnoses are believed to represent stages of normal cardiovascular development. Few data gleaned from routine echocardiographic screening to determine the prevalence of congenital cardiovascular malformations in normal children are currently available for comparison.

Possible Etiologic Mechanisms

A report of a pericardial effusion diagnosed prenatally at 28 weeks gestation demonstrated the potential for relatively early cardiac involvement in the fetus of an HIV-infected woman.[28] More recently,

Table 7-1. Congenital Cardiovascular Malformations in Children of HIV-Infected Mothers

Italian Multicenter Study[20]
  Shunt Lesions (6/10)
    1 Patent foramen ovale
    1 Atrial septal defect
    2 Ventricular septal defect
    2 Patent ductus arteriosus
  Right-Sided Flow Lesions (3/10)
    2 Pulmonary artery stenosis
    1 Peripheral pulmonary stenosis
  Left-Sided Flow Lesions (1/10)
    1 Left superior vena cava
NHLBI P[2]C[2] Study (Preliminary Data)†
  Cyanotic Lesions (2/79, 2.5%)
    1 Total anomalous pulmonary venous return
    1 Ventricular septal defect with pulmonary stenosis
  Shunt Lesions (38/79) 48.1%)
    12 Patent foramen ovale
    7 Atrial septal defect
    10 Ventricular septal defect
    9 Patent ductus arteriosus
  Right-Sided Flow Lesions (28/79, 35.4%)
    6 Valvar pulmonary stenosis
    13 Supravalvar pulmonary stenosis
    9 Branch pulmonary artery stenosis
  Left-Sided Flow Lesions (6/79, 7.5%)
    3 Bicommissural aortic valve
    1 Mitral valve prolapse
    1 Double orifice mitral valve
    1 Left superior vena cava
  Miscellaneous (5/79, 6.3%)
    4 Coronary arteriovenous fistula
    1 Dilated main pulmonary artery

*Data from Ref. 20.
†Data from Ref. 27.

Hornberger and colleagues reported that fetuses of HIV-infected mothers had increased left and right ventricular end-diastolic wall thickness and increased placental vascular resistance. Increases in peak atrioventricular valve velocities, semilunar valve velocities, and both tricuspid and mitral peak A:E velocity ratios were seen (see Chapter 6).[29] The fetal population studied was part of the group used to describe the postnatal prevalence of congenital cardiovascular malformations in the NHLBI P[2]C[2] Study noted above.[27]

Alterations in flow and vascular resistance or impedance may play important roles in the normal and abnormal development of the fetal heart.[30] The interplay between these forces and molecular defects underlying congenital cardiovascular malformations is only now being more fully appreciated.[31] Although alterations in fetal flow patterns may be present, the question of whether or not maternal HIV infection plays a significant role in the development of congenital cardiovascular malformations remains unresolved.

Teratogenic Effect of Other Maternal Risk Factors

In a large cohort study, almost half of the pregnant HIV-infected women used cocaine (or crack), heroin, methadone, or marijuana. Moreover, women underreported their drug use by 29% in that study, suggesting that other studies with self-reporting as the mechanism of detection may be unreliable.[24] One study demonstrated an increased risk of congenital cardiovascular malformations in infants prenatally exposed to cocaine.[32] The maternal HIV-infected population is also at risk for increased alcohol use and poor nutrition, factors that may significantly affect fetal organogenesis.

Zidovudine, which has been shown to reduce the mother–infant transmission rate, is now routinely prescribed for HIV-infected pregnant women. When administered starting at 14 to 34 weeks gestation and continued throughout pregnancy, zidovudine was associated with a decreased infant hemoglobin concentration at birth, but the incidence of structural abnormalities was unchanged.[3] There is one report on the adverse effect of zidovudine on in vitro human fetal lung maturation.[33]

Comparison to Population-Based Congenital Cardiovascular Malformation Prevalence Data

Population-Based Prevalence of Congenital Cardiovascular Malformations

The prevalence of congenital cardiovascular malformations is generally quoted as 8 per 1,000 live births, or 0.8%, from population-based studies, both historical and recent. Based on a large number of studies involving populations from around the world, the reported range of cardiovascular malformation prevalence is relatively narrow (from 4 to 14 per 1,000 live births). Most studies fall into the middle of this range.[34–39] Several recent studies have demonstrated a small increase in the prevalence of congenital cardiovascular malformations during the 1980s. This trend was attributed to improved methods of detection. In particular, the detection of ventricular septal defects increased significantly with the greater availability and use of echocardiography.[40–43]

Ferencz and colleagues[44] have pointed out the difficulties in comparing studies of congenital cardiovascular malformation prevalence. Variables that must be factored into the comparison include study population characteristics, case ascertainment methods, categorization, and diagnostic definitions.[44] Studies on mother–infant HIV transmission in the United States have historically enrolled large numbers of black and Hispanic patients. In the Baltimore–Washington Infant Study, subgroup analysis revealed white–black differences in certain cardiovascular malformations. There was an excess of white infants among cases with Ebstein anomaly, aortic stenosis, pulmonary atresia, and transposition of the great arteries. There was an excess of black infants among cases of pulmonary stenosis and heterotaxy syndrome. Socioeconomic factors affected the variation in some diagnostic groups: attenuating the excess of whites among cases with Ebstein anomaly, disclosing an excess for *l*-transposition of the great arteries, and revealing that the excess of white infants with aortic stenosis was limited to low and middle socioeconomic strata.[45] Another study conducted in Dallas County, Texas demonstrated differences in prevalence rates of specific cardiac defects among white, black, and Mexican-American children. White children had higher prevalence rates for endocardial cushion defect, ventricular septal defect, and aortic stenosis. Prevalence rates were not affected by socioeconomic status in this study.[46]

Other important differences in population characteristics may exist. In the Baltimore–Washington Infant Study population, chromosomal disorders were found in 12.5% of the patients with a cardiovascular malformation.[47] A significant difference in the proportion of patients with chromosomal disorders in a study population may have a small but measurable effect on the prevalence and distribution of congenital cardiovascular malformations.

Effect of HIV on Prevalence of Congenital Cardiovascular Malformations

Population characteristics may account for small differences in cardiovascular malformation prevalence between studies, but the greatest variable appears to be the use of routine screening echocardiograms for case ascertainment. Using this technique, the NHLBI P^{2}C^2 Study preliminarily reported a prevalence of 12.3% in children of HIV-infected mothers,[27] while the Italian Multicenter Study, which presumably used a standard method of case ascertainment, reported a prevalence of 1.1%.[20] As mentioned above, postnatal HIV infection status does not appear to affect the prevalence of congenital cardiovascular malformations in children of HIV-infected mothers.

Two recent studies have examined the prevalence of muscular ventricular septal defects in normal neonates by the use of routine echocardiography. Hirashi and colleagues[48] found a prevalence of 2.0% in 1,028 neonates with a 76% spontaneous closure rate by 12 months of age. Roguin and colleagues[49] found a prevalence of 5.3% in 1053 neonates, with an 89% spontaneous closure rate by 10 months of age; in their study, 50 of the 56 cases (89%) were clinically silent at the time of echocardiographic diagnosis.[49] Examination of the preliminary NHLBI P^{2}C^2 Study data reveals a 2% prevalence of ventricular septal defects in a population of children of HIV-infected mothers,[27] a rate comparable to that found in the two studies of normal children. Additional normal population studies are needed to allow for valid comparisons of the rates of other cardiovascular malformations as determined by routine screening echocardiograms.

Based on the information currently available, prenatal cardiac development in the presence of maternal HIV infection does not appear to significantly increase congenital cardiovascular malformation prevalence. The reported prevalence of congenital cardiovascular malformations in children of HIV-infected mothers varies widely, depending on whether routine echocardiograms are used as the method of case ascertainment. Postnatal HIV infection status does not appear to influence the prevalence of caardiovascular congenital malformations in children of HIV-infected mothers.

Surgical Considerations

Immunologic abnormalities have been seen in patients following cardiac surgery. Two factors have been implicated: multiple blood transfusions and the use of cardiopulmonary bypass. Patients who receive multiple blood transfusions have depressed natural killer cell function but normal CD4+:CD8+ lymphocyte ratios.[50] In patients who undergo cardiopulmonary bypass, decreases in CD3+ (pan-T lymphocyte), CD4+, and CD8+ lymphocyte populations, and total lymphocyte count occur regardless of transfusion status.[51,52] A decline in CD4+:CD8+ lymphocyte ratio may be sustained through the sixth postoperative day.[53] These abnormalities in immune system regulation have led to the speculation that cardiopulmonary bypass may increase the risk of HIV infection from contaminated blood products administered in the perioperative period.

Standard antibody testing for HIV-1 became available in June 1985. To my knowledge, the first published report of HIV infection in a child who underwent cardiac surgery appeared in 1986.[54] The effect of cardiac surgery and cardiopulmonary bypass on children with HIV infection and congenital cardiovascular malformations is unknown. Anecdotally, children with HIV infection have survived surgery to correct congenital cardiovascular malformations. To date, there are no published morbidity and mortality data. The most relevant studies involve adult patients with infective endocarditis secondary to intravenous drug use. These patients underwent cardiac surgery with cardiopulmonary bypass to have their valves repaired or replaced. Some investigators raised concerns about worsened surgical outcome and potential acceleration of infection to AIDS.[55,56] Several other groups investigating these concerns concluded that there was no difference in surgical outcome and progression to AIDS in HIV-infected patients undergoing cardiac surgery and cardiopulmonary bypass.[57–59] In the largest study to date, Aris and collegues[59] analyzed the clinical course of 40 HIV-infected patients with a mean age of 30 years; 34 patients (85%) were intravenous drug-abusers. Hospital mortality was 20%. With a mean follow-up period of 21 months, 4 patients (12.5%) progressed to AIDS and 8 patients (25%) died. Actuarial progression to AIDS was 5% (±5%) at 1 year, 20% (±10%) at 2 years, and 40% (±19%) at 5 years. Actuarial survival was 79% (±8%) at 1 year, 60% (±11%) at 2 years, and 45% (±14%) at 5 years.[59] The extent to which this experience is applicable to HIV-infected children undergoing surgery for congenital cardiovascular malformations is unknown.

At this time, it appears reasonable to recommend corrective cardiac surgery for HIV-infected children with significantly symptomatic or life-threatening congenital cardiovascular malformations for which no effective nonsurgical therapy is available. Palliative surgery without cardiopulmonary bypass or an interventional procedure in the catheterization laboratory may be preferable options for a patient with HIV infection, depending on the circumstances of the case. Treatment decisions often must take into account abnormalities of other organ systems secondary to HIV infection. As always, recommendations must be tailored to the needs of the individual patient. Additional data on the effect of cardiopulmonary bypass on children with HIV infection undergoing surgery for congenital cardiovascular malformations will be needed before more specific recommendations can be made.

References

1. Mofenson LM. Epidemiology and determinants of vertical HIV transmission. *Semin Pediatr Infect Dis* 1994;5:252–265.

2. Mayaux MJ, Blanche S, Rouzioux C, et al., for the French Pediatric HIV Infection Study Group. Maternal factors associated with perinatal HIV 1 transmission: the French cohort study: 7 years of follow-up observation. *J Acquir Immune Defic Syndr Hum Retrovirol* 1995;8:188–194.

3. Conner EM, Sperling RS, Gelber R, et al., for the Pediatric AIDS Clinical Trials Group Protocol 076 Study Group. Reduction of maternal-infant trans-

mission of human immunodeficiency virus type 1 with zidovudine treatment. *N Engl J Med* 1994;331: 1173–1180.

4. Boyer PJ, Dillon M, Navaie M, et al. Factors predictive of maternal-fetal transmission of HIV 1: preliminary analysis of zidovudine given during pregnancy and/or delivery. *JAMA* 1994;271:1925–1930.

5. Moore KL. *The Developing Human,* 3rd ed. Philadelphia: WB Saunders, 1982:298–343.

6. Lewis SH, Reynolds Kohler C, Fox HE, Nelson JA. HIV 1 in trophoblastic and villous Hofbauer cells and haematological precursors in eight week fetuses. *Lancet* 1990;335:565–568.

7. Brossard Y, Aubin JT, Mandelbrot L, et al. Frequency of early in utero HIV 1 infection: a blind DNA polymerase chain reaction study on 100 fetal thymuses. *AIDS* 1995;9:359–366.

8. Ehrnst A, Lindgren S, Dictor M, et al. HIV in pregnant women and their offspring: evidence for late transmission. *Lancet* 1991;338:203–207.

9. Courgnaud V, Laure F, Brossard A, et al. Frequent and early in utero HIV 1 infection. *AIDS Res Hum Retrov* 1991;7:337–341.

10. Lyman WD, Kress Y, Kure K, et al. Detection of HIV in fetal central nervous system tissue. *AIDS* 1990;4:917–920.

11. Soeiro R, Rubinstein A, Rashbaum WK, Lyman WD. Maternofetal transmission of AIDS: frequency of human immunodeficiency virus type 1 nucleic acid sequences in human fetal DNA. *J Infect Dis* 1992;166:699–703.

12. Luzuriaga K, McQuilken P, Alimenti A, et al. Early viremia and immune responses in vertical human immunodeficiency virus type 1 infection. *J Infect Dis* 1993;167:1008–1013.

13. Rouzioux C, Costagliola D, Burgard M, et al., and the HIV Infection in Newborns French Collaborative Study Group. Estimated timing of mother to child human immunodeficiency virus type 1 (HIV 1) transmission by use of a Markov model. *Am J Epidemiol* 1995;142:1330–1337.

14. Marion RW, Wiznia AA, Hutcheon G, Rubinstein A. Human T cell lymphotropic virus type III (HTLV III) embryopathy. *Am J Dis Child* 1986;140: 638–640.

15. Marion RW, Wiznia AA, Hutcheon RG, Rubinstein A. Fetal AIDS syndrome score. Correlation between severity of dysmorphism and age at diagnosis

of immunodeficiency. *Am J Dis Child* 1987;141: 429–431.

16. Iosub S, Bamji, M, Stone RK, et al. More on human immunodeficiency virus embryopathy. *Pediatrics* 1987;80:512–516.

17. Embree JE, Braddick M, Datta P, et al. Lack of correlation of maternal human immunodeficiency virus infection with neonatal malformations. *Pediatr Infect Dis J* 1989;8:700–704.

18. Qazi QH, Shiekh TM, Fikrig S, Menikoff H. Lack of evidence for craniofacial dysmorphism in perinatal human immunodeficiency virus infection. *J Pediatr* 1988;112:7–11.

19. Nair P, Alger L, Hines S, et al. Maternal and neonatal characteristics associated with HIV infection in infants of seropositive women. *J AIDS* 1993;6: 298–302.

20. Italian Multicentre Study. Epidemiology, clinical features and prognostic factors of paediatric HIV infection. *Lancet* 1988;2:1043–1046.

21. Blanche S, Rouzioux C, Guihard Moscato ML, et al., and the HIV Infection in Newborns French Collaborative Study Group. A prospective study of infants born to women seropositive for human immunodeficiency virus type 1. *N Engl J Med* 1989; 320:1643–1648.

22. Hutto C, Parks WP, Lai S, et al. A hospital based prospective study of perinatal infection with human immunodeficiency virus type 1. *J Pediatr* 1991;118: 347–353.

23. The European Collaborative Study. Mother-to-child transmission of HIV infection. *Lancet* 1988;2: 1039–1042.

24. Rodriguez EM, Mendez H, Rich K, et al. Maternal drug use in perinatal HIV studies: the women and infants transmission study. *Ann NY Acad Sci* 1993; 693:245–248.

25. Vogel RL, Alboliras ET, McSherry GD, et al. Congenital heart defects in children of human immunodeficiency virus positive mothers. [Abstract]. *Circulation* 1988;78:II–17.

26. Tripp ME, McKinney RE, Katz SL. Cardiac complications of human immunodeficiency virus (HIV) infection in children. [Abstract]. *Pediatr Res* 1993; 22:185A.

27. Lai WW, Lipshultz S, Easley K, et al., for the P^{2}C^2 Study Group, NHLBI, Bethesda, MD. Prevalence of congenital cardiovascular malformation in children of HIV-infected mothers: the prospective P^{2}C^2 study. [Abstract]. *Circulation* 1995;92:I–581.

28. Rudin C, Meier D, Pavic N, et al., and the Swiss Collaborative Study Group "HIV and Pregnancy." Intrauterine onset of symptomatic human immunodeficiency virus disease. *Pediatr Infect Dis J* 1993; 12:411–414.

29. Hornberger LK, Lipshultz SE, Easley KA, et al., for the P^{2}C^2 Study Group. Cardiac structure and function in fetuses of human immunodeficiency virus infected mothers: the prospective NHLBI P^{2}C^2 study. [Abstract]. *J Am Coll Cardiol* 1995; (Feb):30A.

30. Clark EB. Morphogenesis, growth, and biomechanics: mechanisms of cardiovascular development. In: Emmanouilides GC, Riemenschneider TA, Allen HD, Gutgesell HP (eds). *Moss and Adams Heart Disease in Infants, Children, and Adolescents: Including the Fetus and Young Adult,* 5th Ed. Baltimore: Williams & Wilkins, 1995:1–16.

31. Payne RM, Johnson MC, Grant JW, Strauss AW. Toward a molecular understanding of congenital heart disease. *Circulation* 1995;91:494–504.

32. Lipshultz SE, Frassica JJ, Orav EJ. Cardiovascular abnormalities in infants prenatally exposed to cocaine. *J Pediatr* 1991;118:44–51.

33. DiMaio MF, Ting A, Hsu MT, et al. Effect of zidovudine on human fetal lung development. *Pediatr AIDS HIV Infect Fetus Adolesc* 1995;6:83–90.

34. Mitchell SC, Korones SB, Berendes HW. Congenital, heart disease in 56,109 births: incidence and natural history. *Circulation* 1971;43:323–332.

35. Ferencz C, Correa Villasenor A. Epidemiology of cardiovascular malformations: the state of the art. *Cardiol Young* 1991;1:264–284.

36. Hoffman JIE. Incidence of congenital heart disease: I. Postnatal incidence. *Pediatr Cardiol* 1995;16: 103–113.

37. Ferencz C, Boughman JA. Teratology, genetics, and recurrence risks. *Cardiol Clin* 1993;11:557–567.

38. Fixler DE, Pastor P, Chamberlin M, et al. Trends in congenital heart disease in Dallas County births: 1971–1984. *Circulation* 1990;81:137–142.

39. Samanek M, Slavik Z, Zborilova B, et al. Prevalence, treatment, and outcome of heart disease in live born children: a prospective analysis of 91,823 live born children. *Pediatr Cardiol* 1989;10: 205–211.

40. Martin GR, Perry LW, Ferencz C. Increased prevalence of ventricular septal defect: epidemic or improved diagnosis. *Pediatrics* 1989;83:200–203.

41. Meberg A, Otterstad JE, Froland G, Sorland S. Children with congenital heart defects in Vestfold

1982–88: increase in the incidence resulting from improved diagnostic methods. *Tidsskr Nor Laegeforen* 1990;110:354–357.

42. Tikanoja T. Effect of technical development on the apparent incidence of congenital heart disease. [Letter]. *Pediatr Cardiol* 1995;16:100–101.

43. Wilson PD, Correa-Villasenor A, Loffredo CA, Ferencz C, and the Baltimore–Washington Infant Study Group. Temporal trends in prevalence of cardiovascular malformations in Maryland and the District of Columbia, 1981–1988. *Epidemiology* 1993;4:259–265.

44. Ferencz C, Czeizel A, Lys F. The problem of comparative analysis of birth prevalence of congenital cardiovascular malformations. *Acta Paediatr Hung* 1990;30:169–189.

45. Correa-Villasenor A, McCarter R, Downing J, Ferencz C, and the Baltimore–Washington Infant Study Group. White-black differences in cardiovascular malformations in infancy and socioeconomic factors. *Am J Epidemiol* 1991;134:393–402.

46. Fixler DE, Pastor P, Sigman E, Eifler CW. Ethnicity and socioeconomic status: impact on the diagnosis of congenital heart disease. *J Am Coll Cardiol* 1993;21:1722–1726.

47. Ferencz C, Rubin JD, McCarter RJ, et al. Cardiac and noncardiac malformations: observations in a population based study. *Teratology* 1987;35: 367–378.

48. Hirashi S, Agata Y, Nowatari M, et al. Incidence and natural course of trabecular ventricular septal defect: two-dimensional echocardiography and color Doppler flow imaging study. *J Pediatr* 1992; 120:409–415.

49. Roguin N, Du ZD, Barak M, et al. High prevalence of muscular ventricular septal defect in neonates. *J Am Coll Cardiol* 1995;26:1545–1548.

50. Gascon P, Zoumbos NC, Young NS. Immunologic abnormalities in patients receiving multiple blood transfusions. *Ann Intern Med* 1984;100:173–177.

51. DePalma L, Yu M, McIntosh CL, et al. Changes in lymphocyte subpopulations as a result of cardiopulmonary bypass: the effect of blood transfusion. *J Thorac Cardiovasc Surg* 1991;101:240–244.

52. Ide H, Kakiuchi T, Furuta N, et al. The effect of cardiopulmonary bypass on T cells and their subpopulations. *Ann Thorac Surg* 1987;44:277–282.

53. Pollock R, Ames F, Rubio P, et al. Protracted severe immune dysregulation induced by cardiopulmonary bypass: a predisposing etiologic factor in blood

transfusion-related AIDS? *J Clin Lab Immunol* 1987;22:1–5.

54. Schaffer MS, Langendorfer SI, Campbell DN. AIDS related–complex following infant cardiac surgery. [Letter]. *Pediatr Cardiol* 1986;6:335–336.

55. Yee ES . Accelerating HIV infection by cardiopulmonary bypass-case reports. *Vasc Surg* 1991;25: 725–731.

56. Uva MS, Jebara VA, Fabiani JN, et al. Cardiac surgery in patients with human immunodeficiency virus infection: indications and results. *J Cardiovasc Surg* 1992;7:240–244.

57. Frater RWM, Sisto D, Condit D. Cardiac surgery in human immunodeficiency virus (HIV) carriers. *Eur J Cardiothorac Surg* 1989;3:146–151.

58. Lemma M, Vanelli P, Beretta L, et al. Cardiac surgery in HIV-positive intravenous drug addicts: influence of cardiopulmonary bypass on the progression to AIDS. *Thorac Cardiovasc Surgeon* 1992;40:279–282.

59. Aris A, Pomar JL, Saura E. Cardiopulmonary bypass in HIV-positive patients. *Ann Thorac Surg* 1993;55:1104–1108.

8

Left Ventricular Hypertrophy in HIV Disease

Michelle A. Grenier, M.D., and Steven E. Lipshultz, M.D.

Among the cardiovascular manifestations of patients infected with the human immunodeficiency virus (HIV) is the disease referred to as "cardiomyopathy," a term implying intrinsic abnormality of the myocardium. HIV cardiomyopathy results in cardiac dysfunction and congestive heart failure, which has been well described and has been associated with increased morbidity and mortality in both adult and pediatric populations.[1-5] The dysfunction of HIV cardiomyopathy may be a direct result of inadequate ventricular hypertrophy, which does not allow for compensation and normalization of peak wall stress, the overall increase in left ventricular mass for body surface area, or both. Because a wide spectrum of cardiovascular disease is categorized as HIV cardiomyopathy, and the cause of this entity is thought to be multifactorial,[6] the understanding and treatment of this potentially lethal complication of HIV are difficult.

This chapter compares HIV cardiomyopathy with dilated cardiomyopathy, another disease state of abnormal ventricular hypertrophy. The question is asked, Is HIV cardiomyopathy just a variant of dilated cardiomyopathy? Factors influencing the disease state in HIV-infected and noninfected patients with cardiomyopathy are compared. The mechanics of ventricular hypertrophy in the noninfected patient are compared with those of the HIV-

infected host, with a discussion of the relations of inadequate ventricular hypertrophy and of increased left ventricular mass to increased morbidity and mortality. Several disease states consisting of abnormalities of ventricular hypertrophy are discussed.

A brief overview presents the molecular biology of ventricular hypertrophy and how it might relate to the disease state in the HIV-infected patient. Growth factors, endothelin, stress or heat-shock proteins (HSPs), mechanical stress (stretch), the renin-angiotensin system, catecholamines, hormonal influences, and nitric oxide (NO) are reviewed, with discussions as to how each might influence myocardial cell growth in the HIV-infected patient.

The role of patient nutrition in myocardial growth is briefly discussed. Abnormalities of programmed cell death (apoptosis) are briefly discussed and are considered to influence ventricular hypertrophy in the HIV-infected patient. This chapter concludes with a speculation that the HIV-infected patient may not be able to mount the usual response to the barrage of disease factors and in fact may be affected by premature senility. Ultimately, there is no single cause of HIV cardiomyopathy, although there are many influencing factors. This chapter is based largely upon speculation, given

111

the present knowledge of the factors and mechanics involved in myocardial cell growth.

Is HIV Cardiomyopathy Just A Variant of Dilated Cardiomyopathy?

HIV cardiomyopathy shares similarities with the dilated cardiomyopathy of HIV-negative patients, but it also may differ substantially. There is heterogeneity of ventricular hypertrophy, resulting in a remodeling process that may be lethal. Both disease entities share an abnormality of ventricular hypertrophy, and it is this abnormality that may relate to the increased morbidity and mortality seen with both conditions.

Dilated cardiomyopathy in the HIV-negative host commonly consists of remodeling: specifically, biventricular dilatation, often with dilated atria and associated dilated mitral and tricuspid annuli. The pathology includes varying degrees of interstitial fibrosis and occasional small clusters of lymphocytes. The total heart weight for body surface area is usually increased, and there is remarkable hypertrophy and concomitant degeneration of the myocytes.[7] In spite of this hypertrophy, the maximal thickness of the septum and free wall are normal—as a result of dilatation. There is an abnormal thickness:dimension ratio (thickness being somewhat less than dimension), resulting in an inadequate ventricular hypertrophic response. The dilated chambers are predisposed to lethal arrhythmias.

Dilated cardiomyopathy in the HIV-negative patient, is a disease of the myocyte thought to be related to familial or genetic factors; metabolic, energetic or contractile abnormalities, or immune abnormalities. The histology of this disease is remarkable for a loss of cardiac myofilaments with subsequent loss of contractility and function, which in some cases may represent the end of the spectrum of viral myocarditis.[7]

HIV cardiomyopathy is more complex than the dilated cardiomyopathy of HIV-negative patients. At one end of the spectrum, an HIV-positive patient may manifest a thinned, dilated myocardium, and at the other end of the spectrum, another HIV-positive host will manifest a hypertrophic cardiomyopathy. The hypertrophic response in HIV cardiomyopathy represents the heterogeneity of hypertrophy that accounts for variation in the spectrum of disease.[8] The myocardium is diseased, and it may be too thick or too thin for a given ventricular dimension. Both conditions may be manifested at different times in the same patient. The primary abnormality, left ventricular dysfunction, may not be due only to decreased contractility.[9] The natural history of HIV cardiac disease in children often consists of progressive left ventricular dilatation, which results in excess ventricular afterload, thereby reducing left ventricular function. Up to 93% of children with HIV infection have abnormal ventricular function by echocardiography, with only 26% of these actually having depressed contractility.[10,11]

HIV cardiac muscle disease may be associated with increased cardiac growth, which may represent a form of remodeling. Remodeling consists of the myocardial response to a cardiac insult. The classic example of remodeling is that of ischemic heart disease, where infarction of one specific portion of the myocardium has occurred. Side-to-side slippage of myocytes and hypertrophy of myocytes, results in progressive cardiac dilatation at the expense of ejection fraction.[12] Subsequently, there is an increase in left ventricular mass due to an increase in protein content of the myocytes. This "compensatory" phenomenon results in a stiffer ventricle with higher filling pressures. The resultant congestive heart failure may be due to this remodeling process rather than to a more general systolic or diastolic dysfunction. As the HIV-infected patient is subjected to many insults, the remodeling concept may be applicable to HIV cardiomyopathy.

Autopsy studies in HIV cardiomyopathy have shown hypertrophy and enlargement in weight or size, with increased diameters of myocardial fibers, nuclear enlargement, and left ventricular endocardial thickening.[13-15] In children, the heart weight may be up to 184% of that predicted from the basal surface area.[10,11,16,17] Although there are similarities, HIV cardiomyopathy may differ substantially from dilated cardiomyopathy in the HIV-negative patient.

Research into the pathogenesis of dilated cardiomyopathy has shown such familial causes as autosomal dominance for the angiotensin-converting enzyme (ACE) DD genotypes, Xp21 locus of the dystrophin gene, and a prevalence of human leukocyte antigen (HLA) II DR, DQ, DR4, and DQW4 antigens.[18,19] Immune dysregulation may be present, with activated T lymphocytes and heart muscle-specific autoantibodies (against adrenergic receptors, mitochondrial antigens, ATP carrier proteins, and cardiac myosin heavy chains) that are capable of altering and destroying myocytes.[20] There may also be decreased activity of natural lymphocyte killer cells and suppressor lymphocytes. These factors may contribute to the dilated cardiomyopathic state, which is speculated to be the end result of viral myocarditis in most cases.

In accordance with that theory, early research on the etiology of HIV cardiomyopathy focused on myocarditis as a precursor to dilated cardiomyopathy. One study reported that patients infected with HIV had a 52% prevalence of myocarditis at autopsy.[21] Similarly, a focal lymphocytic myocarditis was found in 26 consecutive HIV-infected patients who died.[22] Although initially it seemed that the myocardial dysfunction seen in HIV-infected patients might be explained by myocarditis, endomyocardial biopsies have routinely shown only patchy mononuclear inflammation, with no conclusive evidence of disease. Frequently there is inflammation with myocyte necrosis, inflammation without myocyte necrosis, and myocyte necrosis without inflammation.[6] Biopsy findings have been largely unreliable for the diagnosis of HIV cardiomyopathy.

Since these initial hypotheses regarding myocarditis as a cause of HIV cardiomyopathy, several more regarding the etiology of this disease have been elaborated. Dilated cardiomyopathy may be considered one variant of HIV cardiomyopathy. HIV cardiomyopathy may represent damage not only to the cardiomyocyte but to the nonmyocytic structures as well. Where dilated cardiomyopathy may part ways with the cardiomyopathy of the HIV-infected patient, is that the patient with dilated cardiomyopathy may have a familial predisposition, a defined immunologic abnormality, or a metabolic, energetic, or contractile predisposition for cardiomyopathy. The HIV-infected patient, on the other hand, who also may have a familial predisposition, a defined immunologic abnormality, or a metabolic, energetic, or contractile predisposition for cardiomyopathy, may be affected by additional factors (Table 8-1). Thus, dilated cardiomyopathy appears to be a variant of HIV cardiomyopathy.

Factors Influencing the HIV-Infected Patient with HIV Cardiomyopathy

Patients infected by HIV are compromised by lymphocytic abnormalities that predispose them to a variety of opportunistic infections. These infections may cause a myocarditic picture leading to cardiac dysfunction and cardiomyopathy. In addition, the myocytes themselves may be infected by HIV,[23,24] inducing myocardial dysfunction. Various soluble factors, such as tumor necrosis factor α (TNF-α), interferon alfa (IFN-α), interferon gamma, interleukins (IL)-1, -6, -8, and -11, and other circulating factors, such as transforming growth factor β (TGF-β), platelet-derived growth factor (PDGF), fibroblast growth factor (FGF), endothelin-1 (ET-1), bradykinin, NO, stress proteins or HSPs, circulating immunoglobulins, and cortisols, may cause a secondary cardiomyopathy whereby the heart is injured during a mounted immune response or a lack thereof (Table 8-2 and Figure 8-1).

Infections may cause fluctuating states of hyperthermia and hypothermia, which may elicit stress proteins or other factors. Infection may cause hyperglycemia or hypoglycemia, thereby producing varying insulin levels in the blood and inducing insulin growth factors. There may be total body volume extremes due to diarrhea, emesis, or anemia, or a malfunctioning renin–angiotensin system secondary to renal disease. These mechanical effects may influence myocardial growth and function by distortion of the cytoskeleton of the cardiomyocyte, which induces growth signals.

HIV affects a variety of organ systems. The relative hypoxia caused by HIV pulmonary disease may also elicit stress proteins that may affect the heart, or it may induce compensatory right ventricular hypertrophy. Renal disease may alter total body volume, change peripheral vascular resistance, and influence the renin–angiotensin system. Endocrine abnormalities may include pancreatic dysfunction, thyroid disease, and malfunction of the adrenocortical axis.

The malnutrition of HIV-infected patients is well documented. Malnourished patients who have not been infected with HIV will typically show diminished left ventricular volume, ventricular function, and blood pressure.[25,26] The cardiomyopathy of

Table 8-1. Factors Involved in the Preservation of Normal Cardiac Function and the Evolution of Cardiomyopathies

Preservation of Normal Function and Architecture	Malfunctions in Dilated Cardiomyopathy* (A disease of the myocyte)	Abnormal Growth in Cardiac Muscle in HIV-infected patients† (A disease of all components, myocytic and nonmyocytic)
Autonomic nervous system	Familial predisposition/genetic factors	Predisposition to opportunistic infection (abnormal lymphocytes)
Mechanical-stretch mechanisms	ACE DD genotypes, Xp21 dystrophic, HLA II, DR, DQ, DR$_4$, DQW$_4$Ag	Primary HIV infection of heart muscle
Renin-angiotensin system	Metabolic disease	Secondary cardiomyopathy: soluble factors (TNF-α; IFN-γ; IL-1, -2, -6, -8; ET-1; TGF-β; FGF; PDGF; stress proteins)
Endothelins (ET-1)	Energetics (mitochondrial)	Bradykinins
ANF	Contractile abnormalities	Hypothermia/hyperthermia → heat shock/stress proteins
Prostaglandins	Immune abnormalities (Activated system and cells and heart muscle-specific antibodies)	Hyperglycemia/ hypoglycemia → IGF-I/growth hormone
NO	Hypervolemia/hypovolemia → mechanical stretch/renin-angiotensin II	
Normal programmed cell death	Autonomic nervous system → abnormalities of the central and peripheral nervous system	
Normal pulmonary/renal/endocrine systems	Malnutrition → glucose/IGF-I → endocrine abnormalities	
	Endocrine → pancreatic/ growth hormone/thyroid/adrenocortical axis	
	Hypoxia (secondary to pulmonary disease) → stress proteins	
	Renal disease	
	Iatrogenic factors → antiretroviral/other medications	

TNF-α, tumor necrosis factor-α; PDGF, platelet-derived growth factor; IFN-γ, interferon-γ; IGF-I, insulinlike growth factor; IL-1, -2, -6, -8, interleukins; NO, nitric oxide; ET-1, endothelins; ANF, atrial natriuretic factor; TGF-β, transforming growth factor-β; ACE, angiotensin-converting enzyme; FGF, fibroblast growth factor; HLA, human leukocyte antigen.

*A disease of the myocyte.

†A disease of all components, myocytic and nonmyocytic.

HIV, with its increased mass, is typically different from that of HIV-negative malnourished patients, who typically show decreased mass, heart rate, and blood pressure. Some workers have described a myocardial atrophy in response to the wasting associated with HIV infection. Patients who were free of overt opportunistic infections or clinical evidence of heart disease had a significantly decreased left ventricular mass by echocardiography, even when it was corrected for body surface area.[27] There was no documentation of a decline in blood pressure or diminishment in ventricular volume. The importance of adequate nutrition for optimal cardiac performance is illustrated by hearts that have been severely stunned from any of a variety of causes. Myocardial function after stunning may be restored by infusion of glucose and insulin.[28] This implies that hearts deprived of adequate glucose stores and appropriate insulin regulation, as in the malnutrition of HIV disease, may be predisposed to dysfunction.

HIV cardiomyopathy may be iatrogenically induced. The antiretroviral medications used to treat HIV have been reported to cause mitochondrial dystrophy by a direct toxic effect,[29] due to a proposed DNA gamma polymerase mechanism.[30] These medications may exert an effect on the cardiac disease process seen in HIV-infected patients.

Table 8-2. Factors Involved in Hypertrophy

Factor	Mechanism	Effect	Pharmacologic Intervention
Catecholamines	Bind with cardiovascular α- and β-adrenergic receptors	May have a direct effect on myocytes	β-Blockers, hydralazine, ACE inhibitors to prevent "neuro-humoral storm"
	Chronotropic and inotropic effects	May affect mechanical/loading conditions	
	May interact with TGF-β and ANF	May act as second messengers, inducing protein synthesis	
Angiotensin II and mechanical load	Acts on cardiac cytoskeleton; second messenger in the stretch-mediated response	Ventricular hypertrophy/remodeling through calcium reserves	ACE inhibitors
	Affects sarcoplasmic reticulum	Increased protein synthesis	
	Stress signaling through autocrine/paracrine routes		
Endothelin-1	Affects vascular tone and mechanical stretch	Upregulation of protein synthesis. Interaction with NO	Block NO
	Also found in myocardium, signals early immediate genes		
Bradykinin	Vascular tone effects; signals early immediate genes	May downregulate protein synthesis	Antiinflammatory drugs
ANF	Through early immediate genes	Upregulation of β-MHC, skeletal α-actin; downregulation of α-MHC, cardiac α-actin	
Peptide growth factors	May affect cytoskeleton, vascular system, cardiomyocytes	Increase protein content	
Cytokines	May inhibit cellular response, induce stress proteins, induce NO synthase (100–1,000×)	Up- or down-regulation of proteins	Anti-inflammatory drugs
NO	Vascular effects, as well as maintenance of diastolic tone in the endomyocardium	Affects myocytic and nonmyocytic growth, increased or decreased protein Chronotropic/inotropic effects	

See Table 8-1 for abbreviations.

It has also been noted that left ventricular dysfunction occurs independently of zidovudine therapy.[31] A significant increase in left ventricular wall thickness after zidovudine therapy has been reported, which may actually be beneficial in decreasing peak systolic wall stress. The role of antiretroviral medications in the induction of HIV cardiomyopathy remains ambiguous.

There is an association between increased cardiac morbidity and mortality and the presence of encephalopathy.[4] The encephalopathy of HIV has been well described and may be attributed to direct infection of the central nervous system.[32] It may be that encephalopathy induces an autonomic neuropathy in HIV, or the two may be separate entities. Early cardiovascular disturbance has been described, in the form of bradycardia, hypotension, syncope, and ultimately cardiopulmonary arrest.[33] Autonomic dysfunction might explain the sinus tachycardia frequently seen in HIV-infected patients. Sympathetic overdrive appears to be common in patients manifesting congestive heart failure. Research regarding the presence of catecholamine excess in HIV-infected patients would be helpful.

The HIV-infected patient is subjected to a bar-

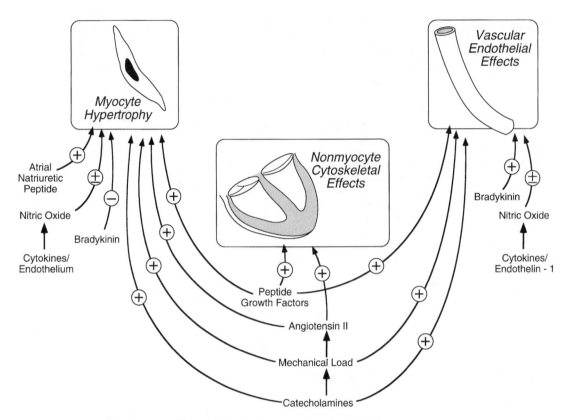

Figure 8-1. Effects on cardiac hypertrophy.

rage of biochemical and physiologic abnormalities that complicate the search for a single cause of cardiovascular dysfunction. The constant stress of HIV infection, with associated growth factors and stress proteins, may cause the host to revert to the embryologic or neonatal program, with induction of the immediate early gene (IEG) responses. Alternatively, HIV itself may induce a state of early senility in which the host cannot respond by reversion to the embryologic or neonatal program and fetal myocyte isoforms.

The strong association of HIV with cellular growth factors and cytokines,[34] the association of TNF-α and the ILs,[35,36] and their presence in the HIV cardiomyopathic state in the adult[37] underline the contribution of these cytokines and growth factors to HIV-associated myocardial disease. In addition, the blunted response to the increased afterload seen in these patients[38] may be directly attributable to a defect in the normal reexpression of the neona-

tal genetic program crucial to the development of an appropriate hypertrophic response.

Thus, the HIV-infected patient is exposed to a barrage of physiologic, nutritional, and disease states. There may be extreme variation in loading conditions. All of these factors may influence the cardiomyocyte growth patterns.

Cardiac Growth: Left Ventricular Mass and Hypertrophy

Does Hypertrophy Equal Increased Mass?

The terms "mass" and "hypertrophy" are used interchangeably in the literature. Both terms have been used to describe a thickening of the left ventricle that is out of proportion to the patient's weight or basal surface area. In fact, hypertrophy refers to the ratio of the wall thickness to the end-diastolic dimension, as this echocardiographic parameter is related to a physiologic condition of increased myocyte mass. Hypertrophy may be concentric, with the entire left ventricle thickened symmetrically; or eccentric, with thickening confined to the ventricular free wall or septum. Mass encompasses the total dimension and involves calculations based on the entire cardiac structure. Devereux devised a formula that accurately calculates ventricular mass, as confirmed by heart weights from autopsy data.[39,40] The initial formula was designed to assess left ventricular hypertrophy. Hypertrophy was then shown to correlate with the degree of chronic overload with extreme hypertrophy, yielding a very poor diagnosis. When HIV cardiomyopathy is considered, the question comes to mind, Which is worse prognostically, increased mass (estimated total heart weight) or severe hypertrophy? Can myocardial remodeling alone account for the increased morbidity and mortality associated with HIV cardiomyopathy?

The Normal Hypertrophic Response

In a normal person, the size of the cardiac chamber remains proportional to its workload. The degree and type of hypertrophy are influenced by factors such as body weight, growth, and maturation.[41] Hypertrophy is the response of the mature heart to such environmental factors as volume or pressure overload (workloads), excess catecholamines or hormones, cytokines, peptide growth factors or soluble factors, and ischemia.[42] The type of workload may determine the form of hypertrophy. Volume overload typically results in increased ventricular cavity volume in proportion to mass, that is, eccentric hypertrophy. Pressure overload results in increased left ventricular mass out of proportion to volume, that is, concentric hypertrophy.[41]

The mechanics of the hypertrophic response to an increased hemodynamic load consists of either a decline in the ratio of left ventricular thickness:dimension or an increase in pressure with an increase in peak systolic wall stress. Peak stress (the loading condition) mediates mechanically induced hypertrophy by a variety of factors. Hypertrophy of the ventricle continues until the peak systolic wall stress returns to normal, thereby inhibiting any further hypertrophic response. An attenuated hypertrophic response to pressure and volume overload occurs with age.[41]

From a molecular standpoint, hypertrophy results in an increase in total cell size and volume, usually through an increase in cell protein content. Activation of the IEGs by an environmental stimulus results in the accumulation of individual contractile proteins, which are then organized into sarcomeres. The transcriptional activation and translation of these embryonic genes and the constitutive expression of contractile proteins are responsible for hypertrophy.[42]

Depending on the stimulus and the individual's response, hypertrophy may be either a compensatory response that is quite functional or a response that exacerbates the underlying condition and increases morbidity and mortality.

Hypertrophic Response in the HIV-Infected Patient

As previously mentioned, the HIV-infected patient is subjected to a variety of conditions that, working together, will affect the overall remodeling or hypertrophic response, yielding a form of hypertrophy that typically differs from that of an HIV-negative person. In zidovudine-treated HIV-infected children, progressive dilatation from unknown, and possibly multiple, causes induced wall thinning, resulting in a diminished thickness:dimension ratio, which increased peak systolic and end-systolic wall stress (afterload).[31] Increased afterload was associated with decreased ventricular performance, as indicated by the fractional shortening index. When loading conditions were maintained constant, left ventricular contractility was unimpaired. The rise in afterload further exacerbated left ventricular dilatation, resulting in thinning of the left ventricular wall. The resultant increase in peak systolic wall stress due to left ventricular dilatation induced a hypertrophic response to normalize the thickness:dimension ratio. Left ventricular masses, which were 184% of normal,[10,11,16,17] increased significantly but failed to keep pace with ventricular dimension. The thickness:dimension ratio diminished. The result was inadequate compensatory hypertrophy but a significant

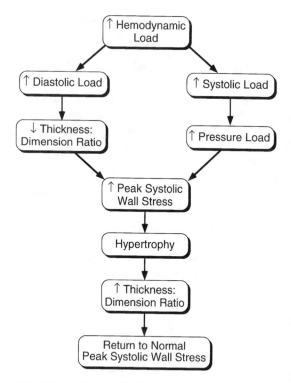

Figure 8-2. Compensatory left ventricular hypertrophy in the normal person.

increase in left ventricular mass (Figure 8-2). The HIV-infected patient appears to manifest an abnormal hypertrophic response for the type of myocardial stimulus involved, resulting in increased morbidity and mortality.[43,44]

Which Is Worse, Increased Total Mass or Severe Hypertrophy?

The association between death and increased left ventricular mass is remarkable. It has recently been reported that children infected with HIV have significantly increased heart weights standardized for body mass on postmortem examination.[45] The patients' heights and weights are significantly decreased for age, reflecting poor somatic growth, likely due to malnutrition. Malnourished patients typically have dilated hearts with decreased mass,[25,26] as shown by a study of HIV-infected adults that documented decreased ventricular mass for body surface area.[27] Conversely, symptomatic

HIV-infected children had hypertrophied hearts that did not function well and were overly large for calculated body size. Another study of cardiac dysfunction in HIV-infected children, using univariate analysis, found that the factors predictive of increased mortality were a decrease in fractional shortening, an increase in left ventricular afterload, an increase in wall thickness, and an increase in left ventricular mass.[44] The pattern of increased left ventricular mass with diminished body surface area is ominous.

It appears that the HIV-infected patient does not manifest a "normal" hypertrophic response, and that mass is out of proportion for height and weight. Hypertrophy may be compensatory for the HIV-negative person, but it is largely inadequate, and it may be a predictive factor for increased morbidity and mortality in the HIV-infected patient. Increased left ventricular mass is associated with increased morbidity and mortality in HIV-infected patients.

Increased Myocardial Cell Growth: a Double-Edged Sword

Many researchers have pondered the question, "Is cardiac hypertrophy a useful adaptation or a pathologic process?"[46,47] Accelerated myocardial growth is a response of the myocardium to stress, with peak systolic wall stress being the impetus for growth. When is cardiac hypertrophy or accelerated cell growth "well-compensated accelerated growth," and when is it a pathologic condition?[48] Conversely, what is the consequence of inadequate hypertrophy for the given loading condition?

The following is a discussion of increased myocardial cell growth resulting in ventricular hypertrophy or increased ventricular mass in various clinical settings. Each individual setting may depict myocardial cell growth as either an adaptive or pathologic response, which may or may not relate to patient outcome. Each clinical setting may be compared to the heterogeneous hypertrophy of HIV cardiomyopathy, where inadequate ventricular hypertrophy and increased ventricular mass are detrimental.

Accelerated Myocardial Cell Growth in the Setting of Dilated Cardiomyopathy

Early studies of prognostic factors in cardiomyopathy indicated that, at least for this disease, ventricular hypertrophy was a beneficial compensatory response that was associated with increased length of survival.[49,50] Several mechanisms are involved in myocardial cell growth. One early preliminary study found that thickening was accelerated by exogenous growth hormone.[51] Administration of growth hormone increased left ventricular muscle mass, thereby improving left ventricular ejection fraction and increasing isovolumic relaxation time.[51] Recent studies have shown improved hemodynamic measurements, decreased myocardial oxygen consumption, efficient energy use, and overall improved functional capacity. It seemed that inducing mechanisms of hypertrophy would be a panacea, but these preliminary studies make a case for cautious optimism.[52] Acromegaly is an example of a condition in which inappropriate hypertrophy results in cardiomegaly and diastolic abnormalities, leading to overt congestive heart failure or worse.

An example of the detrimental effects of increased myocardial cell growth comes from one study that found that children with dilated cardiomyopathy had a worse outcome if there was any evidence of significant ventricular hypertrophy.[53] Increased left ventricular mass in children, but not in adults, has been associated with poor contractility and increased wall stress, resulting in exacerbated symptoms of congestive heart failure. Children with dilated cardiomyopathy without ventricular hypertrophy had a much better outcome. These researchers speculated that the observed hypertrophy may have resulted in coronary insufficiency and poor diastolic function.

Accelerated Myocardial Cell Growth in the Setting of Ischemic Heart Disease

Many studies have shown a correlation between sudden death and left ventricular hypertrophy in adults.[54-58] Patients with left ventricular hypertrophy without coronary artery disease have poorer survival than those with coronary artery disease without hypertrophy,[59] indicating that hypertrophy is an inciting factor. That is, not all sudden death can be explained by coronary artery disease, although the hypertrophic process may itself narrow the coronary arteries.

Accelerated Myocardial Cell Growth in the Setting of Hypertension

As well as narrowing the coronary arteries, hypertrophy appears to have some effect on systemic blood pressure. Normotensive adults with increased left ventricular mass and wall thickness may develop hypertension later.[60] Therefore, it appears that hypertrophy and increased left ventricular mass may be independent risk factors for sudden death. The presence of left ventricular hypertrophy or increased left ventricular mass represents myocardial remodeling and is ominous. It is invariably associated with a poor outcome.

Sex and Body Weight Differences in Accelerated Myocardial Cell Growth

When mass is indexed for basal surface area, it is greater in males than females, increases in females with increasing age (due to their increasing basal surface area with age), and is significantly correlated with body size.[61] Increased body size results in increased left ventricular mass. Obesity, in particular, correlates with increased left ventricular mass.[62] In this form of increased left ventricular mass, heart weight increases in proportion to body mass, with a concomitant increase in body size, an increase in the size and diameter of the myocytes, but no degeneration or fibrosis of the myocytes.[63] The increased morbidity and mortality seen with left ventricular hypertrophy and increased left ventricular mass is even more significant for women, independently of the presence or absence of coronary artery disease.[58] This is thought to be due to increasing body fat content with age in women. The Bogalusa Heart Study showed that left ventricular hypertrophy or increased left ventricular mass was significantly correlated with obesity in children.[64] Sudden death is a well-known consequence of morbid obesity[63] and may have some correlation with increased left ventricular mass.

If increased left ventricular mass correlates with increased body surface area, then weight reduction should result in decreased left ventricular mass and an overall improved prognosis. With reversal to normal loading conditions, that is, weight loss, and relief of the hemodynamic load, there is reversal of the hypertrophic state.[65] Obese people, whether hypertensive or normotensive, can modify their left ventricular mass by weight reduction.[66] The overall prognosis for these people is unknown, as there are still conflicting data regarding whether a decline in left ventricular mass is truly beneficial.[67,68] The speculation is that decreased left ventricular mass and reduction in left ventricular hypertrophy should result in improvement in morbidity and mortality.

Hypertrophic Cardiomyopathy and Accelerated Myocardial Cell Growth

Hypertrophic cardiomyopathy has entered the jargon of laypeople as the media have reported sudden death in young athletes.[69] Sudden death has been attributed to myocardial thickening, which may or may not be associated with arrhythmias and myocardial scarring secondary to ischemic disease. Hypertrophic cardiomyopathy is a particularly devastating disease, as it tends to strike adolescents and young adults. The incidence of sudden death associated with this condition is well known.[70–72]

In addition to hypertrophic cardiomyopathy, concentric left ventricular hypertrophy secondary not to mutations in β-myosin heavy chains, but rather to conditioning, is also associated with an increase in the risk of sudden death in young athletes.[71,72] The prognostic implications of left ventricular hypertrophy in young athletes are not known.[73,74] Physiologic hypertrophy results in young athletes results in marked alterations in left ventricular loading conditions, with resulting changes in systolic performance.[75] Left ventricular contractility is normal in these young athletes when loading conditions are held constant; however, there is markedly increased left ventricular mass.

Concentric or physiologic left ventricular hypertrophy is likely to be a "compensatory" response to increased dynamic load. By contrast, in the histo-logically abnormal hypertrophic cardiomyopathy there is fibromuscular disarray based on an abnormal cytoskeletal structure that results in a ventricular septum one and a half times as thick as the left ventricular free wall. Hypertrophic cardiomyopathy, or asymmetric hypertrophy, is recognized by the hallmark disorganization of the cardiac muscle cells, with extreme disarray of myocardial structure extending through the interventricular septum and free wall, abnormal intramural coronary arteries, and myocardial fibrosis. This histology and architecture is found in hypertrophic cardiomyopathy in cats and dogs, as well as in humans.[76] Stress-induced hypertrophy may show cellular shape changes with alterations in the capillary luminal volume and surface, as well as the mitochondrial: myofibril ratio.[48]

The mechanism of sudden death in left ventricular hypertrophy remains elusive. Changes in left ventricular hypertrophy include the appearance of coronary tunnels, coronary insufficiency resulting in ischemia, arrhythmias, increased myocardial oxygen consumption, and overall inadequate growth adaptation of structures responsible for oxygenation and energy production. It has been postulated that hypertrophy of the myocyte with its multiple intercalated disks facilitates current flow and reentry, perpetuating arrhythmia and leading to sudden death.[63] Myocardial fibrosis and collagen compartment remodeling may result in less useful cardiac muscle.[59] Fibrosis may cause ineffective transmission electrical impulses. One speculative cause of sudden death is myocardial ischemia due to decreased myocardial vascularity. In sheep, adults showed a paucity of coronary perfusion of the myocardium, while young sheep adapted to a hypertrophic state with appropriate angiogenesis.[77] Young sheep exhibited angiogenesis in proportion to their hypertrophy, which resulted in well-compensated capillary density and conductance. These observations have been made in humans, where the capillary density is higher in infants, decreasing with increasing heart weight during normal growth in early childhood.[78] Therefore, the capillary density in increased myocardial mass is likely to depend on the age of onset or the cause of the hypertrophic condition.

Congenital Diseases Associated with Accelerated Myocardial Cell Growth

Increased ventricular mass is a complication of several other disease states, resulting in increased morbidity and mortality. These conditions include a rapidly obstructive cardiomyopathy in infants with Noonan syndrome,[79,80] hypertrophic cardiomyopathy during corticotropin therapy for infantile spasms,[81] a hypertrophic cardiomyopathy induced by twin-to-twin transfusion in infants,[82] and cardiac septal hypertrophy in hyperinsulinemic infants.[83] Interest in the hypertrophic cardiomyopathy seen in infants of diabetic mothers peaked with reports of death from severe hypertrophy.[84] There are also iatrogenic forms of increased left ventricular mass. Left ventricular mass increases significantly in the first month after cardiac transplantation in children.[85] Although the absolute cause is unknown, it is speculated that this initial hypertrophy is due to the use of steroids. These forms of increased left ventricular mass and hypertrophy result in increased morbidity and possibly mortality.

Hormonally Induced Accelerated Myocardial Cell Growth

Left ventricular hypertrophy or increased ventricular mass due to steroid use has been reported in premature infants with bronchopulmonary dysplasia treated with dexamethasone.[86–89] This form of hypertrophic cardiomyopathy is reversible on discontinuation of the steroids. The morbidity and mortality in these infants due to the hypertrophic state are unknown, as other variables are involved, including their chronic lung disease. This entity is more consistent with a transient concentric left ventricular hypertrophy than with true hypertrophic cardiomyopathy. The myocytes in the iatrogenic state are diffusely hypertrophied and not disarrayed as they are in hypertrophic cardiomyopathy.[90] In fact, the iatrogenic hypertrophic cardiomyopathy or transient concentric left ventricular hypertrophy may be nothing more than an exaggerated neonatal myotropic response. In one study, newborns and infants had a higher ratio of end-diastolic mass:end-diastolic volume than older children.[91]

Dexamethasone-induced hypertrophic cardio-myopathy also occurs in neonatal rat models.[92] The changes in rats were similar to those in humans, showing a thickened interventricular septum and left ventricular free wall, with diminished left ventricular chamber diameter. Dexamethasone reduced survival and retarded growth in neonatal rats. Overall, the heart weights were diminished when compared with controls; however, when adjusted for rat basal surface area, there was a remarkable increase in heart weight adjusted for body size. This state is similar to that seen in HIV-infected children.

HIV-Infected Children: "Abnormal" Cell Growth?

Children infected with HIV appear to have an abnormality of left ventricular hypertrophy[11,17,38,42] and increased ventricular mass, which correlates with increased morbidity.[45] These HIV-infected children typically have stunted somatic growth but have 184% expected left ventricular mass for age and body size.[10,11,16,17] Their hypertrophic response to increased peak systolic wall stress is inadequate, yet the increase in left ventricular mass is greatly exaggerated. It is difficult to factor out which feature contributes more to increased morbidity and mortality: inadequate hypertrophy (compensatory response) or increased ventricular mass (bigger is not always better). As in all of the previously mentioned clinical situations, the myocardial hypertrophic response in these children is abnormal.

From the Womb to Adulthood and Back Again: Is it Necessary to Revert to Infancy?

The fetus and the neonate have an ability to proliferate myocytes. This state of hyperplastic growth is accounted for by an increase in cell number through the meiotic process of nuclear division or replication of DNA.[42] In early postnatal life the well-orchestrated program of hyperplasia declines, and the mature organism is left with a fixed number of cardiomyocytes. Through proliferation of protein, the cardiomyocyte increases in cell mass, length and volume. During normal physiologic hypertrophy, there is a well-balanced response, including proportionate angiogenesis compensated to adequately supply the enlarging myocardium.[78] There are sufficient numbers of mitochondria to supply oxidative energy and proportional subcellular components, such as myofibrils and sarcoplasmic reticulum, to provide normal contractile expansion. Growth is usually proportional with a normal cytoskeletal structure. The transition from the fetal to the adult state involves an initial increase in volume on both sides of the heart, then a preferential increase on the left. Chamber growth is linearly correlated with age. In normal physiologic hypertrophy, there is a substantial increase in wall stress in the first few years of life. Although children show increased contractility, there is a natural increase in afterload and a decrease in systolic function with age.[93]

The hypertrophy seen in the adult state, which involves an increase in myocyte length and diameter, is not proportional. Growth is not well compensated. There may be side-to-side slippage of myocytes. Wall thickness is increased at the expense of the cellular and subcellular levels of organization, resulting in inefficient energy production, utilization, and expenditure. There is a paucity of capillary volume and a decreased mitochondrial and myofibrillar volume ratio. This condition of remodeling makes the adult hypertrophied heart vulnerable to contractile abnormalities, increased systolic wall stress, decreased diastolic function, and ischemia. Therefore, although physiologic hypertrophy may result in improved cardiac performance, the stress-induced hypertrophy representative of remodeling may actually be maladaptive. The trophic response diminishes with advancing age.[93]

During normal development of terminally differentiated cardiomyocytes, the fetal proteins are downregulated. The growth of many cell types involves the suppression of the adult phenotype and the reexpression of the fetal pattern. The increase in size of the cardiomyocytes is the end result of complex genetic expression. Stress stimuli, such as adrenergic regulation, soluble factors, hormones, peptide growth factors and resultant nitric oxide synthase with its induced and constitutive components, heat shock or stress proteins, and shear stretch or strain on the myocte, may cause reexpres-

sion of the protooncogenes. The protooncogenes (IEGs, embryonic genes, contractile protein genes) are mediators of cell growth through their actions in the regulatory signaling cascade that is likely mediated by protein kinase C.[94] The cascade of secondary messages, leading either to cell death or to hypertrophy, is mediated by the ubiquitous tyrosine kinase pathways.[12] These pathways are crucial to mitogenic responses and the hypertrophic response of the cardiomyocyte to stretch and humoral stimulation. Take, for example, the rat heart, which upregulates the IEGs—c-*myc*, c-*jun*, b-*jun*, *Erg* 1, *nur* 7, and c-*fos*—in response to an environmental stress stimulus. The overexpression of c-*myc* is important in causing hypertrophy of the heart by production of protein.

During these gene-induced states, there may be a release of growth factors, such as ET-1, PDGF, heparin-binding FGF, TGF-β, and insulinlike growth factor (IGF). The peptide growth factors are a series of regulatory protein families with inhibitory or inducing effects. They are interdependent with other embryonic programming events. Two major sets of growth factors involved in cardiomyocyte growth are the FGF family and the TGF-β family. The TGF-β family are the first set of growth factors expressed in the developing heart and seem to be involved in development of the outflow tract, septation, and formation of the cardiac valves.[95] FGF transcripts function in the proliferation and multilayering of cardiogenic cells in cardiac morphogenesis, influence myocyte terminal differentiation in culture, and are abundant in the endocardial cushion.[96] Myocyte growth becomes FGF-independent after the second week of embryogenesis.[97] The FGF receptors are still present in the adult heart. The long isoform is abundant in the embryo, and the short isoform is abundant in the adult.[95] This indicates a functional role of FGF in the adult myocardium. Note that the IGF family has anabolic actions and suppresses degradation of proteins in the adult myocardium.[98] ET-1, also found in adult myocardium, is produced both by endothelial cells and by cardiomyocytes. It is not only a potent vasoconstrictor peptide but maintains chronotropy and inotropy in heart failure and induces hypertrophy through expression of a fetal gene program.[99]

Introduction of virus into a cardiomyocyte induces remarkable changes in the shape and function of the cardiomyocyte (S.E. Lipshultz, personal communication, 1996).[100] Any virus can conceivably rearrange the oncogenes contained within the cardiomyocyte, cause a point mutation altering expression of any of these protooncogenes, or alter the interacting growth factors and other cytokines. HIV itself, or any other virus, such as cytomegalovirus or Epstein-Barr virus, might target a protooncogene to provide up- or downregulation of any of the aforementioned genes or gene products, resulting in an abnormality in left ventricular hypertrophy. For example, in congenitally acquired HIV infection, the retrovirus may target one of the early regulatory genes, such as the nestin gene, which independently controls the production of intermediate filaments in muscle and nerve cells.[100] A point mutation would modify this gene, causing a defective myocardial growth program for the life span of the host. In addition, there is now evidence that some of the growth factors, such as TGF-β, may play a role in HIV infection.[101]

Consider how the fluctuations in the physiologic state of the HIV host might affect the cellular milieu and the neonatal program. A dramatic rise in intracellular pH by the removal of protons from the intracellular environment has been noted to increase the efficiency of translation of the genetic program.[42] This might result in a small increase in calcium, which would allow binding to calmodulin, initiating cell motility and DNA synthesis. The calmodulin gene is linked to a promotor for atrial natriuretic factor (ANF), known to cause hypertrophy. One might speculate that the persistent acidosis common to the septic state or decreased renal function manifested by patients infected with HIV would have an effect on the genetic program responsible for cardiac hypertrophy. See Figure 8-3.

Growth Factors and Induction of Hypertrophy in HIV Cardiomyopathy

Growth factors are families of peptides that stimulate or inhibit chemotaxis, mitogenesis, or differentiation of cells. FGF and TGF-β work antagonistically or synergistically. Both influence extracellular matrix accumulation. The FGFs influence early cell differentiation, such as DNA proliferation and synthesis, expression of fetal myosin heavy chain, increase in skeletal α-actin, and decrease in adult α-myosin heavy chain, as well as capillary angiogenesis.[102] They do so by binding heparin, which binds to the proteoglycans in the extracellular matrix encircling the cardiomyocyte. Heparin has been shown to promote angiogenesis in the pressure-overload hypertrophied heart, regardless of the age of the myocardium.[103] Stretch and strain on the myocyte may influence gene expression through this deformation of the extracellular matrix.

Specific ventricular cell types at distinct developmental stages appear to be responsive to ventricular myocyte-derived α-FGF[102] and β-FGF.[104] As the organism matures, ventricular capillary angiogenesis is facilitated by a release of cardiomyocyte-derived FGF into the surrounding extracellular matrix, with a subsequent increase in capillary angiogenesis.[105] The early expression of FGF may explain why physiologic hypertrophy is well compensated with capillary perfusion, but stress hypertrophy that occurs in the adult is not. The paucity of capillary perfusion in ventricular hypertrophy is a well-documented cause of ischemia, which may lead to sudden death. As reported by Flanagan and colleagues, "Young age confers advantages in the coronary adaptation to left ventricular pressure overload hypertrophy including angiogenesis maintaining left ventricular capillary density . . . Age-related changes are paralleled by changes in β-FGF."[104]

The TGF-β family has been reported to be overexpressed in HIV infection.[101] TGF-β is thought to result in chronically increased viral replication through its interference with the host defense mechanism. The TGF-β family are potent inhibitors of leukocyte activation, are chemoattractants for fibroblasts and monocytes (which might affect the myocardial cytoskeleton), decrease B lymphocyte responses, and reduce IL-2 receptor expression on T lymphocytes.[101] In monocytes, TGF-β inhibits the production of NO (known to both inhibit and induce a hypertrophic response), and inhibits INF-α and the subsequent expression of HLA-DR. The HLA-DR and -DQB1 genes and antigens have been implicated in the development of dilated cardiomyopathy.[19] The perpetuation of HIV infection with de-

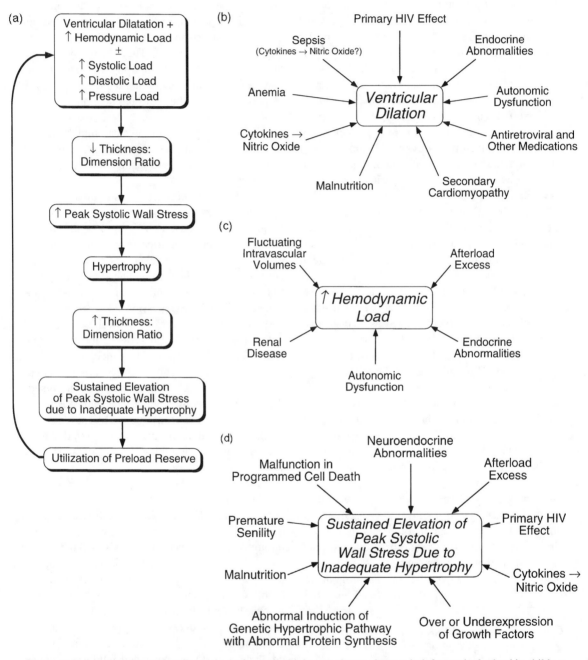

Figure 8-3. **a:** Compensatory left ventricular hypertrophy in response to changes in left ventricular load in children with symptomatic HIV infection. **b:** Non-cardiac factors that potentially influence left ventricular dilation in HIV-infected patients. **c:** Non-cardiac factors that potentially influence increased hemodynamic load in HIV-infected patients. **d:** Non-cardiac factors that potentially influence sustained elevation of peak systolic wall stress due to inadequate hypertrophy in HIV-infected patients.

creasing cellular and humoral immunity can itself perpetuate a cardiomyopathic response but may, in addition, affect the host's normal compensatory hypertrophic response.

HIV induces the expression in monocytes of a cellular protein that induces TGF-β production. In addition, IL-1 and IL-6 induce TGF-β production in mesenchymal cells.[102] The specific cell response is dependent on the cellular milieu, consisting of cell density, other growth factors, and the three-dimensional orientation of the cell. Although TGF-β is not able to stimulate protein synthesis directly, as a multifunctional regulatory protein it can stimulate or inhibit protein synthesis and growth in various cell types, including the cardiomyocyte. TGF-β has an inducible hypertrophic effect,[106] which may be partially through rearrangement of the cytoskeleton, as well as function and hypertrophy of the cardiomyocyte.

As previously mentioned, the TGF-β family are present early in myocardiogenesis,[107–109] and, although their roles change during development in the mature myocardium, they are crucial in the repair of myocardial damage, such as ischemia and reperfusion injuries. TGF-β is upregulated during hemodynamic stress and induces the expression of skeletal α-actin, a primitive component of cardiomyocytes,[107] and also increases the number of contractile and noncontractile muscle cells to three to seven times those of cells not exposed to TGF-β.[108] This stimulation may have a great effect upon the myocardial cytoskeleton, further influencing hypertrophy. The immunoreactive TGF-β family are intrinsic intracellular components of cardiomyocytes and are therefore greatly influenced by the immunologic status of the host. Thus, TGF-β regulation is highly influenced by the HIV state and may account for the abnormal hypertrophy seen in HIV-infected patients.

It is unknown what influence the retroviruses and other infectious agents might have on such growth factors as FGF, PDGF, and IGF. IGF, a paracrine and/or autocrine factor, directly activates protein synthesis in cardiomyocytes by stimulating the accumulation of inositol-1,4-biphosphate and inosine triphosphate (IP3), which regulates cardiac protein metabolism, resulting in hypertrophy.[106] It

is a vital growth factor in cellular proliferation and differentiation during development.[110] IGF-1 stimulates myocardial hypertrophy in rats in, and, and influences ventricular remodeling after an induced ischemic event.[111] PDGF is associated with macrophages and is located predominantly in the interstitium of globally ischemic hearts. PDGF induces c-*myc* and c-*fos* RNA in smooth muscle cells, has potent mitogenic activity in fibroblasts, and may therefore have a role in compensatory hypertrophy.[112] The roles of these growth factors in the development of abnormal ventricular hypertrophy in HIV cardiomyopathy remain to be elucidated.

Myocardial Vasculature and the Effects of ET-1 in HIV Cardiomyopathy

The vascular system is an integral part of the cardiac system. The effects of preload, afterload, vessel capacitance, and vessel conductance transmit force to the heart, inducing physiologic responses. Any factor that affects the vasculature, in particular the endothelium, could have a role in myocardial hypertrophy.

ET-1, a 21-amino acid peptide, is a potent vasoconstrictor that is elaborated by vascular endothelial cells[113] and cardiac myocytes.[114] It may be induced by pressure overload,[115] pulmonary hypertension,[116] shear,[117] or pulsatile stretch[118] and is elaborated during congestive heart failure.[119] ET-1 seems to affect gene expression and subsequently cell growth. ET-1 induces hypertrophy and expression of the fetal gene program in cultured cardiac myocytes,[113,116] with reduced expression of adult genes such as sarcoplasmic reticulum calcium ATPase (SRCA). In addition, ET-1 is important for collagen synthesis and degradation. In this respect, ET-1 may play a vital role in determining the configuration of the cytoskeleton, which influences the architecture of the myocardium, and subsequent myocyte growth and distribution. In addition, its importance in collagen synthesis, distribution, and degradation would be expected to induce interstitial fibrosis with resultant abnormal diastolic properties, impaired oxygenation, and impaired delivery of nutrients to the myocytes.

Although the role of ET-1 in HIV disease is yet

to be determined, the various factors influencing the HIV-infected patient would likely be sufficient to elaborate ET-1 from endothelial cells and myocytes: hypovolemia or hypervolemia, autonomic dysfunction, and opportunistic infection. ET-1 seems to be a powerful mediator of cell growth and myocardial function, as it affects SRCA and controls chronotropy and inotropy during congestive heart failure.[119] Fluctuations in pressure and volume would have variable effects on the production of ET-1 and its subsequent induction of hypertrophy.

The Role of Heat-Shock and Stress Proteins in HIV Cardiomyopathy

The TGF-β family regulates heat-shock or stress proteins (HSPs), particularly in embryonic cells.[120,121] The heat-shock or stress proteins are a family of highly conserved constitutive proteins that are elaborated by cells during stressful periods. They are thought to have a protective effect on the cellular milieu, and research into their cardioprotective effect, particularly following ischemic events, is ongoing.[122–124] HSP 70 has been elaborated during the evolution of stress-induced hypertrophy, after the proliferation of the protooncogenes c-*fos* and c-*myc*.[125] HSP 70 has been elaborated secondary to stretch,[126] which is compatible with its presence during cardiac hypertrophy.

Many factors are known to induce HSPs: retroviruses, insulin, long- term anoxia, low pH, 2-deoxyglucose, glucosamine, and anything that causes calcium deprivation. Cell synthesis induces HSPs. Cells undergoing myogenesis also induce HSPs.[127] Small mammalian HSPs are rapidly phosphorylated in response to stress and mitogenic signals and thereby affect the polymerization of actin.[128] Phosphorylation of HSP-27 is related to cellular growth and differentiation.[129] Overexpression of HSP-27 prevents actin depolymerization,[130] with the potential of affecting both cardiomyocytes and other cells. The role of HSPs in normal myocardiogenesis and in hypertrophy is yet to be elucidated, but they are constitutively expressed. Up- or downregulation by factors such as retroviral infection, anoxia, starvation, or malnutrition, or even excess thyroid hormone, may affect the normal cardiac hypertrophic response.

The Effect of Stretch on the Myocardium and Its Relation to HIV Cardiomyopathy

The HIV-infected patient experiences a great variation in loading conditions, which are transmitted through the heart. A patient may experience a low output state due to gastroenteric losses, anemia, malnutrition, or poor intake. Renal disease may induce a hypervolemic state. Intermittent sepsis may cause decompensated shock due to decreased systemic vascular resistance. These external loading conditions determine cardiac muscle mass and its phenotype. Mechanical stretch activates multiple signal transduction pathways in the cardiomyocytes, probably through autocrine and paracrine mechanisms.[106,131–135]

Alterations of the load on the cardiomyocytes have been shown to induce rapid and reversible changes in cardiac structure, composition, and function.[136] Cell length may increase by 10%, cell surface area by 8%, and sarcomere length by 7%. Stretch up to 20% induces hypertrophy in neonatal cardiomyocytes and hyperplasia in nonmyocytes by induction of the IEGs: c-*myc*, c-*fos*, c-*jun*, and *Egr*-1. Stretch may be transmitted to the nucleus of the cardiac myocyte through some mechanism other than electrical or direct mechanical transduction.[132]

Under mechanical load, angiotensin II is released, activating angiotensin receptors.[106] This increases the number of endothelin receptors and initiates the release of ET-1, which stimulates protein kinase C and subsequent protein synthesis. Some of the proposed mediators include the aforementioned tyrosine kinases, p21ras, mitogen-activated protein, protein kinase C, S6 kinases (pp90RSK), tyrosine kinase enzymes, and phospholipases C, D, A2, and P450.[131] There may also be stretch-activated cation channels, stimulation of cyclic AMP, and hydrolysis of inositol.[34] Activation of the tyrosine kinase pathway may initiate a cascade of secondary messages that lead to hypertrophy and occasionally to cell death. The tyrosine kinase pathways are involved in the mitogenic response to growth factors in cell lines capable of division, and are responsible for hypertrophy within the cardiomyocyte in response to stretch and humoral stimulation.[12] There is subsequent proliferation of skeletal α-actin,

ANF, and β-myosin heavy chain, which are normally expressed in the embryonic system. The stretch response can be mediated by cell medium transferred to nonstretched cells, which subsequently react by induction of the IEGs, indicating an autocrine/paracrine role in stretch-induced hypertrophy.[42]

For the stretch pathways to transmit their messages to induce hypertrophy, the IEGs and fetal protein production must be intact. The stretch transduction signal is not yet known. HIV recurrent episodes of sepsis, temperature lability, and hemodynamic instability are suspected to trigger the mechanical regulatory cascade inducing hypertrophy, but the mechanisms involved are unknown. It is speculated that the heterogeneous load distribution in the infarcted ventricle caused by abnormal shape changes in the chambers results in regional myocardial remodeling, leading to "greater elongation in noninfarcted myocardium adjacent to the infarct border."[12] This accounts for a variant of ventricular hypertrophy in ischemia. This type of remodeling in HIV cardiomyopathy remains to be explained.

The Renin–Angiotensin System in HIV Cardiomyopathy

Angiotensin II affects myocardial contractility and metabolism, as well as hypertrophic growth.[137] In hypertensive left ventricular hypertrophy, there is progressive interstitial and perivascular fibrosis, resulting in abnormal myocardial stiffness. This is attributed to enhanced growth of cardiac fibroblasts and synthesis of collagen,[138] which may represent the influence of the nonmyocyte components of the cardiac interstitium, important determinants of pathologic ventricular hypertrophy. The ventricular remodeling and compensatory hypertrophy commonly seen after a myocardial infarction are associated with the local increase in the production of angiotensin.[138]

The ACE inhibitors, which inhibit the products of the renin–angiotensin system, have been shown to reduce left ventricular mass while preserving its function. The improvement in diastolic function in these patients is not attributed to a decline in blood pressure, since there is no change in afterload.[138] In fact, chronic infusion of angiotensin II into rats

increased left ventricular mass, even when the pressor activity of the angiotensin was blocked.[139] There are similar findings with volume in spontaneously hypertensive rats that are salt-sensitive.[140] Rats pretreated with an ACE inhibitor and subsequently exposed to volume overload did not develop left ventricular hypertrophy, but in fact showed marked regression of hypertrophy.

In addition to its effects on the cardiac cytoskeleton, angiotensin acts as a second messenger in the stretch-mediated response. Such stimuli as sodium depletion, β-adrenergic agonists, and calcium-channel blockade suppress total cellular renin, whereas glucocorticoids, estrogens, and thyroid hormone markedly increase levels of angiotensin mRNA in the atria and ventricles. Nephrectomy has no effect on levels of angiotensin mRNA in the heart,[139] implying that the cardiac system itself is responsible for activation of the angiotensin response independently of the kidneys. It is the hemodynamic load that mediates the stretch stimulus, inducing the entire hypertrophy cascade. If the hemodynamic load is altered in HIV-infected patients, the angiotensin hypertrophy cascade may be initiated. It is unknown whether the retrovirus or any infectious agent targets the cardiac angiotensin system.

The ACE inhibitors are thought to "prevent the neurohumoral storm"[140] of typical congestive heart failure. With activation of catecholamines and the renin–angiotensin system, there is marked collagen I and II expression, with decreased α-myosin heavy chain and heart α-actin, and increased β-myosin heavy chain and skeletal α-actin. There is upregulation of TGF-β. If ACE inhibitors prevent the neurohumoral storm of heart failure, thereby preventing pathologic hypertrophy, there may be a role for them in the modulation and prevention of HIV cardiac muscle disease, depending on the renin–angiotensin system response in HIV-infected patients.

Catecholamines in HIV Cardiomyopathy

HIV directly infects the central nervous system, resulting in encephalopathy.[32] An HIV-associated autonomic neuropathy resulting in syncope and sudden death has been described.[33] The sinus tachycardia seen in HIV-infected patients has frequently been attributed to this autonomic dysfunction. In HIV-infected children, encephalopathy is correlated with increased morbidity and mortality from heart disease.[4]

The usual course of congestive heart failure involves an upregulation of circulating catecholamines, with a concomitant increase in the number of myocardial adrenergic receptors. The overall increase in the sympathetic tone of the failing heart serves to increase myocardial contractility, preserving cardiac function. In addition, increased sympathetic activity induces ventricular hypertrophy.[42,106] β-Adrenergic agonists induce increased protein synthesis, thereby increasing cell size and cellular protein mass.

According to some researchers, this system does not have a direct effect on hypertrophy, as increased sympathetic tone merely increases workload, which may itself induce ventricular hypertrophy.[42] It has been reported that α_1-adrenoreceptor transcription factors, extracellular signal factors such as ANF and TGF-β, and structural proteins such as β-myosin heavy chain are upregulated.[106]

The proteins that are induced are preferentially expressed during the fetal state of development. When cardiac growth is still occurring by myocyte proliferation, β-adrenergic stimulation inhibits division of myocytes. It subsequently promotes hypertrophy in a heart that has made the transition to growth by myocyte hypertrophy.[141] Several investigators have demonstrated the hypertrophic effects due to reexpression of the fetal program secondary to catecholamine stimulation.[142–145] In fact, it has been shown that norepinephrine may stimulate TGF-β, which in turn stimulates ANF, thereby inducing hypertrophy.

It seems likely that any autonomic disturbance created by the HIV infection should have an impact on neural and circulating catecholamines, which might in turn have an impact on the hypertrophic response. The sympathetic nervous system is another component of the hypertrophic response that might malfunction in HIV-infected patients.

Hydralazine and β-adrenergic antagonists, such as carvedilol, have been shown to prevent remodeling.[146] Blocking βII- and α_2-adrenergic receptors appears to prevent ventricular hypertrophy or reverse remodeling. This type of pharmacotherapy may have a role in the prevention of increased left ventricular mass in HIV cardiomyopathy.

Hormones and Their Effects in HIV Cardiomyopathy

Cytoplasmic intracellular receptors may be activated by a superfamily of related genes that includes estrogen, progesterone, mineralocorticoids, glucocorticoids, thyroxine, aldosterone, and retinoic acid. Any condition in an HIV-infected patient affecting growth factors or any of the superfamily of hormones could cause an abnormality in ventricular hypertrophy due to abnormal cell growth.

A condition that produces hyperthyroidism, for example, would induce a hypertrophic state. Thyroid hormone increases the mass of the heart by increasing the size of the cardiac myocyte. Thyroxine may act at the cellular level, where it binds to a nuclear receptor for thyroid hormone, c-*Erb*. There is then binding of the thyroid response element, with subsequent activation of genes to induce a myosin heavy chain and repression of the genes, that inhibit β-myosin heavy chain. Conversely, β-myosin heavy chain is expressed in the hypothyroid state. Thyroxine can also induce sodium and potassium ATPases, enzymes involved in diastolic relaxation. It activates calcium as a second messenger, with increases in calcium ATPase.[147,148]

The levels of circulating catecholamines are normal to decreased in hyperthyroidism and increased in hypothyroidism. Both chronotropy and inotropy are enhanced, suggesting that sensitivity to catecholamines increases in the hyperthyroid state. These effects, however, may be more related to increased sodium pump density and enhancement of sodium and potassium permeability. In hyperthyroidism, diastolic relaxation is enhanced, because of induction of the sodium-potassium pump ATPase and the SRCA. This causes the heart to function at its limit of contractile reserve. An increase in chronotropy and inotropy, coupled with an increase in total blood volume, creates a hemodynamic load that stresses the myocardium. The altered loading condition of the heart (increased preload with decreased afterload) induces the stretch response. Protooncogenes are induced, and the result is a stimulation of specific changes in the myosin isoforms and stimulation of myocardial protein synthesis due to an increased workload.[147,148]

HIV infection and associated opportunistic infections may affect thyroid function, resulting in state of thyroid abnormality. This condition would subsequently result in a state of cardiac hypertrophy, either appropriately or inappropriately.

Recently, growth hormone, a counterregulatory hormone opposing the action of insulin on carbohydrate and lipid metabolism and thereby maintaining muscle mass, has been used to treat dilated cardiomyopathy, with a focus toward increasing left ventricular mass.[51] It increased left ventricular function and improved isovolumic relaxation time. Other workers have found evidence that provision of IGF-I plus growth hormone causes only minor remodeling in pretreated rats that have had myocardial infarctions, with improvement in left ventricular index and performance.[149] Because these growth factors are nonspecific, they also caused body growth, a side effect that might be beneficial in cachectic HIV-infected patients.

It is notable that the mRNA for growth hormone receptors is expressed in mammalian myocytes.[52] The administration of growth hormone increases IGF-I in myocytes and induces expression of mRNA for IGF-I in the cardiomyocyte. IGF-I is a paracrine factor that directly activates protein synthesis in cardiomyocytes, thereby inducing hypertrophy.[106] A lack or aberrancy of growth hormone due to HIV infection, malnutrition, or endocrinologic diseases secondary to the HIV state would cause an abnormality of cardiomyocytes.

Glucocorticoids may induce hypertrophy. Dexamethasone used for the treatment of bronchopulmonary dysplasia in premature infants induces concentric ventricular hypertrophy.[86–89] The effects are reversible and seem to mimic the increase in left ventricular mass seen in the HIV-infected patient, although the neonatal heart may respond to steroids somewhat differently from the mature myocardium. Certainly steroids are crucial to the treatment programs of patients affected by lupus, asthma, or organ transplantation and may have variable effects on the myocardium. It may be that HIV-infected persons are transiently exposed to bursts of endogenous steroids due to fluctuating cortisol levels secondary to intermittent episodes of sepsis, which results in abnormal hypertrophy and mass out of proportion to body weight and size.

Other Factors Involved in HIV Cardiomyopathy

HIV-infected patients develop hypergammaglobulinemia. Retroviral-specific DNA is integrated into the genome, where it is dormant for a period of time. Upon reactivation, the virus assumes control of the genetic and biochemical machinery, causing a hyperactivation process, with a massive release of cytokines. This induces growth of T-lymphocytes and production of differentiation factors, which in turn stimulate B lymphocytes. The end result is hypergammaglobulinemia, which, although termed dysfunctional, may be functional in ventricular hypertrophy.

Left ventricular structure and function appear to be more normal in HIV-infected children who have received intravenous immunoglobulin (IVIG) treatment than in those children with higher endogenous IgG levels.[150] There is a significant increase in wall thickness and reduction in peak wall stress with IVIG and elevated IgG levels. The IVIG appears to somehow normalize left ventricular hypertrophy, which implies that left ventricular dysfunction may be immunologically mediated and responsive to immunomodulatory therapy.

In children with Kawasaki disease who have been given a therapeutic course of IVIG, left ventricular contractility has been shown to improve markedly.[151] This improvement has been seen as one of contractility rather than normalization of left ventricular hypertrophy. However, Kawasaki disease appears to be immune-modulated, with elevated TNF-α, IL-6, and IL-8,[152] and the IVIG likely plays a role in inhibiting the autoimmune aspect of this disease. In addition, IVIG may have a role in the treatment of myocarditis.[153,154] IVIG therapy completely obliterated the acute viremic stage in mice exposed to coxsackie virus B3, with a subsequent antiinflammatory effect in the aviremic stage of the disease. Thus the role of immunoglobulins in restoring ventricular function is likely to be that of suppression of cellular growth factors and cytokines. Natural IgG has been shown to inhibit TNF-α and IL-1$_\alpha$ production.[155]

TNF-α and IL-6 have been associated with HIV.[34,36] TNF-α, a proinflammatory cytokine and negative inotrope, is commonly found in states of septic shock, reperfusion injuries, congestive heart failure, and acute myocarditis.[156] It may be localized to the myocardium, where it is a potential signaling pathway. Cytomegalovirus transcripts have been shown to upregulate TNF-α production[157] and have been subsequently localized in the hearts of HIV-infected patients.[158] The ILs, particularly IL-1, induce the IEGs, c-*fos* and c-*jun* through different signaling transduction pathways.[159] These are the genes responsible for myocyte protein production and, ultimately, hypertrophy. Any alteration in induction of these pathways from any cytokine or growth mediators will affect ventricular hypertrophy.

HIV primary isolates that are resistant to INF-α, and seem to correlate with disease progression have been demonstrated in HIV-infected patients.[160] The IFNs are vital to the host response to viral infection and inhibit HIV retroviral replication within certain cell lines. In the early stages of viral replication, IFN represses HIV expression. Once there is progression to symptomatic HIV disease, IFN loses its efficacy in preventing HIV replication. This loss of efficacy may have a direct impact on the heart. For example, IFN has been used successfully to treat coxsackievirus myocarditis by reducing viral replication, with a distinct improvement in function.[161] The repression of this particular cytokine may have implications for the interaction with various growth factors within the cardiomyocytes.

Cardiomyopathy may be accompanied by a reactivation of genes expressed in fetal heart development. The cytokines IL-2 and IL-6, oncostatin M, ciliary neurotrophic factor, leukemia inhibiting factor, and cardiotrophin 1 have been shown to be expressed.[162] Cardiotrophin 1 appears to activate the hypertrophic response by inducing the immediate early genes: c-*fos*, c-*jun*, c-*myc*, and *Egr*-1, with reexpression of the ANF. ANF is one of the most prominent biologic markers of the hypertrophic response. This pathway may be instrumental in cardiac hypertrophy.

Cytokines and growth factors are proliferated in abundance in HIV infection in response to both the retrovirus itself and its accompanying opportunistic infections. These various factors mediate the hypertrophic response, and any inhibition or overexpression of any step will influence the production of a "normal" hypertrophic response to stress stimulus.

Does It All Come Down to Nitric Oxide?

Nitric oxide (NO) is a ubiquitous factor with a variety of functions in many organ systems. L-Arginine, through nitric oxide synthase, forms L-citrulline, releasing NO. This reaction may reverse, reforming L-arginine at the expense of ATP and guaranteeing a constant supply of NO, as long as ATP is provided. NO interacts with the heme prosthetic group of cytosolic guanylate cyclase (cGMP), which translates the actions of NO.[163]

NO has been implicated in maintaining vascular tone, affects macrophage tumoricidal and bactericidal activities, and affects signal transduction, cellular dysfunction, and, ultimately, death. How and where NO is produced depends on its cellular location, the activating factors, and the form of NO synthase (NOS). There are three forms of NOS: cNOS, the constitutive form of the enzyme present in endothelium; bNOS, the enzyme present in neurologic tissues, such as the sinoatrial and atrioventricular nodes; and iNOS, the inducible form of the enzyme.[164] Whereas the constitutive and neurologic forms of NOS are important in maintaining vascular tone as well as myocardial contractility and chronotropy, the inducible NOS may have devastating effects. "Physiologic" elevation of cGMP by NO may preserve myocardial function, whereas great increases in NO depress myocardial function.[165] NO produced by iNOS may be cytotoxic, if not lethal. The iNOS is cytokine-inducible and calcium-independent.[166] It is becoming increasingly apparent that NO is mediated by many cytokines and growth factors, including TNF-α, IL-1β, IFN-γ, IL-6, TGF-β, ET-1, prostaglandin E_2 (PGE$_2$), and prostaglandin I_2 (PGI$_2$).[166–169] TNF and NO are expressed in dilated cardiomyopathy, septic shock, allograft rejection, and viral myocarditis.[170] NO may be the common pathway for many cascades. Inflammatory cytokines such as IL-1, IFN-γ, and TNF-α, may induce 100 to 1000 times the levels of NOS that cells might usually produce.[171] At best, there is evidence of myocardial dysfunction and diminished protein production in myocytes and nonmyocytes. At worst, there is myocyte necrosis and cell death. In fact, one study of dilated cardiomyopathy found that in addition to its negative inotropic effect, the NO resulting from TNF-stimulated iNOS was cytotoxic and likely resulted in cell death.[170] In this study, iNOS was produced most strongly in myocytes and less intensely in the endothelial cells.

In endotoxemia and septic shock, NO is overproduced as a result of expression of iNOS. The same state is noted in allograft rejection.[171] NO is liberated during transplant rejection by CD4+ and CD8+ lymphocytes[167]; this form of iatrogenically induced immunosuppression closely mimics that in HIV infection. Although the cytokines and growth factors, the stimuli inducing these factors, and the mechanisms by which NO is elaborated vary, the common pathway is NO. If NO is a common point, can its production be regulated so that only levels that are not cytotoxic are produced? NO is likely to play a major role in the protein synthesis involved in ventricular hypertrophy. Given that fact that the HIV-infected state induces cytokine production, NO must be present in various quantities in various organ systems throughout the host.

The State of Malnourishment and its Relation to HIV Cardiomyopathy

Malnutrition is common at all ages and at various stages of HIV infection.[6] In the HIV-negative patient, malnutrition is accompanied by ventricular dilatation, an overall decrease in blood pressure, and loss of ventricular mass.[25,26] The inadequate nutrition may contribute to a subnormal hypertrophic response; however, the overall left ventricular mass for body surface area was still 184% of normal.[10,11,16,17] Factors other than malnutrition are implied in the development of HIV cardiomyopathy.

There is a known association between insulin resistance, hypertension, and left ventricular hypertrophy. Hypertrophy may precede the development of hypertension. Insulinomas have been shown to cause a form of hypertrophic cardiomyopathy, and

the literature is replete with reports of concentric hypertrophy in the infants of diabetic mothers who are exposed to relative hyperinsulinemic states.[83]

Insulin stimulates the uptake and metabolism of glucose in regulatory cells, which inhibits the regulatory cells in the brainstem. The sympathetic regulatory centers in the brainstem are disinhibited, which increases sympathetic activity.[172] It may be the increased sympathetic tone in hyperinsulinemic states that induces hypertrophy indirectly, or the direct effect of insulin on the IGF systems may produce hypertrophy. The IGFs have been shown to increase protein synthesis in cardiomyocytes,[106] but their role in hypertrophy remains ill-defined.

Researchers using Langendorf-perfused rat hearts have shown that myocardial function during states of depressed myocardial contractility can improved by perfusing a combination of glucose and insulin.[29] Glucose provides the necessary energy substrates to the heart, while insulin improves uptake. The actual effects on the hypertrophic pathways and normalization of peak systolic wall stress remain to be explored. If the HIV host is consistently malnourished, the energy substrates, glucose utilization, and insulin levels are bound to be subnormal, thereby affecting overall cardiac contractility and the hypertrophic state.

Neonatal Expression Versus Senility in HIV Cardiomyopathy

If reexpression of the neonatal program is crucial to ventricular hypertrophy, then premature senescence, with a resultant attenuated response to hypertrophy, would change the expected hypertrophic response of the myocardium, greatly reducing the cardiac adaptive response to stress. Overall protein synthesis would be diminished, which would preclude immediate replacement of contractile myofibers and damaged mitochondria.

Common age-associated myocardial changes in humans include an increase in the size of the myocytes with an increase in the rate of degenerative changes; increased deposition of lipid, elastic tissue, and collagen; increased deposition of lipofuscin, representing oxidized lipid pigments derived from mitochondrial membranes; a decrease in oxidative phosphorylation; and an increase in tubular dilatation.[173] In spite of the increase in myocyte volume and nuclear size, the number of myocytes diminishes, resulting in an increase in wall thickness but no change in overall heart size.

The hearts of aged rats have a decreased capacity to develop left ventricular hypertrophy in response to stress.[174] This is due to a decreased production of the protooncogenes c-*fos* and c-*jun*. There is also a delayed response in switching from the production of β-myosin heavy chain to α-myosin heavy chain, steps that are necessary to induce proper hypertrophic growth of the cardiomyocytes. The pattern of gene expression in aged rats is quantitatively and qualitatively different from that in younger rats. It is possible that HIV-infected patients manifest a form of premature senescence that induces a deficiency in reexpression of the fetal gene program, precluding a normal hypertrophic state. The inconsistency lies in the fact that HIV-infected children manifest greatly increased left ventricular mass for age and size, in spite of inadequate left ventricular hypertrophy for level of stress.

Programmed Cell Death in HIV Cardiomyopathy

Cells have developed a sort of programmed housekeeping known as apoptosis. Cellular degeneration is not a passive necrotic process, but rather an endogenous, physiologically regulated cell pathway. With the exception of embryonic blastomeres, cells undergo apoptosis when they are deprived of exogenous signals or cell contacts; induction of apoptosis must be repressed and expressed appropriately.[175] Normal cardiac embryogenesis relies on controlled apoptosis, allowing proper resorption of structures and connections no longer required for the mature organism. Apoptosis controls the destruction of cells, structures, and tissues that are no longer required by the organism. The inhibition of apoptosis may also result in the immortalization of cells.

Structures that have become hypertrophied may not regress or degenerate appropriately if the process of apoptosis is impaired. HIV causes inappropriate apoptosis by inducing the expression of host genes that regulate this process.[175] The virus or other infectious agent may impair intracellular and intercellular signaling, resulting in inappropriate death of infected and uninfected cell populations. Cell depletion caused by expression of host genes may promote atrophy, thereby impairing a "normal" hypertrophic response.

HIV is a disease in which retroviral interference, or mediated interference with apoptosis at different times in different cell populations, may result simultaneously in premature cell death and immortalization.[175] The result might be concomitant cell death and cell proliferation, which would induce an abnormal or deficient cardiac hypertrophic response while causing overall increased ventricular mass. The role of apoptosis in HIV cardiomyopathy remains to be investigated.

Summary

There is a primary abnormality of cardiac growth in HIV-infected patients, with increased left ventricular mass corrected for body surface area, yet inadequate ventricular hypertrophy to compensate for increased systolic wall stress induced by the increased afterload common to these patients. The patients are subject to increased morbidity and mortality due to the abnormal cardiac growth. HIV cardiac muscle disease has a multifactorial etiology, with a primary abnormality in the reexpression of the neonatal program for proper induction of cardiac hypertrophy. Malnutrition, cytokines and growth factors, varying hemodynamic states, fluctuating endocrinologic states, autonomic neuropathy, temperature instability, possible early senility, and abnormalities of the apoptotic response all interact in the cardiac hypertrophic abnormalities. Pharmacologic interventions, such as β-adrenergic antagonism, hydralazine, and ACE inhibition, have potential in the regulation of hypertrophy. NO is a common pathway of cardiac demise, and regulation of its production may be key to preserving the myocardium in the disease milieu. To target therapy more effectively, it will be necessary for future researchers to find the common pathway through which all of these factors are funneled.

Acknowledgments

We are indebted to Dr. Michael Flanagan, Dr. Carol Kasten-Sportès, and Dr. Douglas Mann for critical review of this chapter.

References

1. Fink L, Reichek N, Sutton MG. Cardiac abnormalities in acquired immunodeficiency syndrome. *Am J Cardiol* 1984;54:1161–1163.

2. Lipshultz SE, Chanock S, Sanders S, et al. Cardiovascular manifestations of human immunodeficiency virus in infants and children. *Am J Cardiol* 1989;63:1489–1497.

3. Kavanaugh-McHugh A, Ruff AJ, Rowe SA, et al. Cardiovascular abnormalities. In: Pizzo PA, Wilfert CM (eds). *Pediatric AIDS*. Baltimore: Williams & Wilkins, 1991:355–372.

4. Luginbuhl LM, Orav EJ, McIntosh K, Lipshultz SG. Cardiac morbidity and related mortality in children with HIV infection. *JAMA* 1993;296:2869–2875.

5. Frenkel Z, Serianda G. Perinatal HIV infection and AIDS. *Clin Perinatol* 1994;21:95–107.

6. Lipshultz SE. Cardiovascular problems. In: Pizzo PA, Wilfert CM (eds). *Pediatric AIDS*. Baltimore: Williams & Wilkins, 1994:355–372.

7. Dec GW, Fuster V. Idiopathic dilated cardiomyopathy. *N Engl J Med* 1994;331:1564–1578.

8. Lipshultz SE, Bancroft EA, Boller AM. Cardiovascular manifestations of HIV infection in children. In: Bricker JT (ed). *The Science and Practice of Pediatric Cardiology,* 2nd Ed. Baltimore: Williams & Wilkins, 1996.

9. Lipshultz SE, Orav JE, Sanders SP, et al. Limitations of fractional shortening as an index of contractility in pediatric patients infected with human immunodeficiency virus. *J Pediatr* 1994;125:563–570.

10. Lipshultz SE, Chanock S, Sanders SP, et al. Cardiac manifestations of pediatric HIV infection. [Abstract] *Circulation* 1987;76:IV-515.

11. Lipshultz SE, Sanders SP, Colan SD, et al. Does the increased myocardial mass seen in pediatric HIV result from direct infection of cardiocytes? [Abstract]. *Circulation* 1989;80:II-322.

12. Melillo G, Lima JAC, Judd RM, et al. Intrinsic myocyte dysfunction and tyrosine kinase pathway activation underlie the impaired wall thickening of adjacent regions during postinfarct left ventricular remodeling. *Circulation* 1996;93:1447–1458.

13. Joshi VV, Gadol C, Connor E, et al. Dilated cardiomyopathy in children with acquired immunodeficiency syndrome: pathologic study of five cases. *Hum Pathol* 1988;19:69–73.

14. Bharati S, Joshi VV, Connor EM, et al. Conduction system in children with acquired immunodeficiency syndrome. *Chest* 1989;96:406–413.

15. Joshi VV. Pathology of childhood AIDS. *Pediatr Clin North Am* 1991;38:97–120.

16. Lipshultz SE, Miller TL, Orav EJ, McIntosh K. Exaggerated myocardial hypertrophic responses in pediatric HIV infection. [Abstract]. *Circulation* 1990;82:111.

17. Lipshultz SE, Orav EJ, Sanders SP, et al. Progressive abnormalities of cardiac structure and function in HIV-infected children treated with AZT. [Abstract]. *Pediatr Res* 1992;31:169A.

18. McMinn TR, Ross U. Hereditary dilated cardiomyopathy. *Clin Cardiol* 1995;18:7–15.

19. Limas CJ, Limas C, Goldenberg IF, Blair R. Possible involvement of the HLA–DQB1 gene in susceptibility and resistance to human dilated cardiomyopathy. *Am Heart J* 1995;129:1141–1144.

20. Latif N, Baker CS, Dunn MJ, et al. Frequency and specificity of antiheart antibodies in patients with dilated cardiomyopathy detected using SDS-PAGE and Western blotting. *J Am Coll Cardiol* 1993;22:1378–1384.

21. Anderson DW, Virmani R, Reilly JM, et al. Emerging patterns of heart disease in HIV. *Hum Pathol* 1990;21:253–259.

22. Baroldi G, Corallo S, Moroni M, et al. Focal lymphocytic myocarditis in AIDS: a correlative and morphologic and clinical study in 26 fatal cases. *J Am Coll Cardiol* 1988;12:463–469.

23. Lipshultz SE, Fox CH, Perez-Atayde AR, et al. Identification of human immunodeficiency virus-1 RNA and DNA in the heart of a child with cardiovascular abnormalities and congenital acquired immune deficiency syndrome. *Am J Cardiol* 1990;66:246–250.

24. Rodriguez ER, Nasim S, Hsia J, et al. Cardiac myocytes and dendritic cells harbor HIV in infected patients with and without cardiac dysfunc-

tion: detection by multiplex, nested, polymerase chain reaction in individually microdissected cells from right ventricular endomyocardial biopsy tissue. *Am J Cardiol* 1991;68:1511–1520.

25. Webb JG, Kiebs MC, Chan-Yan CC. Malnutrition and the heart. *Can Med Assoc J* 1986;135:753.

26. Alden PB, Madoff RD, Stahl TJ, et al. Cardiac function in malnutrition. In: Watson RR (ed). *Nutrition and Heart Disease.* Boca Raton, FL: CRC Press, 1987;2:71–81.

27. Samaan SA, Foster A, Raizada V, et al. Myocardial atrophy in acquired immunodeficiency syndrome-associated wasting. *Am Heart J* 1995;130: 823–827.

28. Taegtmeyer H. Energy metabolism of the heart: from basic concepts to clinical applications. *Curr Prob Cardiol* 1994;19:57–116.

29. Arnaudo E, Dalakas M, Shanske S, Moraes C. Depletion of muscle mitochondrial DNA in AIDS patients with zidovudine-induced myopathy. *Lancet* 1991;377:508–510.

30. Lewis W, Simpson JF, Meyer RR. Cardiac mitochondrial DNA polymerase–gamma is inhibited competitively and noncompetitively by non-phosphorylated zidovudine. *Circ Res* 1994;74: 344–348.

31. Lipshultz SE, Orav EJ, Sanders SP, et al. Cardiac structure and function in children with human immunodeficiency virus infection treated with zidovudine. *N Engl J Med* 1992;327:1260–1265.

32. Epstein LG, Sharer LR, Oleske JM, et al. Neurologic manifestations of human immunodeficiency virus infection in children. *Pediatrics* 1986:78: 678–687.

33. Craddock C, Pasvol G, Bull R, et al. Cardiorespiratory arrest and autonomic neuropathy in AIDS. *Lancet* 1987:16–18.

34. Matsuyama T, Kobayashi N, Yamamoto N. Cytokines and HIV infection: is AIDS a tumor necrosis factor disease? *AIDS* 1991;5:1405–1417.

35. Rautonen J, Rautonen N, Martin NL, et al. Serum interleukin-6 concentrations are elevated and associated with tumor necrosis factor-α and immunoglobulin G and A concentrations in children with HIV infection. *AIDS* 1991;5:1319–1325.

36. Odeh J. Tumor necrosis factor-α as a myocardial depressant substance. *Int J Cardiol* 1993;42: 231–238.

37. Herskowitz A, Willoughby S, Wu TC, et al. Immunopathogenesis of HIV-1-associated cardiomyopathy. *Clin Immunol Immunopathol* 1993;68: 234–241.

38. Lipshultz SE, Chanock S, Sanders SP, et al. Cardiovascular manifestations of human immunodeficiency virus infection in infants and children. *Am J Cardiol* 1989;63:1489–1497.

39. Devereux RB, Reichek N. Determination of left ventricular mass in man. *Circulation* 1977;55: 613–618.

40. Devereux RB, Alonso DR, Lutas EM, et al. Echocardiographic assessments of left ventricular hypertrophy: comparison to necropsy findings. *Am J Cardiol* 1986;57:450–458.

41. Frohlich ED, Apstein C, Chobanian A, et al. The heart in hypertension. *N Engl J Med* 1992;327: 988–1007.

42. Mann DL, Roberts R. The molecular basis for hypertrophic growth of the adult heart. In: McCall D, Rahimtoola SH (eds). *Heart Failure.* New York: Chapman and Hall, 1995:67–88.

43. Grenier MA, Karr SS, Rakusan TA, Martin GR. Cardiac disease in children with HIV: relationship of cardiac disease to HIV symptomatology. *Pediatr AIDS HIV Infect Fetus Adolesc* 1994;5: 174–178.

44. Lipshultz SE for the Pediatric Pulmonary and Cardiovascular Complications of Vertically Transmitted HIV P^{2}C^2 Study. Cardiac dysfunction predicts mortality in HIV-infected children: the prospective NHLBI P^{2}C^2 study. [Abstract]. *Proc Conf Retrov Opportun Infect* 1996;130.

45. Kearney DL for the Pediatric Pulmonary and Cardiovascular Complications of Vertically Transmitted HIV P^{2}C^2 Study. Postmortem cardiomegaly correlates with premortem measurements of left ventricular size in malnourished HIV-infected children . [Abstract] *Proc Conf Retrov Opportun Infect* 1996;133.

46. Grossman W, Jones D, McLaurin LP. Wall stress and patterns of hypertrophy in the human left ventricle. *J Clin Invest* 1975;56:56–64.

47. Grossman W. Cardiac hypertrophy: useful adaptation or pathologic process? *Am J Med* 1980; 69:576.

48. Anversa P, Ricci R, Olivetti G. Quantitative structural analysis of the myocardium during physiologic growth and induced cardiac hypertrophy: review. *J Am Coll Cardiol* 1986;7:1140–1149.

49. Oakley C. Ventricular hypertrophy in cardiomyopathy. *Br Heart J* 1971;33:179–186.

50. Field BJ, Baxley WA, Russel RO, et al. Left ventricular function and hypertrophy in cardiomyopathy with depressed ejection fraction. *Circulation* 1973;47:1027–1031.

51. Fazio S, Sabatini D, Capaldo B, et al. A preliminary study of growth hormone in the treatment of dilated cardiomyopathy. *N Engl J Med* 1996;334:809–814.

52. Loh E, Swain JL. Growth hormone for heart failure: cause for cautious optimism. *N Engl J Med* 1996;334:856–857.

53. Kimball TR, Daniels SR, Meyer RA, et al. Left ventricular mass in childhood dilated cardiomyopathy: a possible predictor for selection of patients for cardiac transplantation. *Am Heart J* 1991;122:126–131.

54. Kannel NB, Gordon T, Offutt D. Left ventricular hypertrophy by ECG. Prevalence, incidence, and mortality in the Framingham study. *Ann Intern Med* 1969;71:89–105.

55. Messerli FH, Ventura HO, Elizardi DJ, et al. Hypertension and sudden death: increased ventricular ectopic activity in left ventricular hypertrophy. *Am J Med* 1984;77:18–22.

56. Casale PR, Devereux RB, Millner M, et al. Value of echocardiographic measurement of left ventricular mass in predicting cardiovascular morbid events in hypertensive man. *Ann Intern Med* 1986;105:173–178.

57. McLenachan JM, Henderson E, Morris KI, Dargie MJ. Ventricular arrhythmias in patients with hypertensive left ventricular hypertrophy. *N Engl J Med* 1987;317:787–792.

58. Liao Y, Cooper RS, Mensa GA, McGee DL. Left ventricular hypertrophy has a greater impact on survival in women than in men. *Circulation* 1995;92:805–810.

59. Ghali JK, Liao Y, Simmons B, et al. The prognostic role of left ventricular hypertrophy in patients with or without coronary artery disease. *Ann Intern Med* 1992;117:831–836.

60. Post WS, Larson MG, Levy D. Impact of left ventricular structure on the incidence of hypertension: the Framingham Heart Study. *Circulation* 1994;90:179–185.

61. Shub C, Klein A, Zachariah PK, et al. Determination of left ventricular mass by echocardiography in a normal population: effect of age and sex in addition to body size. *Mayo Clin Proc* 1994;69:205–211.

62. Lauer MS, Anderson KM, Kanner WB, Levy D. The impact of obesity on left ventricular mass and geometry: the Framingham Study. *JAMA* 1991;266:231–236.

63. Duflou J, Virmani R, Rabin I, et al. Sudden death as a result of heart disease in morbid obesity. *Am Heart J* 1995;130:306–313.

64. Urbina EM, Gidding SS, Bao W, et al. Effect of body size, ponderosity, and blood pressure on left ventricular growth in children and young adults in the Bogalusa Heart Study. *Circulation* 1995;91:2400–2406.

65. Cooper G. Cardiocyte adaptation to chronically altered load. *Annu Rev Physiol* 1987;49:501–518.

66. Himeno E, Nishino K, Nakashima Y, et al. Weight reduction regresses left ventricular mass regardless of blood pressure level in obese subjects. *Am Heart J* 1996;131:313–319.

67. Frohlich ED. The heart in hypertension: unresolved conceptual challenges. *Hypertension* 1988;11:I-19–I-24.

68. Fouad FM, Tarazi RC, Liebson RR. Echocardiographic studies of regression of left ventricular hypertrophy in hypertension. *Hypertension* 1987;9:11-65–11-68.

69. Maron BJ. Sudden death in young athletes. *N Engl J Med* 1993;329:55–57.

70. Topaz O, Edwards JE. Pathologic features of sudden death in children, adolescents and young adults. *Chest* 1985;87:476–482.

71. Maron BJ, Epstein SE, Roberts WC. Causes of sudden death in competitive athletes. *J Am Coll Cardiol* 1986;7:204–214.

72. Burke AP, Farb A, Virmani R, et al. Sports-related and non-sports-related sudden cardiac death in young adults. *Am Heart J* 1991;121:568–575.

73. Epstein SE, Maron BJ. Sudden death and the competitive athlete: perspectives on preparticipation screening studies. *J Am Coll Cardiol* 1986;7:220–230.

74. Maron BJ, Bodison SA, Wesley YE, et al. Results of screening a large group of intercollegiate competitive athletes for cardiovascular disease. *J Am Coll Cardiol* 1987;10:1214–1221.

75. Colan SD, Sanders SP, Boron KM. Physiologic hypertrophy: effects of left ventricular systolic mechanics for athletes. *J Am Coll Cardiol* 1987;9:776–783.

76. Liu SK, Roberts WC, Maron BJ. Comparison of morphologic findings in spontaneously occurring

hypertrophic cardiomyopathy in humans, cats and dogs. *Am J Cardiol* 1993;72:944–951.

77. Flanagan MF, Aoyagi T, Currier JJ, et al. Effect of young age on coronary adaptations to left ventricular pressure overload hypertrophy in sheep. *J Am Coll Cardiol* 1994;24:1786–1796.

78. Rakusan K, Flanagan MF, Geva T, et al. Morphometry of human coronary capillaries during normal growth and the effect of age in left ventricular pressure-overload hypertrophy. *Circulation* 1992; 86:38–46.

79. Hirsch HD, Gelband H, Garcia O, Gottlieb S. Rapidly progressive obstructive cardiomyopathy in infants with Noonan syndrome. *Circulation* 1975;52:1161–1165.

80. Van Der Hauwaert LG, Fryns JP, Dumoulin M, Logghe N. Cardiovascular malformations in Turner's and Noonan's syndrome. *Br Heart J* 1978; 40:500–509.

81. Bobele GB, Ward KE, Bodensteiner JB. Hypertrophic cardiomyopathy during corticotropin therapy for infantile spasms: a clinical and echocardiographic study. *Am J Dis Child* 1993;147:223–228.

82. Zosmer N, Bajoria R, Wejner E, et al. Clinical and echocardiographic features of in utero cardiac dysfunction in the recipient twin in twin-twin transfusion syndrome (TTTS). *Br Heart J* 1994; 72:74–79.

83. Breitweser JA, Meyer RA, Sperling MA, et al. Cardiac septal hypertrophy in hyperinsulinemic infants. *J Pediatr* 1980;96:535–539.

84. McMahon JN, Berry PJ, Joffe HS. Fatal hypertrophic cardiomyopathy in an infant of a diabetic mother. *Pediatr Cardiol* 1990;11:211–212.

85. Kimball TR, Witt SA, Daniels SR, et al. Frequency and significance of left ventricular thickening in transplanted hearts in children. *Am J Cardiol* 1996;77:77–80.

86. Werner JC, Sicard RE, Hansen TWR, et al. Hypertrophic cardiomyopathy associated with dexamethasone therapy for bronchopulmonary dysplasia. *J Pediatr* 1992;120:286–291.

87. Israel BA, Sherman FS, Guthrie RD. Hypertrophic cardiomyopathy associated with dexamethasone therapy for chronic lung disease in preterm infants. *Am J Perinatol* 1993;10:307–310.

88. Ohning BL, Fyfe DA, Riedel PA. Reversible obstructive hypertrophic cardiomyopathy after dexamethasone therapy for bronchopulmonary dysplasia. *Am Heart J* 1993;125:253–256.

89. Evans N. Cardiovascular effects of dexamethasone in the preterm infant. *Arch Dis Child* 1994; 70:F25-F30.

90. Silver MM, Silver MD. Left ventricular hypertrophy vs. hypertrophic cardiomyopathy. [Editorial]. *J Pediatr* 1992;12:500–501.

91. Vogel M, Staller W, Buhlmeyer K. Left ventricular mass determined by cross-sectional echocardiography in normal newborns, infants, and children. *Pediatr Cardiol* 1991;12:143–149.

92. Sicard RE, Werner JC. Dexamethasone induces a transient relative cardiomegaly in neonatal rats. *Pediatr Res* 1992;31:359–363.

93. Colan SD, Parness IA, Spevak PJ, Sanders SP. Developmental modulation of myocardial mechanics: age- and growth-related alterations in afterload and contractility. *J Am Coll Cardiol* 1992;19:619–629.

94. Chien K, Knowlton K, Zhu H, Chien S. Regulation of cardiac gene expression during myocardial growth and hypertrophy: molecular studies of an adaptive physiologic response. *FASEB J* 1991;5: 3037–3046.

95. Pasumarthi KBS, Jin Y, Bock ME, et al. Characteristics of fibroblast growth factor receptor/RNA expression in the embryonic mouse heart. *Ann NY Acad Sci* 1995;752:406–416.

96. Sugi Y, Sasse J, Barron M, Lough J. Developmental expression of fibroblast growth factor receptor-1 (cek-1fg) during heart development. *Dev Dynam* 1995;202:115–125.

97. Mima T, Veno H, Fischman DA, et al. Fibroblast growth factor receptor is required for in vivo cardiac myocyte proliferation of early embryonic stages of heart development. *Proc Natl Acad Sci USA* 1995;92:467–471.

98. Florini JR, Enton DJ, Magri KA. Hormones, growth factors, and myogenic differentiation. *Annu Rev Physiol* 1991;53:201–216.

99. Sakai S, Miyauchi T, Sakurai T, et al. Endogenous endothelin-1 participates in the maintenance of cardiac function in rats with congestive heart failure. *Circulation* 1996;93:1214–1222.

100. Kachinsky AM, Dominov JA, Miller JB. Intermediate filaments in cardiac myogenesis: nestin in the developing mouse heart. *J Histochem Cytochem* 1995;43:843–847.

101. Lotz M, Seth P. TGF β and HIV infection. *Ann NY Acad Sci* 1993;685:501–511.

102. Saunders KB, D'Amore PA. FGF and TFG β-actions and interactions in biological systems. *Crit Rev Euk Gene Exp* 1991;1:157–172.

103. Flanagan MF, Aoyagi T, Fujii AM, et al. Effects of heparin on coronary vasculature with pressure overload hypertrophy. [Abstract]. *Circulation* 1994;90:1378.

104. Flanagan MF, Aoyagi T, Arnold L, et al. Age, bFGF and coronary adaptations to left ventricular pressure overload hypertrophy. [Abstract]. *J Am Coll Cardiol* 1994;93A.

105. Engelmann GL, Boehm KD, Birchenall-Roberts MC, Ruscetti FW. Transforming growth factor-β in heart development. *Mech Dev* 1992;38:85–98.

106. Schluter KD, Millar BC, McDermott BJ, Piper HM. Regulation of protein synthesis and degradation in adult ventricular cardiomyocytes. *Am J Physiol* 1995;269:C1347–C1355.

107. MacLellan WR, Brand T, Schneider MD. Transforming growth factor-β in cardiac ontogeny and adaptation. *Circ Res* 1993;73:783–791.

108. Slager HG, Van Inzen W, Freund E, et al. Transforming growth factor-β in the early mouse embryo: implications for the regulation of muscle formation and implantation. *Dev Genet* 1993;14:212–224.

109. Roberts AB, Roche NS, Winokur TS, et al. Role of transforming growth factor-β maintenance of function of cultured neonatal cardiac myocytes. *J Clin Invest* 1992;90:2056–2062.

110. Powell-Braxton L, Hollingshead P, Warburton C, et al. IGF-1 is required for normal embryonic growth in mice. *Genes Dev* 1993;12B:2609–2617.

111. Duerr R, Huang S, Miraliakbar HR, et al. Insulin-like growth factor 1 enhances ventricular hypertrophy and function during the onset of experimental cardiac failure. *J Clin Invest* 1995;95:619–627.

112. Shaddy RE, Hammond EH, Yowell RL. Immunohistochemical analysis of platelet-derived growth factor in cardiac biopsy and autopsy specimens of heart transplant patients. *Am J Cardiol* 1996;77:1210–1215.

113. Yangisawa M, Kurihara H, Kimura S, et al. A novel potent vasoconstrictor peptide produced by vascular endothelial cells. *Nature* 1988;332:411–415.

114. Suzuki T, Kumazaki T, Mitsui Y. Endothelin-1 is produced and secreted by neonatal rat cardiac myocytes in vitro. *Biochem Biophys Res Commun* 1993;191:823–830.

115. Yorikane R, Sakai S, Miyauchi T, et al. Increased production of ET-1 in the hypertrophied rat heart due to pressure overload. *FEBS Lett* 1993;332:31–34.

116. Miyauchi T, Yorikane I, Sakai S, et al. Contribution of endogenous ET-1 to the progression of cardiopulmonary alterations in rats with monocrotaline-induced pulmonary hypertension. *Circ Res* 1993;73:887–897.

117. Yoshizumi M, Kurihara H, Sugiyama T, et al. Hemodynamic shear stress stimulates endothelin production by cultured endothelial cells. *Biochem Biophys Res Commun* 1989;161:859–864.

118. Sumpio BE, Widman MD. Enhanced production of endothelium-derived contracting factors by endothelial cells subjected to pulsatile stretch. *Surgery* 1990;108:277–281.

119. Sakai S, Miyauchi T, Sakurai T, et al. Endogenous endothelin–1 participates in the maintenance of cardiac function in rats with congestive heart failure. *Circulation* 1996;93:1214–1222.

120. Takenaka IM, Hightower LE. Transforming growth factor-β1 rapidly induces HSP 70 and HSP 90 chaperones in cultured chicken embryo cells. *J Cell Physiol* 1992;152:568–577.

121. Takenaka IM, Hightower LE. Regulation of chicken Hsp 70 and Hsp 90 family gene expression by transforming growth factor-β1. *J Cell Physiol* 1993;155:54–62.

122. Williams RS, Benjamin IJ. Stress proteins and cardiovascular disease. *Mol Biol Med* 1991;8:197–206.

123. Marber MS. Stress proteins and myocardial protection. *Clin Sci* 1994;86:375–381.

124. Mestril R, Dillman WH. Heat shock proteins and protection against myocardial ischemia. *J Mol Cell Cardiol* 1995;27:45–52.

125. Knowlton AA. The role of heat shock proteins in the heart. *J Mol Cell Cardiol* 1995;27:121–131.

126. Knowlton AA, Eberli FR, Brecher P, et al. A single myocardial stretch or decreased systolic fiber shortening stimulates the expression of heat shock protein 70 in the isolated, erythocyte-perfused rabbit heart. *J Clin Invest* 1991;88:2018–2025.

127. Atkinson BG. Synthesis of heat shock proteins by cells undergoing myogenesis. *J Cell Biol* 1981;89:666–673.

128. Benndorf R, Hayess K, Ryazantsev S, et al. Phosphorylation and supramolecular organization of

murine small heat shock protein Hsp25 abolish its actin polymerization-inhibiting activity. *J Biol Chem* 1994;269:20780–20784.

129. Mehlen P, Arrigo AP. The serum-induced phosphorylation of mammalian HSP 27 correlates with changes in its intracellular localizations and levels of oligomerization. *Eur J Biochem* 1994;221: 327–334.

130. Lavoie JU, Hickey E, Weber LA, et al. Modulation of actin microfilament dynamics and fluid phase pinocytosis by phosphorylation of HSP 27. *J Biol Chem* 1993;263:24210–24214.

131. Sadoshima JI, Izumo S. Mechanical stretch rapidly activates multiple signal transduction pathways in cardiac myocytes: potential involvement in an autocrine/paracrine mechanism. *EMBO J* 1993; 12:1681–1692.

132. Sadoshima JI, Takahashi T, Jahn L, Izumo S. Roles of mechanosensitive channels, cytoskeleton, and contractile activity in stretch-induced immediate-early gene expression and hypertrophy of cardiac myocytes. *Proc Natl Acad Sci USA* 1992;89:9905–9909.

133. Sadoshima JI, Jahn L, Takahashi T, et al. Molecular characterizations of the stretch-induced adaptation of cultured cardiac cells. *J Biol Chem* 1992; 267:10551–10560.

134. Komoro I, Kaida T, Shibazaki Y, et al. Stretching cardiac myocytes stimulates protooncogene expression. *J Biol Chem* 1990;265:3595–3598.

135. Komoro I, Katoh Y, Kaida T, et al. Mechanical loading stimulates cell hypertrophy and specific gene expression in cultured rat cardiac myocytes: possible role of protein kinase C activation. *J Biol Chem* 1991;266:1265–1268.

136. Mann DC, Kent RL, Cooper GN. Load regulation of the properties of adult feline cardiocytes: growth induction by cellular deformation. *Circ Res* 1989;64:1079–1090.

137. Weber KT, Brilla CG. Pathological hypertrophy and cardiac interstitial fibrosis and renin-angiotensin aldosterone system. *Circulation* 1991;83: 1849–1865.

138. Orev S, Grossman E, Frohlich E. Reduction in left ventricular mass in patients with systemic hypertension treated with enalapril, lisinopril, fosenopril. *Am J Cardiol* 1996;77:93–96.

139. Baker KM, Booz GW, Dostal DE. Cardiac actions of angiotension II: role of an intracardiac renin-angiotensin system. *Annu Rev Physiol* 1992;54: 227–241.

140. Bing O. Presentation at symposium on "Hypertrophy and Remodeling: From the Molecule to the Myocardium." April 24, 1996, Boston.

141. Love TC, Tucker DC. Timing of sympathetic innervation affects growth of myocardium in oculo. *Am J Physiol* 1995;269:H140–H148.

142. Iwaki K, Sukhatme VP, Shubeita HE, Chien KR. α- and β-Adrenergic stimulation induces distinct patterns of immediate early gene expression in neonatal rat myocardial cells. *J Biol Chem* 1990; 265:13809–13817.

143. Dunnmon PM, Iwaki K, Henderson SA, et al. Phorbolesters induce immediate-early genes and activate cardiac gene transcription in neonatal rat myocardial cells. *J Mol Cell Cardiol* 1990;22: 901–910.

144. Bishopric NH, Kedes L. Adrenergic regulation of the skeletal α-active gene promotor during myocardial cell hypertrophy. *Proc Natl Acad Sci USA* 1991;88:2132–2136.

145. Bishopric NH, Jayasena V, Webster KA. Positive regulation of the skeletal α-actin gene by *fos* and *jun* in cardiac myocytes. *J Biol Chem* 1992;267: 25535–25540.

146. Cohn J. Presentation at symposium: "Hypertrophy and Remodeling: From the Molecule to the Myocardium." April 24, 1996. Boston.

147. Polikar R, Burger A, Scherrer V, Nicod P. Thyroid and the heart. *Circulation* 1993;87:1435–1450.

148. Woeber KA. Thyrotoxicosis and the heart. *N Engl J Med* 1992;327:94–98.

149. Duerr RL, McKirnan D, Gim RD, et al. Cardiovascular effects of insulin-like growth factor-1 and growth hormone in chronic left ventricular failure in the rat. *Circulation* 1996;93:2188–2196.

150. Lipshultz SE, Orav EJ, Sanders SP, Colan SD. Immunoglobulins and left ventricular structure and function in pediatric HIV infection. *Circulation* 1995;92:2220–2225.

151. Newburger JW, Sanders SP, Burns JC, et al. Left ventricular contractility and function in Kawasaki syndrome: effect of intravenous gamma-globulin. *Circulation* 1989;19:1237–1246.

152. Lin Cy, Lin CC, Hwang B, Chiang BN. Cytokines predict coronary aneurysm formation in Kawasaki disease patients. *Eur J Pediatr* 1993;152:309–312.

153. Drucker NA, Colan SD, Lewis AB, et al. Immunoglobulin treatment of acute myocarditis in the pediatric population. *Circulation* 1994;89:252–257.

154. Takada H, Kishimoto L, Hiraoka Y. Therapy with immunoglobulin suppresses myocarditis in a murine coxsackievirus B3 model. *Circulation* 1995; 92:1604–1611.

155. Horiuchi A, Abe Y, Miyake M, et al. Natural human IgG inhibits the production of tumor necrosis factor-α and interleukin-1-α through the Fc portion. *Surg Today* 1993;23:241–245.

156. Torre-Amione G, Kapadia S, Lee J, et al. Expression and functional significance of tumor necrosis factor receptors in human myocardium. *Circulation* 1995;92:1487–1493.

157. Geist LJ, Monick MM, Stinski MF, Hunninghake GW. The immediate early genes of human cytomegalovirus upregulate tumor necrosis factor-α expression. *J Clin Invest* 1994;93:474–478.

158. Wu T-C, Pizzorno MC, Hayward GS, et al. In situ detection of human cytomegalovirus immediate early gene transcripts within cardiac myocytes of patients with HIV-associated cardiomyopathy. *AIDS* 1992;6:777–785.

159. Munoz E, Zubiaga A, Huber B. Interleukin–1 induces *c fos* and *c jun* gene expression in T helper type II cells through different signal transmission pathways. *Eur J Immunol* 1992;22:2101–2106.

160. Kunzi MS, Farzadegan H, Margolick JB, et al. Identification of human immunodeficiency virus primary isolates resistant to interferon-α and correlation of prevalence to disease progression. *J Infect Dis* 1995;171:822–828.

161. Herzum M, Schafer A, Mahr P, et al. Improvement of cardiac function in acute murine coxsackievirus B3 myocarditis by interferon-2α [Abstract].

162. Pennica D, King KL, Shaw KJ, et al. Expression cloning of cardiotrophin-1, a cytokine that induces cardiac myocyte hypertrophy. *Proc Natl Acad Sci USA* 1995;92:1142–1146.

163. Maulik N, Engelman DT, Watanabe M, et al. Nitric oxide signaling in ischemic heart. *Cardiovasc Res* 1995;30:593–601.

164. Bing RJ. Nitric oxide. *Cardiovasc Res* 1995;30:203–205.

165. Mohan P, Sys SU, Brutsaert DL. Positive inotropic effect of nitric oxide in myocardium. *Int J Cardiol* 1995;50:233–237.

166. De Belder A, Moncada S. Cardiomyopathy: a role for NO? *Cardiovasc Res* 1995;30:263–268.

167. Finkel MS, Oddis CV, Jacob TD, et al. Negative inotropic effect of cytokines on the heart mediated by nitric oxide. *Science* 1992;257:387–389.

168. Finkel MS, Hoffman RA, Shen, et al. Interleukin-6 (IL-6) as a mediator of stunned myocardium. *Am J Cardiol* 1993;71:1231–1232.

169. Pinsky DJ, Cai B, Yang X, et al. The lethal effects of cytokine-induced nitric oxide on cardiac myocytes are blocked by nitric oxide synthase antagonism on transforming growth factor β. *J Clin Invest* 1995;95:677–685.

170. Habib FM, Springal DR, Davies GJ, et al. Tumour necrosis factor and inducible nitric oxide synthase in dilated cardiomyopathy. *Lancet* 1996;347:1151–1155.

171. Shah AM, Prendergast BD, Grocott-Mason R, et al. The influence of endothelium-derived nitric oxide on myocardial contractile function. *Cardiovasc Res* 1995;30:225–231.

172. Reaven GM, Lithell H, Landsberg L. Hypertension and associated metabolic abnormalities: the role of insulin resistance and the sympathoadrenal system. *N Engl J Med* 1996;334:374–381.

173. Wei JY. Age and the cardiovascular system. *N Engl J Med* 1992;327:1735–1739.

174. Takahashi T, Schunkert H, Isoyama S, et al. Age-related differences in the expression of protooncogene and contractile protein genes in response to pressure overload in the rat myocardium. *J Clin Ivest* 1992;89:939–946.

175. Amiesen JC, Estaquier J, Idziorer T, DeBels F. The relevance of apoptosis to AIDS pathogenesis. *Trends Cell Biol* 1995;5:27–32.

9

Left Ventricular Dysfunction in HIV-Infected Infants and Children

*Steven E. Lipshultz, M.D., Steven D. Colan, M.D.,
and Michelle A. Grenier, M.D.*

Infants and children with human immunodeficiency virus (HIV) infection are a rapidly expanding population.[1] As many as 10 million infected children are projected worldwide by the year 2000.[2] In addition, HIV has become one of the leading causes of symptomatic heart disease.[3] There is a 20% cumulative incidence of transient and chronic congestive heart failure in HIV-infected infants and children,[2] which appears to occur both early[4] and late[2] in the course of infection.

The spectrum of echocardiographic abnormalities associated with congestive heart failure in HIV-infected infants and children includes hyperdynamic left ventricular function, depressed left ventricular contractility, left ventricular dilatation, inadequate left ventricular hypertrophy, increased left ventricular mass, pericardial effusion, and other structural abnormalities[2,5–12] (Figure 9-1). As HIV-infected children live longer, virtually all of them show progressive left ventricular dilatation with inadequate hypertrophy,[4] resulting in excessive left ventricular afterload, which reduces left ventricular function and may contribute to the increased morbidity and mortality seen in these patients.[2,4,13–15] Most HIV-infected children with congestive heart failure have significant abatement of clinical symptoms and improvement of ventricular function with

appropriate therapeutic interventions, especially if they are initiated early.[2,6,8–12,15]

The high incidence of symptomatic heart disease in HIV-infected infants and children requires a better understanding of the significance and limitations of commonly used noninvasive techniques to assess left ventricular function. Fractional shortening is the most common measurement of left ventricular performance, but abnormal fractional shortening does not necessarily mean that the patient has sustained clinically significant myocardial damage or has depressed contractility. A variety of factors unrelated to the health of the heart muscle cells can cause abnormal fractional shortening, necessitating measurements that can discriminate between muscle cell (myocardial) damage and other (ventricular) factors. Load-dependent-ejection phase indices such as fractional shortening do not provide direct information about the intrinsic contractile state of the left ventricle independent of preload and afterload, the conditions under which the ventricle is working.[16,17]

This chapter reviews the correlation between echocardiographic measurements, discusses the magnitude of discrepancy between these measurements, and evaluates the clinical impact of the discrepancy in assessing the natural history of the disease.

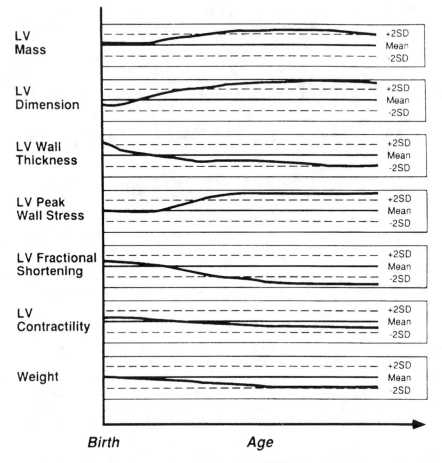

Figure 9-1. Changes in left ventricular structure and function in HIV-infected children as a function of age. For each parameter, z scores are used that indicate the position of each measurement relative to the normal population, expressed as SD from the population mean. Reporting data as z scores adjusts for effects of variation in age and body size. Body weight is listed as a noncardiac marker of stage of HIV disease. Data represent an assimilation of available information.

Factors Affecting Measurement of Left Ventricular Function

Preload

Preload is the extent of filling of the left ventricle before the onset of contraction; it is the force needed to attain the precontraction length needed to generate systolic force. Preload is influenced by factors that affect the central circulating volume, such as anemia and dehydration, or left ventricular distensibility, such as left ventricular relaxation and compliance, myocardial hypertrophy, fibrosis, valvular abnormalities, or pericardial effusion and con-

straint. Preload may be determined by adjusting the fractional shortening for afterload and subtracting for contractility.

Afterload

Afterload is the force that the myofibers must overcome to shorten and eject the blood during systole. The extent and velocity of fiber shortening are inversely related to the force acting on the muscle fiber. Afterload is a function of blood pressure, left ventricular diameter, and left ventricular wall thickness. It may be elevated by conditions that lead to left ventricular dilatation, such as cardiomyopathy and acute changes in blood pressure. Afterload is affected by factors extrinsic to the myocardium, such as blood pressure, arterial compliance, and left ventricular outflow tract obstruction. It is also affected by intrinsic factors, such as inadequate hypertrophy, excess hypertrophy, and left ventricular dilatation.[18] It may be measured as the left ventricular meridional end-systolic wall stress according to the formula[16,17]

$$\text{Afterload} = \frac{(0.3375)(p_{es})\ (D_{es})}{(h_{es})\ [1 + (h_{es}/D_{es})]}$$

where p_{es} is the end-systolic pressure in millimeters of mercury, D_{es} is the end-systolic dimension in centimeters, and h_{es} is the end-systolic posterior wall thickness in centimeters.

An altered inotropic state, through secondary effects on left ventricular geometry and chamber pressure, may alter both preload and afterload.[18]

Fractional Shortening Versus Contractility in Assessing Left Ventricular Function

Left ventricular fractional shortening and contractility are not equivalent. Contractility of the left ventricle, defined as the force-generating property of cardiac myocytes, is an important measurement of both the extent of the impact of HIV on myocardial function and the response to therapeutic interventions.[2,5–9] It is a better measure of cardiac health than fractional shortening, as it represents the intrinsic ability of the myocardium. Contractility alone does not reliably estimate ventricular systolic performance, which can only be estimated by the intrinsic ability of the myocardium, the loading conditions under which the heart is working, and the heart rate.[19–22] It may be calculated by dividing fractional shortening by the rate-adjusted ejection time (measured from the carotid pulse tracing and divided by the square root of the heart rate, determined as the time from one R wave to the next), thus creating a heart rate-adjusted velocity of fiber shortening.

Cardiac performance reflects all the determinants of ventricular function, not just contractility. These commonly used indices do not differentiate contractility changes from alterations in loading conditions.[17,19–25] When the heart rate, left ventricular preload, and left ventricular afterload are all normal, the trends observed by using these load-dependent indices may approximate those observed for left ventricular contractility (Figure 9-2a).

Fractional shortening is calculated by determin-

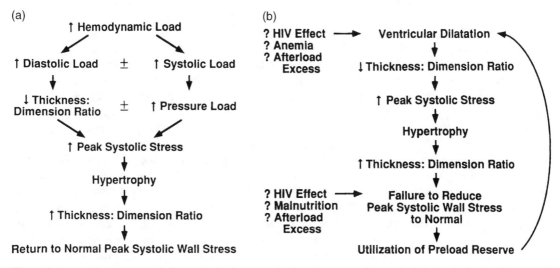

Figure 9-2. **a:** Compensatory left ventricular hypertrophy in response to changes in left ventricular load in normal children without HIV infection. **b:** Compensatory left ventricular hypertrophy in response to changes in left ventricular load in children with symptomatic HIV infection.

ing the difference between the left ventricular dimension at the end of diastole and at the end of systole, divided by the left ventricular end-diastolic dimension. Measurements of fractional shortening cannot be made independently of loading conditions, contractility, or heart rate.

For children with HIV infection, some of the factors contributing to differences between load-dependent fractional shortening and contractility include anemia, fever, volume infusions, medications, sepsis, central nervous system disease (including seizures), autonomic imbalance, renal failure, and malnutrition (Figure 9-2b). For example, fever causes tachycardia and cutaneous vasodilatation, resulting in reduced systemic resistance, preload, and afterload. Under these conditions, even an abnormal left ventricle might have a normal fractional shortening. Conversely, renal failure, by causing high blood pressure and increased intravascular volume, raises both afterload and preload. In this case, even a normal left ventricle may have a low fractional shortening, not because of cardiomyopathy, but because of excessive load on the left ventricle. Moreover, the absence of hypertension, fever, or anemia does not necessarily make fractional shortening a reliable measure of contractility. For example, healthy long-distance runners, who would be expected to have normal fractional shortening at rest, have a significantly reduced preload, even though their contractility is normal.[26]

In addition to contractility, nearly all published investigations examining left ventricular performance in HIV-infected patients have used measurements dependent on both preload and afterload. These measurements have been used to determine the need for endomyocardial biopsy in symptom-free children,[10] to assess the success of experimental cardiac interventions,[27,28] and to screen for cardiac toxic effects of experimental therapy.[29–31] Moreover, fractional shortening is used to define HIV cardiomyopathy in many AIDS Clinical Trials Group protocols conducted by the National Institutes of Health. Consequently, fractional shortening may determine who is treated on such protocols and how a patient's cardiac status is classified. Numerous studies have documented that fractional shortening may not be a sufficiently reliable indicator of intrinsic myocardial function in HIV-infected infants and children.[5–9,32]

The Natural History of Left Ventricular Dysfunction in HIV-Infected Infants and Children

Lipshultz and colleagues[6] described the cardiovascular manifestations of HIV infection in infants and children in a retrospective study by evaluating the shape, wall motion, valve morphology, and function of the left ventricle. Left ventricular performance was evaluated by the shortening fraction, afterload by the end-systolic wall stress, and contractility by the relation between the end-systolic wall stress and the rate-corrected velocity of shortening. The marked variation in loading conditions necessitated the use of a load-independent index of contractility.

When these parameters were used, two patterns of left ventricular function abnormalities became apparent: hyperdynamic left ventricular performance with enhanced contractility and reduced afterload, and diminished contractility associated with symptomatic cardiomyopathy. In 89% of patients, serial echocardiographic evaluations revealed changes from the original levels of ventricular function, afterload, and contractility. This initial study first implicated left ventricular dysfunction as a likely cause of cardiac symptoms and even death.

Similarly, a retrospective study by Grenier and colleagues[13] was notable for a strong correlation between increased morbidity and mortality and evidence of left ventricular dysfunction in HIV-infected infants and children. The patients with severe left ventricular dysfunction were most likely to die.

Luginbuhl and colleagues,[2] in a historical cohort study, determined the cumulative incidence and clinical predictors of HIV cardiac disease in children. They noted chronic congestive heart failure in 10% of patients. One-third of the children who died during this study had significant cardiac dysfunction, as determined by fractional shortening; these were the children with advanced HIV disease. Encephalopathy and Epstein-Barr virus coinfection identified children at extremely high risk of increased cardiac morbidity and mortality.

Domanski and colleagues,[33] reporting on the effects of zidovudine and didanosine on heart function in HIV-infected children, substantiated the fact that advanced HIV infection is associated with poor cardiac outcome. Cardiomyopathy, or left ventricular dysfunction, was defined as a fractional shortening of 25% or less. By this definition, there was a decline in left ventricular function over time.

Although it has become apparent that HIV-infected infants and children manifest echocardiographic abnormalities of cardiac structure and function, it has remained unclear how these abnormalities are attributable to left ventricular dysfunction, cardiomyopathy, and increased morbidity and mortality. An echocardiographic study of 24 children with symptomatic HIV infection before, during, and after treatment with zidovudine found remarkable progressive left ventricular dilatation with compensatory hypertrophy, which was inadequate to maintain peak systolic wall stress within the normal range[4] (Figures 9-1 and 9-2b). There was progressive elevation of ventricular afterload due to dilatation, which resulted in depressed ventricular performance, even though ventricular contractility remained normal. Zidovudine did not appear to worsen or to ameliorate these cardiac changes.[4] Left ventricular contractility seemed to have no predictive value in the HIV-infected pediatric population. However, diminished wall thickness (ventricular hypertrophy) and progressive increase in ventricular afterload due to left ventricular dilatation (thickness:dimension ratio) resulted in depressed ventricular function and seemed to have a positive predictive value for symptomatic HIV cardiac disease. The fractional shortening of the left ventricle was significantly decreased.

This study by Lipshultz and colleagues[4] was the first to describe the progressive abnormalities of left ventricular size and function in children with HIV infection (both before and after receiving zidovudine). The study is most notable for two findings, which have since been replicated in the HIV-infected pediatric population:

1. Progressive left ventricular dilatation with associated wall thinning, resulting in a decreased ratio of thickness to dimension, with a resultant increase in both peak systolic and end-systolic wall stress (increase in afterload without effect on contractility)
2. And a significant increase in left ventricular mass, which failed to keep pace with ventricular dilatation, resulting in inadequate hypertrophy (Figure 9-2b)

Other studies[14,15] support the findings: abnormal thickness:dimension ratio due to left ventricular dilatation and inadequate hypertrophy associated with increased left ventricular mass and increased patient morbidity and mortality. Abnormalities of left ventricular structure and function are apparent in the infants of HIV-infected mothers.[34] In a study of 208 infants, fractional shortening was found to be depressed in both infected and uninfected infants exposed to HIV. Although there was significant improvement in fractional shortening in the uninfected infants over time, function remained depressed in both the infected and uninfected infants at 4 months of age compared with the general population.[34] In both groups, the left ventricular end-diastolic dimensions were significantly greater, and the left ventricular wall thicknesses were significantly diminished. These parameters changed significantly toward normal over time, but the question of the relation of these abnormalities to the later development of congestive heart failure remains to be answered.

Diastolic abnormalities are thought to occur before the development of systolic dysfunction in patients infected with HIV.[35] In a study of 51 adult patients, diastolic function was significantly altered, even in the early stages of the disease. In a retrospective analysis of 37 HIV-infected pediatric patients, which used the corrected velocity of fractional shortening to assess systolic function and the isovolumic relaxation time to assess diastolic dysfunction, approximately half the patients with normal fractional shortening values manifested diastolic dysfunction, which declined further with time.

In a longitudinal prospective study of HIV-infected infants and children, the clinical significance of left ventricular dysfunction was questioned. Left ventricular abnormalities in 197 HIV-infected children were examined to determine whether they predicted mortality (n = 43 deaths). Univariate analysis revealed that depressed fractional shortening and increased left ventricular afterload, mass, and wall thickness at enrollment were all related to an increased risk of death.[14] Multivariate analyses showed that fractional shortening was a significant cardiac predictor of mortality after adjusting for age, height, CD4+ lymphocyte count, z score, and progressive neurologic disease. The survival experience of those

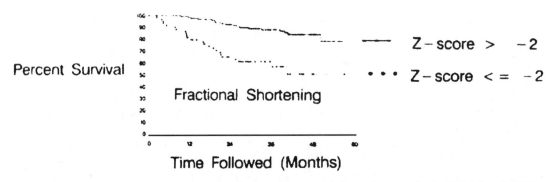

Figure 9-3. Depressed left ventricular fractional shortening as a risk factor for mortality in HIV-infected children independently of depressed CD4+ lymphocyte counts and progressive neurologic disease.

children whose fractional shortening indices were > 2 SD below normal revealed that depressed left ventricular fractional shortening is a risk factor for mortality in HIV-infected children independently of depressed CD4+ lymphocyte count and progressive neurologic disease[1] (Figure 9-3).

Progressive left ventricular dilatation is common in infants and children exposed to or infected with HIV. It may be preceded by diastolic dysfunction and may be a harbinger of congestive heart failure. Although there are limitations to the use of fractional shortening as a predictor of morbidity and mortality in HIV-infected infants and children, diminished fractional shortening has been associated with increased cardiac morbidity and mortality.

Do Echocardiographic Parameters Predict Morbidity and Mortality in HIV-Infected Infants and Children?

To determine the predictive value of fractional shortening in HIV-infected infants and children, Lipshultz and colleagues[36] obtained 212 echocardiograms in 81 consecutive patients between 1984 and 1990 (Figure 9-4). The median age at first evaluation was 1.9 years (range: 2.4 months to 22.6 years), and the mean fractional shortening from 193 studies was 32.8% (range: 10.0–53.5%). Although a fractional shortening of 32.8% would typically be considered on the high side of normal, the mean z score for fractional shortening after adjustment for age was 1.58 SD below normal (range: −11.5 to 6.3). This discrepancy resulted from the fact that

almost all normal children under 5 years of age had fractional shortening greater than 32%, but nearly half the HIV-infected children had fractional shortening less than 32%. Contractility on 178 studies gave a mean z score of −0.02 SD (range: −8.19 to 11.04 SD).

The overall preload was abnormally high in 11 studies (6%) and abnormally low in 26 (15%). The afterload was abnormally high in 69 studies (39%) and abnormally low in 6 (3%).

The overall correlation coefficient (r) between age-adjusted fractional shortening and contractility was 0.70, which is statistically significant but indicates only moderate agreement (Figure 9-5). Among the 65 echocardiograms for children less than 2 years of age, the correlation was weaker ($r = 0.52$) than among the 112 echocardiograms for older children ($r = 0.84$). Of 177 echocardiograms, fractional shortening and contractility differed by >1 SD for 119 and by >2 SD for 63.

Alternatively, when fractional shortening was considered without adjustment for age, and studies were divided into those showing depressed (<28%), enhanced (>34%), and normal ranges, contractility was incorrectly classified on 46% of echocardiograms. Of the 42 echocardiograms with depressed fractional shortening, 18 (43%) showed either normal or enhanced contractility. Moreover, 16% of the echocardiograms with normal fractional shortening showed depressed contractility. Enhanced fractional shortening predicted enhanced contractility in only 36% of the echocardiograms (Figure 9-5).

Depressed cardiac function was defined as con-

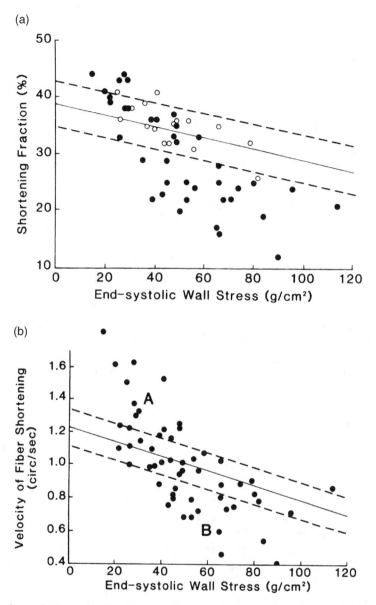

Figure 9-4. **a:** Left ventricular shortening fraction and end-systolic wall stress in 30 pediatric patients with HIV (54 studies). The *Y*-axis shows shortening fraction (normal range for our laboratory, 31% + 3%), and the *X*-axis shows end-systolic wall stress (normal range for our laboratory, 40 to 60 g/cm^2). The *closed circles* represent patients with symptomatic infection. The *broken lines* indicate 95% confidence limits for preload-dependent left ventricular contractility. **b:** Relation between heart rate-corrected velocity of fiber shortening and end-systolic wall stress in 30 patients with HIV (54 studies). The *broken lines* indicate 95% confidence limits for left ventricular contractility. *A*, patients with enhanced contractility and normal or low end-systolic wall stress. *B*, patients with depressed contractility and normal to elevated end-systolic wall stress.

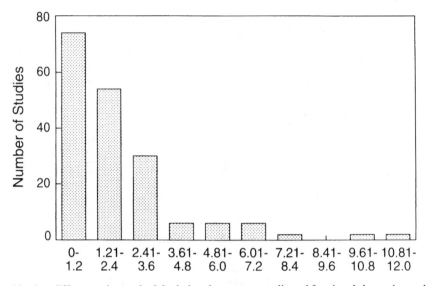

Figure 9-5. Absolute differences in standard deviations between age-adjusted fractional shortening and contractility *z* scores. The *Y*-axis shows the number of studies in which the absolute difference between *z* scores for fractional shortening and contractility was in a range as shown on the *X*-axis.

tractility >2 SD below normal. Depressed fractional shortening accurately discriminated between studies with and without depressed contractility. Sensitivity, specificity, and positive and negative predictive values for contractility of three conventional cutoff points for fractional shortening, as well as for fractional shortening adjusted for age or body surface area, were compared. Of all definitions of depressed cardiac function, fractional shortening <27% resulted in the highest positive predictive value (61%), but the lowest sensitivity (69%). The basal surface area-adjusted fractional shortening resulted in the greatest sensitivity (100%), detecting all 32 echocardiograms with depressed contractility, but provided the lowest positive predictive value: 41% of echocardiograms with depressed basal surface area-adjusted fractional shortening showed depressed contractility (Figure 9-6).

There was a tradeoff between the sensitivity (the proportion of children with depressed contractility who had values below a chosen cutoff point for fractional shortening) and the specificity (the proportion of children with normal or elevated contractility who had values above the chosen cutoff point for fractional shortening) of various cutoff points for fractional shortening to define depressed contractility (Figure 9-6). With a cutoff point of frac-

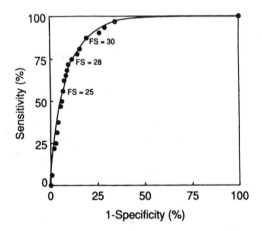

Figure 9-6. Curve illustrating how changing the definition for depressed fractional shortening changes our ability to use fractional shortening as a marker of depressed contractility. The *X*-axis shows the probability of depressed fractional shortening when contractility is normal, while the *Y*-axis shows the probability of depressed fractional shortening when contractility is depressed.

tional shortening ≤25%, 56% of the echocardiograms revealed depressed contractility (a sensitivity of 56%) and 93% of the echocardiograms revealed normal or elevated contractility (1 − specificity = 100% − 7%). A cutoff point ≤30% increased the sensitivity to 82% but reduced the specificity to 81%.

In this study, age-adjusted fractional shortening was, on average, 1.5 SD lower than contractility. The discrepancies between these two measures could be partially explained by preload ($P = .0001$), afterload ($P = .0001$), and age ($P = .0001$) in a multiple regression model. Assuming constant preload and afterload, fractional shortening and contractility were more concordant among older children than among younger children. For children at the same HIV stage, each year of increasing age reduced the discrepancy between fractional shortening and contractility by 0.08 SD.

The discrepancy between fractional shortening and contractility was magnified by preload and afterload. Higher preload was found for echocardiograms in which fractional shortening exceeded contractility ($P = .002$). Higher afterload was found when contractility exceeded fractional shortening ($P < .001$).

Because HIV-infected children tend to progress to the acquired immunodeficiency syndrome (AIDS) as they grow older, reduction in the discrepancy from increasing age is generally counteracted by disease progression.

In the aforementioned study,[36] 16% (12/76) of the population had clinical congestive heart failure; 6 of them had transient heart failure, and 6 had chronic heart failure. All patients had fractional shortening <25%. Four of them had normal contractility, indicating that the depressed fractional shortening was related to abnormal loading conditions. Afterload was abnormally elevated in patients with heart failure, but contractility was normal.

Determination of Left Ventricular Dysfunction and Therapeutic Improvement

Left ventricular function is the product of the intrinsic systolic properties of the myocardium (contractility), the loading conditions under which the myocardium is working, and, to a lesser extent, the heart rate. Ejection-phase indices of left ventricular function, such as fractional shortening or ejection fraction, reflect all the determinants of left ventricular function, not just contractility. In healthy subjects, such indices may reliably reflect the contractile state of the myocardium because the loading conditions and the heart are normal. However, in people with abnormal loading conditions, standard indices of function are not reliable. The magnitude of the discrepancy between fractional shortening and contractility was exemplified by the study of Lipshultz and colleagues,[36] who examined the frequency with which fractional shortening is inadequate as an index of contractility. More importantly, the study examined the magnitude of the discrepancy between the two indices in infants and children with HIV infection, especially in relation to age and stage of disease.

Children and infants infected with HIV have a high incidence of abnormal loading status, resulting in contractility and fractional shortening discrepancies greater than 2 SD in more than a third of cases. Although the sensitivity and specificity of fractional shortening for detecting depressed contractility are dependent on the value chosen to define depressed fractional shortening, the use of the typical value of <28% resulted in a sensitivity of only 75% and a specificity of 88%. In the Lipshultz study, 43% of the echocardiograms showed normal or elevated contractility. The predictive capacity of the fractional shortening index was not improved by changing the definition of depressed, or by adjusting for age or basal surface area. Fractional shortening and contractility are particularly dissimilar in children less than 2 years of age because somatic growth and increasing age are associated with alterations in myocardial mechanics.[37] In the face of HIV infection, the discrepancy between fractional shortening and contractility appears to be a greater problem for children than for adults. If afterload and preload measurements are not available, information on disease stage and age may be clinically useful in interpreting the discrepancy between fractional shortening and contractility.

The clinical state of congestive heart failure has a more specific relation to ventricular function than to myocardial function, as illustrated by the fact that ventricular function, as assessed by fractional shortening, tends to be depressed in patients with congestive heart failure.[36] In some patients, this depression in fractional shortening may be attributed to abnormal contractility, although in others it may be due to excessive afterload. Contractility was found to be normal in the one-third of the HIV-infected children studied who had congestive heart failure.[36]

It is particularly important to discriminate between abnormal contractility and abnormal loading conditions when considering the etiology, prognosis, and, to a lesser extent, treatment of heart disease in children infected with HIV. In general, the presence of cardiomyopathy implies some intrinsic abnormality of the myocardium. The patient's age and the stage of HIV disease affect the loading conditions and result in values of fractional shortening that poorly reflect contractility. Because fractional shortening does not discriminate between intrinsic and extrinsic effects on ventricular function, it has serious limitations for detecting cardiomyopathy.[18,31,38] The use of fractional shortening to detect cardiomyopathy in HIV-infected patients may result in a misunderstanding of the potential cardiac effects of therapies and in the denial of potential therapeutic interventions. Depressed left ventricular function has been noted in 54% to 72% of adults with AIDS and in 62% to 64% of children with HIV infection when load-dependent indices are used,[10] leading some investigators to cite an incidence of cardiomyopathy as high as 70%.

By contrast, depressed left ventricular function was present in only 26% of HIV-infected children when load-independent indices were used.[6] In one study, half the reported patients who had depressed fractional shortening did not have depressed contractility.[36] Conversely, one-quarter of the patients in the same study had depressed contractility but normal fractional shortening, which suggests that depressed contractility is incompletely captured on the basis of fractional shortening alone.

Both the overreporting and the incomplete capture of depressed contractility may be clinically relevant. The reported incidence of cardiomyopathy depends on which definition of contractility is used. In addition, diastolic dysfunction, as determined by isovolumic relaxation time, may precede any evidence of systolic dysfunction, as indicated by a decline in fractional shortening.[35] There must be further research into the area of diastolic dysfunction and its relationship to systolic dysfunction in HIV-infected infants and children.

In spite of its limitations in predicting cardiomyopathy, fractional shortening remains a clinically important index. In the prospective National Heart, Lung, and Blood Institute P^2C^2 study of 197 HIV-infected children, univariate analysis revealed that depressed fractional shortening and increased left ventricular afterload, mass, and wall thickness at enrollment were all related to an increased risk of death.[14] Multivariate analysis showed that fractional shortening was a significant cardiac predictor of mortality after adjusting for age, height, CD4+ lymphocyte count, z score, and progressive neurologic disease (per 2 SD drop in fractional shortening: RR = 1.81; $P < .001$; 95%CI: 1.58–2.07). Depressed left ventricular fractional shortening is a risk factor for mortality in HIV-infected children, independently of depressed CD4+ lymphocyte count and progressive neurologic disease.[14] Fractional shortening was found to be depressed in infants of HIV-infected mothers, an abnormality that persisted over the first 4 months of life. In addition, these infants manifested increased left ventricular end-diastolic volume and decreased left ventricular wall thickness.[33]

In some settings, the use of load-independent contractility more accurately predicted the clinical course of cardiac dysfunction, and thereby influenced clinical management, than did load-independent measurements such as fractional shortening.[19,39–43] Measurements of load-independent contractility and specific loading conditions allow a more accurate determination of clinical status and may lead to better clinical management of HIV-infected infants and children. However, recent data support the prognostic role of fractional shortening in the management of HIV cardiomyopathy in infants and children.

References

1. Chin J. Current and future dimensions of the HIV/AIDS pandemic in women and children. *Lancet* 1990;336:221–224.
2. Luginbuhl LM, Orav EJ, McIntosh K, Lipshultz SE. Cardiac morbidity and related mortality in children with HIV infection. *JAMA* 1993:269:2869–2875.

3. Kasper EK, Agema WRP, Hutchins GM, et al. The causes of dilated cardiomyopathy: a clinicopathologic review of 673 consecutive patients. *J Am Coll Cardiol* 1994;23:586–590.

4. Italian Register for HIV Infection in Children. Features of children perinatally-infected with HIV-1 surviving longer than 5 years. *Lancet* 1994;343: 191–195.

5. Lipshultz SE, Orav EJ, Sanders SP, et al. Cardiac structure and function in children with human immunodeficiency virus treated with zidovudine. *N Engl J Med* 1992;327:1260–1265.

6. Lipshultz S, Chanock S, Sanders SP, et al. Cardiac manifestations of human immunodeficiency virus in infants and children. *Am J Cardiol* 1989;63: 1489–1497.

7. Lipshultz SE, Fox CH, Perez-Atayde AR, et al. Identification of human immunodeficiency virus–1 RNA and DNA in the heart of a child with cardiovascular abnormalities and congenital acquired immune deficiency syndrome. *Am J Cardiol* 1990;66: 246–250.

8. Chanock SJ, Luginbuhl LM, McIntosh K, Lipshultz SE. Life-threatening reactions to trimethoprim/sulfamethoxazole in pediatric human immunodeficiency virus infection. *Pediatrics* 1994;93:519–521.

9. Lipshultz SE. Cardiovascular problems. In: Pizzo PA, Wilfert CM (eds.). *Pediatric AIDS: The Challenge of HIV Infection in Infants, Children, and Adolescents*, 2nd Ed. Baltimore: Williams & Wilkins, 1994:483–511.

10. Kavanaugh-McHugh A, Ruff AJ, Rowe SA, et al. Cardiovascular abnormalities. In: Pizzo PA, Wilfert CM (eds.). *Pediatric AIDS: The Challenge of HIV Infection in Infants, Children, and Adolescents*. Baltimore: Williams & Wilkins, 1991:355–372.

11. Stewart JM, Kaul A, Gromisch DS, Reyes E, et al. Symptomatic cardiac dysfunction in children with human immunodeficiency virus infection. *Am Heart J* 1988;117:140–144.

12. Steinherz L, Brochstein S, Robins J. Cardiac involvement in congenital acquired immune deficiency syndrome. *Am J Dis Child* 1986;140:1241–1244.

13. Grenier MA, Karr SS, Rakusan TA, Martin GR. Cardiac disease in children with HIV: relationship of cardiac disease to HIV symptomatology. *Pediatr AIDS HIV Infect: Fetus Adolesc* 1994;5:174–178.

14. Lipshultz SE, for the Pediatric Pulmonary and Cardiovascular Complications of Vertically Transmitted HIV (P^{2}C^2) Study. Cardiac dysfunction predicts mortality in HIV-infected children- the prospective NHLBI P^{2}C^2 study. [Abstract]. *Proc Conf Retrov Opportun Infect* 1996;130.

15. Kearney DL, for the Pediatric Pulmonary and Cardiovascular Complications of Vertically Transmitted HIV (P^{2}C^2) Study. Postmortem cardiomegaly correlates with premortem measurements of left ventricular size in malnourished HIV-infected children. [Abstract]. *Proc Conf Retrov Opportun Infect* 1996;133.

16. Colan SD, Sanders SP, Inglefinger JR, Harmon W. Left ventricular mechanics and contractile state in children and young adults with end-stage renal disease: effect of dialysis and renal transplantation. *J Am Coll Cardiol* 1987;10:1085–1094.

17. Colan SD, Borow KM, Neumann A. Left ventricular end-systolic wall stress-velocity of fiber shortening relation: a load-independent index of myocardial contractility. *J Am Coll Cardiol* 1984;4: 715–724.

18. Borow KM, Neumann A, Marcus RH, et al. Effects of simultaneous alterations in preload and afterload on measurements of left ventricular contractility in patients with dilated cardiomyopathy: comparisons of ejection phase, isovolumetric and end-systolic force velocity indexes. *J Am Coll Cardiol* 1992;20: 787–795.

19. Ross J Jr. Control of cardiac performance. In: Berne RM, Sperelakis N, Geiger SR (eds.). *Handbook of Physiology: The Cardiovascular System*, Vol 1. Baltimore: Williams & Wilkins, 1979:533–580.

20. Ross J Jr. Afterload mismatch and preload reserve: a conceptual framework for the analysis of ventricular function. *Prog Cardiovasc Dis* 1976;18:255–264.

21. Weber KT, Janicki JS. The heart as a muscle-pump system and the concept of heart failure. *Am Heart J* 1979;98:371–384.

22. Borow KM. Clinical assessment of contractility in the symmetrically contracting left ventricle. *Mod Concepts Cardiovasc Dis* 1988;57:29–34.

23. Parmley WW. Pathophysiology and current therapy of congestive heart failure. *J Am Coll Cardiol* 1989; 13:771–785.

24. Peterson KL, Skloven D, Ludbrook P, et al. Comparison of isovolumic and ejection phase indices of myocardial performance in man. *Circulation* 1974; 49:1088–1101.

25. Kass DA, Maughan LW, Zhong MG, et al. Comparative influence of load versus inotropic state on

indexes of ventricular contractility: experimental and theoretical analysis based on pressure-volume relationships. *Circulation* 1987;76:1422–1436.

26. Colan SD, Sander SP, Borow KM. Physiologic hypertrophy: effects on left ventricular systolic mechanics in athletes. *J Am Coll Cardiol* 1987;9: 776–783.

27. Wilkins CE, Sexton DJ, McAllister HA. HIV-associated myocarditis treated with zidovudine (AZT). *Tex Heart Inst J* 1989;16:44–45.

28. Kavanaugh-McHugh AL, Ruff A, Perlman E, et al. Selenium deficiency and cardiomyopathy in acquired immunodeficiency syndrome. *J Parenter Enteral Nutr* 1991;15:347–349.

29. Herskowitz A, Willoghby SB, Baughman KL, et al. Cardiomyopathy associated with antiretroviral therapy in patients with HIV infection: a report of six cases. *Ann Intern Med* 1992;116:311–313.

30. Brown DL, Sather S, Cheitlin MD. Reversible cardiac dysfunction associated with foscarnet therapy for cytomegalovirus esophagitis in an AIDS patient. *Am Heart J* 1993;125:1439–1441.

31. Deyton LR, Walker RE, Kovacs JA, et al. Reversible cardiac dysfunction associated with interferon alfa therapy in AIDS patients with Kaposi's sarcoma. *N Engl J Med* 1989;329:1246–1249.

32. Lipshultz SE, Sanders SP, Colan SD. Cardiac structure and function in HIV-infected children [Letter]. *N Engl J Med* 1993;328:513–514.

33. Domanski MJ, Sloas MM, Follman DA, et al. Effect of zidovudine and didanosine treatment on heart function in children infected with human immunodeficiency virus. *J Pediatr* 1995;127:137–146.

34. Lipshultz SE, Easley K, Kaplan S, et al. Abnormal left ventricular structure and function shortly after birth in infants of HIV-infected mothers-the prospective NHLBI P^2C^2 Study [Abstract]. *Circulation* 1995;92:I–581.

35. Coudray N, de Zuttere D, Force G, et al. Left ventricular diastolic function in asymptomatic and symptomatic human immunodeficiency virus carriers: an echocardiographic study. *Eur Heart J* 1995; 16:61–67.

36. Lipshultz SE, Orav JE, Sander SP, et al. Limitations of fractional shortening as an index of contractility in pediatric patients infected with human immunodeficiency virus. *J Pediatr* 1994;125:563–570.

37. Colan SD, Parness IA, Spevak PJ, Sanders SP. Developmental modulation of myocardial mechanics: age- and growth-related alterations in afterload and contractility. *J Am Coll Cardiol* 1992;19:619–629.

38. Lipshultz SE, Colan SD. The use of echocardiography and Holter monitoring in the assessment of anthracycline-treated patients. In: Bricker JT, Green DM, D'Angio GJ. (eds.) *Cardiac Toxicity After Treatment for Childhood Cancer.* New York: Wiley-Liss, 1993:45–62.

39. Ricci DR. Afterload mismatch and preload reserve in chronic aortic regurgitation. *Circulation* 1982; 66:826–834.

40. Wisenbaugh T, Booth D, DeMaria A, et al. Relationship of contractile state to ejection performance in patients with chronic aortic valve disease. *Circulation* 1986;73:47–53.

41. Wisenbaugh T, Spann JF, Carabello BA. Differences in myocardial performance and load between patients with similar amounts of chronic aortic versus chronic mitral regurgitation. *J Am Coll Cardiol* 1984;3:916–923.

42. Zile MR, Gaasch WH, Levine HJ. Left ventricular stress-dimension-shortening relations before and after correction of chronic aortic and mitral regurgitation. *Am J Cardiol* 1985;56:99–105.

43. Dorn GW, Donner R, Assey ME, et al. Alterations in left ventricular geometry, wall stress, and ejection performance after correction of congenital aortic stenosis. *Circulation* 1988;78:1358–1364.

10

Autonomic Abnormalities and Arrhythmias

J. Philip Saul, M.D., and Roy Freeman, M.D.

This chapter discusses both the autonomic and the arrhythmic complications and manifestations of HIV infection. Although these two topics can certainly be dissociated in some patients, the nearly ubiquitous role of the autonomic nervous system in abnormalities of cardiac rhythm has been recognized for some time in the field of cardiac electrophysiology.[1,2] When the myocardial substrate for arrhythmias exists, changes in autonomic activity can often both enhance and reduce the likelihood of an arrhythmic event. A classic example, which has some applicability to patients with human immunosufficiency virus (HIV) infection, is that of torsades de pointes in patients with the long QT syndrome, where an underlying abnormality of repolarization due to either genetic or drug-induced changes in membrane ionic channels is catalyzed by changes in cardiac sympathetic activity to produce the life-threatening arrhythmia.[3,4] The existing data suggest that HIV infection produces a similar syndrome in which both the myocardial substrate and the autonomic milieu are modified by the disease to produce a state of increased risk.

Autonomic Dysfunction

The systemic migration of HIV-infected mononuclear phagocytes underlies the potential spread of the virus to all areas of the body, including the central nervous system and most neurons.[5,6] Thus, HIV can produce a spectrum of neurologic diseases that involves every level of the neuraxis.[7–9] In addition, the opportunistic infections and neoplasms that result from HIV can lead to a similar range of abnormalities. These problems may manifest at any stage of the infection, from initial seroconversion to established AIDS. In retrospective reports, 10% of patients with AIDS have neurologic symptoms at presentation, 40% develop neurologic symptoms during the course of the illness, and 75% to 95% have evidence of central or peripheral nervous system pathology at autopsy.[7–9] Thus, as expected from these data, the symptoms of autonomic dysfunction are common, particularly in well-established cases of the acquired immunodeficiency syndrome (AIDS). However, the prevalence of dysautonomia accompanying HIV infection is unknown.

Lin-Greenberg and Taneja-Uppal[10] first drew attention to the association of HIV infection with autonomic dysfunction. They described a patient with AIDS who had orthostatic hypotension, impotence, and anhidrosis. Several additional case reports expanded upon their description, and have included patients with orthostatic hypotension, syncope and presyncope, proximal body hyperhidrosis, diminished sweating, diarrhea, bladder dysfunction, and impotence.[10–15]

Cardiac Syndromes

Cohen and associates[16] reported five HIV-infected patients with orthostatic hypotension, four of whom had AIDS and one of whom had AIDS-related complex. Concurrent infection, severe vomiting, and diarrhea were not present, and the patients did not have a significant tachycardia with postural change. However, a variety of neurologic signs were noted, including cognitive abnormalities, extrapyramidal dysfunction, reduced coordination, and peripheral neuropathy. Autonomic evaluation of these patients revealed abnormal heart rate variation with deep breathing in four patients and an abnormal quantitative sudomotor axonal reflex test in three patients. All patients improved on therapy with fludrocortisone, and four of the five remained asymptomatic when fludrocortisone was discontinued, suggesting a transient cause of the orthostatic hypotension, at least in those patients. Orthostatic hypotension also frequently occurs when a tricyclic antidepressant is introduced as therapy for a painful neuropathy or depression. Optimum hydration alone with patient monitoring of urine color and frequency may be adequate therapy; however, when orthostatic symptoms persist, the addition of fludrocortisone or a pressor agent is usually sufficient to control all symptoms. Unfortunately, the painful peripheral neuropathy usually precludes the use of support stockings to minimize venous pooling.

Hypotension in HIV infection may also be a manifestation of adrenal insufficiency.[17,18] Characteristically, these patients have low plasma cortisol levels with a blunted plasma cortisol response to ACTH stimulation,[17,18] and the hypotension may be associated with weakness, weight loss, mucocutaneous pigmentation, and hyponatremia.

Hemodynamic lability, consisting of hypotension, hypertension, or both, has also been reported in HIV-infected patients.[19] Luginbuhl and colleagues[19] drew attention to the presence of episodic hypotension in 20%, episodic hypertension in 19%, and episodes of both in 11% of their cohort of HIV-infected children. Heart rate and rhythm abnormalities, including resting tachycardia (64%), sinus bradycardia (11%), marked sinus arrhythmia (17%), ventricular tachycardia, and torsades de pointes, were also observed.[19]

Finally, from a cardiovascular standpoint, when Lipshultz and coworkers[20] examined left ventricular function with a simultaneous measure of afterload, as many as 93% of children with HIV infection were found to have abnormalities, regardless of stage. Importantly, these abnormalities included both changes in left ventricular performance, which were manifest as either hyperdynamic (62%) or reduced (29%) function, and changes in afterload, either decreased (48%) or increased (29%). Some patients were found to progress from hyperdynamic to reduced cardiac function with symptoms of congestive heart failure during the course of their illness, leading to speculation that prolonged sympathetic activation may lead to cardiac decompensation. These observed changes in cardiac function may also help explain the variety of hemodynamic symptoms found in HIV-infected patients.

Episodic hypotension may result either from an inability to raise cardiac output in response to an increased demand or from abnormal peripheral vascular responses, including both inadequate vasoconstriction and inappropriate vasodilatation, in response to a reduction in cardiac output, such as that which occurs with postural changes. Patients with HIV infection who demonstrate hyperdynamic function may be at risk for both of these responses, similar to patients with the common form of neurocardiogenic syncope, who exhibit a reflex withdrawal of sympathetic efferent activity in response to a hypothesized stimulation of left ventricular mechanoreceptor afferents.[21] Although the precise afferent stimulus for this form of syncope in non-HIV-infected patients is incompletely resolved, it is clear that either enhanced left ventricular function or the inotropic agent isoproterenol markedly enhances the likelihood of a syncopal or presyncopal response during tilt-table testing,[21] supporting a causative role for hyperdynamic function in producing hypotension in some patients with HIV infection. Alternatively, in patients with reduced cardiac function and left ventricular dilatation, hypotension may result from the inability of cardiac output to increase with demand.

Noncardiac Syndromes

Despite the high prevalence of autonomically mediated cardiac problems in HIV-infected patients, gastric and bowel autonomic symptoms may be even more common. HIV-infected patients frequently report bowel, bladder, and erectile dysfunction,[22] with diarrhea being particularly troublesome. Using electron microscopy, Griffin and colleagues[23,24] documented structural abnormalities of the axons and Schwann cells of the autonomic nerves of the jejunal mucosa, suggesting that autonomic denervation of the jejunum might be responsible for nonpathogen-caused diarrhea in some patients. As further evidence of structural autonomic damage, Batman and colleagues[25] used the neuron-specific polyclonal antibody PGP 9.5 to quantify the depletion of autonomic axons in the villi and lamina propria of the jejunum. These histologic abnormalities were present at all stages of HIV infection, including in asymptomatic patients. Abnormalities of the rectal autonomic nerves have also been documented on rectal biopsy.[26] Alternatively, nonpathogen-caused diarrhea may also result from functional autonomic changes, such as increased efferent parasympathetic nervous activity to the gut.[27] Incontinence of bowel and bladder is characteristically a late symptom of AIDS, which is typically associated with a severe neuropathy, myelopathy, or polyradiculopathy and may be exacerbated by an accompanying dementia.

Tests of Autonomic Function

Autonomic testing of seropositive patients and patients with AIDS patients has been the subject of several reports and case studies.[10,12–14,16,28–30] In a controlled study, Freeman and coworkers[31] used multiple tests primarily of the cardiovascular autonomic nervous system to demonstrate significant differences in autonomic function between controls and HIV-infected patients. A steady decline in autonomic function was noted across diagnostic groups (controls, AIDS-related complex, AIDS), with the most severe autonomic dysfunction found in patients with AIDS. The abnormalities were also correlated with signs of HIV-associated nervous system disease. In fact, the three patients with the most severe autonomic dysfunction all had evidence of dementia, myelopathy, and distal sensory neuropathy.

The autonomic abnormalities were most prominent for tests of heart-rate variation. These tests, which principally assess vagus nerve function, included the expiratory-inspiratory ratio (E:I ratio), the standard deviation of heart rate (SD HR), the heart rate mean square successive difference (MSSD), and the maximum–minimum heart rate difference on deep respiration (MAX–MIN) (Figure 10-1 and Table 10-1). Resting heart rates were significantly higher in patients with AIDS than in control subjects, probably because of vagal neuropathy and unopposed cardiac sympathetic activity, similar to that sometimes seen in diabetic patients.[32] None of the patients had clinical findings or symptoms, such as dehydration or cardiac failure, which might have explained the resting tachycardia. There was also a low correlation between the resting heart rate and the fall in blood pressure with orthostatic change, a finding that would not be expected to occur if hemodynamic factors were solely responsible for the resting tachycardia. However, since echocardiographic data were not available, the possibility that subclinical myocardial dysfunction or myocarditis might be partially responsible could not be ruled out.[20,33,34] A resting tachycardia might be expected with either of the left ventricular performance abnormalities described by Lipshultz and colleagues,[20] that is, hyper- or hypodynamic function. Comparison of the heart rate response to postural change (30:15 ratio) and the Valsalva ratio between controls and patients with AIDS also revealed a trend toward declining autonomic function in the patients with AIDS (see Figure 10-1 and Table 10-1).

Sympathetic nervous system function was also found to be abnormal in the HIV-infected patients.[31] Patients with AIDS-related complex in particular had the most abnormal arterial pressure responses to standing, with mean pressure falling far more in patients with AIDS-related complex than in either controls or patients with AIDS (Table 10-1). These somewhat unexpected findings of worse function in patients with AIDS-related complex may be con-

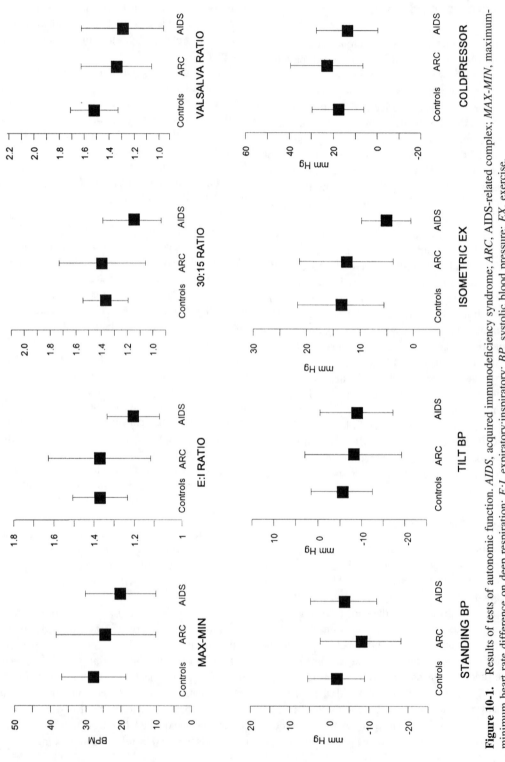

Figure 10-1. Results of tests of autonomic function. *AIDS*, acquired immunodeficiency syndrome; *ARC*, AIDS-related complex; *MAX-MIN*, maximum-minimum heart rate difference on deep respiration; *E:I*, expiratory:inspiratory; *BP*, systolic blood pressure; *EX*, exercise.

Table 10-1.　Results of Tests of Autonomic Function*

Test	Controls	ARC	AIDS
E:I ratio	1.37 ± 0.14*,**	1.37 ± 0.27	1.20 ± 0.13
MAX–MIN	27.3 ± 9.12	24.47 ± 15.03	21.17 ± 10.19
SD HR	3.79 ± 1.33**	3.41 ± 1.62	2.60 ± 1.70
MSSD	3385 ± 3181.5*,**	2725.6 ± 3527***	413.1 ± 652.3
30/15 ratio	1.31 ± 0.23	1.39 ± 0.36	1.25 ± 0.24
Valsalva ratio	1.48 ± 0.25	1.33 ± 0.30	1.38 ± 0.35
ST MAP	4.59 ± 9.51	1.63 ± 3.78	5.20 ± 9.77
ST SBP	−2.95 ± 7.63	−7.75 ± 10.85	−4.20 ± 7.57
Tilt MAP	5.36 ± 6.57*,**	−1.63 ± 6.80	0.39 ± 6.89
Tilt SBP	−5.23 ± 7.09	−8.38 ± 11.70	−8.72 ± 8.63
Isometric exercise	13.57 ± 8.35*,**	−12.43 ± 9.47***	5.17 ± 4.79
Cold pressor	17.90 ± 12.02	23.00 ± 17.94	13.71 ± 14.48

AIDS, acquired immunodeficiency syndrome; ARC, AIDS-related complex; E:I, expiratory–inspiratory; MAX-MIN, maximum-minimum heart rate difference on deep respiration; SD HR, standard deviation of the heart rate; MSSD, heart rate mean square successive difference; ST MAP, standing mean arterial pressure; Tilt MAP, mean arterial pressure on tilt-table testing; SBP, systolic blood pressure.

†Mean ± SD; *$P<0.05$ (ANOVA); **$P<0.017$ (Bonferroni corrected t test-controls to AIDS); ***$P<0.017$ (Bonferroni corrected t test-AIDS TO ARC).

sistent with the data described above of hyperdynamic left ventricular function and reduced afterload in some asymptomatic patients with HIV infection. One might hypothesize either that the sympathetic activation that leads to hyperdynamic function leaves little reserve for further reflex activation under stress, or the maneuvers that further enhance sympathetic activity stimulate ventricular afferents and induce reflex vasodilatation and hypotension. In fact, one patient with AIDS who was taking fludrocortisone for the treatment of symptomatic orthostatic hypotension and three patients with AIDS-related complex exhibited pathologic falls of more than 20 mmHg systolic blood pressure in response to standing or passive tilting. None of the controls showed comparable declines in blood pressure.

A mean autonomic deviation score was computed from the sample z scores (units of standard deviation) of two tests of sympathetic function (the systolic blood pressure responses to tilt-table testing and isometric exercise) and two tests of parasympathetic function (the E:I ratio and the Valsalva ratio), using the mean and standard deviation of the controls to establish the normal population variability. The mean autonomic deviation scores were −0.005, −0.321, and −0.823 in the control, AIDS-related complex, and AIDS subgroups, respectively ($P = .001$ by analysis of variance). Further analysis

of the intergroup comparisons revealed that this difference largely stemmed from abnormalities in the patients with AIDS, whose mean autonomic deviation score differed significantly from that of controls ($P < .005$). Eight of the 10 most abnormal scores were in patients with AIDS, and two in patients with AIDS-related complex, with none in the controls (Figure 10-2).

Similar results to those described by Freeman and associates[31] have been found in other studies.[15,29,30,35] Two of these studies had the opportunity to use HIV-negative intravenous drug users as controls for HIV-positive drug users, finding 5.6% and 33.3% incidences of abnormal autonomic tests in the HIV-negative controls.[15,30]

In summary, the results of test of autonomic function are often abnormal in patients with HIV infection, with parasympathetic function most abnormal in patients with AIDS, and sympathetic function more often perturbed in patients with AIDS-related complex. The findings are also consistent with clinical syndromes of autonomic dysfunction in these two groups.

Natural History

Although autonomic dysfunction appears to occur more frequently and with greater severity in patients with AIDS, several reports suggest that

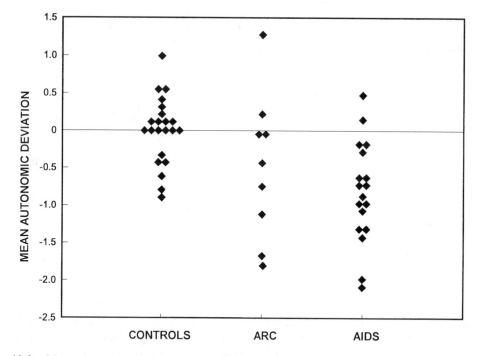

Figure 10-2. Mean autonomic deviation scores. *AIDS,* acquired immunodeficiency syndrome; *ARC,* AIDS-related complex.

seropositive patients and patients in the early stages of infection exhibit evidence of dysautonomia.[14,15,29,30,36,37] This observation is probably not surprising, since both peripheral and central neurologic signs may be the presenting or sole manifestation of HIV infection.[38,39] The appearance of autonomic dysfunction in the early stage of infection, before the appearance of opportunistic infections and tumors, implicates HIV or a virus–host interaction in the causation of the dysautonomia. However, autonomic dysfunction also appears to constitute a continuum from the early to the later stages of HIV infection,[15,31,37,40] suggesting that toxins, medications, vitamin deficiency, malnutrition, and opportunistic infections play a role in the manifestations of this syndrome in the later stages of illness.

One particularly interesting aspect of the HIV-related autonomic dysfunction is that for some parameters, particularly those related to parasympathetic control (e.g., MAX–MIN heart rate change to deep inspiration, E:I ratio, and MSSD), there is a progressive decrease in function with disease progression to AIDS-related complex and AIDS;

however, for some of the tests related to sympathetic activity (e.g., standing blood pressure, cold pressor), the AIDS-related complex population stands out as the most abnormal (Table 10-1 and Figure 10-2).[31] The patients with AIDS-related complex were a heterogeneous group, with a large variance and several results exhibiting a bimodal distribution (Figure 10-2). Several patients in the AIDS-related complex group showed exaggerated supranormal responses to autonomic testing. These findings are consistent with the demonstration by others that tachycardia, marked heart rate variability, and cardiac arrest are associated with mildly symptomatic HIV infection.[19]

Two small longitudinal studies of autonomic function have been performed in patients with HIV infection.[30,41] In one study of patients in the early stages of infection (seropositive or persistent generalized lymphadenopathy), 12 subjects underwent repeated autonomic testing over the course of 9 to 18 months, during which no patient had a significant deterioration in autonomic function, possibly reflecting either the early stage of HIV infection, the short duration of the follow-up period, or both.[41] By contrast, in a longitudinal study of more advanced HIV infection, progression of autonomic test abnormalities occurred in nine of 17 patients retested after an average of 11.2 months,[37] a period when only two of the patients changed their Centers for Disease Control stage.

Neuropathologic Basis of Autonomic Dysfunction

The underlying neuroanatomic cause of the dysautonomia accompanying HIV infection is not established; however, it is known that HIV can involve the central and peripheral nervous system at multiple sites. Thus, in a given patient there is likely to be more than one cause of the dysautonomia. The presence of nonautonomic neurologic signs might have been a useful guide to the location of autonomic deficits; however, because there has been no correlation between specific neurologic signs and autonomic abnormalities, one must use the available data to speculate on the anatomic regions and neurologic syndromes most likely to be responsible.

Central Nervous System

The neurologic and autonomic syndromes identified in HIV-infected patients, combined with data from biopsies and autopsies, indicate that abnormalities are likely to arise from one of three areas of the central nervous system: the cerebrum, the hypothalamus, and the spinal cord with its cauda equina.

The AIDS dementia complex, characterized most frequently by psychomotor slowing, poor attention, apathy, and memory loss, in association with various motor abnormalities,[42] involves subcortical cerebral regions, such as the basal ganglia, subcortical white matter, thalamus, and other deep brain nuclei.[38] Dysfunction of these structures could constitute a central neuroanatomic basis for the dysautonomia. The central nervous system may also be affected by opportunistic infections and neoplasms, whose clinical manifestations will depend on the specific sites of involvement. Although these disorders have no predilection for central autonomic structures, the autonomic nervous system may, nevertheless, be involved.

On the basis of animal studies demonstrating that central vasopressin and oxytocin play a role in the expression of autonomic functions such as eating, cardiovascular regulation, nociception, and thermoregulation, Purba and coworkers[43] hypothesized that changes in the hormone-secreting neurons from the paraventricular nucleus of the hypothalamus might be the basis for part of the neuroendocrine, autonomic dysfunction, and vegetative symptoms in AIDS. Using immunocytochemical methods to analyze vasopressin and oxytocin neurons in the paraventricular nucleus of the hypothalamus, they noted that the number of oxytocin-expressing neurons was 40% lower in patients with AIDS than in controls; however, there was no difference between the two groups in the number of vasopressin-expressing neurons.

No specific association has been found between neurologic abnormalities of the spinal cord in HIV-infected patients and cardiovascular autonomic dysfunction. However, symptoms of bladder and bowel dysfunction, including urinary retention and loss of sphincter control, are often a feature of a polyradiculomyelopathy seen in patients with AIDS. Pathologic examinations have revealed vacuolation of the myelin sheath (vacuolar myelopathy) in some cases,[44–46] and documented cytomegalovirus infection in others.[9,47] The vacuolar myelopathy tends to involve the posterior and lateral columns of the middle and lower thoracic spinal cord, although cytomegalovirus inclusions have been noted on neuropathologic examination of the lumbosacral nerve roots and lower spinal cord. A similar clinical picture may occur with other opportunistic infections of the lumbosacral nerve roots and spinal cord, such as *Toxoplasma gondii*,[48,49] herpes simplex virus type 2,[50] neurosyphilis,[51,52] and leptomeningeal spread of systemic lymphoma.[53]

Peripheral Nervous System

The peripheral nervous system is involved clinically in up to 80% of patients with AIDS, with 95% involvement post mortem.[54] Although there are fewer direct data on the specific involvement of the autonomic components of the peripheral nerves in HIV-infected patients, pathologic examination of the sympathetic and sensory ganglia has revealed a mild ganglionitis, consisting of macrophages, T lymphocytes, and an increase in the amount of major histocompatibility complex class II antigen expression.[55] In addition, HIV p24 core protein antigen and HIV gp41 envelope protein antigen have been found within macrophages in the ganglia of HIV-infected subjects.[55] These findings were present in many HIV-positive patients but were most prominent in patients with clinical AIDS.

More peripheral pathologic changes have included loss of myelinated and unmyelinated fibers, wallerian degeneration, and a mononuclear inflammatory infiltrate.[54,56–58] Griffin and colleagues[24] described extensive loss of unmyelinated fibers in two patients with AIDS who died shortly after the onset of neuropathic pain, supporting the notion that the distal sensorimotor neuropathy of AIDS may be a cause of autonomic dysfunction.

Medications and Toxins

Several medications commonly used to treat AIDS-related complications have recognized neurologic side effects.[59] Thus, treatment with these agents may produce symptoms of autonomic dysfunction or may be responsible for some of the abnormalities in autonomic testing. Vincristine, a component of the drug regimen prescribed for Kaposi's sarcoma, is associated with orthostatic hypotension[60]; however, in a prospective study in non-HIV-infected cancer patients, only one of 26 patients treated with vincristine suffered from orthostatic hypotension.[61] Pentamidine,[62,63] zidovudine,[64] and trimethoprim–sulfamethoxazole[65] have also been associated with orthostatic hypotension. The antiretroviral nucleoside analogues 2′,3′-dideoxyinosine (ddI or didanosine),[66,67] 2′,3′-dideoxycytidine (ddC or zalcitabine),[68,69] and 2′,3′-dihydro 3′-deoxythymidine (d4T or stavudine)[70,71] all have known peripheral nervous system neurotoxic effects, yielding the potential for autonomic effects; however, dysautonomia has not yet been associated with use of these agents.

Cardiac Arrhythmias

On the basis of the above observations concerning autonomic abnormalities, and the literature on myo-

cardial involvement in this patient population,[33] one would speculate that a combination of influences, including myocarditis, proarrhythmia from medications, and cardiac sympathetic activation, could lead to arrhythmias in HIV-infected patients. In fact, a variety of cardiac arrhythmias and possible arrhythmia-related events have been described in patients with HIV infection.[12,20,33,72–77] Although many of these reports have been specific to an association between administration of intravenous pentamidine for *Pneumocystis carinii* infection and the development of torsades de pointes,[78–82] there have been a few reports surveying the occurrence of other arrhythmias or cardiac conduction abnormalities in HIV-infected patients.

Adults

In one of the only studies to assess the prevalence of cardiac rhythm disturbances in HIV-infected adults, Cardoso et al.[83] examined Holter, electrocardiographic (ECG), and echocardiographic data in 21 patients with various stages of HIV infection. Although most patients had some type of rhythm disturbance, no patient had a clinically significant abnormality on Holter or surface ECG. Extrasystolic disturbances, included isolated atrial and ventricular ectopy (66% each), ventricular couplets (4.8%), and nonsustained supraventricular tachycardia (14.3%), but no ventricular tachycardia was seen. Four patients (19%) had conduction disturbances which included one with intermittent second-degree atrioventricular block (Mobitz 1-Wenkebach), two with occasional 2:1 atrioventricular block rhythm abnormalities, and one with bifascicular block. No patient had bradyarrhythmias, ischemic changes, or any cardiac symptoms at the time of monitoring, but the one patient with persistent bifascicular block later developed complete atrioventricular block and syncope, and underwent pacemaker implantation. Thus, in their small population of young adults, ECG abnormalities were common, but few were clinically significant.

Children

Luginbuhl and colleagues[19] examined a group of 81 children with HIV infection (median age 1.5 years). In contrast to the findings of Cardoso,[83] Luginbuhl and colleagues found an abnormally high prevalence of benign rhythm disturbances and, importantly, ventricular tachycardia in two patients and ventricular fibrillation in one. Benign rhythm abnormalities occurred widely, including atrial ectopy (25%), junctional ectopy (4%), and isolated ventricular ectopy (15%), as well as sinus tachycardia (64%), sinus bradycardia (11%), and marked sinus arrhythmia, defined as greater than 50 beats per minute variations in rate (17%). One of the patients with ventricular tachycardia had torsades de pointes during pentamidine administration and later died suddenly, with myocarditis, pericarditis, and conduction system inflammation diagnosed at autopsy. Seven other patients also had cardiorespiratory arrest, but none died. Importantly, rhythm abnormalities could be associated with other manifestations of the HIV infection. Marked sinus arrhythmia was strongly associated with many outcome variables, including AIDS-related complex, lymphocytic interstitial pneumonitis, encephalopathy, and cytomegalovirus infection. Tachycardia, bradycardia, and cardiac arrest were also associated with many of these diagnoses, but the specific classes of ectopy were not included in the risk analysis. Thus, it appears that abnormalities of heart rate control, which probably reflect neurologically mediated autonomic dysfunction, and premature beats, which probably reflect a combination of myocardial and autonomic abnormalities, are both common in HIV-infected children and are associated with the clinical manifestations of the disease.

Conduction System

Much of the data documenting conduction system abnormalities in patients with HIV infection must be drawn from more general reports on the cardiac complications of HIV. However, Bharati and coworkers[77] specifically examined the entire cardiac conduction system in six children who died of AIDS, using about 1,400 to 2,500 serial sections per heart. The sinoatrial and atrioventricular node and their approaches, the penetrating atrioventricular bundle, and the left and right bundle branches were all examined in detail. Marked abnormalities of the conduction system, including vasculitis, myocarditis, and fragmentation of the conduction

fiber bundles with lobulation and fibrosis, were seen in all cases, but the locations of the changes were highly variable between patients. These authors also noted that the changes in the surrounding myocardium were generally worse than those in the conduction system. A dominant observation for both conduction tissue and the remainder of the myocardium was a vasculitis of both the arteries and veins of almost every size, occasionally resulting in thrombosis. There were no data to suggest whether the changes were due to the direct effects of the HIV virus, the autoimmune response, or opportunistic infections. Although the findings were only associated with a prior ECG abnormality in one case (a left hemiblock), other reports have documented clinically apparent conduction changes on the surface ECG in HIV-infected patients.[83]

Torsades de Pointes and Pentamidine

There are numerous case reports describing the phenomenon of QT prolongation and torsades de pointes in HIV-infected patients receiving pentamidine;[19,79,82,84–88] however, there are few reports of pentamidine and torsades in non-HIV-infected patients,[89] suggesting strongly that it is the combination of HIV-related cardiomyopathy, nutritionally based electrolyte disturbances, and the drug that leads to the arrhythmogenicity. Given the role of sympathetic activation in producing torsades in the congenital form of the long QT syndrome,[4] it also seems likely that the dysautonomia of AIDS plays a role in the generation of the arrhythmia. In fact, one patient with penatamidine-induced torsades reported by Luginbuhl[19] was specifically noted to have marked autonomic dysfunction.

To further document the causal influence of pentamidine on the QT interval and on torsades in HIV-infected patients, Eisenhauer and colleagues[80] performed a prospective evaluation of these effects in 14 HIV-infected patients receiving intravenous pentamidine for *P. carinii* pneumonia. Of the 14 subjects, three developed torsades de pointes, which was associated with prolongation of the corrected QT interval (QT_c) to more than 0.48 second in all three. Two other patients who did not develop torsades also had QT_c prolongation to more than 0.48 second, while the remaining nine patients had only minimal changes in QT_c (mean increase: 0.03 second). Thus, QT prolongation was significantly associated with both pentamidine therapy and the development of torsades.

Role of the Autonomic Nervous System

As noted above, the autonomic nervous system plays a role as a trigger in many arrhythmias in patients with or without HIV infection.[1,2] Thus, one might expect that a disease that produces autonomic dysfunction, particularly reduced cardiac vagal and enhanced cardiac sympathetic control, would be associated with an increased prevalence of arrhythmias. Indeed, as discussed above, such is the case for HIV infection. However, some data suggest that the link between malignant arrhythmic deaths and the autonomic dysfunction associated with HIV infection may be even tighter. Villa and associates[90] found that the corrected QT interval was at least 0.44 second in 24 of 37 HIV-positive patients (64.8%) with autonomic neuropathy, but in only 5 of 20 HIV-positive patients (25%) without autonomic neuropathy. There were no clinical signs of cardiac disease in any of these patients, although echocardiographic studies were not performed. Such observations may partially underlie the predisposition of HIV-infected patients to cardiac arrhythmias such as ventricular tachycardia and torsades de pointes, and the observed incidence of unexpected cardiorespiratory arrest.[12,19,78,80–82]

Conclusion

Autonomic dysfunction is a common and disabling complication of AIDS. Arrhythmias are less common, but often have devastating consequences, including sudden death. Characteristic features of the autonomic dysfunction include syncope and pre-syncope, blood pressure and heart rate lability, cardiac arrhythmias, impotence, bowel dysfunction, bladder dysfunction, incontinence, and anhidrosis. A broad array of arrhythmias have been identified in HIV-infected patients, with the most serious ones usually being a consequence of either conduction system disease or administration of toxic drugs, such as pentamidine. Many others are probably

related to the myocarditis found in a high percentage of infected patients. Importantly, it is likely that the underlying autonomic dysfunction in these patients interacts in a multiplicative way with the myocarditis, which is often present to produce more severe cardiac rhythm disturbances. To date, there has been no large prospective study of autonomic failure or cardiac rhythm in patients with AIDS. Thus, our knowledge of the prevalence of these disorders, their association with neurologic and nonneurologic complications of AIDS, and their relation to therapeutic interventions using potentially neurotoxic agents is still limited. Ongoing prospective studies and trials should help address these questions.

References

1. Ben-David J, Zipes DP. Autonomic neural modulation of cardiac rhythm. Part 1: Basic concepts. *Mod Concepts Cardiovasc Dis* 1988;57:41–46.

2. Zipes DP, Ben-David J. Autonomic neural modulation of cardiac rhythm, part 2: mechanisms and examples. *Mod Concepts Cardiovasc Dis* 1988;57:47–52.

3. Roden DM, George AL, Jr., Bennett PB. Recent advances in understanding the molecular mechanisms of the long QT syndrome. *Cardiovasc Electrophysiol* 1995;6:1023–1031.

4. Schwartz PJ, Bonazzi O, Locati E, et al. Pathogenesis and therapy of the idiopathic long QT syndrome. *NY Acad Sci* 1992;644:112–141.

5. Ho DD, Rota TR, Schooley RT, et al. Isolation of HTLV-III from cerebrospinal fluid and neural tissues of patients with neurological syndromes related to the acquired immunodeficiency syndrome. *N Engl J Med* 1985;313:1493–1499.

6. Levy JA, Shimabukuro J, Hollander H, et al. Isolation of AIDS associated retroviruses from the cerebrospinal fluid and brains of patients with neurological symptoms. *Lancet* 1985;2:586–588.

7. Bredesen DE, Levy RM, Rosenblum ML. The neurology of human immunodeficiency virus infection. *Q J Med* 1988;68:665–677.

8. Levy RM, Bredesen DE, Rosenblum ML. Neurological manifestations of the acquired immunodeficiency syndrome (AIDS): experience at UCSF

and review of the literature. *Neurosurgery* 1985;62: 475–495.

9. McArthur JC. Neurologic manifestations of AIDS. *Medicine* 1987;66:407–437.

10. Lin-Greenberger A, Taneja-Uppal N. Dysautonomia and infection with the human immunodeficiency virus. [Letter]. *Ann Intern Med* 1987;106:167.

11. Cornblath DR, McArthur JC, Kennedy PGE, et al. Inflammatory demyelinating peripheral neuropathies associated with human-cell lymphotropic virus type III infection. *Ann Neurol* 1987;21:32–40.

12. Craddock C, Pasvol G, Bull R, et al. Cardiorespiratory arrest and autonomic neuropathy in AIDS. *Lancet* 1987;2:16–18.

13. Evenhouse M, Haas E, Snell E, et al. Hypertension infection with the human immunodeficiency virus. [Letter]. *Ann Intern Med* 1987;107:598–599.

14. Mulhall B, Jennens I. Testing for neurological involvement in HIV infection. [Letter]. *Lancet* 1987;2:1531.

15. Ruttimann S, Hilti P, Spinas GA, Dubach UC: High frequency of human immunodeficiency virus-associated autonomic neuropathy and more severe involvement in advanced stages of human immunodeficiency virus disease. *Arch Intern Med* 1991; 151:2441–2443.

16. Cohen JA, Miller L, Polish L. Orthostatic hypotension in human immunodeficiency virus infection may be the result of generalized autonomic nervous system dysfunction. *J Acquir Immune Defic Syndr* 1991;4:31–33.

17. Klein RS, Mann DN, Friedland GH, Surks MI. Adrenocortical function in the acquired immunodeficiency syndrome. [Letter]. *Ann Intern Med* 1983;99:566.

18. Membreno L, Irony I, Dere W, et al. Adrenocortical function in acquired immunodeficiency syndrome. *J Clin Endocrinol Metab* 1987;65:482–487.

19. Luginbuhl LM, Orav EJ, McIntosh K, Lipshultz SE. Cardiac morbidity and related mortality in children with HIV infection. *JAMA* 1993;269:2869–2875.

20. Lipshultz SE, Chanock S, Sanders SP, et al. Cardiovascular manifestation of human immunodeficiency virus infection in infants and children. *Am J Cardiol* 1989;63:1489–1497.

21. Kosinski D, Grubb BP, Temesy-Armos P. Pathophysiological aspects of neurocardiogenic syncope: current concepts and new perspectives. [Abstract]. *PACE* 1995;18:716–724.

22. Ali ST, Shaikh RN, Siddiqi A. HIV-1 associated neuropathies in males; impotence and penile electrodiagnosis. *Acta Neurol Belg* 1994;94:194–199.

23. Griffin GE, Miller A, Batman P, et al. Damage to jejunal intrinsic autonomic nerves in HIV infection. *AIDS* 1988;2:379–382.

24. Griffin JW, Crawford TO, Tyor WR, et al: Predominantly sensory neuropathy in AIDS: distal axonal degeneration and unmyelinated fiber loss. *Neurology* 1991;41:374

25. Batman PA, Miller AR, Sedgwick PM, Griffin GE. Autonomic denervation in jejunal mucosa of homosexual men infected with HIV. *AIDS* 1991;5:1247–1252.

26. Blanshard C, Ellis DS, Tovey G, Gazzard BG. Electron microscopy of rectal biopsies in HIV-positive individuals. *J Pathol* 1993;169:79–87.

27. Coker RJ, Horner P, Bleasdale-Barr K, et al. Increased gut parasympathetic activity and chronic diarrhoea in a patient with the acquired immunodeficiency syndrome. *Clin Auton Res* 1992;2:295–298.

28. Cohen JA, Laudenslager M. Autonomic nervous system involvement in patients with human immunodeficiency virus infection. *Neurology* 1989;39: 1111–1112.

29. Villa A, Cruccu V, Foresti V, et al. HIV related functional involvement of autonomic nervous system. *Acta Neurol* 1990;12:14–18.

30. Villa A, Foresti V, Confalonieri F. Autonomic neuropathy and HIV infection. [Letter]. *Lancet* 1987; 1:915

31. Freeman R, Roberts MS, Friedman LS, Broadbridge C. Autonomic function and human immunodeficiency virus infection. *Neurology* 1990;40: 575–580.

32. Wheeler T, Watkins PJ. Cardiac denervation in diabetics. *BMJ* 1973;4:584–586.

33. Anderson DW, Virmani R, Reilly JM. Prevalent myocarditis at necropsy in the acquired immunodeficiency syndrome. *J Am Coll Cardiol* 1988;11: 792–799.

34. Cohen IS, Anderson DW, Virmani R, et al. Congestive cardiomyopathy in association with the acquired immunodeficiency syndrome. *N Engl J Med* 1986;315:628–630.

35. Welby SB, Rogerson SJ, Beeching NJ. Autonomic neuropathy is common in human immunodeficiency virus infection. *J Infect* 1991;23:123–128.

36. Kumar M, Morgan R, Szapocznik J, Eisdorfer C. Norepinephrine response in early HIV infection. *J Acquir Immune Defic Syndr* 1991;4:782–786.

37. Villa A, Foresti V, Confalonieri F. Autonomic nervous system dysfunction associated with HIV infection in intravenous heroin users. *AIDS* 1992;6: 85–89.

38. Navia BA, Cho ES, Petito CK, Price RW. The AIDS dementia complex: II. Neuropathology. *Ann Neurol* 1986;19:525–535.

39. Smith T, Jakobsen J, Trojaborg W. Symptomatic polyneuropathy in human immunodeficiency virus antibody seropositive men with and without immune deficiency: a comparative electrophysiological study. *J Neurol Neurosurg Psychiatry* 1990;53: 1056–1059.

40. Gastaut JL, Pouget J, Valentin P, et al. [Study of sensory involvement and dysautonomia in HIV infected patients: a prospective study of 55 cases]. [French]. *Neurophysiol Clin* 1992;22:417–430.

41. Scott G, Piaggesi A, Ewing DJ. Sequential autonomic function tests in HIV infection. *AIDS* 1990;4: 1279–1281.

42. Navia BA, Jordan BD, Price RW. The AIDS dementia complex. I. Clinical features. *Ann Neurol* 1986;19:517–524.

43. Purba JS, Hofman MA, Portegies P, et al. Decreased number of oxytocin neurons in the paraventricular nucleus of the human hypothalamus in AIDS. *Brain* 1993;116:795–809.

44. Dal Pan GJ, Glass JD, McArthur JC. Clinicopathologic correlations of HIV-1-associated vacuolar myelopathy: an autopsy-based case-control study. *Neurology* 1994;44:2159–2164.

45. Petito CK, Navia BA, Cho E, et al. Vacuolar myelopathy pathologically resembling subacute combined degeneration in patients with the acquired immunodeficiency syndrome. *N Engl J Med* 1985; 312:874–879.

46. Tan SV, Guiloff RJ, Scaravilli F. AIDS-associated vacuolar myelopathy: a morphometric study. *Brain* 1995;118:1247–1261.

47. Eidelberg D, Sotrel A, Vogel H, et al. Progressive polyradiculopathy in acquired immune deficiency syndrome. *Neurology* 1986;36:912–916.

48. Kayser C, Campbell R, Sartorious C, Bartlett M. Toxoplasmosis of the conus medullaris in a patient with hemophilia A-associated AIDS: case report. *J Neurosurg* 1990;73:951–953.

49. Overhage JM, Greist A, Brown DR. Conus medullaris syndrome resulting from *Toxoplasma gondii* infection in a patient with the acquired immunodeficiency syndrome. *Am J Med* 1990;89:814–815.

50. Wiley CA, VanPatten PD, Carpenter PM, et al. Acute ascending necrotizing myelopathy caused by herpes simplex virus type 2. *Neurology* 1987;37: 1791–1794.

51. Berger JR. Spinal cord syphilis associated with human immunodeficiency virus infection: a treatable myelopathy. *Am J Med* 1992;92:101–103.

52. Lanska MJ, Lanska DJ, Schmidley JW. Syphilitic polyradiculopathy in an HIV-positive man. *Neurology* 1988;38:1297–1301.

53. Klein P, Zientek G, VandenBerg SR, Lothman E. Primary CNS lymphoma: lymphomatous meningitis presenting as a cauda equina lesion in an AIDS patient. *Can J Neurol Sci* 1990;17:329–331.

54. de la Monte SM, Gabuzda DH, Ho DD, et al. Peripheral neuropathy in the acquired immunodeficiency syndrome. *Ann Neurol* 1988;23:485–492.

55. Esiri MM, Morris CS, Millard PR. Sensory and sympathetic ganglia in HIV-1 infection: immunocytochemical demonstration of HIV-1 viral antigens, increased MHC class II antigen expression and mild reactive inflammation. *J Neurol Sci* 1993; 114:178–187.

56. Fuller GN, Jacobs JM. Axonal atrophy in the painful peripheral neuropathy in AIDS. *Acta Neuropathol* 1990;81:198–203.

57. Leger JM, Bouche P, Bolgert F, et al. The spectrum of polyneuropathies in patients infected with HIV. *J Neurol Neurosurg Psychiatry* 1989;52:1369–1374.

58. Mah V, Vartavarian LM, Akers MA, Vinters HV. Abnormalities of peripheral nerve in patients with human immunodeficiency virus infection. *Ann Neurol* 1988;24:713–717.

59. Simpson DM, Tagliati M. Nucleoside analogue-associated peripheral neuropathy in human immunodeficiency virus infection. *J Acquir Immune Defic Syndr Hum Retrovirol* 1995;9:153–161.

60. Carmichael SM, Eagleton L, Ayers CR, Mohler D. Orthostatic hypotension during vincristine therapy. *Arch Intern Med* 1970;126:290–293.

61. DiBella NJ. Vincristine-induced orthostatic hypotension: a prospective clinical study. *Cancer Treat Rep* 1980;62:359–360.

62. Helmich CG, Green JK. Pentamidine-associated hypotension and route of adminstration. *Ann Intern Med* 1985;103:480

63. Siddiqui MA, Ford PA. Acute severe autonomic insufficiency during pentamidine therapy. [Letter]. *South Med J* 1995;88:1087–1088.

64. Loke RH, Murray-Lyon IM, Carter GD. Postural hypotension related to zidovudine in a patient infected with HIV. *BMJ* 1990;300:163–164.

65. Kelly JW, Dooley DP, Lattuada CP, Smith CE. A severe, unusual reaction to trimethoprim-sulfamethoxazole in patients infected with human immunodeficiency virus. *Clin Infect Dis* 1992;14:1034–1039.

66. Cooley TP, Kunches LM, Saunders CA, et al. Once-daily administration of 2'3'-dideoxyinosine (ddI) in patients with the acquired immunodeficiency syndrome or AIDS-related complex: results of a phase I trial. *N Engl J Med* 1990;322:1340–1345.

67. Lambert JS, Seidlin M, Reichman RC, et al. 2',3'-Dideoxyinosine (EYE) in patients with the acquired immunodeficiency syndrome or AIDS-related complex: a phase I trial. *N Engl J Med* 1990;322:1333–1340.

68. Berger AR, Arezzo JC, Schaumburg HH, et al. 2',3'-Dideoxycytidine (ddC) toxic neuropathy: a study of 52 patients. *Neurology* 1993;43:358–362.

69. Dubinsky RM, Varchoan R, Dalakas M, Broder S. Reversible axonal neuropathy from the treatment of AIDS and related disorders with 2',3'-dideoxycytidine (ddC). *Muscle Nerve* 1989;12:856–860.

70. Skowron G. Biologic effects and safety of stavudine: overview of phase I and II clinical trials. *J Infect Dis* 1995;171(Suppl:2):S113–117.

71. Sommadossi JP. Comparison of metabolism and in vitro antiviral activity of stavudine versus other 2',3'-dideoxynucleoside analogues. *J Infect Dis* 1995;171(Suppl. 2):S88–92.

72. Brady MT, Reiner CB, Singley C, et al. Unexpected death in an infant with AIDS: disseminated cytomegalovirus infection with pancarditis. *Pediatr Pathol* 1988;8:205–214.

73. Kovacs A, Hinton D, Wong W, et al. HIV infection of myocytes and sudden death in pediatric AIDS. [Abstract]. *Pediatr Res* 1992;31:167.

74. Lipshultz SE, Luginbuhl L, Saul JP, McIntosh K. Dysrhythmias, unexpected arrest, and sudden death in pediatric HIV infection. [Abstract]. *Circulation* 1991;84:660.

75. Anderson DW, Virmani R. Emerging patterns of heart disease in human immunodeficiency virus infection. *Hum Pathol* 1991;21:253–259.

76. Reilly JM, Cunnion RE, Anderson DW. Frequency of myocarditis, left ventricular dysfunction, and ventricular tachycardia in the acquired immune deficiency syndrome. *Am J Cardiol* 1988;62:789–793.

77. Bharati S, Joshi VV, Connor EM, et al. Conduction system in children with acquired immunodeficiency syndrome. *Chest* 1989;96:406–413.

78. Cohen AJ, Weiser B, Afzal Q, Fuhrer J. Ventricular tachycardia in two patients with AIDS receiving ganciclovir (DHPG). *AIDS* 1990;4:807–809.

79. Cortese LM, Gasser RA Jr, Bjornson DC, et al. Prolonged recurrence of pentamidine-induced torsades de pointes. *Ann Pharmacother* 1992;26:1365–1369.

80. Eisenhauer MD, Eliasson AH, Taylor AJ, et al. Incidence of cardiac arrhythmias during intravenous pentamidine therapy in HIV-infected patients. *Chest* 1994;105:389–395.

81. Stein KM, Haronian H, Mensah GA, et al. Ventricular tachycardia and torsades de pointes complicating pentamidine therapy of *Pneumocystis carinii* pneumonia in the acquired immunodeficiency syndrome. *Am J Cardiol* 1990;66:888–889.

82. Wharton JM, Demopulos PA, Goldschlager N. Torsade de pointes during administration of pentamidine isethionate. *Am J Med* 1987;83:571–576.

83. Cardoso J, Mota-Miranda A, Cruz A, et al. Dysrhythmic profile of human immunodeficiency virus infected patients. *Int J Cardiol* 1995;49:249–255.

84. Bibler MR, Chou T, Toltzis RJ, Wade PA. Recurrent ventricular tachycardia due to pentamidine-induced cardiotoxicity. *Chest* 1988;94:1303–1306.

85. Pujol M, Carratala J, Mauri J, Viladrich P. Ventricular tachycardia due to pentamidine isethionate. *Am J Med* 1988;84:980

86. Mitchell P, Dodek P, Lawson L, et al. Torsades de pointes during intravenous pentamidine isethionate therapy. *Can Med Assoc J* 1989;140:173–174.

87. Loescher T, Loescher K, Niebel J. Severe ventricular arrhythmia during pentamidine treatment of AIDS-associated *Pneumocystis carinii* pneumonia. [Abstract]. *Infection 15* 1987;45:455.

88. Balslev U, Berild D, Nielsen TL. Cardiac arrest during treatment of *Pneumocystis carinii* pneumonia with intravenous pentamidine isethionate. *Scand J Infect Dis* 1992;24:111–112.

89. Quadrel MA, Atkin SH, Jaker MA. Delayed cardiotoxicity during treatment with intravenous pentamidine: two case reports and a review of the literature. *Am Heart J* 1992;123:1377–1379.

90. Villa A, Foresti V, Confalonieri F. Autonomic neuropathy and prolongation of QT interval in human immunodeficiency virus infection. *Clin Auton Res* 1995;5:48–52.

11

Pulmonary Disease and Therapy in HIV Infection

Suzanne Steinbach, M.D., and Janice Hunter, R.N., M.S.

Pulmonary disease remains a frequent presenting complication and the most common cause of mortality in human immunodeficiency virus (HIV)-infected patients. It is responsible for 50% of deaths in children[1] and 65% of serious illness in adults[2] with acquired immunodeficiency syndrome (AIDS). The high incidence of pulmonary complications results both directly from infection of the lung by HIV and secondarily from immunocompromise, including impairment of local and systemic macrophage and lymphocyte function. When immune defenses deteriorate, the respiratory tract serves as the primary portal of entry for many infectious agents.[3-6] Reflecting the intimate relation between the respiratory and cardiovascular systems, primary pulmonary diseases, by either their severity or their chronicity, may lead to cardiovascular abnormalities or masquerade as such. It is imperative that the cardiac clinician be aware of the many pulmonary disorders associated with HIV infection.

Pulmonary complications in HIV-infected patients may be infectious or noninfectious. The most common life-threatening infectious complication is *Pneumocystis carinii* pneumonia.[7,8] Upper and lower airway infection with pyrogenic bacterial organisms such as *Haemophilus influenzae* and *Streptococcus pneumoniae* is also common and can appear as early as the first year of life.[9,10] Other bacterial infections such as *Mycobacterium tuberculosis* and *Mycobacterium avium-intracellulare* complex are also prevalent. Viruses (cytomegalovirus, herpes simplex, varicella-zoster, influenza, respiratory syncytial virus), fungi (*Histoplasma capsulatum, Cryptococcus, Candida, Aspergillus*), and parasites (*Toxoplasma, Cryptosporidium*) also contribute to the pulmonary pathology. Noninfectious causes of respiratory disease include Kaposi's sarcoma and non-Hodgkin's lymphoma, both more common in adults. Nonspecific interstitial pneumonitis and lymphoid interstitial pneumonitis (pulmonary lymphoid hyperplasia [PLH]) are more common in children. Diseases affecting the airway, such as upper airway obstruction or chronic obstructive sleep apnea, vasculitis, and asthma, are also seen in patients with HIV disease. Each of these entities, either directly or through side effects of therapy, may have cardiovascular consequences.

Pulmonary Disease of Infectious Origin

Bacterial Pneumonia

Next to upper respiratory infection, bacterial pneumonia from pathogens responsible for ordinary community-acquired pneumonia is the most com-

mon respiratory complication in HIV-infected patients. Chest x-ray findings may be atypical, resembling those in a variety of other pathologic
conditions, so that radiographic observations are an
unreliable basis for specific diagnosis. Pneumonia
caused by *S. pneumoniae* is most frequent and is
often accompanied by bacteremia. Since pneumococcal pneumonia is frequent in HIV infection,
Pneumovax has been recommended for all HIV-
infected patients; however, at least half will fail to
mount a protective antibody response to vaccine.[11]
Therefore, pneumococcal pneumonia must remain
high on the differential diagnosis, even in vaccinated patients. Other bacterial pathogens frequently
involved in HIV-related pneumonia include *H. influenzae, Moraxella catarrhalis, Klebsiella pneumoniae*, and *Neisseria meningitidis*. Severely debilitated patients may develop aspiration pneumonia
caused by anaerobic organisms; their heightened
susceptibility to this complication relates both to
gastroesophageal reflux and to failure to protect the
airway from aspiration of oral secretions. In patients
with severe immunologic compromise, *Staphylococcus aureus* is a recognized respiratory pathogen
associated with a mortality rate of 38%.[12] By contrast, indolent bronchopulmonary infection caused
by *Pseudomonas aeruginosa* has been described,
resembling the slowly progressive process in cystic
fibrosis.[13] Both *S. aureus* and *P. aeruginosa* may
have multiple antibiotic resistance, leading to significant infection control concerns.

Microscopic examination and culture of expectorated sputum may reveal the pathogen responsible
for pneumonia. Even in children, sputum induction
with 3% saline nebulization is often effective in
demonstrating the presence of *P. carinii* or other
pathogens.[14] After attempts to obtain sputum, empirical antibiotic therapy is usually begun. Patients
who fail to improve promptly will require bronchoscopy with bronchoalveolar lavage or open lung biopsy. Fiberoptic bronchoalveolar lavage effectively
retrieves a variety of bacterial, viral, fungal, and
protozoal pathogens with very low complication
rates (0.95%).[15] In one series of HIV-infected patients with pneumonia, bronchoalveolar lavage was
positive for specific microorganisms in 84% of
cases. Bacteria were retrieved in 57% of cases, fungi
in 42%, viruses in 29%, *P. carinii* in 11%, *M. avium-*

intracellulare complex in 22%, and *M. tuberculosis*
in 3%.[15] Bronchoalveolar lavage is generally preferred over fine-needle aspiration of the lung, particularly since syncopal reactions with hypotension,
arrhythmias, and cardiorespiratory arrest have occurred after the latter procedure, presumably as a
consequence of autonomic neuropathy.[16]

Although initial therapy for pneumonia usually
elicits a favorable response, relapse is frequent,
and complications such as abscess or empyema
formation are not uncommon.[17] Pleural effusion
was reported in 27% of AIDS-related hospital admissions; 66% of cases involved pulmonary infection (*P. carinii* 15%, *M. tuberculosis* 9%, *M. avium
intracellulare* complex 2%, bacterial 31%, *Nocardia* 3% and *Cryptococcus* 3%, septic embolism
3%).[18] In the remaining one-third of the cases with
pleural effusion, there was no identifiable underlying pulmonary infection; of these, 19% had hypoalbuminemia and 2% had Kaposi's sarcoma. In this
series, only 5% of the patients with pleural effusion
were found to have congestive heart failure as the
primary cause,[18] suggesting that an infectious cause
will usually be the initial presumption and that a
high index of suspicion will be required to achieve
this diagnosis.

Viral Pneumonia

Whenever the response to antibiotic therapy for
pneumonia is slow, the possibility of a concomitant
infection with a second pathogen such as *P. carinii*
or a virus must be considered. Common viral pathogens, including respiratory syncytial virus, parain-
fluenza virus, influenza virus, and adenovirus, may
cause lower respiratory tract infection in patients
with AIDS. Respiratory syncytial virus infection in
children with AIDS is associated with less wheezing but with an increased incidence of viral pneumonia, or concomitant infection with other pathogens such as *P. aeruginosa* and *P. carinii*, and with
markedly increased mortality.[19] Prolonged respiratory syncytial virus shedding in the patient not
known to be HIV-infected may serve as an initial
clue to this diagnosis. Increased severity of respiratory syncytial virus infection and prolonged viral
shedding have led to recommendations for ribavirin
aerosol therapy for HIV-infected children.[20]

Less commonly, other viral pathogens, such as cytomegalovirus, varicella-zoster virus, Epstein-Barr virus, and measles virus, may cause disseminated disease with severe pulmonary involvement in patients with AIDS.[21] Underlying lymphoid interstitial pneumonitis or concomitant *P. carinii* or bacterial infection may aggravate the severity of the viral process. Definitive diagnosis may require bronchoalveolar lavage or, in the case of cytomegalovirus, open-lung biopsy. Although cytomegalovirus may be isolated by bronchoalveolar lavage in up to 20% of cases,[15] open-lung biopsy demonstrating viral inclusion bodies is preferred to achieve the diagnosis of cytomegalovirus pneumonitis. Many patients with a positive bronchoalveolar lavage for cytomegalovirus are only colonized with the viral organism and improve without specific antiviral therapy. Specific therapy available for certain viral infections includes ganciclovir and foscarnet for cytomegalovirus, ribavirin for respiratory syncytial virus and influenza virus, amantadine for influenza virus, and acyclovir for varicella-zoster virus and herpes simplex virus. Yearly influenza vaccine is recommended for prophylaxis of influenza lower respiratory tract infection in patients with AIDS.

Pneumocystis carinii Pneumonia

With the advent of effective prophylaxis, primarily with trimethoprim–sulfamethoxazole, the proportion of AIDS-related hospital admissions due to *P. carinii* pneumonia has declined from 58% to 29% according to one Canadian report.[22] Despite this trend, *P. carinii* pneumonia remains a common complication among HIV-infected individuals. *P. carinii* is the first sign of HIV infection in 48% to 64% of cases among infants and young children.[23,24] The mortality rate from *P. carinii* pneumonia is higher in children than in adults probably because of immaturity of their immune systems and because *P. carinii* pneumonia in children is a primary infection rather than the reactivation of a latent infection as it is in adults.[23–27] Patients ultimately proven to have *P. carinii* pneumonia usually present with cough and varying degrees of tachypnea and hypoxia. In infants and young children the onset is usually acute, but there may be a history of nonproductive cough and increasing tachypnea over a period of weeks. An insidious and prolonged onset is more common in adult patients with AIDS, or those with secondary or breakthrough *P. carinii* pneumonia.[7,28,29]

On chest auscultation, decreased breath sounds, rales, and wheeze may be noted. Laboratory findings are consistent with the degree of hypoxia. PO_2 values are often less than 50 mmHg and the AaO_2 gradient is usually increased. Lactate dehydrogenase (LDH) may be a useful diagnostic tool; it is more often elevated in adults than in children.[30]

Chest x-rays in *P. carinii* pneumonia most commonly reveal diffuse, bilateral air space filling infiltrates, but occasionally nodular infiltrates, focal consolidation, or even cystic lucencies are noted. Thus, the overlap in radiologic findings between *P. carinii* pneumonia and other pulmonary processes in AIDS is large, and chest radiographs should not be relied upon for definitive diagnosis. Moderate to large pleural effusions and hilar or mediastinal lymphadenopathy, if seen in the chest radiograph, should strongly suggest alternative diagnoses, such as tuberculosis, Kaposi's sarcoma, or lymphoma.[17] Cystic areas on chest radiographs have been noted in association with *P. carinii* pneumonia and may lead to pneumothorax during acute episodes or, less commonly, following the acute phase. Up to 10% of patients with *P. carinii* pneumonia develop a pneumothorax, which may be recurrent.[31]

Clinical, laboratory, and radiographic findings are merely suggestive of *P. carinii* pneumonia. A definitive diagnosis can only be made by identification of the organism. In young children this usually requires bronchoalveolar lavage in which a yield of 75% has been reported.[32] In older children and adults, induced sputum with a yield of 55% to 90% is often sufficient for diagnosis.[33–35]

The recommended first-line therapy for *P. carinii* pneumonia is trimethoprim–sulfamethoxazole. The side effects of this medication include rash, nausea and vomiting, neutropenia, and thrombocytopenia (Table 11-1). For unknown reasons the side effects of trimethoprim–sulfamethoxazole are more severe in HIV-infected patients than in those not infected. These reactions can be life-threatening, requiring aggressive intensive care management.[36,37] Of those infected, only 15% of children

Table 11-1. Side Effects of Medications Commonly Employed to Treat Pulmonary Disease in HIV Infection

Agent	Indication	Toxicity	Monitoring Laboratory Tests
Pentamidine	PCP	Dysrhythmias	EKG, blood glucose, calcium
		Renal dysfunction	BUN, creatinine
		Liver dysfunction, hypocalcemia, dysglycemia	Liver function tests
Chloroquine	LIP	Hypotension	Blood pressure
		EKG abnormalities, dysrhythmias	EKG
Corticosteroids	PCP/LIP	Cardiomyopathy	Echocardiogram
		Hypertension	Blood pressure monitoring
Acyclovir	Varicella, herpes	Renal dysfunction	BUN, creatinine
Ganciclovir	CMV	Bone marrow suppression	CBC, retics, platelets,
		Liver dysfunction	Albumin, transferrin
Foscarnet	CMV	Hypocalcemia	Serum calcium
Ribavirin	RSV, influenza	Fluid overload	Serum osmolarity
Amantadine	Influenza	Renal dysfunction	BUN, creatinine
		Behavioral changes	
Ethionamide	MAIC	Abdominal pain	
		Anorexia	
		Depression	
Cycloserine	MAIC	Neurologic: headaches, seizures, drowsiness	Serum drug levels
		Psychological: psychosis, memory loss	Neurophysiologic exam
Clofazimine	MAIC	Rash	
		Abdominal pain	
		Nausea, vomiting	
		Skin discoloration	
Ethambutol	MAIC	Abdominal pain	
		Decreased visual ocuity	
Rifabutin	MAIC	Rash	
		Nausea, vomiting	
		Hepatotoxicity	
Streptomycin	MAIC	Nephrotoxicity	
		Ototoxicity	
Multidrug therapy	Tuberculosis	Stevens-Johnson syndrome	
Isoniazid	Tuberculosis	Hepatitis, rash/pruritus	Liver function tests
Rifampin	Tuberculosis	Rash/pruritus, nausea, vomiting, hepatotoxicity	
Primaquine	PCP	Rash, hemolysis	G6PD assay, CBC
Clindamycin	PCP	Rash	
Ampicillin	Bacterial pneumonia	Rash	
TMP-SMX	PCP	Rash, nausea/vomiting, neutropenia, thrombocytopenia	
Sulfadiazine	Toxoplasmosis	Acute hemolytic anemia, pancytopenia	CBC
		Rash, serum sickness	BUN, creatinine
		Hepatotoxicity, nephrotoxicity	Liver function tests
Amikacin	MAIC	Renal	BUN, creatinine
		Ototoxicity	Audiologic evaluation
Ciprofloxacin	MAIC	Nausea, vomiting, abdominal pain, rash, headache	

Modified from Refs. 21 and 61.

PCP, *P. carinii* pneumonia; LIP, lymphocytic interstitial pneumonitis; BUN, blood urea nitrogen; CBC, complete blood count; CMV, cytomegalovirus; RSV, respiratory syncytial virus; MAIC, *M. avium-intracellulare* complex.

experience side effects compared to 40% to 60% of adults. Furthermore, in adults, complications are seen primarily in the white population.[29,38,39]

The second line of therapy for patients intolerant of trimethoprim–sulfamethoxazole is pentamidine, administered either intravenously or by aerosol inhalation in patients older than 6 years. Pentamidine has a greater toxicity than trimethoprim–sulfamethoxazole, which may cause renal and liver dysfunction, hypocalcemia (especially when the drug is given in combination with foscarnet), dysglycemia, and cardiac dysrhythmias.

A commonly reported cardiac effect of intravenous pentamidine therapy is prolongation of the QT_c interval, which on occasion has reportedly led to torsades de pointes. Furthermore, recurrent dysrhythmias have been noted to last days after termination of therapy. Therefore, patients receiving intravenous pentamidine should have a baseline electrocardiogram performed and should be carefully monitored during and at least 5 to 7 days following therapy.[40]

Tuberculosis

The steady decline in the incidence of tuberculosis in the United States dating back to 1953 was reversed in 1985. By 1992, the number of known tuberculosis cases exceeded prior predictions by 55,000.[41,42] The HIV epidemic has contributed to this trend by providing both susceptible patients and infected individuals to disseminate the tubercle bacillus. Tuberculosis in immunocompromised patients presents as a more aggressive disease; one study found that tuberculosis developed in 14% of persons infected with HIV, who were purified protein derivative (PPD)-positive, within 2 years.[43] Case-control studies indicate that more opportunistic infections occur in patients with AIDS who have active tuberculosis, and they face a higher risk of death, suggesting that tuberculosis may act as a cofactor, accelerating the progression of HIV.[44] In vitro, mycobacteria and their metabolic products transform latent HIV infection of monocytes to active release of viral particles.[45]

The diagnosis of tuberculosis in patients with HIV infection is difficult because the tuberculin test results are often negative, even in active tuberculosis,[46,47] and the results of the sputum smear are less often positive than in patients without HIV infection.[48–50] The chest radiograph may lack typical features of tuberculosis, such as upper lobe opacities and cavities, and is more likely to show hilar adenopathy, pleural effusion, and miliary infiltrates than in patients without HIV infection.[46,47,51] Extrapulmonary disease is more common in HIV-infected patients with tuberculosis. In one large series of cases, 16 (8%) of 206 patients had tuberculous pericarditis.[50] The response to standard 9-month, three-drug therapy (isoniazid (INH), rifampin, pyrazinamide) for drug-sensitive tuberculosis is usually good, although to prevent relapse, INH is recommended for the duration of the patient's life.[52] Adverse reactions to therapy for tuberculosis, including liver dysfunction, hearing and visual impairment, pruritus, rash, and Stevens-Johnson syndrome, occur in 18% to 27% of patients with HIV infection.[47,49,53] Stevens-Johnson syndrome has been reported to occur in up to 3% of HIV-positive patients receiving therapy for tuberculosis.[50] Although it is often difficult to identify the precise causative factor of an adverse drug reaction in patients receiving multiple agents, rash with pruritus was linked to INH in two of six patients and to rifampin in the other four.[49]

Increasingly, with the appearance of multidrug-resistant tuberculosis strains among HIV-infected patients, tuberculosis becomes a threat to other patients and to health-care workers.[54,55] The prognosis for individuals infected with multidrug-resistant tuberculosis is poor regardless of HIV status.[56,57] Suggested treatment protocols combine isoniazid and rifampin with pyrazinamide, ethambutol, and ciprofloxacin.[58] In New York City, between 1992 and 1994, the observance of appropriate infection control guidelines and the imposition of supervised or directly observed therapy resulted in a decrease in the number of reported cases of tuberculosis.[59]

Mycobacterium avium-intracellulare Complex

Disseminated disease with atypical mycobacteria is the most common bacterial infection in late-stage AIDS, particularly when CD4+ lymphocyte counts decline to very low levels ($<50/mm^3$), and eventually arises in 30% to 50% of patients.[60–62] *M. avium-intracellulare* accounts for 85% of these cases. Arising in highly compromised patients, *M.*

avium-intracellulare correlates with a markedly increased risk of death.[63] *M. avium-intracellulare* is more a systemic than a localized pulmonary disease, typically presenting with symptoms such as fever, night sweats, weight loss, diarrhea, and anemia. Focal pneumonic consolidation or endobronchial lesions are occasionally observed.[61] *M. avium-intracellulare* may be confused with tuberculosis when acid-fast bacilli are isolated in clinical specimens.[17] Skin testing is to no avail, since *M. avium-intracellulare*-infected patients are anergic, but isolation of the organism from blood or tissue biopsy specimens enhances diagnostic sensitivity.[61] In contrast to tuberculosis, disseminated nontuberculous mycobacterial infection is believed to be a primary infection, not the reactivation of an old infection. *M. avium-intracellulare* is uniformly resistant to standard antituberculous agents; therapeutic regimens have been devised, including combinations of rifabutin, ethambutol, clarithromycin, rifampin, clofazamine, amikacin, and ciprofloxacin.[64,65] The use of rifabutin (Ansamycin) to prevent dissemination after initial colonization has proved effective in clinical trials.[66]

Fungal Infection

Several fungal pathogens may be responsible for pulmonary infection, particularly late in the disease and in the setting of disseminated infection. Histoplasmosis may be seen in endemic areas or after a travel-related exposure. *Cryptococcus neoformans* infection may be diagnosed rapidly by detecting cryptococcal antigen titers in blood or bronchoalveolar lavage fluid.[17] Disseminated candidiasis may respond better to fluconazole than ketoconazole, with amphotericin B reserved for severe infection. Administration of liposomal amphotericin reduces the risk of side effects.[67]

Pulmonary Disease of NonInfectious Origin

Interstitial Lung Disease

Lymphocytic Interstitial Pneumonitis

Lymphocytic interstitial pneumonitis (pulmonary lymphoid hyperplasia) is characterized by a diffuse lymphocytic infiltration of the lung parenchyma. Lymphocytes form nodules with occasional germinal centers but without evidence of necrosis. Areas involved include the alveolar and interlobar septae, typically sparing the airways, vessels, and lymph nodes. Histologically, the pulmonary infiltrate consists of a preponderance of CD8+ lymphocytes.[68-70] This process may eventually lead to interstitial fibrosis. Lymphocytic interstitial pneumonitis can be viewed as part of a generalized benign lymphoproliferative process that tends to occur more commonly in children, affecting up to 30% to 50% of those perinatally infected with HIV.[71,72] Early clinical symptoms may include nonproductive cough, diffuse crackles, lymphadenopathy, hepatosplenomegaly, and parotid gland enlargement. Chest radiographs commonly show interstitial reticulonodular infiltrates with or without alveolar infiltration. The radiologic findings of lymphocytic interstitial pneumonitis have been noted to become less marked as total lymphocyte and CD4+ lymphocyte counts decline in the peripheral circulation. Lymphocytic interstitial pneumonitis in children can progress to severe chronic respiratory compromise with tachypnea, retractions, digital clubbing, hypoxemia, and oxygen dependence. Chronic hypoxia may lead to the development of cor pulmonale if oxygen therapy is neglected.

Several hypotheses have been suggested to explain the mechanism of lymphocytic interstitial pneumonitis, but as yet the pathogenesis remains unclear. One theory suggests that an interaction between Epstein-Barr virus and HIV accounts for lymphocytic interstitial pneumonitis.[73-77] Isolation of Epstein-Barr viral DNA from lung biopsy specimens of affected children supports this theory.[73] Other theories propose a direct effect of the HIV virus or nonspecific stimulation of the immune system itself.[71,78]

Treatment of lymphocytic interstitial pneumonitis traditionally consists of systemic steroid therapy ($2 \text{ mg kg}^{-1} \text{ day}^{-1}$ tapering to every other day) along with gamma globulin.[77] Cardiovascular side effects of chronic corticosteroid therapy include hypertension and, in small children, myocardial hypertrophy. Recently in a small, uncontrolled study, the use of chloroquine ($10 \text{ mg kg}^{-1} \text{ day}^{-1}$) has been reported to be both safe and efficacious in children with lymphocytic interstitial pneumonitis related to HIV as well as those with primary idiopathic lymphocytic interstitial pneumonitis.[79] Infrequent, cardiovascular effects related to chloroquine use that require vigilant monitoring include hypotension, and ECG changes, particularly T-wave depression and widening of the QRS complex. Coexisting lung disease in some patients with lymphocytic interstitial pneumonitis has been documented and could add to the degree of pulmonary pathology, increasing the predisposition to secondary cardiac symptoms. For example, Amorosa and colleagues[72] report four cases in which HIV-infected children with prior lymphocytic interstitial pneumonitis developed bronchiectasis unassociated with episodes of recurrent viral or bacterial infections. Bronchiectasis, a cylindrical or beaded dilatation of small airways, usually results from the destruction of airway integrity by infection. In the absence of prior lower respiratory tract infection, bronchiectasis may result from lymphocytic release of inflammatory mediators injurious to airway components.

Nonspecific Interstitial Pneumonitis

Nonspecific interstitial pneumonitis consists histologically of diffuse alveolar damage with an interstitial chronic inflammatory infiltrate, chiefly macrophages and lymphocytes in the absence of microbial pathogens; this pattern was identified in 34% to 50% of patients with AIDS and pneumonitis undergoing lung biopsy.[17,80] Often idiopathic, this entity may be related to prior illicit drug use or prescribed medical therapies. It may also be related to Kaposi's sarcoma or *P. carinii* infection, both of which must be excluded.[17] Presentation may be with cough, fever, and dyspnea or simply an abnormal chest radiograph in the absence of symptomatic disease. The course may be mild with spontaneous improvement; as in lymphocytic interstitial pneumonitis, corticosteroid therapy may prove beneficial in cases with progressive symptoms.

Evlogias and colleagues[81] report a case of chronic interstitial pulmonary disease resulting from chronic *P. carinii* infection causing extensive pulmonary fibrosis and calcification in a 3-year-old HIV-positive boy. Interestingly, bronchoalveolar

lavage was negative for *P. carinii*, and the diagnosis was made only on lung biopsy. The authors point out that chronic interstitital lung disease in HIV infection should not automatically be assumed to represent lymphocytic interstitial pneumonitis.[81]

Bronchiectasis, Bronchiolitis Obliterans, and Bullous Lung Disease

Holmes and coworkers[82] described bronchiectasis in seven HIV-infected adult patients. Chronic focal crackles on chest auscultation, chronic productive cough, and exacerbation of respiratory symptoms prompted chest computed tomography (CT) scans, which confirmed the presence of bronchiectasis. In these cases, culture of expectorated sputum yielded *S. pneumoniae, H. influenzae*, or *Pseudomonas aeruginosa*. McGuinness and colleagues,[83] in a retrospective report, described the appearance of bronchiectasis on CT scans of HIV-positive patients with a variety of underlying pulmonary pathologies and concluded that bronchiectasis should be considered as one of the pulmonary manifestations of AIDS. Bronchiectasis has been reported to develop in pediatric patients with HIV infection after lymphocytic interstitial pneumonitis or lower respiratory tract infection.[84] In these cases, persistent basilar rales, often suggestive of congestive heart failure, instead resulted from bronchiectasis as revealed on chest CT scan. Figure 11-1 shows the plain film and chest CT scan findings in a 10-year-old child with perinatally acquired HIV infection, prior biopsy-proven lymphocytic interstitial pneumonitis, and a 6-month history of productive cough. Sputum culture yielded both *S. pneumoniae* and *H. influenzae*. Periodic courses of oral or parenteral antibiotic therapy have prevented disease progression and controlled symptoms sufficiently to permit a normal lifestyle over a 2-year observation period.

Bronchiolitis obliterans with organizing pneumonia has only recently been recognized as occurring in patients with AIDS. Bronchiolitis obliterans with organizing pneumonia represents obliteration of the respiratory bronchioles as a result of an inflammatory and fibrotic process.[85,86] Bronchiolitis obliterans with organizing pneumonia is typically diagnosed on biopsy, and since it is often responsive

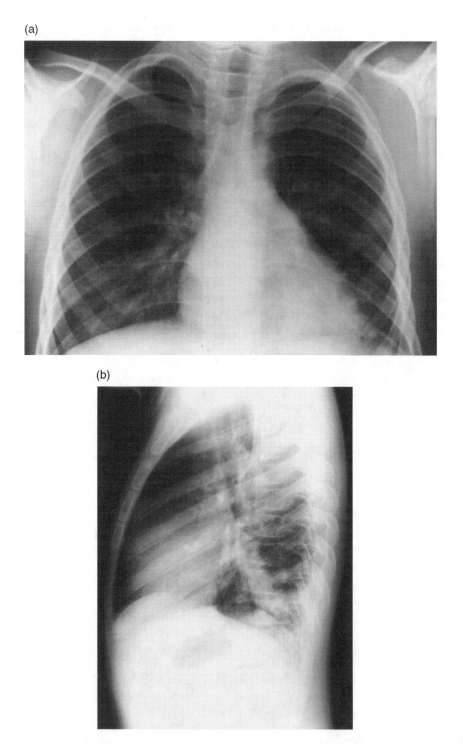

Figure 11-1. Bronchiectasis in a 10-year-old child with HIV infection. **a, b:** Posteroanterior and lateral views on chest x-ray films of a child with perinatally acquired HIV infection and a 6-month history of productive cough. Note staples at lingula from prior open-lung biopsy performed in early childhood, which confirmed lymphocytic interstitial pneumonitis. Plain films demonstrate left lower lobe infiltrate and suggest a cystic component. These findings had been present on plain films for at least 1 year before to the onset of chronic respiratory symptoms.

(c)

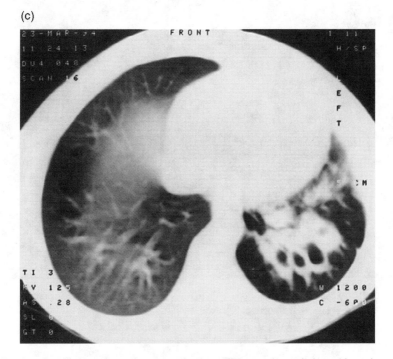

Figure 11-1. *Continued* **c:** Chest computed tomography scan (CT) reveals cystic bronchiectasis confined to the left lower lobe. These findings were unchanged both on plain films on repeat chest CT scan 2 years later (data not shown).

to corticosteroid treatment, the establishment of a definitive diagnosis is important.

Another form of interstitial lung disease reported in patients with AIDS is cystic disease associated with chronic *P. carinii* infection. Bullous lung disease and emphysema have been described in the presence of HIV infection; despite normal plain chest x-ray studies, these findings were present in 42% of a series of 55 patients with AIDS who underwent CT scans.[87]

Neoplastic Disease

Although Kaposi's sarcoma is the most common secondary neoplasm in HIV infection, non-Hodgkin's lymphoma also occurs at high frequencies. As T-lymphocyte function declines and immune surveillance wanes, B lymphocytes infected by the Epstein-Barr virus proliferate with an increased risk of malignant differentiation. In one series of 35 patients with AIDS-related lymphoma, 11 had intrathoracic disease, consisting of pleural effusions, pulmonary infiltrates, parenchymal masses, or me-

diastinal or hilar lymphadenopathy.[88] Primary intrathoracic lymphoma is considered exceedingly rare in HIV infection but has been observed even in young children. Figure 11-2 demonstrates the chest CT scans and gross pathologic findings in a 2.5-year-old child with a primary esophageal T-lymphocyte lymphoma that ultimately perforated the posterior tracheal wall. Although it remains unclear whether the incidence of primary pulmonary carcinoma is increased in HIV-infected patients, cumulative evidence indicates that HIV-positive patients with lung cancer present at younger ages and with more extensive and aggressive disease, strongly associated with a history of smoking.[17]

Upper Airway Obstruction, Obstructive Sleep Apnea, and Central Apnea

Recent reports suggest that infants and young children perinatally exposed to the HIV virus, whether infected or not, may be more prone to periods of apnea, hypoventilation, and upper airway obstruction. Woo and colleagues[89] described 10

(a)

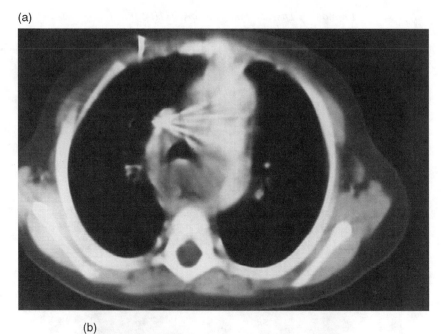

(b)

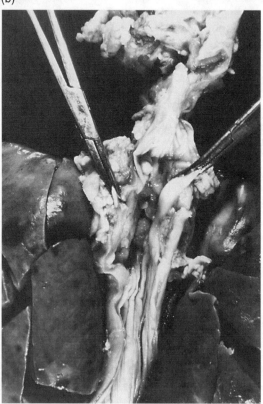

Figure 11-2. **a:** Intrathoracic T-lymphocyte lymphoma in a young child with HIV infection. Computed tomography scan of chest. Note lesion between the esophagus and trachea. **b:** Postmortem finding of the same child: gross pathology. Posterior view of the esophagus showing a mass perforating the anterior wall into the tracheal lumen, which was the ultimate cause of death in this child.

children born to HIV-positive mothers, 7 HIV-negative and 3 HIV-positive, who developed hypoxemia when sedated for infant pulmonary function tests. During overnight polysomnography, 7 of these children had hypoxemia; 3 also had abnormal periodic breathing, and 1 required an emergency airway due to severe obstructive apnea.[89] Children born to HIV-infected mothers appear to be at greater risk for sleep-related breathing disorders; contributing factors may include lymphoid hyperplasia of tonsils and adenoids encroaching on the airway or airway mucosal responses to allergens or irritants in their surroundings, such as environmental tobacco smoke. Adenotonsillar hyperplasia has also been described in adults with HIV infection. In a neuroimaging research study, France and coworkers[90] noted adenoidal enlargement in 60% of 55 adult males undergoing cranial magnetic resonance imaging (MRI). In 12% (7/55) the hyperplasia was of gross or moderate proportions; the remainder were rated as mild.[90]

Hypoxia during periods of airway obstruction induces pulmonary vasoconstriction, leading to increased pulmonary artery pressure, and right ventricular hypertrophy (Figure 11-3). As a result, the development of cor pulmonale may be seen. Further, during episodes of upper airway obstruction, the patient is forced to generate high negative intrathoracic pressures in inspiration to overcome the obstruction. This causes marked pressure swings that may increase venous return and induce pulmonary edema from fluid transudation out of pulmonary capillaries.[91] Case reports have described HIV-negative children with obstructive sleep apnea who presented with signs of congestive heart failure, including dyspnea, orthopnea, cardiomegaly, hepatosplenomegaly, and peripheral edema. Chest radiographs demonstrated cardiomegaly, pulmonary infiltrates, and pleural effusions.[91,92] In these cases, obstructive sleep apnea initially masqueraded as primary heart disease. Guilleminault and colleagues[93] studied 400 patients not known to be HIV-infected but with sleep apnea and found that cardiac arrythmias and conduction abnormalities were common. Cor pulmonale was present in 55% of children with obstructive sleep apnea in a referral clinic population.[94] Burack[95] studied 25 HIV-negative patients with known hypersomnia sleep apnea

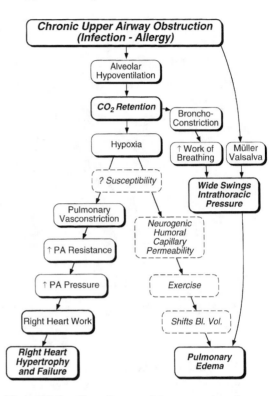

Figure 11-3. Flow diagram of the progression of upper airway obstruction leading to right heart failure and pulmonary edema. (From Ref. 91, with permission.)

syndrome; of these, 14 had symptoms of cardiac disease, including atrial fibrillation, Wolff-Parkinson-White syndrome, cardiomyopathy, myocardial infarction, or arrhythmias. Systemic hypertension has also been reported with chronic upper airway obstruction.[96] Cardiorespiratory arrest with seizures and death occurred in some cases.[92,96]

Lateral neck films allow a subjective estimation of adenotonsillar hypertrophy and distention of the hypopharynx, a correlate of upper airway obstruction.[97,98] When cor pulmonale is suspected, electrocardiography may be suggestive (Figure 11-4), while echocardiography provides useful documentation of right ventricular hypertrophy and right atrial dilatation with reduced right ventricular ejection fraction and permits noninvasive follow-up after relief of upper airway obstruction.[99] Although home oximetry provides a useful screening step for identifying clinically significant obstructive sleep apnea,[100] sleep polysomnography remains the gold

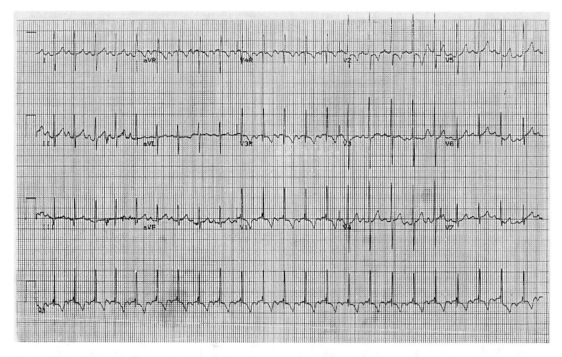

Figure 11-4. Electrocardiogram in a 2-year-old child with HIV infection. Findings are indicative of right ventricular hypertrophy and presumed to result from severe tonsillar hypertrophy with obstructive sleep apnea.

standard. Sudden relief of upper airway obstruction has been linked to pulmonary edema.[101]

Upper airway obstruction has also been reported to occur in adults with HIV infection as a result of bacterial tracheitis [102] and in children due to both bacterial and fungal (candidal) tracheitis.[103] Kaposi's sarcoma affecting the trachea with or without cutaneous involvement has also led to upper airway obstruction.[104,105]

In advanced HIV-related neurodegenerative disease, peripheral muscle weakness has been observed to lead to head droop with kinking of the neck and airway, resulting in stridorous or obstructive apneic episodes. Appropriate neck supports readily alleviate this problem.

In infants, apnea may be the first sign of ominous underlying respiratory disease. Olopoenia and colleagues[106] report a case of an infant eventually discovered to have *P. carinii* pneumonia who presented with apnea and cyanosis. When acute respiratory failure syndrome supervenes in AIDS, mortality rates are high compared to rates in children not infected with HIV.[107] Experience indicates a dismal prognosis for adults who have respiratory

failure while receiving antibiotics and corticosteroid therapy, with 82% mortality despite institution of ventilatory assistance.[108]

Vasculitis

Vasculitic syndromes with pulmonary involvement have been described in HIV infection. One survey documented vasculitis in 23% of 148 HIV-infected patients through biopsy of muscle, peripheral nerve, or skin[109]; 11 of these cases could be classified as a distinct type; the remainder showed nonspecific findings. These included four with polyarteritis nodosa, three with necrotizing angiitis, one with Henoch-Schönlein purpura, and six with hypersensitivity vasculitis. Medications were implicated as a precipitant in four of the six cases of hypersensitivity vasculitis, including penicillin, trimethoprim–sulfamethoxazole, and amoxicillin, the most commonly implicated agents in drug hypersensitivity among AIDS patients.[39,76]

In the granulomatous angiitis group, one of the distinct types of vasculitis, lymphomatoid granulomatosis, falls within a spectrum of disorders referred to as angiocentric immunoproliferative lesions; one of three HIV-infected patients reported with lymphomatoid granulomatosis had vascular involvement extending beyond the central nervous system to the lung. Another HIV-infected patient developed progressive angiitis of the muscles and nerves and lymphoid interstitial disease of the heart, lung, and kidney.[110] Angiocentric immunoproliferative lesions in HIV may arise through HIV-induced immune dysregulation leading to uncontrolled proliferation of T-lymphocyte lineages with angiocentric orientation. Within the systemic necrotizing vasculitis group, several cases of polyarteritis nodosa-like syndromes predominantly affecting the skin and gastrointestinal tract and a single case of Churg-Strauss syndrome, allergic granulomatosis with massive eosinophilia and active lung involvement, have been described.[111,112] Polyarteritis nodosa-like vasculitis typically presents with either peripheral neuropathy or digital ischemic changes combined with several constitutional symptoms. Productive cough and basilar rales have also been described.[113] Chest radiographs may show patchy bilateral interstitial infiltrates, especially of the lower lobes, which are sometimes described as reticulonodular. Diagnosis is achieved by angiogram of the extremities showing tubular narrowing or occlusion and beading of arterioles. Systemic corticosteroid therapy produced prompt response with resolution of respiratory symptoms.

Although vasculitis is not documented in all cases, cutaneous drug reactions are common in HIV-infected patients, occurring in 188 of 684 individuals followed over a 3-year period. Sensitivity to trimethoprim–sulfamethoxazole affected 43% of patients, and sensitivity to sulfadiazine was similarly prevalent. Aminopenicillins (ampicillin) induced reactions in 93 of 1,000 patients (Table 11-1). The likelihood of a cutaneous drug reaction increased as HIV disease advanced in severity, but remarkably, no adverse reactions were reported to result from drug rechallenge in this series.[114]

Asthma

Recent pediatric data indicate that asthma is no more common in HIV-infected patients than it is among appropriate control subjects exposed to similar environmental factors.[9] Lymphocytic bronchiolitis was demonstrated by biopsy in an adult with chronic dyspnea and a combined restrictive-obstructive pattern on pulmonary function testing[115]; lack of response to bronchodilators would help to separate this entity from true asthma. HIV-infected patients with cardiomyopathy may have "cardiac asthma" manifested by wheezing with respiratory distress, particularly at night, small airway obstruction on pulmonary function tests, and improvement in pulmonary function with diuresis.[116,117]

Pulmonary Effects of Cardiomyopathy

Specific discussion of the impact of HIV-related cardiomyopathy on pulmonary function in HIV infection is lacking. Clinical experience and case reports demonstrate that patients with fulminant cardiomyopathy may demonstrate predominantly respiratory symptoms such as tachypnea, retractions, grunting, expiratory wheezing, and evidence of pulmonary edema.[118] Case reports of patients with HIV-related cardiomyopathy stress that respiratory findings figure prominently in their presentation. Dyspnea on exertion is often the first symptom, followed by orthopnea. Physical examination findings may include basilar rales on chest auscultation. Chest radiograph reveals progressive cardiomegaly and eventually pericardial or pleural effusions, with interstitial lung changes that are easily misinterpreted as interstitial pneumonitis but that actually are consistent with congestive heart failure.[110,119,120] Thorough cardiac evaluation is thus essential for HIV-infected patients presenting with progressive dyspnea. Aggressive use of echocardiography in the acute care setting has been recommended to facilitate the recognition of pericarditis and cardiomyopathy in HIV-infected patients with dyspnea disproportionate to pulmonary infiltrates.[121] Cardiac catheterization excludes primary pulmonary hypertension as the basis for right heart failure in this setting. Although treatment with digoxin and diuretics may induce remission of respiratory symptoms, intercurrent, nonrespiratory illnesses may aggravate cardiac dysfunction, with fatal consequences.[119,120,122] Chronic pulmonary edema may compromise pulmonary immune defenses, resulting in increased frequency and severity of pneumonia.

One may extrapolate from the well-studied circumstance of congenital heart disease in pediatric patients without HIV infection to predict possible pulmonary consequences of myocardial dysfunction. In infants with increased pulmonary blood flow due to congenital heart disease, pulmonary compliance is significantly reduced; the degree of abnormality correlates with the elevation in mean pulmonary arterial pressure rather than with left atrial pressure. The respiratory rate and pulmonary resistance also increase in relation to elevated pulmonary blood flow.[123] In analogous fashion, with myocardial dysfunction and decreased contractility, pulmonary vasculature and, ultimately, the interstitial space may become engorged, with resultant declines in pulmonary compliance. Hordof and colleagues[124] described obstructive lung disease in 10 infants with ventricular septal defect and large left-to-right shunts; their airway disease resolved with surgical correction of the ventricular septal defect. Wheezing may result from large airway compression by enlarged pulmonary arteries or cardiac chambers, from small airway compression by peribronchiolar fluid, from edema of the bronchial wall due to increased systemic and pulmonary venous pressure, or from reflex bronchoconstriction. In malnourished children with chronic disease, such as HIV infection, hypoalbuminemia will increase the tendency to form pulmonary interstitial and bronchial wall edema. Cabanes and associates[125] outlined another mechanism possibly contributing to the wheezy dyspnea of patients with congestive heart failure and decreased left heart function; 9 of 10 patients studied had bronchial hyperresponsiveness to methacholine, a cholinergic agonist. Dilatation of bronchial vessels appeared likely to be responsible for the airway obstruction present in these patients.

Pulmonary Effects of Chronic Hypoxia

The numerous HIV-related chronic pulmonary disorders associated with hypoxia, especially lymphocytic interstitial pneumonitis and other interstitial lung disease, may precipitate pulmonary heart disease (cor pulmonale). Right ventricular hypertrophy may arise as a consequence of hypoxia resulting from intrinsic pulmonary disease, upper airway obstruction, or from secondary vasculitis when hypoxia induces chronic pulmonary vasoconstriction and hypertension. Electrocardiographic changes will provide initial indications of cor pulmonale (Figure 11-4). Echocardiography will strongly suggest the diagnosis of cor pulmonale, although primary pulmonary hypertension may be difficult to exclude without cardiac catheterization. Hypoxia may be reversed by nocturnal or continuous supplemental oxygen therapy.

Primary Pulmonary Hypertension

Several case reports and small case series demonstrate that primary pulmonary hypertension can arise in HIV infection. This topic is discussed in detail in Chapter 12 and will not be reviewed further here.

Conclusion

Early in the epidemic of HIV-related disease, the prevalence and severity of pulmonary complications became apparent. More than a decade later and despite improvements in therapy, the significance and diversity of HIV pulmonary disease remain undisputed. Further, the potential impact of lung impairment and its treatment on cardiac function has come into focus. Additionally, experience has amply demonstrated that cardiac disease in HIV infection may present with respiratory symptoms and masquerade as one of the more common primary lung ailments, deceiving the unwary clinician. Familiarity with the diverse array of lung disorders in HIV infection and their potential cardiovascular impact will serve to enable recognition and appropriate treatment of distinct diagnostic entities affecting these closely intertwined organ systems.

References

1. Marolda J, Paca B, Bonforte RJ, et al. Pulmonary manifestations of HIV infection in children. *Pediatr Pulmonol* 1991;10:231–235.

2. Meduri GU, Stein DS. Pulmonary manifestations of acquired immunodeficiency syndrome. *Clin Infect Dis* 1992;14:98–113.

3. Murray JF, Mills J. Pulmonary infectious complications of human immunodeficiency virus infection (Part I). *Am Rev Respir Dis* 1990;141:1356–1372.

4. Salahuddin SZ, Rose RM, Groopman JE, et al. Human T lymphotropic virus type III infection of human alveolar macrophages. *Blood* 1986;68:281–284.

5. Beck JM, Shellito J. Effects of human immunodeficiency virus on pulmonary host defenses. *Semin Respir Infect* 1989;4:75–84.

6. Marcy TW, Reynolds HY. Pulmonary consequences of congenital and acquired primary immunodeficiency states. *Clin Chest Med* 1989;10:503–519.

7. Murray JF, Mills J. Pulmonary infectious complications of human immunodeficiency virus infection (Part II). *Am Rev Respir Dis* 1990;141:1582–1598.

8. Wallace JM, Vijaya A, Glassroth J, et al. Respiratory illness in persons with human immunodeficiency virus infection. *Am Rev Respir Dis* 1993;148:1523–1529.

9. Kattan M, Pediatric Pulmonary and Cardiovascular Complications of Vertically Transmitted HIV Infection P^2C^2 Study Group. Respiratory disease in children born to HIV-infected mothers in the first year of life. [Abstract]. *Proc Conf Retrov Opportun Infect* 1996.

10. Pitkin AD, Grant AD, Foley NM, Miller RF. Changing patterns of respiratory distress in HIV positive patients in referral centers in the United Kingdom between 1986–1987. *Thorax* 1993;48:204–207.

11. Unsworth DJ, Rowen D, Carne C, et al. Defective IgG response to Pneumovax in HIV seropositive patients. *Genitourin Med* 1993;69:373–376.

12. Levine SJ, White DA, Fels AOS. The incidence and significance of *Staphylococcus aureus* in respiratory cultures from patients infected with HIV. *Am Rev Respir Dis* 1990;141:89–93.

13. Baron AD, Hollander H. *Pseudomonas aeruginosa* bronchopulmonary infection in late human immunodeficiency virus disease. *Am Rev Respir Dis* 1993;148:992–996.

14. Ognibene FP, Gill VJ, Pizzo PA, et al. Induced sputum to diagnose *Pneumocystis carinii* pneumonia in immunosuppressed pediatric patients. *J Pediatr* 1989;115:439–433.

15. Abadco DL, Amaroj-Galvez R, Rao M, Steiner P. Experience with flexible fiberoptic bronchoscopy with bronchoalveolar lavage as a diagnostic tool in children with AIDS. *Am J Dis Child* 1992;146:1056–1059.

16. Craddock C, Pasvol G, Bull R, et al. Cardiorespiratory arrest and autonomic neuropathy in AIDS. *Lancet* 1987;2:16–18.

17. Mitchell DM, Miller RF. New developments in the pulmonary diseases affecting HIV-infected individuals. *Thorax* 1995;294:302.

18. Joseph J, Strange C, Sahn SA. Pleural effusions in hospitalized patients with AIDS. *Ann Intern Med* 1993;118:856–859.

19. Chandwani S, Borkowsky W, Krasinki K, et al. Respiratory syncytial virus infection in human immunodeficiency virus-infected children. *J Pediatr* 1990;117:251–254.

20. Thurn JR, Henry K. Influenza A pneumonitis in a patient infected with the human immunodeficiency virus. *Chest* 1989;95:807–810.

21. Hauger SB. Approach to the pediatric patient with HIV infection and pulmonary symptoms. *J Pediatr* 1991;119:S25-S32.

22. Chien SM, Rawjui M, Mintz S, et al. Changes in hospital admission patterns in patients with HIV infection in the era of *Pneumocystis* prophylaxis. *Chest* 1992;102:1035–1039.

23. Connor E, Bagarazzi M, McSherry G, et al. Clinical and laboratory correlates of *Pneumocystis carinii* pneumonia in children infected with HIV. *JAMA* 1991;265:1693–1697.

24. Simonds RJ, Oxtoby MJ, Caldwell B, et al. *Pneumocystis carinii* pneumonia among US children with perinatally acquired HIV infection. *JAMA* 1993;270:470–473.

25. Rothenberg R, Woefel M, Stoneburner R, et al. Survival with the acquired immunodeficiency syndrome: experience with 5833 cases in New York City. *N Engl J Med* 1987;317:1297–1302.

26. Bernstein LJ, Bye MR, Rubinstein AR. Prognostic factors and life expectancy in children with acquired immunodeficiency syndrome and *Pneumocystis carinii* pneumonia. *Am J Dis Child* 1989;143:775–778.

27. Hughes WT. *Pneumocystis carinii* pneumonia. In: Patrick CC. (ed). *Infections in Immunocompro-*

mised Infants and Children, 1st Ed. New York: Churchill Livingstone, 1992:711–717.

28. Glatt A, Chirgwin K. *Pneumocystis carinii* pneumonia in human immunodeficiency-virus infected patients. *Arch Intern Med* 1990;150:271–279.

29. Kovacs JA, Hiemenz JW, Macher AM, et al. *Pneumocystis carinii* pneumonia: a comparison between patients with the acquired immunodeficiency syndrome and patients with other immunodeficiencies. *Ann Intern Med* 1984;100:663–671.

30. Zaman MK, White DA. Serum lactate dehydrogenase levels and *Pneumocystis carinii* pneumonia. *Am Rev Respir Dis* 1988;137:796–800.

31. McClellan MD, Miller SB, Parsons PE, et al. Pneumothorax with *Pneumocystis carinii* pneumonia in AIDS. *Chest* 1991;100:1224–1228.

32. DeBlic J, Blanche S, Danel C, et al. Bronchoalveolar lavage in HIV-infected patients with interstitial pneumonitis. *Arch Dis Child* 1989;64:1246–1250.

33. Cohn DL, Stover DE, O'Brien RF, Shelhamer JH. Pulmonary complications of AIDS: advances in diagnosis and treatment. *Am Rev Respir Dis* 1988;138:1051–1052.

34. Golden JA, Holander H, Stulbarg MS, Gamsu G. Bronchoalveolar lavage as the exclusive diagnostic modality of *Pneumocystis carinii* pneumonia. *Chest* 1986;90:18–22.

35. Hopewell P. *P. carinii* pneumonia. In: Sande MA Volberding PA (eds). *The Medical Management of AIDS,* 2nd Ed. Philadelphia: WB Saunders, 1990.

36. Chanock SJ, Luginbuhl LM, McIntosh K, Lipshultz SE. Life-threatening reaction to trimethoprim/sulfamethoxazole in pediatric human immunodeficiency virus infection. *Pediatrics* 1994;93:519–521.

37. Bayard PJ, Berger TG, Jacobson MA. Drug hypersensitivity reactions and human immunodeficiency virus disease. *J Acquir Immune Defic Syndr* 1992;5:1237–1257.

38. Centers for Disease Control. Guidelines for prophylaxis against *Pneumocystsis carinii* pneumonia for children infected with human immunodeficiency virus. *MMWR* 1991;40:1–11.

39. Gordin FM, Simon GL, Wofsy CB, et al. Adverse reactions to trimethoprim-sulfamethoxasole in patients with the acquired immunodeficiency syndrome. *Ann Intern Med* 1984;100:495–499.

40. Eisenhauer MD, Eliasson AH, Taylor AJ, et al. Incidence of cardiac arrhythmias during intrave-nous pentamidine therapy in HIV-infected patients. *Chest* 1994;105:389–394.

41. Goodman PC. Tuberculosis and AIDS. *Radiol Clin North Am* 1995;33:707–717.

42. Centers for Disease Control. Tuberculosis morbidity in the United States final data, 1990. *MMWR* 1992;40:23–27.

43. Selwin PA, Hartel D, Lewis BA, et al. A prospective study of the risk of tuberculosis on intravenous drug users with human immunodeficiency virus infection. *N Engl J Med* 1989;320:545–550.

44. Whalen C, Horsburh CR, Hom D, et al. Accelerated course of human immunodeficiency virus infection after tuberculosis. *Am J Respir Crit Care Med* 1995;151:129–135.

45. Lederman MM, Georges D, Zeichner SL, et al. *Mycobacterium tuberculosis* and its purified protein derivative activates expression of the human immunodeficiency virus. *J AIDS* 1994;7:727–733.

46. Jones DS, Malecki JM, Bigler WJ, et al. Pediatric tuberculosis and human immunodeficiency virus infection in Palm Beach County, Florida. *Am J Dis Child* 1992;146:1166–1170.

47. Toma E, Fournier S, Poisson M, et al. Clindamycin with primaquine for *Pneumocystis carinii* pneumonia. *Lancet* 1989;1:1046–1048.

48. Pesanti EL. The negative tuberculin test: tuberculin, HIV, and anergy panels. *Am J Respir Crit Care Med* 1994;149:1699–1709.

49. Chaisson RE, Schecter GF, Thener CP. Tuberculosis as a manifestation of the acquired immunodeficiency syndrome. *Am Rev Respir Dis* 1987;136:570–574.

50. Elliott AM, Luo N, Tembo G, et al. Impact of HIV on tuberculosis in Zambia: a cross-sectional study. *BMJ* 1990;301:412–415.

51. Long R, Maycher B, Scalcini M. The chest roentgenogram in pulmonary tuberculosis patients seropositive for human immunodeficiency virus type 1. *Chest* 1991;99:123–127.

52. Brindle RJ, Nunn PP, Githui W, et al. Quantitative bacillary response to treatment in HIV-associated pulmonary tuberculosis. *Am Rev Respir Dis* 1993;147:958–961.

53. Small PM, Schechter GF, Goodman PC, et al. Treatment of tuberculosis in patients with advanced human immunodeficiency virus infection. *N Engl J Med* 1991;324:289–294.

54. Pearson ML, Jereb JA, Friedan TR, et al. Nosocomial transmission of multidrug-resistant *Myco-*

bacterium tuberculosis: a risk to patients and health care workers. *Ann Intern Med* 1992;117: 191–196.

55. Edlin BR, Tokars JI, Grieco MJ, et al. An outbreak of multidrug-resistant tuberculosis among hospitalized patients with the acquired immunodeficiency syndrome. *N Engl J Med* 1992;326:1514–1521.

56. Fischl MA, Daikos GL, Uttamchandani RB, et al. Clinical presentation and outcome of patients with HIV infection and tuberculosis caused by multiple drug resistance bacilli. *Ann Intern Med* 1992;117: 184–190.

57. Goble M, Iseman MD, Madsen LA, et al. Treatment of 171 patients with pulmonary tuberculosis resistant to isoniazid and rifampin. *N Engl J Med* 1993;328:527–532.

58. Centers for Disease Control. Management of persons exposed to multidrug-resistant tuberculosis. *MMWR* 1992;41:61–71.

59. Frieden TR, Fujiwara PI, Washko RM, et al. Tuberculosis in New York City: turning the tide. *N Engl J Med* 1995;333:229–233.

60. Masur H. Recommendations in prophylaxis and therapy for disseminated *Mycobacterium avium* complex disease in patients infected with HIV. *N Engl J Med* 1993;329:898–904.

61. Horsburgh CR. *Mycobacterium avium* complex infection in the acquired immunodeficiency syndrome. *N Engl J Med* 1991;324:1332–1338.

62. Horsburgh CR, Caldwell MB, Simonds RJ. Epidemiology of disseminated nontuberculous mycobacterial disease in children with acquired immunodeficiency syndrome. *Pediatr Infect Dis J* 1993; 12:219–222.

63. Chaisson RE, Moore RD, Richman DD, et al. Incidence and natural history of *Mycobacterium avium* complex infections in patients with advanced human immunodeficiency virus treated with zidovudine. *Am Rev Respir Dis* 1992;146: 285–289.

64. Kemper CA, Meng TC, Nussbaum J, et al. Treatment of *Mycobacterium avium* complex bacteremia in AIDS with a four drug oral regimen. *Ann Intern Med* 1992;116:466–472.

65. Chiu J, Nussbaum J, Bozzette S, et al. Treatment of disseminated *Mycobacterium avium* complex infection in AIDS with amikacin, ethambutol, rifampin, and ciprofloxacin. *Ann Intern Med* 1990; 113:358–361.

66. Nightingale SD, Cameron DW, Gordin FM, et al. Two controlled trials of rifabutin prophylaxis against *Mycobacterium avium* complex infection in AIDS. *N Engl J Med* 1993;329:828–833.

67. British Society for Antimicrobial Chemotherapy Working Party. Antifungal chemotherapy in patients with AIDS. *Lancet* 1992;340:648–651.

68. Saldana MJ, Mones JM. Pulmonary pathology in AIDS: atypical *Pneumocystis carinii* infection and lymphoid interstitial pneumonia. *Thorax* 1994;49: 461–465.

69. Haller JO, Cohen HL. Pediatric HIV infection: an imaging update. *Pediatr Radiol* 1994;24:224–230.

70. Berdon WE, Mellins RB, Abramson SJ, et al. Pediatric HIV infection in its second decade: the changing pattern of lung involvement. *Radiol Clin North Am* 1993;31:453–464.

71. Pitt J. Lymphocytic interstitial pneumonia. *Pediatr Clin North Am* 1991;38:89–95.

72. Amorosa JK, Miller RW, Laraya-Cuasay L, et al. Bronchiectasis in children with lymphocytic interstitial pneumonia and acquired immune deficiency syndrome. *Pediatr Radiol* 1992;22:603–607.

73. Andiman WA, Eastman R, Martin K, et al. Opportunistic lymphoproliferations associated with Epstein-Barr viral DNA in infants and children with AIDS. *Lancet* 1985;2:1390–1393.

74. Katz BZ, Berkman AM, Shapiro ED. Serologic evidence of active Epstein-Barr virus infection in Epstein Barr virus-associated lymphoproliferative disorders of children with acquired immunodeficiency syndrome. *J Pediatr* 1992;120:228–232.

75. Kramer MR, Saldana MJ, Ramos M, Pitchenik AE. High titers of Epstein-Barr virus antibodies in adult patients with lymphocytic interstital pneumonitis associated with AIDS. *Respir Med* 1992; 86:49–52.

76. Battegay M, Opravil M, Wuthrich B. Rash with amoxicillin-clavulanate therapy in HIV-infected patients. [Letter]. *Lancet* 1989;2:1100.

77. Rubinstein A, Bernstein LJ, Charytan M, et al. Corticosteroid treatment for pulmonary lymphoid hyperplasia in children with the acquired immune deficiency syndrome. *Pediatr Pulmonol* 1988;4: 13–17.

78. Teirstein AS, Rosen MJ. Lymphocytic interstial pneumonia. *Clin Chest Med* 1988;9:467–471.

79. Campos JM, Simonetti JP. Treatment of lymphoid interstitial pneumonia with chloroquine. *J Pediatr* 1993;122:50–53.

80. Suffredini A, Ognibene F, Lack E. Non-specific interstitial pneumonitis: a common cause of pulmonary disease in the acquired immunodeficiency syndrome. *Ann Intern Med* 1987;107:7–13.

81. Evlogias NE, Leonidas JC, Rooney J, Valderama E. Severe cystic pulmonary disease associated with chronic *Pneumocystis carinii* infection in a child with AIDS. *Pediatr Radiol* 1994;24:606–608.

82. Holmes AH, Trotman-Dickenson B, Edwards A, et al. Bronchiectasis in HIV disease. *Q J Med* 1992;85:875–882.

83. McGuinness G, Naidich DP, Garay S, et al. AIDS-associated bronchiectasis: CT features. *J Comp Tomogr* 1993;17:260–266.

84. Holmes AH, Pelton S, Steinbach S, et al. HIV-related bronchiectasis. [Letter]. *Thorax* 1995;50:1227–1228.

85. Joseph J, Harley RA, Frye MD. Bronchiolitis obliterans with organizing penumonia in AIDS. *N Engl J Med* 1995;332:273.

86. Leo Y, Pitchon HE, Messler G, Meyer RD. Bronchiolitis obliterans organizing pneumonia in a patients with AIDS. *Clin Infect Dis* 1994;18:921–924.

87. Kuhlman JE, Knowles MC, Fishman EK, et al. Premature bullous pulmonary damage in AIDS: CT diagnosis. *Radiology* 1989;173:23–26.

88. Sider L, Weiss AJ, Smith MD, et al. Varied appearance of AIDS-related lymphoma in the chest. *Radiology* 1989;171:629–632.

89. Woo MS, Wong WY, Fukushimna L, et al. Unsuspected hypoxemia during infant pulmonary function testing in children of HIV-infected mothers. *Am Rev Respir Dis* 1995;151:235.

90. France AJ, Kean DM, Douglas RHB. Adenoidal hypertrophy in HIV-infected patients. [Letter]. *Lancet* 1988;2:1076.

91. Luke MJ, Mehrizi A, Folger GM, et al. Chronic nasopharyngeal obstruction as a cause of cardiomegaly, cor pulmonale, and pulmonary edema. *Pediatrics* 1966;37:762–768.

92. Cayler GG, Johnson EE, Lewis BE, et al. Heart failure due to enlarged tonsils and adenoids: the cardiorespiratory syndrome of increased airway resistance. *Am J Dis Child* 1969;118:708–717.

93. Guilleminault C, Connolly SJ, Winkle RA. Cardiac arrhythmia and conduction disturbances during sleep in 400 patients with sleep apnea syndrome. *Am J Cardiol* 1983;52:490–494.

94. Brouillette RT, Fernbach SK, Hunt CE. Obstructive sleep apnea in infants and children. *J Pediatr* 1982;100:31–40.

95. Burack B. The hypersomnia-sleep apena syndrome: its recognition in clinical cardiology. *Am Heart J* 1984;107:543–548.

96. Ross RD, Daniels SR, Loggie JMH, et al. Sleep apnea-associated hypertension and reversible left ventricular hypertrophy. *J Pediatr* 1987;111:253–255.

97. Capitanio MA, Kirkpatrick JA. Obstructions of the upper airway in children as reflected on the chest radiograph. *Radiology* 1973;107:159–161.

98. Fernbach SK, Brouillette RT, Riggs TW, et al. Radiologic evaluation of adenoids and tonsils in children with obstructive sleep apnea: plain films and fluoroscopy. *Pediatr Radiol* 1983;13:258–265.

99. Sofer S, Weinhouse E, Tal A, et al. Cor pulmonale due to adenoidal or tonsillar hypertrophy or both in children: noninvasive diagnosis and follow-up. *Chest* 1988;93:119–122.

100. Gyulay S, Olson LG, Hensley MJ, et al. A comparison of clinical assessment and home oximetry in the diagnosis of obstructive sleep apnea. *Am Rev Respir Dis* 1993;147:50–53.

101. Feinberg AN, Shabino CL. Acute pulmonary edema complicating tonsillectomy and adenoidetomy. *Pediatrics* 1985;75:112–114.

102. Valor RR, Polnitxky CA, Tains DJ, Sherter CB. Bacterial tracheitis with upper airway obstruction in a patient with the acquired immunodeficiency syndrome. *Am Rev Respir Dis* 1992;146:1598–1599.

103. Hass A, Hyatt AC, Kattan M, et al. Hoarseness in immunocompromised children: association with invasive fungal infection. *J Pediatr* 1987;111:731–733.

104. Roy TM, Dow FT, Puthuff DL. Upper airway obstruction from AIDS-related Kaposi's sarcoma. *J Emerg Med* 1991;9:23–25.

105. Chin R, Jones DF, Pegram PS, Haponik EF. Complete endobronchial occlusion by Kaposi's sarcoma in the absence of cutaneous involvement. *Chest* 1994;105:1581–1582.

106. Olopoenia L, Jayam-Trouth A, Barnes S, et al. Clinical apnea as an early manifestation of *Pneumocystis carinii* pneumonia in an infant with perinatal HIV-1 infection. *J Natl Med Assoc* 1992;834:79–80.

107. DeBruin W, Notterman DA, Magid M, et al. Acute hypoxemic respiratory failure in infants and children: clinical and pathologic characteristics. *Crit Care Med* 1992;20:1223–1234.

108. Staikowsky F, Lafon B, Guidet B, et al. Mechanical ventilation for *Pneumocystis carinii* pneumonia in patients with AIDS. *Chest* 1993;104:756–762.

109. Gherardi R, Belec L, Mhiri C, et al. The spectrum of vasculitis in human immunodeficiency virus-infected patients. *Arthritis Rheum* 1993;36:1164–1174.

110. Calabrese LH, Proffitt MR, Yen-Liberman B, et al. Congestive cardiomyopathy and illness related to the acquired immunodeficiency syndrome (AIDS). *Ann Intern Med* 1987;107:691–692.

111. Cooper LM, Patterson JAK. Allergic granulomatosis and angiitis of Churg Strauss: case report in a patient with antibodies to HIV and hepatitis B virus. *Int J Dermatol* 1989;23:597.

112. Calabrese LH. Vasculitis and infection with the human immunodeficiency virus. *Rheum Dis Clin North Am* 1991;17:131–147.

113. Libman BS, Quismorio FP, Stimmler MM. Polyarteritis nodosa-like vasculitis in human immunodeficiency virus infection. *J Rheumatol* 1995;22:351–355.

114. Coopman SA, Johnson RA, Platt R, Stern RS. Cutaneous disease and drug reactions in HIV infection. *N Engl J Med* 1993;328:1670–1674.

115. Ettensohn EB, Mayer KH, Kessimian N, Smith PS. Lymphocytic bronchiolitis associated with HIV infection. *Chest* 1988;93:201–202.

116. Fishman AP. *Pulmonary Diseases and Disorders,* 2nd Ed. New York: McGraw-Hill, 1988.

117. Peterman W, et al. Heart failure and airway obstruction. *Int J Cardiol* 1987;17:207–209.

118. McLain LG, Torres A, Fisher E, Winters G. Respiratory distress in an 11-month old infant. *J Pediatr* 1990;116:148–152.

119. Cohen IS, Sanderson DW, Virmani R, et al. Congestive cardiomyopathy in association with the acquired immunodeficiency syndrome. *N Engl J Med* 1986;315:628–630.

120. Kamisuka PK. Abrupt development of cardiac enlargement and respiratory distress in a 31-year-old man with AIDS. *N Engl J Med* 1992;327:790–799.

121. Venable RS, Yanda RL. Cardiopulmonary manifestations in HIV-infected patients. *Top Emerg Med* 1994;16:17–23.

122. Scully RE, Mark EJ, McNeely WF, Kamitsuka PF. Case records of the MGH: weekly clinicopathological exercises. *N Engl J Med* 1992;327:790–799.

123. Bancalari E, Jesse MJ, Gelband H, Garcia O. Lung mechanics in congenital heart disease with increased and decreased pulmonary blood flow. *J Pediatr* 1977;90:192–195.

124. Hordof AJ, Mellins RB, Gersony WM, Steeg CN. Reversibility of chronic obstructive lung disease in infants following repair of ventricular septal defect. *J Pediatr* 1977;90:187–191.

125. Cabanes LR, Weber SN, Matran R, et al. Bronchial hyperresponsiveness to methacholine in patients wth impaired left ventricular function. *N Engl J Med* 1989;320:1317–1322.

12

Pulmonary Hypertension in Patients Infected with HIV

Arwa Saidi, M.B., B.Ch., and J. Timothy Bricker, M.D.

It is well known that the human immunodeficiency virus (HIV) can cause dilated cardiomyopathy, myocarditis, a depression in left ventricular function, pericarditis, and endocarditis. It is also well known that cor pulmonale due to chronic lung disease may complicate infection by HIV. The primary effect of this virus on the right ventricle and pulmonary vasculature is less clear. A primary association of HIV and pulmonary hypertension has been difficult to determine because of other frequently associated conditions that may also increase pulmonary pressure, such as recurrent pulmonary infections and illicit drug use.

Pulmonary hypertension is not a disease but a manifestation of a disorder of the pulmonary vascular bed that causes obstruction to pulmonary blood flow, resulting from increased resistance in a pulmonary vascular bed with normal or decreased blood flow or increased blood flow through a vascular bed.[1] Pulmonary hypertension usually develops secondary to underlying pulmonary disease, cardiovascular disease , connective tissue disease, thromboembolic disease or portal hypertension. Primary pulmonary hypertension is a diagnosis of exclusion, if the elevated pulmonary pressure cannot be explained by any underlying conditions.

Definition

The normal mean pulmonary artery pressure is 18–20 mmHg with a pressure gradient of 9 mmHg across the lungs (mean pulmonary artery pressure minus the wedge or left atrial pressure).

$P = QR$
P = pressure (mmHg)
Q = flow (l/min)
R = resistance (mmHg $.l^{-1}$ min^{-1} or Wood units)

Therefore, arteriolar resistance is calculated by the following equation:

$$R = P \div Q$$

To convert Wood units to another commonly used nomenclature, the cgs system (dynes s^{-1} cm^{-5}), Wood units are multiplied by a factor of 80.[2] The normal pulmonary arteriolar resistance is less than 4 Wood units. In pulmonary hypertension the mean pulmonary artery pressure is greater than 25 mmHg at rest and 30 mmHg during exercise. The gradient across the lungs increases to 10 to 12 mmHg and the pulmonary vascular resistance is greater than 4 Wood units with exercise.[3]

The diagnosis of pulmonary hypertension is often difficult to make or is delayed, but it must be considered if the patient presents with dyspnea or hypoxia out of proportion to the chest examination or radiograph.

Several definitions have been used for cor pulmonale. Cor pulmonale has been defined as right heart failure or right ventricular hypertrophy or dilatation in patients who do not have primary cardiac disorder. It is usually a terminal event in patients with long-standing pulmonary hypertension or is caused by an acute increase in pulmonary artery pressure.

Clinical Features

Even patients with significant pulmonary hypertension may be asymptomatic. The initial presentation may be syncope, exercise-induced dyspnea, or palpitations. Fatigue and cough are occasional presentations. Cough develops because of pressure on the bronchi by the dilated pulmonary arteries.

Patients may have signs of low cardiac output, dyspnea, and tachypnea. There may be signs of right heart failure with an elevated jugular venous pressure, hepatomegaly, and peripheral edema. In the absence of right heart failure, the jugular venous pressure is not elevated, but there is an increase in the A wave and a large V wave from tricuspid regurgitation. The right ventricular impulse is increased, with an increase in the intensity of the second heart sound. An ejection click may be heard, with a short systolic murmur. A high-frequency diastolic decrescendo murmur of pulmonary regurgitation (Graham-Steell) murmur is heard in 10% to 15% of patients, and a high-pitched pansystolic tricuspid regurgitation murmur is heard in 40% to 71% of patients. A fourth heart sound is frequently heard over the right ventricle, and occasionally a third heart sound. Premature ventricular contractions and supraventricular tachycardias may be present.[1]

On the electrocardiogram, there is right atrial enlargement and right ventricular hypertrophy with right axis deviation. There may be an incomplete right bundle branch block pattern, reflecting mild right ventricular hypertrophy early in the course.

Chest radiography usually shows a normal-sized heart and a prominent pulmonary artery segment with dilated prominent right and left arteries. The peripheral pulmonary vascular markings may be decreased. On the lateral radiograph there may be retrosternal fullness.

Echocardiogram

Echocardiography is useful in estimating pulmonary pressure and evaluating changes in pulmonary artery pressure in response to therapy. The pulmonary valve opening velocity is increased, with partial closure of the valve in midsystole. There is flattening of the E to F slope during diastole on the M mode.

The ratio of the right ventricular preejection time to the right ventricular ejection time has been used in evaluating the patients with an elevated pulmonary pressure. The right ventricular systolic time intervals can be calculated from the motion of the pulmonary valve or by valve opening with Doppler. The normal ratio of the right ventricular preejection time to the right ventricular ejection time is less than 0.26. An increase in this ratio to greater than 0.3 suggests pulmonary hypertension.[4] Systolic time intervals are nonspecific and can vary with a change in heart rate, ventricular contractility, and bundle branch block. Serial changes are of very limited use in following the course or response to treatment.

Isobe and colleagues[5] noted that the ratio of right ventricular preejection period to the acceleration time (measured from the onset of the flow to the peak velocity of flow on the Doppler tracing) was an echocardiographic predictor of pulmonary hypertension. A ratio >1.1 is seen in 93% of the patients with pulmonary hypertension studied; 97% of patients with normal pulmonary hypertension had a ratio <1.1.[5] Factors such as age, heart rate, and right ventricular preload, and right ventricular function affect these Doppler time intervals.

The velocity of the tricuspid regurgitation jet, if present, is an estimate of right ventricular pressure and therefore pulmonary pressure. By using the modified Bernoulli equation [four times the (tricuspid regurgitation velocity in meters per second)^2] the pressure difference between the right ventricle and atrium can be estimated. Right ventricular systolic pressure as a percentage of systemic pressure can be estimated by evaluating the septal curvature. If the right ventricular pressure is supresystemic, the ventricular septum curves toward the left ventricle.[6]

Cardiac Catheterization

Cardiac catheterization is useful in confirming the diagnosis of pulmonary hypertension. The measurement of the pulmonary artery pressure and cardiac output is used for the calculation of the pulmonary vascular resistance. This helps to define the degree of the pulmonary vascular disease and is of prognostic value. The degree of the pulmonary vascular disease can be assessed by doing multiple wedge angiograms. The reactivity of the pulmonary vasculature to oxygen and short-acting intravenous vasodilators (e.g., nitroprusside, adenosine, prostacycline) or nitric oxide can be evaluated during the cardiac catheterization and can aid in the therapeutic decisions. Palliative balloon atrial septostomy at catheterization may be therapeutic in pulmonary hypertension and will be discussed further under treatment.

The risk to the operator of carrying out a heart catheterization on an HIV-positive patient is low but must be considered. There have been no reports of needle-stick injuries with HIV-positive blood during a cardiac catheterization. The use of double gloves and meticulous precautions during cardiac catheterization is recommended to minimize the risk to the operators.

Primary Pulmonary Hypertension

Pulmonary hypertension is classified as primary if there is no known heart or lung disease to account for the elevation in the pulmonary vascular resistance. It is associated with various connective tissue diseases, liver disease, ingestion of aminorex, and

various hematologic conditions, but most cases are not found to have a specific cause. Several cases of primary pulmonary hypertension in patients infected by HIV have been reported since the first description by Kim and Factor in 1987.[7] According to a recent review of the literature, 61 patients who were HIV-positive had pulmonary hypertension, and 20 of this group had AIDS.[8] These patients presented most commonly with symptoms of progressive dyspnea as well as cough, right heart failure, fatigue, or presyncope. The most distinguishing clinical feature in one report of six men was right ventricular hypertrophy on the electrocardiogram.[9] This was present in all the patients and was often the initial finding that suggested a diagnosis of pulmonary hypertension. In children, pulmonary hypertension is a rare presentation of HIV infection. However, a case of a 10-year-old girl who presented with cor pulmonale secondary to congenitally acquired HIV infection has been reported.[10]

A case of a 2-year-old child with mild pulmonary parenchymal disease and severe pulmonary hypertension has also been reported. This patient had a favorable response to home oxygen, which suggests that some of the elevated pulmonary pressure was due to a reversible pulmonary vasoconstriction. This reversibility has not been a prominent feature in adult patients.[11]

In patients using injected drugs, the possibility arises of pulmonary hypertension being secondary to microemboli, such as from talc injection. Tomashefski and Hirsch[12] reviewed autopsy results from 70 patients with a history of intravenous drug abuse and concluded that there was no risk of developing foreign-body granulomas that could lead to pulmonary hypertension unless the injected drug consisted of crushed oral medication.[12]

Etiology

Various speculations regarding the possible cause of primary pulmonary hypertension in patients with HIV have been considered. Primary pulmonary hypertension is characterized by progressive narrowing of the microvasculature in the pulmonary vascular bed. Endothelin 1, a vasoconstrictor derived from endothelial cells, is usually cleared from the blood during passage through the lung. This clearance appears to be reduced in patients with primary pulmonary hypertension.

Coplan and coworkers[13] suggested that growth factors produced by a virus or by virally infected T lymphocytes may cause the proliferation of pulmonary endothelium thus leading to pulmonary hypertension. In support of this hypothesis, pulmonary arteriopathy was documented in 19 of 85 monkeys who died from infection by the simian immunodeficiency virus.[14]

Nakamura and colleagues[15] identified a growth factor elaborated by retrovirus-infected T lymphocytes that stimulates and maintains the growth of human vascular endothelial cells in cell culture.

Mette and colleagues[16] attempted to identify the HIV-1 in the vascular endothelial cells of affected vessels by electron microscopy and immunohistochemical techniques with monoclonal antibodies directed against several HIV-1 proteins. There was no evidence of direct HIV-1 infection of the vascular endothelium. There was also no evidence of HIV-1 genome or p24 HIV-1 major core protein detected by polymerase chain reaction or in situ hybridization.[16] However, in a separate report, HIV-1 RNA and DNA were detected in the heart of a 13-month-old patient who died from respiratory failure. The viral RNA was detected by in situ hybridization and the HIV-1 proviral DNA was determined after polymerase chain reaction amplification of DNA in the tissue section.[17]

The presence of primary pulmonary hypertension in five hemophiliac patients who were HIV-positive was initially reported by Goldsmith and coworkers,[18] and later by Schulman and coworkers[19] Both these reports suggested that therapy with factor VIII and not infection with HIV was the underlying cause. However, Bray and colleagues[20] reported a case in which an HIV-positive hemophiliac boy who had received minimal infusion with factor VIII developed histologically confirmed primary pulmonary hypertension. These authors considered the HIV infection as the more significant risk factor for developing primary pulmonary hypertension.

Morse and colleagues[21] reported that HIV-associated primary pulmonary hypertension reflects the host response, the HIV, which differs immunogenetically from that in HIV-negative patients with primary pulmonary hypertension, even though the clinical disease is the same. The host response in primary pulmonary hypertension with HIV may be determined by one or more HLA-DR alleles with major histocompatibility loci HLA DR6 and DR52.

Histology

The pathologic pattern seen in primary pulmonary hypertension is usually plexogenic pulmonary arteriopathy. On histologic examination, this is characterized by concentric intimal proliferation and fibrosis with associated medial proliferation and plexiform lesions. A review of 61 HIV-infected patients, who were diagnosed with primary pulmonary hypertension, included 23 patients who had a biopsy or autopsy; 21 had the classic lesions of primary pulmonary hypertension, which include plexiform lesions, intimal fibrosis, and medial hypertrophy.[8]

In three patients with HIV infection, the plexiform lesion contained proliferated endothelial cells as assessed by immunostaining with anti-factor VIII-related antigen and with MIB-1 antibodies that are directed to the Ki-67 antibodies. There was also an increase in the number of chronic inflammatory cells in this region. These findings suggest that pulmonary hypertension associated with HIV has histologic similarities to primary pulmonary hypertension with active endothelial cell proliferation and perivascular inflammation.[22]

A case of primary pulmonary hypertension with a histologic pattern of a thrombotic pulmonary arteriopathy with eccentric intimal fibrosis in a patient with HIV has been reported.[23]

Secondary Pulmonary Hypertension

Pulmonary hypertension is usually secondary to underlying left heart disease or lung disease. In patients infected with HIV, there are many underlying disorders that can lead to pulmonary hypertension. Pulmonary infections by *Mycobacterium tuberculosis*, *Pneumocystis carinii*, and cytomegalovirus are common and may lead to elevated pulmonary artery pressure and right heart failure. Pulmonary cancers that are frequently seen in patients with AIDS, such as Kaposi's sarcoma or lymphoma, may also cause pulmonary hypertension. Talc granulomatosis resulting from intravenous injection of crushed oral medication may elevate pulmonary pressure. Thromboembolic phenomena from indwelling central lines may shed small emboli. Nonbacterial thrombotic endocarditis is associated with chronic wasting disease[24] and may cause right heart valve lesions that can result in pulmonary embolism.

Dilated cardiomyopathy in 30% to 40% of patients with AIDS[25] and myocarditis[26] in 46% of patients with AIDS can cause left atrial hypertension from left ventricular failure and therefore a secondary pulmonary hypertension. Left ventricular dysfunction has been reported secondary to therapy with interferon alfa-2a, pentamidine, and ganciclovir.[27–29]) Doxorubicin for AIDS-related Kaposi's sarcoma may also depress left ventricular function. Cardiac Kaposi's sarcoma[30,31] and malignant lymphoma[32] of the heart have been reported and may cause congestive heart failure with secondary pulmonary hypertension.

Treatment

Home oxygen has been shown to be beneficial in patients with severe dyspnea on exertion and fatigue. This may be delivered continuously or intermittently as needed, for example, before exercise. There has been one report of regression of pulmonary hypertension with the combination of nocturnal oxygen, anticoagulants, and vasodilators.[33]

Right heart failure is a poor prognostic factor and must be treated aggressively with digoxin and diuretics. Vasodilators may be of some benefit if the patient is not hypotensive. Treatment with calcium channel blockers has been shown to reduce the pulmonary artery pressure and pulmonary vascular resistance, with regression of right ventricular hypertrophy.[34] Nifedipine has been shown to improve symptoms and perhaps prolong life in some patients.

Anticoagulants[35] and antiplatelet agents have been used in patients with primary pulmonary hypertension to reduce thrombosis and to blunt the platelet endothelial interaction, respectively. The benefit of anticoagulant therapy to a patient with

HIV who may have an increased risk of bleeding and thrombocytopenia must be weighed.

The response of the pulmonary vascular reactivity to therapy with calcium antagonists may be predicted by response to a trial of 80 ppm of nitric oxide. In a recent study of the pulmonary vascular response to face-mask oxygen, 80 ppm of nitric oxide, and oral calcium antagonists, all patients who responded to oral calcium antagonists responsed to nitric oxide.[36]

The long-term benefit of nitric oxide for pulmonary hypertension remains uncertain, with a risk of rebound pulmonary hypertension after drug withdrawal.[37] Chest pain accompanying pulmonary hypertension is often anginal and has been thought to respond to nitroglycerine by some.

Chronic infusion of intravenous prostacyclin has resulted in an improvement in the pulmonary metabolism of endothelin 1.[38] Therapeutic use of continuous intravenous prostacyclin has been shown by Barst and colleagues[39,40] to provide symptomatic relief and improve quality of life and survival of patients with primary pulmonary hypertension in both adults and children.

Cardiac catheterization has been beneficial for evaluating treatment in some patients with pulmonary hypertension but must be considered carefully. One advantage of cardiac catheterization in patients with elevated pulmonary pressure is to evaluate the reversibility of the pulmonary hypertension with oxygen and short-acting intravenous medications such as adenosine, prostacyclin, nitroprusside, and isoproterenol. If the response is greater than 20 mmHg, therapy with intravenous prostacyclin or oral nifedipine may be beneficial in reducing the pulmonary pressure.

In patients with low cardiac output, right heart failure, or syncope, an atrial septostomy may improve cardiac output and symptoms of congestive heart failure. Creating a right-to-left shunt will cause hypoxemia. Limited size of septostomy with a high-pressure 8- or 10-mm balloon has been used following a transeptal procedure. Progressive balloon diameters are recommended, and the procedure is completed when the cardiac index improves with a minimal decrease in oxygen saturation. At the time of the atrial septostomy, the patient may benefit from a blood transfusion to improve the oxygen carrying capacity. A large septostomy from a blade procedure may result in excessive hypoxemia. The right-to-left shunt created will increase the risk of embolic disease and stroke in the systemic arterial circulation.

Single or double lung transplantation has been used for primary pulmonary hypertension with some success; however, HIV infection has been considered an absolute contraindication to transplantation.

Summary

Secondary pulmonary hypertension in patients infected with HIV is seen in some frequency with pulmonary infections or malignancies or with left ventricular failure. The association of primary pulmonary hypertension with HIV is infrequent and the relationship to HIV disease has been more difficult to establish. There might be underdiagnosis or underreporting of patients with primary pulmonary hypertension. This diagnosis must be considered in all patients with a physical examination suggestive of elevated pulmonary artery pressure or symptoms that appear worse than their clinical examination or chest radiograph.

References

1. Nihill MR. Clinical management of patients with pulmonary hypertension. In: Pine JW Jr (ed). *Heart Disease in Infants, Children and Adolescents,* 5th Ed. Baltimore: Williams & Wilkins, 1995:695–711.

2. Vargo TA. Cardiac catheterization: hemodynamic measurements. In: Garson A, Bricker VT, McNamara DG (eds). *The Science and Practice of Pediatric Cardiology,* 1st Ed. Malvern, PA: Lee & Febiger, 1990:913–945.

3. Weir EK, Reeves JT. *Pulmonary Hypertension.* New York: Futura Publishing, 1984.

4. Hirschfeld S, Meyer R, Schwartz DC, et al. The echocardiographic assessment of pulmonary artery hypertension. *Circulation* 1975;52:642.

5. Isobe M, Yazaki Y, Takaku F, et al. Prediction of pulmonary arterial pressure in adults by pulsed Doppler echocardiography. *Am J Cardiol* 1986;58: 352–356.

6. Lipshultz SE, Sanders SP, Mayer JE, et al. Are routine preoperative cardiac catheterization and angiography necessary before repair of ostium primum atrial septal defect? *J Am Coll Cardiol* 1988; 11:373–378.

7. Kim KK, Factor SM. Membranoproliferative glomerulonephritis and plexogenic pulmonary arteriopathy in a homosexual man with acquired immunodeficiency syndrome. *Hum Pathol* 1987;18: 1293–1296.

8. Weiss JR, Pietra GG, Scharf SM. Primary pulmonary hypertension and the human immunodeficiency virus. *Arch Intern Med* 1995;155:2350–2354.

9. Himelman RB, Dohrmann M, Goodman P, et al. Severe pulmonary hypertension and cor pulmonale in the acquired immunodeficiency syndrome. *Am J Cardiol* 1989;64:1396–1399.

10. Hays MD, Wiles HB, Gillette PC. Congenital acquired immunodeficiency syndrome presenting as cor pulmonale in a 10 year old girl. *Am Heart J* 1991;121:929–931.

11. Rhodes J, Schiller MS, Montoya CH, Fikrig S. Severe pulmonary hypertension without significant pulmonary parenchymal disease in a pediatric patient with acquired immunodeficiency syndrome. *Clin Pediatr* 1992;Oct;31:629–631.

12. Tomashefski JE, Hirsch CS. The pulmonary vascular lesions of intravenous drug abuse. *Hum Pathol* 1980;11:133–145.

13. Coplan NL, Shimony RY, Ioachim HL, et al. Primary pulmonary hypertension associated with human immunodeficiency viral infection. *Am J Med* 1990;89:96–99.

14. Chalifoux LV, Simon MA, Pauley DR, et al. Arteriopathy in macaques infected with simian immunodeficiency virus. *Lab Invest* 1992;67:338–349.

15. Nakamura S, Salahuddin SZ, Biberfeld P, et al. Kaposi's sarcoma cells: long-term culture with growth factor from retrovirus-infected CD4+ T cells. *Science* 1988;242:426–430.

16. Mette SA, Palevsky HI, Pietra GG, et al. Primary pulmonary hypertension in association with human immunodeficiency virus infection. *Am Rev Respir Dis* 1992;145:1196–1200.

17. Lipshultz SE, Fox CH, Perez-Atayde AR, et al. Identification of human immunodeficiency virus-1 RNA and DNA in the heart of a child with cardiovascular abnormalities and congenital acquired immune deficiency syndrome. *Am J Cardiol* 1990;66; 246–250.

18. Goldsmith GH, Bailey RG, Brettler DB, et al. Primary pulmonary hypertension in patients with classic hemophilia. *Ann Intern Med* 1988;108:797–799.

19. Schulman S, Johnson H, Blomqvist S. Pulmonary hypertension in hemophilia. *Ann Intern Med* 1988; 109:759–760.

20. Bray GL, Martin GR, Chandra R. Idiopathic pulmonary hypertension, hemophilia A, and infection with human immunodeficiency virus (HIV). *Ann Intern Med* 1989;111:689–690.

21. Morse JH, Barst RJ, Itescu S, et al. Primary pulmonary hypertension in human immunodeficiency virus infection: an outcome determined by particular major histocompatibility class II alleles. [Abstract]. *Circulation* 1992;I-241:1148.

22. Cool C, Voekel N, Kennedy D, Tuder RM. Pulmonary vascular lesions in scleroderma and AIDS patients contain elements of endothelial cell proliferation and perivascular inflammation. [Abstract]. *Circulation* 1992;I-579:2770.

23. Heron E, Laaban JP, Capron F, et al. Thrombotic primary pulmonary hypertension in an HIV+ patient. *Eur Heart J* 1994;15:394–396.

24. Lopez JA, Ross R, Fishbein M, Siegel RJ. Nonbacterial thrombotic endocarditis: a review. *Am Heart J* 1987;113:773–784.

25. Levy WS, Simon GL, Rios JC, Ross AM. Prevalence of cardiac abnormalities in human immunodeficiency virus infection. *Am J Cardiol* 1989;63: 86–89.

26. Anderson DW, Virmani R, Reilly JM, et al. Prevalent myocarditis at necropsy in the acquired immunodeficiency syndrome. *J Am Coll Cardiol* 1988; 11:792–799.

27. Lipshultz SE, Chanock S, Sanders SP, et al. Cardiovascular manifestations of human immunodeficiency virus infection in infants and children. *Am J Cardiol* 1989;63:1489–97.

28. Cohen AJ, Weiser B, Afzal Q, Fuhrer J. Ventricular tachycardia in two patients with AIDS receiving ganciclovir (DHPG). *AIDS* 1990;4:807–809.

29. Deyton LR, Walker RE, Kovacs JA, et al. Reversible cardiac dysfunction associated with interferon alpha therapy in AIDS patients with Kaposi's sarcoma. *N Eng J Med* 1989;321:1246–1249.

30. Silver MA, Macher AM, Reichert CM, et al. Cardiac involvement by Kaposi's sarcoma in acquired immunodeficiency syndrome (AIDS). *Am J Cardiol* 1984;53:983–985.

31. Levison DA, Semple PA. Primary cardiac Kaposi's sarcoma. *Thorax* 1976;31:595–600.

32. Ziegler J, Beckstead J, Volberding P, et al. Non-Hodgkin's lymphoma in 90 homosexual men: relation to generalized lymphadenopathy in the acquired immunodeficiency syndrome. *N Engl J Med* 1984;311:565–750.

33. Kanemoto M, Yamagushi H, Shiina Y, Goto Y. Reversibility of primary pulmonary hypertension with vasodilator, anticoagulant and nocturnal oxygen therapy. *Jpn Heart J* 1989;30:929–934.

34. Rich S, Brundage BH. High-dose calcium channel-blocking therapy for primary pulmonary hypertension: evidence for long-term reduction in pulmonary arterial pressure and regression of right ventricular hypertrophy. *Circulation* 1987;76;135–141.

35. Fuster V, Steele PM, Edwards WD, et al. Primary pulmonary hypertension: natural history and the importance of thrombosis. *Circulation* 1984;70: 580–587.

36. Landzberg MJ, Graydon E, Fernandes SM, et al. Inhaled nitric oxide in primary pulmonary hypertension: the "perfect" pulmonary vasodilator. [Abstract]. *Circulation* 1992;I-241:1150.

37. Miller OI, Tang SF, Keech A, Celermajer DS. Rebound pulmonary hypertension: a frequent complication of withdrawal from nitric oxide. [Abstract]. *Circulation* 1992;I-241:1151.

38. Langleben D, Long WA, Barst RJ, et al. Prostacyclin infusion improves the balance between pulmonary clearance and production of endothelin-1 in patients with primary pulmonary hypertension. [Abstract]. *Circulation* 1992;I-241:1149.

39. Barst RJ. Pharmacologically induced pulmonary vasodilation in children and young adults with primary pulmonary hypertension. *Chest* 1986;89:497–503.

40. Barst RJ. A comparison of continuous intravenous epoprostenol (prostacyclin) with conventional therapy for primary pulmonary hypertension. *N Engl J Med* 1996;334;296–301.

13

Pericardial Disease in HIV Infection

Robert J. Lederman, M.D., and Melvin D. Cheitlin, M.D.

Pericardial Disease in HIV

Pericardial abnormalities commonly accompany human immunodeficiency virus (HIV) infection. The symptoms and signs may be subtle and difficult to distinguish from those of other, often concurrent, cardiopulmonary disease processes. This chapter reviews the prevalence, etiology, outcome, and therapy of pericardial involvement.

Prevalence and Incidence

Table 13-1 pools the reported literature on the prevalence of subclinical pericardial effusions in HIV-seropositive patients without obvious cardiac pathology. Approximately one-fifth of patients without suspected cardiac disease had pericardial effusion. Of these, approximately one-fifth were large effusions. Pericardial effusions generally were more common in patients with acquired immunodeficiency syndrome (AIDS) than in patients with asymptomatic HIV infection.

Two groups reported serial echocardiography in large cohorts of HIV-infected subjects. Blanchard et al.[1] found that 5 of 44 patients with AIDS or AIDS-related complex developed new pericardial effusions during a 9 ± 3 months follow-up period (annual incidence 15%). Heidenreich and col-

leagues[2] reported an 11% annual incidence of pericardial effusion in patients with AIDS surveyed prospectively over a 2-year period (see Figure 13-1). The majority of these effusions were clinically silent. Only 13% of the effusions developed in HIV-infected patients without AIDS.

Women had a higher incidence of pericardial disease in some reports,[3] yet none of the 40 women who constituted 9% of the population studied by Hsia and coworkers[4] developed pericardial effusions. These discrepancies may reflect the varying proportions of parenteral drug abusers and African immigrants studied.

Pericardial disease in Africa increasingly is related to HIV infection. Cegielski and colleagues[5] found 28 of 42 patients with symptomatic (clinically detected) pericardial disease to be HIV-seropositive. The proportion of seropositive patients apparently increases over time. Taelman and colleagues[6] reported 30 of 37 Rwandan patients with pericardial tamponade to be HIV-seropositive: 10 had proven and 18 had presumptive myocobacterial disease.

Symptomatic Pericarditis

Symptomatic pericarditis is considerably less common than subclinical effusion. Reilly and asso-

Table 13-1. Prevalence of Echocardiographic Pericardial Effusion in Patients Without Suggestive Symptoms or Signs

Ref.	Population	Location	Pericardial Effusion	Size of Effusions
80	Retrospective of patients without significant abnormality on physical examination, echocardiography, or autopsy	Philadelphia	8/15	
105	Consecutive ambulatory inpatients (1 ARC, 11 AIDS)	New Jersey	1/12	
106	Consecutive inpatients with AIDS, no clear signs of heart failure or tamponade	Milan	39/102	30/39 small–medium 9/39 large
3	Subpopulation of patients from 7 hospitals, without clinical evidence of heart disease	Paris, Miami	4/68	4/4 small–medium
107	Homosexual men with AIDS and normal examination, electrocardiography, and cardiac silhouette	New York	7/21	
59	University hospital AIDS clinic inpatients and outpatients	San Francisco	7/70	6/7 small
108	Consecutive inpatients with opportunistic infections and no evident heart disease	Copenhagen	5/24	
31	Prospective study of HIV-seropositive patients	Cologne (Germany)	12/92	12/12 small–medium
109	Consecutive parenteral drug abusers, 80% HIV-seropositive	Valencia (Spain)	27/32 HIV+AIDS– 31/39 HIV+AIDS+	27/58 small–medium 31/58 large
1	Consecutive HIV-seropositive outpatients without symptomatic heart disease	San Diego	11/50 AIDS-ARC 4/20 HIV+	
52	Consecutive HIV-seropositive patients, 74% IVDA, 63% AIDS	Rome	13/72	12/13 small–medium
110	Consecutive HIV-infected patients without apparent opportunistic infections	Denmark	0/60	No effusions>2.0 mm
104	Consecutive HIV-seropositive homosexual men, in- and outpatients	London	44/101 HIV+AIDS+ 2/23 HIV+AIDS-	
4	Prospective study of HIV-seropositive patients, 83% homosexual men	Washington, DC	71/429	58/71 small–medium 13/71 large
2	Prospective study of HIV-seropositive in- and outpatients	San Francisco	15/216	14/15 small–medium 1/15 large
Total **15**			**301/1446** (20.8%)	**60/310** (19.3%) of effusions were large

ciates[7] reviewed the clinical records of 58 consecutive autopsies performed on patients with AIDS at the National Institutes of Health. Two had pericarditis clinically, and seven had pericardial effusion postmortem. These were evenly distributed among patients with and without histopathologic evidence of myocarditis. Malu and coworkers[8] described 17 patients in Kinshasa, Zaire, with clinical pericarditis: 16 had chest pain, 10 a pericardial friction rub, 10 palpitation, 15 an abnormal electrocardiogram, and 11 an enlarged cardiac silhouette; pericardiocentesis in 12 yielded a small amount of exudate, but no pathogen was identified. Heidenreich and colleagues[2] reported that only 2 of 195 HIV-infected patients prospectively observed over 2 years developed clinical pericarditis: 1 asymptomatic HIV-infected patient with no effusion, and 1 AIDS patient with effusion.

Although atrial arrhythmias commonly accompany clinical pericarditis, they have not been reported specifically in association with HIV infection. Pousett and coworkers[9] reported a patient with atrial flutter and cardiac lymphoma not confined to the pericardium. One of 195 HIV-infected patients surveyed by Heidenreich and colleagues[2] developed atrial flutter in association with pericardial effusion.

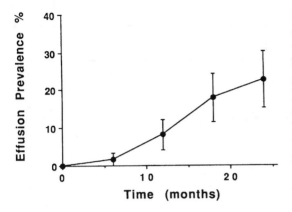

Figure 13-1. Incidence of pericardial effusion in patients with AIDS. (From Ref. 2, with permission.)

Etiology

Table 13-2 lists the diverse causes of pericardial disease described in patients with HIV infection.

Malignant Pericardial Effusions

Kaposi's Sarcoma

Kaposi's sarcoma behaves epidemiologically like a sexually transmitted disease, usually affecting homosexual men with AIDS. Recently it has been associated with human herpesvirus.[10,11] The heart is involved in up to 28% of patients with AIDS dying with Kaposi's sarcoma.[12] Typically the pericardium and epicardial fat are involved, with invasion of subepicardial myocardium and extension along the roots of the great vessels and coronary arteries. When Kaposi's sarcoma involves the heart, it usually also is widely disseminated. Silver and colleagues[12] described autopsies of 18 patients with Kaposi's sarcoma and AIDS, 5 of whom had cardiac (epicardial adipose) involvement; all had multiorgan involvement as well. In Lewis' series[13] of 59 autopsies of patients with AIDS and cardiac involvement, 7 had cardiac Kaposi's sarcoma; in only 3 was it confined to the epicardium.

Cardiac Kaposi's sarcoma usually is not recognized clinically. None of the patients in the series by Silver and colleagues[12] had symptoms or electrocardiographic (EKG) or radiographic evidence of cardiac disease antemortem. Remick and colleagues[14] diagnosed pleuropericardial Kaposi's sarcoma antemortem by pericardial biopsy in a man with recurrent pleural and pericardial effusion. Occasionally the heart is involved even without cutaneous or visceral Kaposi lesions. Autran and colleagues[15] describe a Haitian woman with bacterial sepsis and AIDS but no cutaneous or visceral Kaposi's sarcoma and no pericardial effusion; autopsy showed extensive Kaposi's sarcoma involvement of the anterior cardiac surface.

Occasionally Kaposi's sarcoma manifests as pericardial effusion or hemorrhagic tamponade. Stotka and associates[16] described cardiac tamponade in a man with cutaneous and visceral Kaposi's sarcoma lesions and cryptococcal meningitis. Pericardiocentesis yielded exudative fluid with unrevealing cytologic findings. Autopsy revealed Kaposi's sarcoma nodules and plaques confined to the pericardium and pericardial fat, but invading the media and adventitia of the pulmonary trunk and aorta. Steigman and coworkers[17] reported a man with *Pneumocystis carinii* pneumonia who died of acute pericardial tamponade. Autopsy revealed bloody pericardial fluid and coalescent Kaposi nodules in the epicardial fat and root of the great vessels, extensive pulmonary and gastrointestinal involvement, and a solitary endocardial nodule with surrounding myocarditis. Langer and associates[17] described autopsies in two patients with extensive Kaposi's sarcoma dying of pericardial tamponade. Each had hemorrhagic effusions and cardiac infiltration extending along the great vessels and coronary arteries. Others report similar experiences.[3,6,19]

Symptomatic visceral Kaposi's sarcoma may be palliated with radiotherapy or systemic chemotherapy, but the responses are disappointing.[20–24] Liposomal anthracycline formulations may reduce toxicity.[25–27]

Malignant Lymphoma

High-grade extranodal non-Hodgkin's lymphoma is a common opportunistic malignancy in advanced HIV infection.[28,29] As in Kaposi's sarcoma, secondary cardiac involvement is seen in about 20% of patients with lymphoma subject to autopsy.[30] Primary cardiac lymphoma is rare. Antemortem diagnosis is unusual.

Table 13-2. Causes of Pericardial Effusion in HIV Infection

Transmission	Clinical Characteristic	Cause	Ref.
Noninfective	Malignant	Lymphoma	3, 9,31–41
		Kaposi's sarcoma	3,6,12,14–18,106,111
		Adenocarcinoma	42
	Inflammatory	Nonspecific/lymphocytic/fibrinous/idiopathic pericarditis	3,13,56
		Postirradiation	
		Postmyocardial infarction	
		Constrictive pericarditis	
	Uremic		
	Postmyocardial infarction		56
	Hemodynamic	Congestive heart failure	
		Lymphatic obstruction	
		Reduced plasma oncotic pressure, i.e., hypoalbuminemia	
Infective	Purulent		40,54
		Streptococcus pneumoniae	3,5
		Staphylococcus aureus	4,5,43,52,58,111–114
		Chlamydia trachomatis	64
		Nocardia asteroides	63
		Rhodococcus equi	60,61
		Listeria monocytogenes	62
	Mycobacterial	*Mycobacterium tuberculosis*	5,6,31,40,43,54,55,66,69–77, 81–83,115,116
		Nontuberculous mycobacteria, i.e., *Mycobacterium avium* complex	93–95
		Mycobacterium kansasii	92
	Fungal and Protozoal		15
		Cryptococcus neoformans	48,49
		Histoplasma	50
		Toxoplasma gondii	51
	Viral	Cytomegalovirus	44,45
		Herpes simplex viruses	46,47
		Primary human immunodeficiency virus	8

Malignant lymphoma has been reported to involve the pericardium of HIV-infected patients.[3,9,31–41] Most of these had AIDS and relatively abrupt onset of dyspnea, pleuritic, or positional chest pain. Others had nonspecific constitution or other vague symptoms. Usually these symptoms were rapidly progressive. Many had pericardial rubs, supraventricular arrhythmias like atrial fibrillation[36] or flutter[9] signaling pericardial inflammation, or pericardial tamponade. Histology typically showed diffuse large-cell immunoblastic or small-cell noncleaved cells. Typical necropsy findings were pericardial nodules and variable subepicardial infiltration.

Treatment with radiation therapy and chemotherapy has short-term efficacy in AIDS-associated lymphoma involving the pericardium, but longer-term responses are limited.[33,41,42]

Other malignancies involving the pericardium in AIDS have been described rarely. In the series by Flum and coworkers[43] of patients with AIDS undergoing operative pericardial drainage, 2 of 29 had adenocarcinoma of unknown primary source.

Infective Pericarditis

Viral Pericarditis

Human herpesviruses are nearly ubiquitous. Distinguishing infection from colonization can be difficult.

Two reports of cytomegalovirus pericarditis showed evidence of infection. Scott and colleagues[44] reported a man with AIDS treated with ganciclovir for cytomegalovirus retinitis who had vague thoracic symptoms for 1 week and pericardial tamponade. Cytologic examination of pericardial fluid revealed mesothelial cells with inclusion bodies suggesting cytomegalovirus infection. Nathan and colleagues[45] reported a man with AIDS, Kaposi's sarcoma, and cryptococcal meningitis who developed sudden hypotension and tamponade as a first manifestation of moderate pericardial effusion. Autopsy showed fibrinous pericarditis with cytomegalic inclusion bodies, as well as evidence of disseminated cytomegalovirus infection. Successful therapy has not been reported for cytomegalovirus pericarditis.

Two groups reported herpes simplex virus causing pericarditis with HIV infection. Freedberg and colleagues[46] isolated herpes simplex virus 1 and Toma and colleagues[47] isolated herpes simplex virus 2 from pericardial fluid in symptomatic patients; neither distinguished colonization from infection.

Fungal and Protozoal Pericarditis

Fungi are always pathogenic when found in blood or the pericardial space, unlike the Herpesviridae described above. Reports of fungal pericarditis are sparse and probably underrepresent the true incidence in advanced AIDS.

Schuster and associates[48] reported a large pericardial effusion with hemorrhagic tamponade in a pigeon fancier and parenteral drug abuser with AIDS who had 2 weeks of fever, pleuritic chest pain, exertional dyspnea, and orthopnea. Examination of pericardial fluid showed budding yeast and grew *Cryptococcus neoformans*; excised lymph nodes also demonstrated the organism. She improved and fungal antigen titers decreased after treatment with amphotericin and flucytosine. Zuger

and associates[49] reported another case. Cryptococcal pericarditis more often is seen in the context of fungal endocarditis or myocarditis.

Pericardial histoplasmosis has been reported only once complicating HIV infection, although disseminated disease is not unusual. Zakowski and collaborators[50] reported biopsy-proven pericardial *Histoplasma capsulatum* with intense mesothelial proliferation.

Toxoplasma gondii occasionally causes myocarditis but usually is not confined to the pericardium. Guerot and coworkers[51] reported a patient with AIDS and several days of fever and weakness with a large exudative pericardial effusion. *Toxoplasma gondii* grew from pericardial fluid. The patient died of nonspecific pneumonitis; postmortem examination showed lymphocytic pericarditis with mild lymphocytic infiltration of myocardium.

Bacterial Pericarditis

Purulent pericarditis associated with HIV infection resembles purulent pericarditis in other immunocompromised hosts. Usually there is no uncertainty to the diagnosis even before examination of pericardial fluid. Affected patients tend to be severely ill. Pathogens reported in the literature include *Staphylococcus aureus*,[4,5,13,42,52–58] *Streptococcus pneumoniae*,[57,59] *Rhodococcus equi*,[60,61] *Listeria monocytogenes*,[62] *Nocardia asteroides*,[63] *Chlamydia trachomatis*.[64.] *Proteus mirabilis* has been isolated from the pericardial space, but the report does not distinguish bacteremia from pericardial infection.[40]

Tuberculous Pericarditis

Tuberculosis commonly represents primary infection or primary reinfection[65] (rather than reactivation) complicating HIV disease. It involves predominantly extrapulmonary sites.[66,67] Analogous to tuberculous pleuritis, clinical pericarditis may represent an *in situ* delayed-type hypersensitivity reaction.[68]

The setting and clinical manifestations of pericardial tuberculosis vary widely in HIV infection. Usually patients have a prolonged fever with dyspnea, orthopnea, or pleurisy.[69,70] Because *M. tuberculosis* is a relative virulent CD4+ lymphocyte pathogen, it may affect patients with early HIV infection and relatively preserved CD4+ lymphocyte counts and may be the first manifestation of AIDS.[69,71] The initial manifestations may be subacute, although pericardial tamponade may ensue rapidly in patients with large effusions. Serrano-Heranz and coworkers[72] reported three intravenous drug users who developed pericardial tamponade after a subacute febrile illness with chest pain and exertional dyspnea. All had low CD4+ lymphocyte counts (range: 145–200 cells/mm³), enlarged radiographic cardiac silhouettes, and large effusions by echocardiography. All were tachycardic, but not all had pulsus paradoxus, and none were hypotensive. Clues to pericardial involvement included miliary-pattern pulmonary infiltrates in one, and unilateral left pleural effusion in another. Multidrug-resistant tuberculosis also has been reported to cause pericardial tamponade in the setting of miliary disease.[73] Pericardial tuberculosis may progress to constriction (see below) and has been reported to cause cutaneous–pericardial fistula.[74]

In Africa, where tuberculosis and AIDS are closely associated, tuberculosis is responsible for most of the large pericardial effusions in HIV-seropositive patients. All of the 14 HIV-infected, but only 4 of 8 HIV-seronegative, Tanzanian patients reported by Cegielski and colleagues[75] with large pericardial effusions had tuberculosis proven by biopsy and drainage. Elliot and colleagues[66,76] reported a similar experience. In Zimbabwe, tuberculous pericarditis associated with HIV infection usually signaled disseminated tuberculosis.[77] However, an earlier study from Zaire[8] did not find tuberculosis in any of 12 patients undergoing pericardiocentesis for large effusion associated with HIV infection.

Cutaneous anergy is common,[66,74,77] as it is in all tuberculous serositis. However, in one report from Tanzania, where tuberculosis is perhaps seen early in HIV infection, cutaneous anergy was seen only in 1 of 14 patients with tuberculous pericarditis.

Definitive diagnosis of pericardial tuberculosis can be challenging, regardless of HIV status. The yield of microbiologic or histologic examination of pericardial fluid[78,79] or tissue[80] is low. Only 3 of 16 patients in Zimbabwe diagnosed with tuberculous pericarditis had microbiologic or histologic confirmation.[81,82] Gallium[83,84] and indium-leukocyte[84] scintigraphy have localized inflammation to the pericardium of patients with tuberculous pericarditis, but these techniques probably do not add much to the diagnostic armamentarium. Adenosine deaminase, a lymphocyte-specific enzyme, is elevated in the pericardial fluid of patients with tuberculous pericarditis[85,86] and has good diagnostic sensitivity and specificity.[87] Its utility in HIV-infected patients is unknown, although its use has been reported.[72] Serologic diagnosis of extrapulmonary tuberculosis has been possible by the use of specific epitopes.[82] Polymerase chain reaction amplification of tuberculous DNA may increase the sensitivity of pericardial fluid testing[88] and recently has been approved by the U.S. Food and Drug Administration (FDA) for sputum analysis. More often, diagnosis of tuberculous pericarditis is presumptive.

Pericarditis in any patient with active tuberculosis can be ascribed to tuberculosis and generally resolves with antituberculous chemotherapy. Patients with large symptomatic pericardial effusions and HIV infection generally are treated presumptively for tuberculosis if diagnostic pericardiocentesis is not performed (see the section Pericardial Tamponade and Pericardiocentesis below). Patients often respond briskly to antituberculous chemotherapy with defervescence and resolution of both symptoms and effusions.

Delayed complications of pericardial tuberculosis include acute or subacute recurrent effusion with tamponade and subacute or chronic constrictive pericarditis in as many as half the patients.[69,79,89] The former may respond to percutaneous drainage. The latter is suprising in the face of impaired cell-mediated immunity. Both may require surgical pericardiectomy. Both may occur despite antituberculous chemotherapy. Antiinflammatory treatment during the acute phase may prevent these delayed complications. Strang and colleagues[78] reported a prospective placebo-controlled trial of glucocorticoid therapy for tuberculous pericarditis in Transkei, not confined to patients with HIV infection. Patients were randomized to four-drug chemotherapy with or without a 3-month taper of prednisolone beginning at 30 to 60 mg/day. Of 76 patients given prednisolone, 2 (3%) died of pericarditis, compared with 10 patients (14%) of 74 given placebo, who also died of pericarditis, 6 patients (8%) versus 9 (12%) underwent pericardiectomy, 10 patients (14%) versus 24 (33%) required repeat pericardial drainage. Steroid-treated patients improved more rapidly, judged by reduction in jugular vein pressure and heart rate.[88] Initial prednisone doses of 120 mg/day combined with antituberculous chemotherapy led to rapid decrease in the radiographic cardiac silhouette in 10 HIV-seronegative patients after 1 week.[90]

It is unclear whether these benefits extend to patients infected with HIV. Glucocorticoids were associated with increased opportunistic disease in a cohort of patients in Zambia who had AIDS with tuberculosis not specifically involving the pericardium.[91] Of 47 patients receiving glucocorticoids, herpes zoster developed in 6 (13%), compared to 2 of 118 patients (2%) not receiving glucocorticoids. Of the 47 patients receiving glucocorticoids, Kaposi's sarcoma developed in 3, compared to none among matched controls. Since patients were treated with glucocorticoids for specific indications, there may be unrecognized bias in this series. Nevertheless, glucocorticoids have been employed successfully in AIDS-associated tuberculous pericarditis.[70,71]

Other nontuberculous mycobacteria also have been reported to cause pericardial disease. Moreno and coworkers[92] reported three patients with advanced AIDS (CD4+ lymphocytes: 4–33 cells/mm³) and tuberculous pericarditis caused by *Mycobacterium kansasii*. Pericardial cellularity was predominantly granulocytic, in contrast to the typical lymphocyte predominance in *Mycobacterium tuberculosis*. Two responded to antituberculous chemotherapy. *Mycobacterium avium* complex commonly causes disseminated infection in patients with advanced AIDS infection but infrequently leads to death; reports of significant pericardial involvement are few. Woods and Goldsmith[93] reported a patient with autopsy-proven chronic *M. avium* complex pericarditis. Other reports of pericardial effusion and *M. avium* complex infection are difficult to interpret because of the possible coincidence of these two common complications of HIV infection.[3,94–96]

Other Causes of Pericardial Effusion

Autopsy series have identified a number of patients with inflammatory pericarditis in whom no pathogen was identified. Of 25 patients in Nice

dying of AIDS,[53] 3 had "lymphocytic pericarditis" on autopsy without evidence of myocarditis. Each had one or more concurrent opportunistic infections involving other organ systems. In Lewis's[13] large autopsy series from the University of California at Los Angeles (UCLA), 59 of 115 patients with AIDS had cardiac abnormalities post mortem. Of these, 5 had "fibrinous" pericarditis without myocarditis, infarction, antemortem renal insufficiency, or identifiable pathogen. Of 10 French patients undergoing surgical pericardiotomy, 3 had histologically nonspecific pericarditis,[3] characterized by granulocytic and lymphocytic infiltrates and moderate fibrosis.

In Lewis's series,[13] 35 of 59 patients had serous pericardial effusions. Many had concurrent serous ascites or pleural effusions; none had identifiable causes. Two more had serous and fibrinous effusions; none had identifiable causes. Pericardial as well as pleural effusions were common in the Mexican autopsy series by Rosales-Guzman and colleagues[55]: 9 of 51 patients with AIDS had small to moderate pericardial effusions, 7 had pericardial inflammation, 3 of which were fibrinous, 1 tuberculous, and 3 "nonspecific" and presumably serous. Typically HIV-associated pericardial effusions are exudative.[40]

Dilated cardiomyopathy is associated with HIV infection and commonly is associated with pericardial effusion.[2,97] Other contributing mechanisms might include uremia, acute myocardial infarction or postinfarction pericarditis,[56] impaired pericardial lymphatic drainage from mediastinal infection or malignancy, or reduced plasma oncotic pressure related to hypoalbuminemia. Malu and associates[8] speculated that their Zairian patients with clinical pericarditis and small exudative effusions might have had primary HIV pericarditis, a cause not yet demonstrated.

Natural History of Nonspecific Pericardial Effusions Associated With HIV Infection

Nonspecific pericardial effusions tend to resolve without treatment. In the series by Steffen and colleagues,[31] 12 of 92 consecutive AIDS patients in Cologne had subclinical effusions according to echocardiography; 3 resolved spontaneously and 2 resolved after antituberculous chemotherapy. Blanchard and colleagues[1] performed serial echocardiograms on 70 consecutive outpatients in San Diego with HIV infection. Of 9 subclinical effusions detected initially, 7 resolved during a mean 15-month follow-up period; 6 patients developed new effusions. In the series by Hsia and Ross[4] 71 of 429 HIV-infected outpatients had pericardial effusions. Of these 71 patients, 33 underwent serial echocardiography. In 9 of these 33 patients, the effusions spontaneously resolved, and effusion increased in only 3 patients.

Pericardial Tamponade and Pericardiocentesis

Heidenreich and colleagues[2] reported an annual incidence of tamponade of 9% for patients with AIDS with effusions, compared with 1% for all patients with AIDS.

The high prevalence of subclinical pericardial effusion probably reflects a relatively benign and nonspecific process. Symptomatic effusion, as well as large pericardial effusion, often reflects less benign causes.

Fink and collaborators[80] described pericardial tamponade in 3 of 8 patients; 2 of these were unsuspected and led to cardiopulmonary arrest. Examination and culture of pericardial fluid did not establish an etiology. Between 1985 and 1990, Reynolds and coworkers[40] performed 14 pericardiocenteses in patients with AIDS in New York, 7 of whom were parenteral drug abusers. These investigators found echocardiographic evidence of tamponade (right atrial or ventricular collapse) in 10 patients; in 7 of these there was clinical evidence of tamponade (dyspnea, jugular venous distention, and pulsus paradoxus > 10 mmHg, with improvement after pericardiocentesis). All fluid samples were exudative. Pericardial fluid was diagnostic in 3 of 14 (acid-fast bacilli on direct examination, lymphoma on cytologic examination, and culture for *P. mirabilis*). Pericardial biopsy showed granulomata attributed to *M. tuberculosis* in 1 of 14. Of the remaining 10 patients, 4 had concomitant pulmonary tuberculosis and 2 had persistent fevers; all had clinical improvement, defervescence, and no return of effusions with antituberculous chemotherapy. No cause was determined for the remaining 4 patients.

Kwan and colleagues[98] compared tamponade in HIV-infected and non-HIV-infected patients in Brooklyn. Of HIV-infected patients, 85% had dyspnea and 92% enlarged cardiac radiographic silhouettes, but only 62% had tachycardia, 46% pulsus paradoxus, and 15% pericardial rub. These proportions were similar in non-HIV-infected patients: 54% of HIV patients, compared with 17% of non-HIV-infected patients, had coexistent pulmonary infiltrates. On echocardiogram, four patients had right atrial diastolic collapse, three had right ventricular diastolic collapse, and four had both; the remaining two patients had hemodynamic instability, which improved after pericardial decompression. The cause was established in four patients: only two had tuberculosis, and two had pericardial *S. pneumoniae*. However, eight patients were known to have extracardiac tuberculosis.

In the Paris and Miami series, Monsuez and colleagues[3] reported on open pericardiotomy performed on 9 of 18 patients with effusions and cardiac symptoms and 1 asymptomatic patient with tamponade; 5 patients were diagnosed with *M. tuberculosis*, 1 with *M. avium* complex, and 1 with lymphoma. Three cases were declared "nonspecific" pericarditis. No patient had recurrence of effusion postoperatively. The asymptomatic patient had tamponade detected when an enlarged radiographic cardiac silhouette prompted echocardiography. An additional autopsy of a patient dying of pericardial and pleural hemorrhage showed epicardial and myocardial Kaposi's sarcoma.

Pericardial Window and Percutaneous Pericardiostomy

As described above, symptomatic pericardial effusions often recur. Some centers have attempted early operative pericardial drainage and biopsy in all patients with AIDS and symptomatic pericardial effusion. Flum and associates[43] reported on 29 patients undergoing pericardiotomy and biopsy under general anesthesia in New York; 9 of these had tamponade. Pathologic specimens were diagnostic in only 7 patients (3 lymphoma, 2 adenocarcinoma, 1 tuberculosis, 1 purulent); 4 of these 7 patients were considered too ill for specific therapy. Of the study's 29 subjects, 5 required prolonged postoperative mechanical ventilation, and 2 had prolonged postoperative pain. The 2-month mortality was

69%; and all patients were dead by 22 weeks after Kaposi's sarcoma was diagnosed. In light of this experience the authors question the use of operative pericardiotomy in the management of AIDS.

Recently, percutaneous pericardiostomy has been used in the management of patients with recurrent symptomatic pericardial effusions.[99,100] A balloon valvuloplasty catheter is inserted percutaneously over a guidewire into the pericardium and inflated, creating a communication between the pericardial and pleural spaces. The procedure can be performed with limited morbidity and excellent short-term results. The technique has been successfully employed in patients with AIDS at the San Francisco General Hospital (R. J. Lederman and J. S. MacGregor, personal communication) In the future, percutaneous pericardial biopsy may be possible at the time of pericardiocentesis or pericardiostomy using an over-the-wire bioptome.[101–103]

Prognosis

Manifest or subclinical pericardial effusions confer a poor prognosis in HIV infection. Heidenreich and colleagues[2] prospectively surveyed 195 HIV-infected men and 36 controls over 2 years at the University of California at San Francisco. The pericardial effusion contributed directly to death in only one patient, with a large effusion and dilated cardiomyopathy. The average CD4 lymphocyte count and lymphocyte count of patients with AIDS at the time of discovery of pericardial effusion was 59 cells/mm^3 compared to 146 cells/mm^3 for patients with AIDS without effusions on entry into the study. The albumin level also was lower (4.00 vs 4.25 g/dl). This finding was reproduced in one prospective study[1] but not in another retrospective study.[104]

For the 13 patients with AIDS and subsequent effusions, survival was substantially reduced: 36 ± 11 at 6 months, compared with 93 ± 3% in patients with AIDS without effusions on entry to the study (see Figure 13-2). This difference remained statistically significant after correction for possible lead time bias. In multivariate analysis of HIV-infected patients followed prospectively in Philadelphia, death was more frequent in patients with effusions than in those without effusions, corrected for CD4

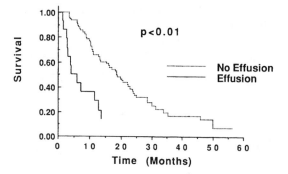

Figure 13-2. Survival of patients with pericardial effusion at time of AIDS diagnosis. (From Ref. 2, with permission.)

lymphocyte count and presence of AIDS.[4] Inpatient mortality was 29% in another series of patients with HIV and pericardial effusions referred for echocardiography.[56]

An Approach to the Evaluation and Management of HIV-Infected Patients With Pericardial Effusion

Patients with incidentally detected pericardial effusions probably should not undergo an exhaustive search for otherwise silent infection or malignancy. Serial physical examination or echocardiography usually demonstrates spontaneous resolution.

Patients with AIDS and unexplained dyspnea, enlarged radiographic cardiac silhouette, or jugular venous distention probably should undergo echocardiography as soon as possible. Large effusions with or without tamponade should be drained, and the fluid should be studied for signs of infection and malignancy. Percutaneous or surgical pericardiostomy and even biopsy can be done as the initial procedure. Patients with symptomatic small or moderate pericardial effusions without evident tamponade can be more challenging to manage. Since such patients are at high risk for tuberculosis, empirical antituberculous chemotherapy often is initiated without diagnostic sampling and regardless of tuberculin skin test results. These patients need to be observed for subacute or chronic pericardial constriction. Pericardial drainage may be deferred as long as serial echocardiography does not demonstrate progression and close follow-up does not suggest tamponade. Those with concurrent cardiomy-opathy usually respond simply to diuresis. Those with persistent or recurrent symptomatic effusions probably should undergo surgical or percutaneous pericardiostomy, the latter particularly in debilitated patients.

Summary

Pericardial disease is common in HIV-infected patients. Pericardial disease usually is subclinical or manifests with vague symptoms and signs. The most common abnormality is pericardial effusion. Subclinical pericardial effusions generally do not have an identifiable cause and often resolve spontaneously. Even so, they are found in patients with more advanced HIV infection and confer a worse prognosis. Large pericardial effusions are less benign, have diverse causes including malignancy and infection, and may progress to tamponade. Curative and palliative therapy is possible with suitably chosen antimicrobial and antineoplastic agents as well as open or percutaneous mechanical interventions.

References

1. Blanchard DG, Hagenhoff C, Chow LC, et al. Reversibility of cardiac abnormalities in human immunodeficiency virus (HIV)-infected individuals: a serial echocardiographic study. *J Am Coll Cardiol* 1991;17:1270–1276.

2. Heidenreich P, Eisenberg M, Kee L, et al. Pericardial effusion in AIDS. *Circulation* 1995;92:3229–3234.

3. Monsuez J, Kinney E, Vittecoq D, et al. Comparison among acquired immune deficiency syndrome patients with and without clinical evidence of cardiac disease. *Am J Cardiol* 1988;62:1311–1313.

4. Hsia J, Ross AM. Pericardial effusion and pericardiocentesis in human immunodeficiency virus infection. *Am J Cardiol* 1994;74:94–96.

5. Cegielski JP, Ramiya K, Lallinger GJ, et al. Pericardial disease and human immunodeficiency virus in Dar es Salaam, Tanzania. *Lancet* 1990;335:209–212.

6. Taelman H, Kagame A, Batungwanayo J, et al. Pericardial effusion and HIV infection [Letter; Comment]. *Lancet* 1990;335:924.

7. Reilly JM, Cunnion RE, Anderson DW, et al. Frequency of myocarditis, left ventricular dysfunction and ventricular tachycardia in the acquired immune deficiency syndrome. *Am J Cardiol* 1988; 62(10 Pt 1):789–793.

8. Malu K, Longo-Mbenza B, Lurhuma Z, Odio W. [Pericarditis and acquired immunodeficiency syndrome]. *Arch Mal Coeur Vaiss* 1988;81:207–11.

9. Pousset F, Le Heuzey JY, Pialoux G, et al. Cardiac lymphoma presenting as atrial flutter in an AIDS patient. *Eur Heart J* 1994;15:862–864.

10. Whitby D, Howard MR, Tenant-Flowers M, et al. Detection of Kaposi's sarcoma associated herpesvirus in peripheral blood of HIV-infected individuals and progression to Kaposi's sarcoma [see comments]. *Lancet* 1995;346:799–802.

11. Moore PS, Chang Y. Detection of herpesvirus-like DNA sequences in Kaposi's sarcoma in patients with and without HIV infection [see comments]. *N Engl J Med* 1995;332:1181–1185.

12. Silver M, Macher A, Reichert C, et al. Cardiac involvement by Kaposi's sarcoma in acquired immune deficiency syndrome (AIDS). *Am J Cardiol* 1984;53:983–985.

13. Lewis W. AIDS: cardiac findings from 115 autopsies. *Prog Cardiovasc Dis* 1989;32:207–215.

14. Remick SC, Hoisington SA, Migliozzi JA. Epidemic Kaposi's sarcoma presenting with pleuropericarditis [see comments]. *NY State J Med* 1992;92:359–360.

15. Autran B, Gorin I, Leibowitch M, et al. AIDS in a Haitian woman with cardiac Kaposi's sarcoma and Whipple's disease. *Lancet* 1983;1:767–768.

16. Stotka JL, Good CB, Downer WR, Kapoor WN. Pericardial effusion and tamponade due to Kaposi's sarcoma in acquired immunodeficiency syndrome. *Chest* 1989;95:1359–1361.

17. Steigman C, Anderson D, Macher A, et al. Fatal cardiac tamponade in acquired immunodeficiency syndrome with epicardial Kaposi's sarcoma. *Am Heart J* 1988;116:1105–1107.

18. Langer E, Mischke U, Stommer P, et al. [Kaposi's sarcoma with pericardial tamponade in AIDS]. *Dtsch Med Wochenschr* 1988;113:1187–1190.

19. Just M, Raventos A, Romeu J, et al. [Cardiac tamponade and Kaposi's sarcoma]. *Med Clin (Barcelona)* 1994;102:495–497.

20. Wang CY, Schroeter AL, Su WP. Acquired immunodeficiency syndrome-related Kaposi's sarcoma. *Mayo Clin Proc* 1995;70:869–879.

21. Ireland-Gill A, Espina BM, Akil B, Gill PS. Treatment of acquired immunodeficiency syndrome-related Kaposi's sarcoma using bleomycin-containing combination chemotherapy regimens. *Semin Oncol* 1992;19:32–37.

22. Meyer JL. Whole-lung irradiation for Kaposi's sarcoma. *Am J Clin Oncol* 1993;16:372–376.

23. Gill PS, Miles SA, Mitsuyasu RT, et al. Phase I AIDS Clinical Trials Group (075) study of adriamycin, bleomycin and vincristine chemotherapy with zidovudine in the treatment of AIDS-related Kaposi's sarcoma. *AIDS* 1994;8:1695–1699.

24. Bakker PJ, Danner SA, ten Napel CH, et al. Treatment of poor prognosis epidemic Kaposi's sarcoma with doxorubicin, bleomycin, vindesine and recombinant human granulocyte-monocyte colony stimulating factor (rh GM-CSF). *Eur J Cancer* 1995;31:188–192.

25. Presant CA, Scolaro M, Kennedy P, et al. Liposomal daunorubicin treatment of HIV-associated Kaposi's sarcoma. *Lancet* 1993;341:1242–1243.

26. Gill PS, Espina BM, Muggia F, et al. Phase I/II clinical and pharmacokinetic evaluation of liposomal daunorubicin. *J Clin Oncol* 1995;13:996–1003.

27. Harrison M, Tomlinson D, Stewart S. Liposomal-entrapped doxorubicin: an active agent in AIDS-related Kaposi's sarcoma. *J Clin Oncol* 1995;13:914–920.

28. Ziegler JL, Beckstead JA, Volberding PA, et al. Non-Hodgkin's lymphoma in 90 homosexual men: relation to generalized lymphadenopathy and the acquired immunodeficiency syndrome. *N Engl J Med* 1984;311:565–570.

29. Pluda JM, Yarchoan R, Jaffe ES, et al. Development of non-Hodgkin lymphoma in a cohort of patients with severe human immunodeficiency virus (HIV) infection on long-term antiretroviral therapy. *Ann Intern Med* 1990;113:276–282.

30. McDonnell P, Mann R, Bulkley B. Involvement of the heart by malignant lymphoma: a clinicopathologic study. *Cancer* 1982;49:944–951.

31. Steffen HM, Muller R, Schrappe-Bacher M, et al. The heart in HIV-1 infection: preliminary results of a prospective echocardiographic investigation. *Acta Cardiol* 1990;45:529–535.

32. Balasubramanyam A, Waxman M, Kazal H, Lee M. Malignant lymphoma of the heart in acquired immune deficiency syndrome. *Chest* 1986;90:243–246.

33. Gill PS, Chandraratna PA, Meyer PR, Levine AM. Malignant lymphoma: cardiac involvement at initial presentation. *J Clin Oncol* 1987;5:216–224.

34. Andress J, Polish L, Clark D, Hossack K. Transvenous biopsy of cardiac lymphoma in an AIDS patient. *Am Heart J* 1989;118:421–423.

35. Goldfarb A, King C, Rosenzweig B, et al. Cardiac lymphoma in the acquired immunodeficiency syndrome. *Am Heart J* 1989;118:1340–1344.

36. Dalli E, Quesada A, Paya R. Cardiac involvement by non-Hodkin's lymphoma in acquired immune deficiency syndrome. *Int J Cardiol* 1990;26:223–225.

37. Helfand J. Cardiac tamponade as a result of American Burkitt's lymphoma of the heart and pericardium. *Conn Med* 1990;54:186–189.

38. Kelsey RC, Saker A, Morgan M. Cardiac lymphoma in a patient with AIDS. *Ann Intern Med* 1991;115:370–371.

39. Holladay AO, Siegel RJ, Schwartz DA. Cardiac malignant lymphoma in acquired immune deficiency syndrome. *Cancer* 1992;70:2203–2207.

40. Reynolds MM, Hecht SR, Berger M, et al. Large pericardial effusions in the acquired immunodeficiency syndrome. *Chest* 1992;102:1746–1747.

41. Aboulafia DM, Bush R, Picozzi VJ. Cardiac tamponade due to primary pericardial lymphoma in a patient with AIDS. *Chest* 1994;106:1295–1299.

42. Levine AM. AIDS-associated malignant lymphoma. *Med Clin North Am* 1992;76:253–268.

43. Flum DR, McGinn JT Jr, Tyras DH. The role of the 'pericardial window' in AIDS. *Chest* 1995;107:1522–1525.

44. Scott PJ, Conway SP, Da Costa P. Cardiac tamponade complicating cytomegalovirus pericarditis in a patient with AIDS. [Letter]. *J Infect* 1990;20:92–93.

45. Nathan PE, Arsura EL, Zappi M. Pericarditis with tamponade due to cytomegalovirus in the acquired immunodeficiency syndrome. *Chest* 1991;99:765–766.

46. Freedberg RS, Gindea AJ, Dieterich DT, Greene JB. Herpes simplex pericarditis in AIDS. *NY State J Med* 1987;87:304–306.

47. Toma E, Poisson M, Claessens MR, et al. Herpes simplex type 2 pericarditis and bilateral facial palsy in a patient with AIDS. [Letter]. *J Infect Dis* 1989;160:553–554.

48. Schuster M, Valentine F, Holzman R. Cryptococcal pericarditis in an intravenous drug abuser. *J Infect Dis* 1985;152:842.

49. Zuger A, Louie E, Holzman RS, et al. Cryptococcal disease in patients with the acquired immunodeficiency syndrome: diagnostic features and outcome of treatment. *Ann Intern Med* 1986;104:234–240.

50. Zakowski MF, Ianuale-Shanerman A. Cytology of pericardial effusions in AIDS patients. *Diagn Cytopathol* 1993;9:266–269.

51. Guerot E, Aissa F, Kayal S, et al. Toxoplasma pericarditis in acquired immunodeficiency syndrome. *Intensive Care Med* 1995;21:229–230.

52. DeCastro S, Migliau G, Silvestri A, et al. Heart involvement in AIDS: a prospective study during various stages of the disease. *Eur Heart J* 1992;13:1452–1459.

53. Hofman P, Michiels JF, Saint Paul MC, et al. [Cardiac lesions in acquired immunodeficiency syndrome (AIDS): apropos of an autopsy series of 25 cases]. *Ann Pathol* 1990;10:247–257.

54. Kwan T, Einhorn A, Nacht R. A large pericardial effusion in a patient with human immunodeficiency virus type 1. *NY State J Med* 1990;90:612–613.

55. Rosales Guzman I, Rosales L, Zghaib A. [The autopsy findings in 51 cases of AIDS with cardiovascular damage]. *Arch Inst Cardiol Mex* 1994;64:485–490.

56. Eisenberg MJ, Gordon AS, Schiller NB. HIV-associated pericardial effusions. *Chest* 1992;102:956–958.

57. Karve MM, Murali MR, Shah HM, Phelps KR. Rapid evolution of cardiac tamponade due to bacterial pericarditis in two patients with HIV-1 infection. *Chest* 1992;101:1461–1463.

58. Stechel RP, Cooper DJ, Greenspan J, et al. Staphylococcal pericarditis in a homosexual patient with AIDS-related complex. *N Y State J Med* 1986;86:592–593.

59. Himelman RB, Chung WS, Chernoff DN, et al. Cardiac manifestations of human immunodeficiency virus infection: a two-dimensional echocardiographic study. *J Am Coll Cardiol* 1989;13:1030–1036.

60. Legras A, Lemmens B, Dequin PF, et al. Tamponade due to *Rhodococcus equi* in acquired immunodeficiency syndrome. *Chest* 1994;106:1278–1279.

61. Lee-Chiong T, Sadigh M, Simms M, Buller G. Case reports: pericarditis and lymphadenitis due to *Rhodococcus equi*. *Am J Med Sci* 1995;310:31–33.

62. Ferguson R, Yee S, Finkle H, et al. *Listeria*-associated pericarditis in an AIDS patient. *J Natl Med Assoc* 1993;85:225–228.

63. Holtz H, Lavery D, Kapila R. Actinomycetales infection in the acquired immunodeficiency syndrome. *Ann Intern Med* 1985;102:203–205.

64. Kroon F, van't Wout J, Weiland H, van Furth R. *Chlamydia trachomatis* pneumonia in an HIV-seropositive patient. *N Engl J Med* 1989;320:806–807.

65. Small PM, Shafer RW, Hopewell PC, et al. Exogenous reinfection with multidrug-resistant Mycobacterium tuberculosis in patients with advanced HIV infection [see comments]. *N Engl J Med* 1993;328:1137–1144.

66. Elliott AM, Halwiindi B, Hayes RJ, et al. The impact of human immunodeficiency virus on presentation and diagnosis of tuberculosis in a cohort study in Zambia. *J Trop Med Hyg* 1993;96:1–11.

67. Small PM, Schecter GF, Goodman PC, et al. Treatment of tuberculosis in patients with advanced human immunodeficiency virus infection. *N Engl J Med* 1991;324:289–294.

68. Ellner JJ, Barnes PF, Wallis RS, Modlin RL. The immunology of tuberculous pleurisy. *Semin Respir Infect* 1988;3:335–342.

69. Dalli E, Quesada A, Juan G, et al. Tuberculous pericarditis as the first manifestation of acquired immunodeficiency syndrome. *Am Heart J* 1987;114:905–906.

70. de Miguel J, Pedreira JD, Campos V, et al. Tuberculous pericarditis and AIDS. [Letter]. *Chest* 1990;97:1273.

71. Pedro-Botet J, Auguet T, Coll J, et al. Tuberculous pericarditis as the first manifestation of AIDS. *Infection* 1993;21:334–335.

72. Serrano-Heranz R, Camino A, Vilacosta I, et al. Tuberculous cardiac tamponade and AIDS. *Eur Heart J* 1995;16:430–432.

73. Horn DL, Hewlett D Jr, Alfalla C, Peterson S. Fatal hospital-acquired multidrug-resistant tuberculous pericarditis in two patients with AIDS. [Letter]. *N Engl J Med* 1992;327:1816–1817.

74. Sunderam G, McDonald R, Maniatis T, et al. Tuberculosis as a manifestation of the acquired im-

munodeficiency syndrome (AIDS). *JAMA* 1986; 256:362–366.

75. Cegielski JP, Lwakatare J, Dukes CS, et al. Tuberculous pericarditis in Tanzanian patients with and without HIV infection. *Tuber Lung Dis* 1994; 75:429–434.

76. Elliott AM, Luo N, Tembo G, et al. Impact of HIV on tuberculosis in Zambia: a cross sectional study [see comments]. *BMJ* 1990;301:412–415.

77. Pozniak AL, Weinberg J, Mahari M, et al. Tuberculous pericardial effusion associated with HIV infection: a sign of disseminated disease. *Tuber Lung Dis* 1994;75:297–300.

78. Strang JI, Kakaza HH, Gibson DG, et al. Controlled clinical trial of complete open surgical drainage and of prednisolone in treatment of tuberculous pericardial effusion in Transkei. *Lancet* 1988;2:759–764.

79. Fowler NO. Tuberculous pericarditis [see comments]. *JAMA* 1991;266:99–103.

80. Fink L, Reichek N, St. John Sutton M. Cardiac abnormalities in acquired immune deficiency syndrome. *Am J Cardiol* 1984;54:1161–1163.

81. Richter C, Ndosi B, Mwammy AS, Mbwambo RK. Extrapulmonary tuberculosis—a simple diagnosis? A retrospective study at Dar es Salaam, Tanzania. *Trop Geogr Med* 1991;43:375–378.

82. Ng TT, Strang JI, Wilkins EG. Serodiagnosis of pericardial tuberculosis. *Q J Med* 1995;88:317–320.

83. Bertolaccini P, Chimenti M, Bianchi S, et al. Gallium-67 scintigraphy in an AIDS patient presenting with tuberculous pericarditis. *J Nucl Biol Med* 1993;37:245–248.

84. Schmidt U, Rebarber IF. Tuberculous pericarditis identified with gallium-67 and indium-111 leukocyte imaging. *Clin Nucl Med* 1994;19:146–147.

85. Isaka N, Tanaka R, Nakamura M, et al. A case of tuberculous pericarditis: use of adenosine deaminase activity (ADA) in early diagnosis. *Heart Vessels* 1990;5:247–248.

86. Martinez-Vazquez JM, Ribera E, Ocana I, et al. Adenosine deaminase activity in tuberculous pericarditis. *Thorax* 1986;41:888–889.

87. Koh KK, Kim EJ, Cho CH, et al. Adenosine deaminase and carcinoembryonic antigen in pericardial effusion diagnosis, especially in suspected tuberculous pericarditis. *Circulation* 1994;89:2728–2735.

88. Strang JI, Kakaza HH, Gibson DG, et al. Controlled trial of prednisolone as adjuvant in treatment of tuberculous constrictive pericarditis in Transkei. *Lancet* 1987;2:1418–1422.

89. Sagrista-Sauleda J, Permanyer-Miralda G, Soler-Soler J. Tuberculous pericarditis: ten year experience with a prospective protocol for diagnosis and treatment. *J Am Coll Cardiol* 1988;11:724–728.

90. Strang JI. Rapid resolution of tuberculous pericardial effusions with high dose prednisone and antituberculous drugs. *J Infect* 1994;28:251–254.

91. Elliott AM, Halwiindi B, Bagshawe A, et al. Use of prednisolone in the treatment of HIV-positive tuberculosis patients. *Q J Med* 1992;85:855–860.

92. Moreno F, Sharkey-Mathis PK, Mokulis E, Smith JA. *Mycobacterium kansasii* pericarditis in patients with AIDS. *Clin Infect Dis* 1994;19:967–969.

93. Woods GL, Goldsmith JC. Fatal pericarditis due to *Mycobacterium avium-intracellulare* in acquired immunodeficiency syndrome. *Chest* 1989;95:1355–1357.

94. Perich J, Ayuso MC, Vilana R, et al. Disseminated lymphatic tuberculosis in acquired immunodeficiency syndrome: computed tomography findings. *Can Assoc Radiol J* 1990;41:353–357.

95. Choo PS, McCormack JG. *Mycobacterium avium*: a potentially treatable cause of pericardial effusions. *J Infect* 1995;30:55–58.

96. Jorup-Ronstrom C, Julander I, Petrini B. Efficacy of triple drug regimen of amikacin, ethambutol and rifabutin in AIDS patients with symptomatic *Mycobacterium avium* complex infection. *J Infect* 1993;26:67–70.

97. Webb JG, Chan-Yan C, Kiess MC. Cardiac dysfunction associated with the acquired immunodeficiency syndrome (AIDS). *Clin Cardiol* 1988; 11:423–426.

98. Kwan T, Karve MM, Emerole O. Cardiac tamponade in patients infected with HIV: a report from an inner-city hospital. *Chest* 1993;104:1059–1062.

99. Palacios IF, Tuzcu EM, Ziskind AA, et al. Percutaneous balloon pericardial window for patients with malignant pericardial effusion and tamponade [see comments]. *Cathet Cardiovasc Diagn* 1991;22:244–249.

100. Ziskind AA, Pearce AC, Lemmon CC, et al. Percutaneous balloon pericardiotomy for the treatment of cardiac tamponade and large pericardial effu-

sions: description of technique and report of the first 50 cases. *J Am Coll Cardiol* 1993;21:1–5.

101. Selig MB. Percutaneous pericardial biopsy under echocardiographic guidance. *Am Heart J* 1991; 122(3 Pt 1):879–882.

102. Selig MB. Percutaneous transcatheter pericardial interventions: aspiration, biopsy, and pericardioplasty [editorial]. *Am Heart J* 1993;125: 269–271.

103. Ziskind AA, Rodriguez S, Lemmon C, Burstein S. Percutaneous pericardial biopsy as an adjunctive technique for the diagnosis of pericardial disease. *Am J Cardiol* 1994;74:288–291.

104. Akhras F, Dubrey S, Gazzard B, Noble MI. Emerging patterns of heart disease in HIV infected homosexual subjects with and without opportunistic infections: a prospective colour flow Doppler echocardiographic study. *Eur Heart J* 1994;15: 68–75.

105. Raffanti SP, Chiaramida AJ, Sen P, et al. Assessment of cardiac function in patients with the acquired immunodeficiency syndrome. *Chest* 1988; 93:592–594.

106. Corallo S, Mutinelli MR, Moroni M, et al. Echocardiography detects myocardial damage in AIDS: prospective study in 102 patients. *Eur Heart J* 1988;9:887–892.

107. Hecht SR, Berger M, Van Tosh A, et al. Unsuspected cardiac abnormalities in the acquired immune deficiency syndrome: an echocardiographic study [see comments]. *Chest* 1989;96:805–808.

108. Lindvig K, Nielsen TL, Videboek R, et al. Echocardiographic screening in 24 consecutive AIDS patients. *Dan Med Bull* 1990;37:449–451.

109. Almenar L, Sotillo J, Osa A, et al. [Doppler echocardiography assessment of cardiac abnormalities in parenteral drug addicts]. *Rev Esp Cardiol* 1992;45:554–559.

110. Thuesen L, Moller A, Kristensen BO, et al. Cardiac function in patients with human immunodeficiency virus infection and with no other active infections. *Dan Med Bull* 1994;41:107–109.

111. Reichert C, O'Leary T, Levens D, et al. Autopsy pathology in the acquired immunodeficiency syndrome. *Am J Pathol* 1983;112:357–382.

112. Hofman P, Michiels JF, Rosenthal E, et al. Acute *Staphylococcus aureus* myocarditis in AIDS. 2 cases. *Arch Mal Coeur Vaiss* 1993;86:1765–1768.

113. Grant A, Pitkin AD, Buscombe JR, et al. *Staphylococcus aureus* pericarditis in a patient with AIDS. [Letter]. *Genitourin Med* 1993;69:324–325.

114. Decker CF, Tuazon CU. *Staphylococcus aureus* pericarditis in HIV-infected patients. *Chest* 1994; 105:615–616.

115. D'Cruz I, Sengupta E, Abrahams C, et al. Cardiac involvement, including tuberculous pericardial effusion, complicating acquired immune deficiency syndrome. *Am Heart J* 1986;112:1100–1102.

116. Houston S, Ray S, Mahari M, et al. The association of tuberculosis and HIV infection in Harare, Zimbabwe. *Tuber Lung Dis* 1994;75:220–226.

14

Vascular Disease in HIV Infection

Thomas J. Starc, M.D., and Vijay V. Joshi, M.D.

Since the onset of the acquired immunodeficiency syndrome (AIDS) epidemic,[1,2] a variety of infectious, degenerative, and neoplastic pathologic lesions have been described in patients infected with the human immunodeficiency virus (HIV).[3,4] These lesions have now become more evident because of the longer survival of these patients due to earlier diagnosis and improvements in therapy. Focal degenerative arterial lesions characterized by medial calcification were first noted at autopsy in isolated organs such as thymus, lungs, and spleen of patients with AIDS (V. V. Joshi, unpublished data). These lesions differed from the vasculitis and perivasculitis seen in HIV-associated encephalopathy. They also differed from other known degenerative vascular lesions and were considered initially to be pathologic curiosities. However, after the report of a myocardial infarction in a child with a coronary artery aneurysm, it became apparent that AIDS-associated arteriopathy can be of clinical relevance.[5]

In addition to this newly described AIDS-associated arteriopathy, a number of other vascular lesions occur in these patients. Strokes, aneurysms, and arteriopathy of the cerebral arteries are now recognized as important manifestations of AIDS-induced vascular abnormalities.[6] The clinicopathologic features and the known or suggested pathogeneses of these vascular lesions are summarized in Table 14-1 [and include degenerative, inflammatory, atherosclerotic, thromboembolic, proliferative, as well as several other miscellaneous lesions.][7–59] The AIDS virus itself has been implicated recently in the pathogenesis of vasculitis/perivasculitis in the brain.[9,10] However, the exact cause of these vascular lesions is not clear. In some cases the AIDS virus may be directly responsible for the lesion, but in others it may act in concert with infectious, nutritional, or other cofactors. Patients with AIDS may be more susceptible to vascular lesions because they suffer from repeated infections or because they are exposed to numerous drugs that themselves can cause vasculitis. Thus, mycotic aneurysms and hypersensitivity vasculitis could result from chronic infection and drug exposure.[16,27]

Of the vascular lesions summarized in Table 14-1, the AIDS arteriopathy affecting the small and medium-sized arteries appears to be a distinctive lesion occurring in children with AIDS and is described in detail below. The lesion has not been described systematically in adults with AIDS, although one of the authors (V.V.J.) has seen it in the arteries of the kidneys and the intestine of a 30-year-old man who died of AIDS (V.V. Joshi, unpublished data).

Table 14.1. Vascular Lesions Associated with HIV Infection

Type of Vascular Lesion	Source	Location	Clinical Manifestations	Pathology	Pathogenesis
Degenerative Lesion					
Arteriopathy	Joshi et al. (5) Park et al. (6) Phillipet et al. (7) Kure et al. (8)	Small and medium-sized arteries of various organs	Usually asymptomatic; clinical manifestations (stroke, myocardial infarct) related to sequelae (aneurysm of cerebral or coronary arteries)	Destruction of elastic tissue, intimal and medial calcification; aneurysm with/without thrombosis	Exposure to endogenous and exogenous elastases due to repeated infections and a role for HIV have been suggested
Inflammatory Lesions					
Vasculitis/perivasculitis in HIV encephalopathy and in retina	Sotrel et al. (9) Reux et al. (10) Yankner et al. (11) Lang et al. (12) Husson et al. (13) Mizusawa et al. (14) Frank et al. (15)	Small blood vessels in affected white matter and basal ganglia	General CNS signs and symptoms related to HIV encephalopathy (delayed development in children, dementia in adults)	Endothelial hyperplasia, thickening of vessel wall, perivascular collection of lymphocytes, macrophages, and occasional multinucleated giant cells containing HIV particles	Lesions induced directly by HIV infection of endothelial cells and vessel wall
Mycotic aneurysm	Destian et al. (16) Dupont et al. (17) Mestres et al. (18) Marks et al. (19) Gouny et al. (20) Sinzobahamvya et al. (21)	Aortic and iliac, femoral, carotid, and subclavian arteries	Epistaxis, abdominal pain, rupture of aneurysm, pulsatile mass, loss of toes	Eccentric adventitial fibrosis, chronic inflammation, granulation tissue, calcification with thinning and destruction of intima, media and elastic tissue, neutrophilic infiltration, thrombosis in lumen, fibroproliferative vascular disease	Hematogenous or local spread of organism (Mycobacterium-avium intracellulare, Staphylococcus, Salmonella, Hemophilus influenzae, M. tuberculosis) to arteries
Opportunistic cerebral vasculopathy	Kieburtz et al. (22)	Cerebral blood vessels	Loss of vision, hemiparesis, headache, vertigo	Sclerotic changes in vessel wall, luminal occlusion by thrombosis	Vascular invasion by opportunistic organisms (Candida and cytomegalovirus) and by CNS lymphoma
Herpes vasculitis of CNS	Engstrom et al. (23)	Details not given	Transient neurologic deficit	Vasculitis (details not given)	Herpes zoster infection
Systemic vasculitis	Calabrese et al. (24) Valeriano et al. (25) Watkins et al. (26) Gherardi et al. (27)	Small blood vessels primarily of muscle, but also of lung, kidney, myocardium	Swelling and pain of feet, weakness in feet	Lymphocytic (CD8+) infiltration around and within vessel wall	?Immunologic reaction caused by HIV

Disease	Reference	Vessel	Clinical features	Pathology	Comments
Polyarteritis-nodosa-like necrotizing vasculitis	Libman et al. (28)	Medium-sized arteries	Digital ischemia and gangrene, peripheral neuropathy	Necrotizing arteritis with infiltration by CD8 by CD8 lymphocytes, and plasma cells	Demonstration of HIV in perivascular mononuclear cells and deposition of IgM, C3, Clq in the affected artery raises the possibility of pathogenesis being related to immune complex deposits (corticosteroids afford short-term benefits)
Hypersensitivity vasculitis	Gherardi et al. (29)	Small blood vessels	Maculopapular skin rash, palpable purpura	Granulocytic or mononuclear infiltration of affected arterioles and venules	Hypersensitivity to drugs, including penicillin, griseofulvin, amitriptyline
Leukocytoclastic vasculitis	Chren et al. (30) Weimer et al. (31) Potashner et al. (32) Veljii et al. (33)	Small dermal blood vessels	Pruritic skin eruption consisting of scattered 2–3 mm erythematous papules	Focal fibrinoid necrosis of vessel wall, granulocytic infiltrate (karyorrhexis of granulocytes), IgM and fibrinogen deposits in capillary walls	HIV antigen demonstrated in the vessel wall suggests a role of HIV in the pathogenesis
Retinal periphlebitis	Rabb et al. (34)	Retinal venules	Visual loss	Histologic examination not done; perivenular infiltrates of retina on ophthalmoscopic examination	Areas of typical cytomegalovirus retinitis were also present. There was response to ganciclovir suggesting a pathogenetic role of cytomegalovirus response to prednisone and heparin
Eosinophilic vasculitis	Schwartz et al. (35)	Temporal arteries	Amaurosis fugax	Focal medial and adventitial inflammation, intimal thickening with eosinophils	Unknown
Kawasaki syndrome	Yoganathan et al. (36) Wolf et al. (37) Viraben et al. (38) Bayrou et al. (39) Nigro et al. (40)	Conjunctival arteries	Fever, conjunctivitis, adenopathy, desquamation, rash		
Atherosclerotic lesions	Paton et al. (41) Tabib et al. (42)	Coronary arteries	Death in unexplained circumstances	Atherosclerosis (eccentric intimal fibrosis) with 80–90% occlusion (thickening of media due to fibrosis also seen)	Viral coinfections (herpesvirus such as cytomegalovirus, herpes simplex virus, and HIV) may be involved in pathogenesis

Continued

Table 14.1. *Continued*

Type of Vascular Lesion	Source	Location	Clinical Manifestations	Pathology	Pathogenesis
Thromboembolic lesions					
Deep vein thrombosis with or without pulmonary embolism	Becker et al. (43)	Deep leg veins, pulmonary arteries	Pain in lower extremity, chest pain	No pathologic studies done, thrombosis and embolism demonstrated by imaging studies and ventilation perfusion lung scan	Active, ambulatory patients with AIDS but without known risk factors for deep venous thrombosis or pulmonary embolism; some evidence suggests that anticardiolipin antibodies or low protein S level are due to HIV infection of endothelium
Superior sagittal sinus thrombosis	Doberson et al. (44)	Superior sagittal sinus and distal superficial cortical veins	Incidental finding at autopsy	Thrombosis detected at autopsy	Unknown
Central retinal vein thrombosis	Ishmail et al. (45) Teich et al. (46)	Central retinal vein	Sudden visual loss	Thrombosis of vein	Unknown
Cutaneous thrombosis	Smith et al. (47)	Digital infarcts	Epider	Epidermal and dermal necrosis chronic inflammatory infiltrate with thrombosis	Unknown, cytomegalovirus positive staining
Proliferative lesions					
Reactive proliferation					
Bacillary angiomatosis	LeBoit et al. (48) Malane et al. (49) Tappero et al. (50) Steeper et al. (51) Rudikoff et al. (52) Axiotis (53)	Capillaries in skin, gastrointestinal tract, respiratory tract, lymph nodes, brain, bone	Erythematous papules, dome shaped skin nodules or nodules of subcutaneous tissue, mucosal nodules, hemorrhage	Capillary proliferation; prominent endothelial cell, neutrophilic infiltrate, and nuclear debris between capillaries, organisms can be demonstrated by Warthin-Starry silver strain and/or by electron microscopy large blood-filled cystic spaces (with fibrosis in the spleen), causative organisms can be demonstrated	*Bartonella henselae* and *B. quintana* are the causative organisms; may be related to pathogenesis
Bacillary peliosis of liver and spleen	LeBoit (48) Koehler et al. (54)	Sinusoids in liver, spleen	Hepatomegaly, splenomegaly with pancytopenia, behavioral disorder, hemorrhage, elevated alkaline phosphatase		*Bartonella henselae* and *B. quintana* are the causative organisms

Neoplastic proliferation				
Kaposi's sarcoma	Martin et al. (55) Sleeper et al. (51) Chang et al. (56)	Capillaries in skin, gastrointestinal tract, lungs, lymph nodes, liver, spleen, adrenal, heart, and kidneys	Macules, papules, nodules of skin, hemoptysis, gastrointestinal hemorrhage, lymphadenopathy (bacillary angiomatosis and Kaposi's sarcoma may occur simultaneously in the skin)	Proliferation of ectatic jagged blood vessels and of spindle cell between the blood vessels, hyaline inclusions in spindle cells, mitotic activity, hemosiderophages, and chronic inflammatory infiltrate	Malignant proliferation of de-differentiated endothelial cells or pluripotential mesenchymal precursor cells in immunosuppressed individuals; cytomegalovirus, HIV and Kaposi's sarcoma associated virus or human herpesvirus 8 have been implicated in the etiology
Miscellaneous lesions				
Telangiectasia	MacFarlane et al. (57)	Dermal small blood vessels	Telangiectasia of skin of upper body	Dilated dermal blood vessels with perivascular lymphoplasmacytic infiltration (no endothelial proliferating)	Not known; may be a direct manifestation of HIV infection
Zidovudine-induced leukocyctoclastic vasculitis	Torres et al. (58)	Dermal capillaries	Pruritic erythematous papules and blisters	Perivascular inflammatory infiltrate consisting of mononuclear cells, occasional neutrophils and eosinophils, and nuclear debris, swelling of endothelial cells	Hypersensitivity to zidovudine: lesion resolved on withdrawal of zidovudine and recurred after rechallenge with the drug
Raynaud's phenomenon	von Gunten et al. (59)	Arteries of fingers	Bluish discoloration, pain, and temperature intolerance of distal portion of fingers	Data not given	Patients had Kaposi's sarcoma, which was treated with bleomycin; bleomycin-related dysfunction of sympathetic nervous system may play a role in the pathogenesis

CNS, central nervous system.

AIDS-Associated Arteriopathy

Pathologic Features

The following histologic features were noted in the small and medium-sized arteries of children dying of AIDS[5]: (1) Intimal fibrosis with concentric or eccentric involvement resulting in variable degrees of luminal narrowing (Figure 14-1); (2) extensive and consistent fragmentation of elastic fibers, sometimes involving the internal elastic lamina (Figures 14-2 and 14-3); and (3) fibrosis and calcification of the media, with the latter occurring particularly in the region of the internal elastic lamina (Figure 14-4). The arterial lesions varied in extent from segmental to circumferential. The fibrocalcific lesions of the intima and the media that resulted in varying degrees of luminal narrowing were present separately or in combination in the same artery in organs such as brain, lungs, kidneys, spleen, thymus, heart, skeletal muscle, and lymph nodes. However, it was rare that both vasculitis and medial calcification involved the same artery in the brain.

Since the affected arteries were of small or medium size, the vascular lesions were evident only on microscopic examination except in one child who died of myocardial infarction. In this child three fusiform aneurysms of the right coronary artery were detected at autopsy (Figure 14-5). The aneurysms involved a 3-cm segment of the proximal right coronary artery and varied from 0.6 to 0.8 cm in diameter. The aneurysms were occluded by a recent thrombus. The walls of the aneurysms had multiple areas of calcification, and there was fragmentation of the elastic tissue with fibrosis of the intima and media. Neither inflammation nor necrosis was seen in any of the numerous sections made from both coronary arteries. The left coronary artery showed similar, but less severe, lesions of the media; however, there was no aneurysm formation. The ventricular septum and the adjoining portion of the wall of the right ventricle contained an area of infarction measuring 2.5 cm in its longest dimension.

Arterial lesions were also present in the brain, thymus, spleen, and lymph nodes and contained one or more of the following lesions: focal necrosis, atrophy, fibrosis (or gliosis), and lymphocyte depletion. Because of the frequent finding of calcification in the arterial lesions, the parathyroids were examined in two typical cases and were found to be normal. Similar arterial lesions have been described

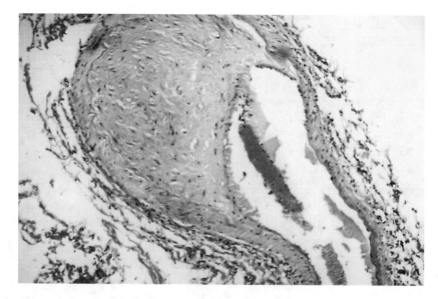

Figure 14-1. Eccentric intimal fibrosis of a medium-sized artery. (Hematoxylin and eosin, ×200.)

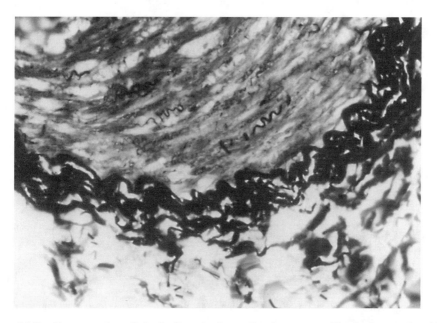

Figure 14-2. Fragmentation of elastic fibers in the media of an artery. (Elastic tissue stain ×400.)

in the arteries of the circle of Willis and meningo-cerebral arteries in children with AIDS who have had strokes.[6] In these cases, focal thrombosis was noted in the aneurysmally dilated arteries of the circle of Willis.

Pathogenesis

The pathogenesis of the arteriopathy in AIDS is unknown. Conditions predisposing to fibrocalcific arterial lesions, such as renal failure, hypervitamin-

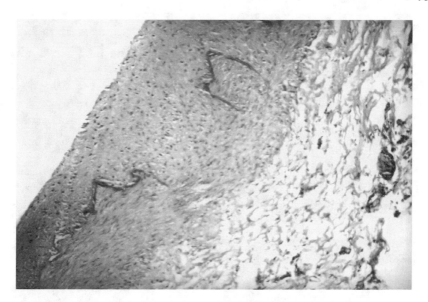

Figure 14-3. An artery showing intimal and medial fibrosis with fragmentation of elastic lamina. (Hematoxylin and eosin, ×200.)

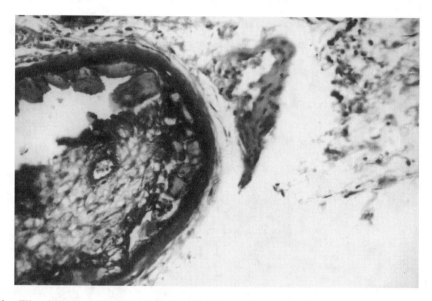

Figure 14-4.   Fibrosis and calcification of media with intimal fibrosis resulting in marked luminal narrowing of a small artery. (Hematoxylin and eosin, ×250.)

osis D, hyperparathyroidism, or exposure to toxins, were not seen in the children who developed arteriopathy.[5,6] Other factors to be considered in the pathogenesis include infection, immune deficiency, and injury of the elastic tissue of the arteries. Intrauter-ine infection caused by rubella is associated with vascular lesions consisting of intimal fibrosis and fragmentation of elastic tissue of the media. This may occur with or without calcification, and can be seen both in the early stage and as a late sequela.[60,61]

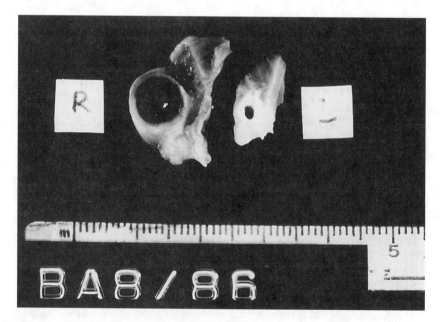

Figure 14-5.   Right and left coronary arteries in a child with AIDS. Note the aneurysmal dilatation with thrombotic occlusion of the right coronary artery. The left coronary artery appears to be unaffected on gross examination.

As in congenital rubella, pediatric AIDS is often a transplacentally transmitted disease, and it is possible that HIV itself can induce vascular lesions.[9,10] Kure and colleagues[8] have shown the presence of HIV antigen (gp41) by immunocytochemical methods in the intima of aneurysmal cerebral arteries in a child with AIDS. HIV-1 RNA has been demonstrated in the retinal blood vessel wall in adults with AIDS.[10] It remains unclear whether the finding of HIV virus in the arteries is a direct effect or merely secondary to injury or thrombosis. It is possible that other viral agents, alone or in synergy with HIV, may be involved. The immunodeficiency present in AIDS patients may have merely made them more susceptible to such viral infection.

It has been suggested that immunodeficiency leads to excessive antigenic stimulation,[62] and thus allergic hypersensitivity and autoimmune phenomena are observed with higher frequency in immunodeficient patients. However, vascular lesions in such a setting are usually of the necrotizing and inflammatory type, and allergic and other related phenomena are unlikely pathogenic mechanisms in AIDS-associated arteriopathy.

Vasospasm has been implicated in the pathogenesis of other vascular lesions, such as segmental arterial mediolysis,[63] to which AIDS-associated arteriopathy bears some resemblance. Hypoxia and shock, often seen in severely ill patients with AIDS, are potent initiators of endothelium-induced vasoconstriction.[64] Dysfunction of the endothelial paracrine system with sustained secretion of endothelin can result in vasospasm and medial necrosis. Lafeuillade et al.[65] have provided evidence of endothelial cell dysfunction manifested by increased antigenic von Willebrand factor and decreased protein S in patients with AIDS, which in turn may lead to abnormal vascular responsiveness. In addition, studies of nail-bed microcirculation demonstrate abnormal end-vessel circulatory patterns suggestive of alterations in vasomotor tone in patients with AIDS.[66]

On microscopic examination of the arterial lesions, the most consistent and impressive changes were found in the elastic tissue of the arterial wall (Figure 14-2). Elastic tissue degeneration and fragmentation (followed by fibrosis and calcification) may thus be of fundamental significance in the pathogenesis of AIDS arteriopathy. The cause of elastic tissue degeneration is not clear. Opportunistic and repeated bacterial infections occurring in children with AIDS may result in increased exposure to endogenous and exogenous elastases.[67] Alternatively, imbalance in the normal inhibitor:elastase ratio may result in increased degradation of elastin.[67] The longer survival of the children with AIDS reported by Joshi and colleagues[4] (average age at death, 40.5 months, versus 20.6 months in their earlier series[3]) may have been associated with more frequent exposure to elastases due to repeated infections. This increased number of infections would thereby provide more time for vascular lesions to increase in severity and become more widespread. The increased length of patient survival seen in recent years because of early diagnosis, aggressive treatment of infections, and specific anti-HIV therapy may lead to an increased incidence of vascular lesions.

Differential Diagnosis

The features of AIDS arteriopathy can usually be distinguished from other vascular lesions such as atherosclerosis, Monckeberg's sclerosis, Takayasu's disease, giant-cell arteritis, and fibromuscular dysplasia. These other lesions occur more commonly in older age groups and can be ruled out on the basis of both intimal and medial involvement, the prominence of the calcification, and the absence of lipid deposition or inflammatory changes such as giant cells. Segmental arterial mediolysis, which may be a precursor lesion of fibromuscular dysplasia,[63] can also be ruled out because of the absence of fibrinous deposits in the media and the presence of medial calcification in the AIDS-associated arteriopathy.

Arterial lesions that occur primarily in the pediatric age group and should be considered in the differential diagnosis of any child with vasculitis include Kawasaki disease and idiopathic arterial calcification of infancy (IACI). Kawasaki's disease and AIDS occur in children and both have similar signs and symptoms such as fever, lymphadenopathy, and mucocutaneous lesions. However, in pediatric AIDS, the mucocutaneous lesions are due to atopic dermatitis, herpes simplex or *Candida* infection. Necrosis and microvascular thrombosis of noninfectious origin, which are seen characteristically in the lymph nodes in Kawasaki disease, are absent in pediatric AIDS.[68] In addition, immunologic abnormalities and HIV antibodies are absent in Kawasaki disease. Kawasaki disease is characterized pathologically by involvement of the major musculoelastic arteries of the viscera of wide distribution, but more particularly of the coronary arteries. Inflammation, necrosis, and aneurysm formation with thrombosis are characteristically present. In the wall of the aneurysm, both necrosis and inflammation are seen.[69] In the regressive stage of aneurysm formation, inflammation and necrosis are absent and scarring with calcification is seen.[70,71] The aneurysms of the coronary artery described above in the child with AIDS were occluded by recent thrombi, indicating an active and not a regressive stage of the disease process. Thus, although there are certain similarities to the arterial lesions of Kawasaki disease, the differences in the clinical, immunologic, and pathologic features indicate that the arterial lesions in children with AIDS are different from those of Kawasaki disease. Of interest are case reports of a child[40] and four adults[36–39] with AIDS who had Kawasaki-like illnesses. They exhibited typical symptoms, including prolonged fever, rash, conjunctivitis, adenopathy, induration of the extremities, and desquamation of the skin. No coronary lesions were reported in these patients. The relation between these two diseases remains unknown; however, one can speculate that if Kawasaki disease is an infectious process, the altered host immunity in patients with AIDS may lead to an increased susceptibility to Kawasaki disease.

Idiopathic arterial calcification of infancy (IACI) is a rare disorder associated with myocardial ischemia secondary to coronary calcification. In IACI death is almost certain, the only exceptions being spontaneous regression in one and response to therapy in several others.[72] In addition to the coronary arteries, lesions affect the arteries of the kidneys, spleen, adrenals, pancreas, lungs, and extremities. Although the microscopic features of IACI are strikingly similar to the arteriopathy seen in children with AIDS,[73] several differences exist: the size of the involved arteries, sparing of arteries of the brain, consistent involvement of coronary arteries,

and younger age at the time of diagnosis in IACI. Moreover, although hypergammaglobulinemia has been described in rare cases, no other immunologic abnormalities have been reported in IACI. In summary, the arterial lesions occurring in children with AIDS occur in a unique clinical, pathologic, and immunologic setting. These differences suggest that it is a new and distinctive arteriopathy.

Clinical Features and Diagnosis

In the series of children with AIDS reported by Joshi and colleagues[5] a direct and well-defined sequela secondary to AIDS arteriopathy, such as infarction, could not be demonstrated in organs other than the heart. Nevertheless, it is possible that the arteriopathy of AIDS is responsible for, or exacerbates, such abnormalities as failure to thrive, respiratory distress, encephalopathy, and the generalized atrophy of lymphoreticular organs (Table 14-2).

The diagnosis of AIDS arteriopathy was made at autopsy.[5,8] The failure to demonstrate calcific arterial lesions, even on retrospective review of various radiographs, may be due to the small size of the involved arteries and the focal distribution of the lesions. In order to make the diagnosis of AIDS arteriopathy, a high index of suspicion will be needed. Belman and colleagues[74] have correlated calcification of the basal ganglia seen on computed tomographic scans with vascular calcification seen in autopsy specimens of brain tissue in children with AIDS. A high degree of awareness regarding the possibility of hypoperfusion of an organ and the judicious use of diagnostic techniques may aid

Table 14-2. Lesions of Organs Possibly Related to Arteriopathy-Associated With AIDS

Organ	Lesion
Thymus	Precocious involution
Spleen	Lymphocytic depletion
Lymph nodes	Atrophy
Lungs	Mild focal interstitial fibrosis
Brain	Atrophy, gliosis, infarction
Kidney	Glomerulosclerosis
Heart	Myocardial infarction, fibrosis
Small intestine	Villous atrophy
Muscles	Atrophy

in the clinical diagnosis of AIDS arteriopathy and aneurysms. Useful investigative techniques will include ultrasound, conventional contrast injection arteriography, magnetic resonance imaging, and magnetic resonance arteriography.

Aneurysmal Lesions

Aneurysms of the small and large arteries have been reported in at least 25 HIV-infected children and adults ranging from 3 to 64 years of age (Table 14-3). They have been described in the coronary and cerebral arteries. In addition they have been reported in almost all major arteries from the ascending aorta to the popliteal artery. In some cases it is difficult to distinguish whether the HIV virus led to the aneurysm, was a cofactor in the pathogenesis of the lesion, or was merely a bystander in a naturally occurring process, for example, atherosclerotic aneurysm of the descending aorta in a patient with atherosclerosis. In other cases, the aneurysms were associated with tuberculosis, salmonella, staphylococcus, or opportunistic infections.[16–21]

Coronary Aneurysms

The previously mentioned child with coronary artery aneurysms died of a myocardial infarction.[5] Other children with dilatation of the coronary arteries and myocardial infarction have also been described.[75,76] Furthermore, the increased incidence of sudden death in children with AIDS[77] suggests that

perhaps coronary lesions are more common than previously suspected.

Cerebral Aneurysms

Numerous cases of cerebral aneurysms have been reported in the right, left and, middle cerebral arteries in both children and adults.[6–8,12,13,16] These lesions vary in size from small to large and have been detected both by angiography and at autopsy. They have often been occluded by thrombus formation and are believed to be associated with neurologic disease and strokes. Several children with cerebral aneurysms have been without obvious neurologic symptoms; however, the majority of patients have suffered some degree of impairment, such as hemiparesis, weakness, or encephalopathy. The true incidence of cerebral vascular involvement is unknown, since these lesions may be silent and only discovered on angiography or autopsy.

Aortic and Other Arterial Aneurysms

Several investigators[16–21] have described aneurysms of large arterial vessels, including the ascending, descending, and abdominal aorta in patients infected with HIV. These have been associated with a variety of infectious agents, such as *Salmonella, Staphylococcus,* and *Mycobacterium avium-intracellulare* complex.

Prospects for Therapy

If a diagnosis of AIDS arteriopathy is made before death, consideration should be given to therapy.

Table 14-3. Aneurysms Associated With HIV Infection

Location/Types	Reported Cases	Age	Infection	Clinical Symptoms	Refs.
Coronary	3	3	No	Myocardial infarction	5,75,76
Cerebral	7	4–12	No	Strokes	7,8,12,13,16
Abdominal aorta	12	26–64	*Salmonella* *Staphylococcus* Tuberculosis	Abdominal pain	17–21
Aortic arch	6	24–38	*Staphylococcus* *Mycobacterium avium-intracellulare* complex	Mass pain	16,18
Other arteries	7	12–46	Yes	Mass pain	18

In IACI, a disease with similar calcific lesions, corticosteroids, estrogens, thyroid hormone, or diphosphonate has been successfully used in some cases with resolution of arterial calcification.[72] Aneurysms should be investigated and a source of infection should be sought. Aneurysms can be often be successfully located by either ultrasound or magnetic resonance imaging. Treatment to prevent thrombus formation or dissolve localized thrombus may be useful in selected cases. Careful consideration should be given to medical and surgical therapies, since recent reports indicate that these aneurysms can be successfully resected and treated.[17-21]

References

1. Gottlieb MS, Schroff R, Schanker HM, et al. *Pneumocystis carinii* pneumonia and mucosal candidiasis in previously healthy homosexual men: evidence of a new acquired cellular immunodeficiency. *N Engl J Med* 1981;305:1425–1431.

2. Oleske J, Minnefor AB, Cooper R, et al. Immune deficiency syndrome in children. *JAMA* 1983;249:2345–2349.

3. Joshi VV, Oleske JM, Minnefor AB, et al. Pathology of suspected acquired immune deficiency syndrome in children: study of eight cases. *Pediatr Pathol* 1984;1:71–87.

4. Joshi VV. Pathology of childhood AIDS. *Pediatr Clin North Am* 1991;38:97–120.

5. Joshi VV, Pawel B, Conner E, et al. Arteriopathy in children with acquired immune deficiency syndrome. *Pediatr Pathol* 1987;7:261–275.

6. Park YD, Belman AL, Kim TS, et al. Stroke in pediatric acquired immunodeficiency syndrome. *Ann Neurol* 1990;28:303–311.

7. Philippet P, Blanche S, Sebag G, et al. Stroke and cerebral infarcts in children with human immunodeficiency virus. *Arch Pediatr Adolesc Med* 1994;148:965–970.

8. Kure K, Park YD, Kim TS, et al. Immunohistochemical localization of an HIV epitope in cerebral aneurysmal arteriopathy in pediatric acquired immunodeficiency syndrome. *Pediatr Pathol* 1989;9:655–667.

9. Sotrel A, Multani P. Pathology of the nervous system in HIV-infected patients. In: Wormser GP (ed).

AIDS and Other Manifestations of HIV Infection, 2nd Ed. New York: Lippicott Raven, 1992:543–584.

10. Reux I, Fillet AM, Fournier JG, et al. In situ hybridization of HIV-1 RNA in retinal vascular wall. *Am J Pathol* 1993;143:1275–1279.

11. Yankner BA, Skolnik PR, Shoukimas GM, et al. Cerebral granulomatous angiitis associated with isolation of human T lymphotropic virus type III from the central nervous system. *Ann Neurol* 1986;20:362–364.

12. Lang C, Jacobi G, Kreuz W, et al. Rapid development of giant aneurysm at the base of the brain in an 8-year-old boy with perinatal HIV infection. *Acta Histochem* 1992;42S:83–90.

13. Husson RN, Saini R, Lewis LL, et al. Cerebral artery aneurysms in children with human immunodeficiency virus. *J Pediatr* 1992;121:927–930.

14. Mizusawa H, Hirano A, Llena JF, Shintakku M. Cerebrovascular lesions in acquired immunodeficiency syndrome (AIDS). *Acta Neuropathol* 1988;76:451–457.

15. Frank Y, Lim W, Kahn E, et al. Multiple ischemic infarcts in a child with AIDS, varicella zoster infection, and cerebral vasculitis. *Pediatr Neurol* 1989;5:64–67.

16. Destian S, Tung H, Gray R, et al. Giant infectious intracavernous carotid artery aneurysm presenting as intractable epistaxis. *Surg Neurol* 1994;41:472–476.

17. Dupont JR, Bonavita JA, DiGiovanni RJ, et al. Acquired immunodeficiency syndrome and mycotic abdominal aortic aneurysms: a new challenge?: report of a case. *J Vasc Surg* 1989;10:254–257.

18. Mestres CA, Ninot S, de Lacy AM, et al. AIDS and salmonella-infected abdominal aortic aneurysm. *Aust NZ J Surg* 1990;60:225–226.

19. Marks C, Kuskov S. Pattern of arterial aneurysms in acquired immunodeficiency disease. *World J Surg* 1995;9:127–32.

20. Gouny P, Valverde A, Vincent D, et al. Human immunodeficiency virus and infected aneurysm of the abdominal aorta: report of three cases. *Ann Vasc Surg* 1992;6:239–243.

21. Sinzobahamvya N, Kalangu K, Hamel-Kalinowski W. Arterial aneurysms associated with human immunodeficiency virus (HIV) infection. *Acta Chir Belg* 1989;89:185–188.

22. Kieburtz KD, Eskin TA, Ketonen L, Tuite MJ. Opportunistic cerebral vasculopathy and stroke in

patients with the acquired immunodeficiency syndrome. *Arch Neurol* 1993;50:430–432.

23. Engstrom JW, Lowenstein DH, Bredesen DE. Cerebral infarctions and transient neurologic deficits associated with acquired immunodeficiency syndrome. *Am J Med* 1989;86:528–532.

24. Calabrese LH, Estes M, Yen-Lieberman B, et al. Systemic vasculitis in association with human immunodeficiency virus infection. *Arthritis Rheum* 1989;32:569–576.

25. Valeriano-Marcet J, Ravichandran L, Kerr LD. HIV associated systemic necrotizing vasculitis. *J Rheumatol* 1990;17:1091–1093.

26. Watkins KV, Ittman MM. Necrotizing vasculitis in a patient with acquired immunodeficiency syndrome. *J Oral Maxillofac Surg* 1992;50:1000–1003.

27. Gherardi R, Belec L, Mhiri C, et al. The spectrum of vasculitis in human immunodeficiency virus-infected patients: a clinicopathologic evaluation. *Arthritis Rheum* 1993;36:1164–74.

28. Libman BS, Quismorio FP Jr, Stimmler MM. Polyarthritis nodosa-like vasculitis in human immunodeficiency virus infection. *J Rheumatol* 1995;22:351–355.

29. Gherardi R, Lebargy F, Gaulard P, et al. Necrotizing vasculitis and HIV replication in peripheral nerves. *N Engl J Med* 1989;321:685–686.

30. Chren MM, Silverman RA, Sorensen RU, Elmets CA. Leukocytoclastic vasculitis in a patient infected with human immunodeficiency virus. *J Am Acad Dermatol* 1989;21:1161–1164.

31. Weimer CE Jr., Sahn EE. Follicular accentuation of leukocytoclastic vasculitis in an HIV-seropositive man: report of a case study and review of the literature. *J Am Acad Dermatol* 1991;24:898–902.

32. Potashner W, Patterson B, Karasik A, Keystone EC. Leukocytoclastic vasculitis with HIV infection. *J Rheumatol* 1990;17:1104–1107.

33. Veljii AM. Leukocytoclastic vasculitis associated with positive HTLV-III serological findings. *JAMA* 1986;256:2196–2197.

34. Rabb M, Jampol L, Fish R, et al. Retinal periphlebitis in patients with acquired immunodeficiency syndrome with cytomegalovirus retinitis mimics acute frosted retinal periphlebitis. *Arch Ophthalmol* 1992;110:1257–60.

35. Schwartz ND, So YT, Hollander H, et al. Eosinophilic vasculitis leading to amaurosis fugax in a patient with acquired immunodeficiency syndrome. *Arch Intern Med* 1986;146:2059–2060.

36. Yoganathan K, Goodman F, Pozniak A. Kawasaki-like syndrome in an HIV positive adult. *J Infect* 1995;30:165–166.

37. Wolf CV, Wolf JR, Parker JS. Kawasaki's syndrome in a man with the human immunodeficiency virus. *Am J Ophthalmol* 1995;120:117–118.

38. Viraben R, Dupre A. Kawasaki disease associated with HIV infection. *Lancet* 1987;1:1430–1431.

39. Bayrou O, Philippoteau C, Artigou C, et al. Adult Kawasaki syndrome associated with HIV infection and anticardiolipin antibodies. *J Am Acad Dermatol* 1993;29:663–664.

40. Nigro G, Pisano P, Krzysztofiak A. Recurrent Kawasaki disease associated with co-infection with parvovirus B19 and HIV-1. *AIDS* 1993;7:288–289.

41. Paton P, Tabib A, Lorie R, Tete R. Coronary artery lesions and human immunodeficiency virus infection. *Res Virol* 1993;44:225–231.

42. Tabib A, Greenland T, Mercier I, et al. Coronary lesions in young HIV-positive subjects at necropsy. *Lancet* 1992;340:730.

43. Becker DM, Saunders TJ, Wispelwey B. Case report: venous thromboembolism in AIDS. *Am J Med Sci* 1992;303:395–397.

44. Dobersen MJ, Kleinschmidt-DeMasters BK. Superior sagittal sinus thrombosis in a patient with acquired immunodeficiency syndrome. *Arch Pathol* 1994;118:844–846.

45. Ismail Y, Nemechek PM, Arsura EL. A rare cause of visual loss in AIDS patients: central retinal vein occlusion. *Br J Ophthalmol* 1993;77:601–602.

46. Teich SA, Sonnabend J. Central retinal vein occlusion in a patient with AIDS. *Arch Ophthalmol* 1988;106:1508–1509.

47. Smith KJ, Skelton HG, Yeager J. Cutaneous thrombosis in human immunodeficiency virus type 1-positive patients with cytomegalovirus viremia. *Arch Dermatol* 1995;131:357–358.

48. Le Boit PE. Bacillary angiomatosis. *Mod Pathol* 1995;8:218–222.

49. Malane MS, Laude TA, Chen CK, Fikrig S. An HIV-1 positive child with fever and a scalp nodule. *Lancet* 1995;346:1466.

50. Tappero JW, Mohle-Boetani J, Koehler JE, et al. The epidemiology of bacillary angiomatosis and bacillary peliosis. *JAMA* 1993;269:770–775.

51. Steeper TA, Rosenstein H, Weiser J, et al. Bacillary epithelioid angiomatosis involving the liver, spleen and skin in an AIDS patient with concurrent

Kaposi's sarcoma. *Am J Clin Pathol* 1992;97: 713–718.

52. Rudikoff D, Phelps RG, Gordon RE, Bottone EJ. Acquired immunodeficiency syndrome-related bacillary vascular proliferation (epithelioid angiomatosis): rapid response to erythromycin therapy. *Arch Dermatol* 1989;125:706–707.

53. Axiotis CA, Schwartz R, Jennings TA, Glaser N. AIDS-related angiomatosis. *Am J Dermatopathol* 1989;11:177–181.

54. Koehler JE, Tappero JW. Bacillary angiomatosis and bacillary peliosis in patients infected with HIV. *Clin Infect Dis* 1993;17:612.

55. Martin RW III, Hood AF, Farmer ER. Kaposi sarcoma. *Medicine* 1993;72:245–261.

56. Chang Y, Cesarman E, Pessin MS, et al. Identification of herpes virus-like DNA sequences in AIDS-associated Kaposi's sarcoma. *Science* 1994;266: 1865–1869.

57. MacFarlane DF, Gregory N. Telangiectases in human immunodeficiency virus-positive patients. *Cutis* 1994;53:79–80.

58. Torres RA, Lin RY, Lee M, Barr MR. Zidovudine-induced leukocytoclastic vasculitis. *Arch Intern Med* 1992;52:850–851.

59. von Gunten CF, Roth EI, Von Roenn JH. Raynaud phenomenon in three patients with acquired immune deficiency syndrome-related Kaposi sarcoma treated with bleomycin. *Cancer* 1993;72:2004–2006.

60. Esterly JR, Oppenheimer EH. Intrauterine rubella infection. *Perspect Pediatr Pathol* 1973;1:313–338.

61. Rosenberg HS, Oppenheimer EH, Esterly JR. Congenital rubella syndrome: the late effects and their relation to early lesions. *Perspect Pediatr Pathol* 1981;6:183–202.

62. Good RA, Yunis E. Association of autoimmunity, immunodeficiency and aging in man, rabbits, and mice. *Fed Proc* 1974;33:2040–2050.

63. Slavin RE, Saeki K, Bhagavan B, Mass AE. Segmental arterial mediolysis: a precursor of fibromuscular dysplasia? *Mod Pathol* 1995;8:287–294.

64. Battistini B, D'Orleans-Juste P, Sirois P. Biology of disease: endothelins: circulating plasma levels and presence in other biologic fluids. *Lab Invest* 1993;68:600–628.

65. Lafeuillade A, Alessi MC, Piozot-Martin I, et al. Endothelial cell dysfunction in HIV infection. *J AIDS* 1992;5:127–131.

66. Xiu RJ, Jun C, Berglund O. Microcirculatory disturbances in AIDS patients-first report. *Microvasc Res* 1991;42:151–159.

67. Werb Z, Banda MJ, McKerrow JH, Sandhaus RA. Elastases and elastin degradation. *J Invest Dermatol* 1982;79 (Suppl):154s–159s.

68. Giesker DW, Pastuszak WT, Farouhar FA, et al. Lymph node biopsy for early diagnosis in Kawasaki disease. *Am J Surg Pathol* 1982;6:493–501.

69. Landing BH, Larson EJ. Are infantile periarteritis nodosa with coronary artery involvement and fatal mucocutaneous lymph node syndrome the same? *Pediatrics* 1977;59:651–652.

70. Amano S, Hazama F, Hamashima Y. Pathology of Kawasaki disease: I. Pathology and morphogenesis of vascular changes. *Jpn Circ J* 1979;43:633–643.

71. Sasaguri Y, Kato H. Regression of aneurysm in Kawasaki disease: a pathologic study. *J Pediatr* 1982;100:225–231.

72. Meradji M, de Villeneuve VH, Huber J, et al. Idiopathic infantile arterial calcification in siblings: radiological diagnosis and successful treatment. *J Pediatr* 1978;92:401–405.

73. Moran JJ. Idiopathic arterial calcification of infancy: clinicopathologic study. *Pathol Annu* 1975; 10:393–417.

74. Belman AL, Lantos G, Horoupian D, et al. AIDS: calcification of the basal ganglia in infants and children. *Neurology* 1986;36:1192–1199.

75. Bharati S, Lev M. Pathology of the heart in AIDS. *Prog Cardiol* 1989;2:261–272.

76. Lipshultz, SE. Cardiovascular problems in pediatric AIDS. In: Pizzo PA, Wilfert CM (eds.), *The Challenge of HIV Infection in Infants, Children and Adolescents,* 2nd Ed. Baltimore: Williams and Wilkins, 1994.

77. Lipshultz SE, Chanock S, Sanders SP, et al. Cardiac manifestations of human immunodeficiency virus infection in infants and children. *Am J Cardiol* 1989;63:1489–1497.

15

Exercise Performance in HIV Infection

Vernat Exil, M.D., Steven D. Colan, M.D., and Michelle A. Grenier, M.D.

Normal Cardiovascular Response to Exercise

The normal cardiovascular response to exercise includes multiple physiologic changes that serve to meet the body's requirement for oxygen. Complex interactions between the cardiovascular system, the pulmonary system, and the skeletal muscles occur so that oxygen, glucose, and fatty acids are supplied to the exercising muscles and the by-products of cell metabolism, such as lactate and CO_2, are eliminated. At any point in this chain of events, normal exercise response may be impaired, and symptoms may occur.[1-4]

Normal cardiovascular changes during exercise include an outpouring of sympathetic activity that results in an increase in cardiac output by increasing the stroke volume and heart rate. During low levels of upright exercise, both heart rate and stroke volume increase as cardiac output rises steadily. Preferential blood flow restricts circulation to the splanchnic bed, the skin, and the kidneys. More blood is redirected to the cardiovascular system and the working muscles. As more blood returns to the heart, the left ventricle increases its end-diastolic volume, and through the Frank-Starling mechanism, the stroke volume increases. As exercise becomes more intense, there is usually no further increase in stroke volume, and additional change in cardiac output depends on the heart rate. Further increase in cardiac output occurs mainly through sympathetic stimulation, resulting in an increase in heart rate and cardiac muscle contractility.[1-4,5]

The right ventricular ejection fraction also increases during exercise, but not to the same extent as does the left ventricular ejection fraction. The right ventricle is working against a fixed, low pulmonary vascular resistance that falls very little during exercise, while the left ventricle is ejecting to a systemic vascular resistance that decreases manifold during exercise.[5] During isotonic exercise, systolic blood pressure increases, but diastolic blood pressure stays the same or increases only slightly. During isometric exercise, both systolic and diastolic pressure increase. The increase in blood pressure is due mainly to an increase in cardiac output, despite a decrease in systemic vascular resistance.[1,2] In the healthy individual, exhaustion occurs when no further increase in cardiac output can be brought about.

Exercise Testing Protocols and the Measurement of Cardiovascular Fitness

Exercise testing is an important tool in the evaluation of the heart and the blood vessels, by indicating the amount of work the heart can perform and revealing when the heart is at risk for adverse events during exercise. It is an important tool in the evaluation of patients with chronic heart disease, because exercise dysfunction may herald cardiac morbidity and mortality.[3] Additionally, exercise testing parameters may assist in monitoring the effectiveness of medical and surgical cardiac treatment. Parameters of different cardiovascular responses to exercise are usually compared with those of healthy age-matched individuals to determine cardiovascular fitness.

Various forms of exercise can be used, including step climbing, treadmill running, recumbent and upright bicycling, and arm cranking. Regardless of the protocol, the blood pressure, heart rate, and electrocardiogram are recorded; arterial oxygen saturation can be measured by pulse oximetry; and breath-by-breath analysis of expired gases can be performed. The data collected are usually expressed as 1-minute averages for heart rate, oxygen consumption ($\dot{V}O_2$), carbon dioxide production ($\dot{V}CO_2$), expired ventilation ($\dot{V}E$), respiratory frequency, and tidal volume. The capacity to exercise, or "fitness," is generally assessed as aerobic power, because exercising muscles performing work mainly depend on aerobic mechanisms of energy production. The best index of fitness or aerobic power is the maximum oxygen consumption that can be achieved during exercise, or $\dot{V}O_{2\,max}$. Maximum oxygen consumption is the plateau of $\dot{V}O_2$ that occurs despite continued work, and requires maximum effort to assess accurately.[1-4] Until this plateau is achieved, the relationships among work, cardiac output (CO), and maximum oxygen consumption ($\dot{V}O_{2\,max}$) are linear, with a relationship of the form: CO = 4 + 0.006 × $\dot{V}O_2$ ml/ kg^{-1} min^{-1}.[6]

As exercise intensifies, oxygen demand outstrips oxygen delivery, with a disproportionate increase in lactate and CO_2 production. Minute ventilation increases in an attempt to maintain eucapnia. Ventilation increases with work due to an increase in both tidal volume and breathing frequency. The relation between minute ventilation ($\dot{V}E$) and work is linear, but the slope of this relation changes abruptly when the ventilatory anaerobic threshold is attained. This point in exercise is called the anaerobic threshold, or ventilatory anaerobic threshold

(VAT), since it is the $\dot{V}O_2$ at which there is a disproportionate increase in minute ventilation ($\dot{V}E$) relative to oxygen uptake. The VAT can also be used as a measure of aerobic power, and it is less dependent on motivation and the need to reach uncomfortable levels of exercise.[1-4] VAT has been calculated to correspond to an increase in blood lactate of 1 to 2 mmol/l, and it usually occurs at 40% to 90% of peak $\dot{V}O_2$.[3]

The anaerobic threshold during exercise can be identified by an abrupt change in the slope of ventilation $\dot{V}E$ and the ventilatory equivalent for O_2 ($\dot{V}E/\dot{V}O_2$), without a concomitant change in the ventilatory equivalent for CO_2 ($\dot{V}E/\dot{V}CO_2$). However, later during exercise, as acidosis becomes more severe, ventilation increases disproportionately to CO_2 production, abruptly changing the slope of $\dot{V}E/\dot{V}CO_2$. At this, point alveolar carbon dioxide tension ($PaCO_2$) and end-tidal CO_2 decrease, and there is respiratory decompensation. For this reason this point has been called the "threshold for decompensated metabolic acidosis."

Fitness can be assessed as the time taken to reach this threshold of decompensated metabolic acidosis. The fit individual reaches maximum heart rate at a greater $\dot{V}O_{2\,max}$ than the unfit individual. Fitness is a state of well-being that is dependent on both the state of cardiovascular health, and the magnitude of prior exercise training. Indices of fitness cannot be interpreted without consideration of both of these factors.

Exercise Intolerance in Patients with Chronic Heart Disease

Exercise intolerance in the patient with chronic heart failure is multifactorial. Intolerance is of interest in patients with chronic heart disease, because it generally correlates with disease severity.[3] Symptoms become manifest during low-level exercise and are related to the decrease in overall exercise capacity. For a given amount of work, patients with chronic heart disease, similar to patients who are poorly conditioned, reach a maximum heart rate more quickly, at a lower work load, and at a lower $\dot{V}O_2$ max. The slope of heart rate to $\dot{V}O_2$ is increased. Patients with chronic heart failure experience a significant deterioration in maximal exercise performance preceding other signs of clinical decompensation.[3] Factors known to contribute to exercise intolerance in patients with chronic heart disease are central hemodynamic factors (systolic and diastolic left ventricular dysfunction, elevated left and right ventricular filling pressures, reduced cardiac output, pericardial restraint, and impaired right ventricular function), peripheral factors (disordered skeletal muscle blood flow, biochemistry, and contractile function), and pulmonary factors (respiratory muscle fatigue, air flow limitations, and hyperpnea).[3]

Elevated right ventricular and left ventricular filling pressures and reduced cardiac output at a given work rate contribute to the presence of symptoms during exercise.[3,5] Cardiac output, the most important of these factors, is the product of heart rate (HR) and stroke volume (SV). It is adversely affected by depressed left ventricular contractility and other factors, including a limited ability to increase left ventricular end-diastolic volume (LVEDV) and the mitral regurgitation fraction.[3] Peak exercise cardiac output and peak Vo_2 in patients with chronic heart failure continue to relate in a linear fashion, but the slope of increase in cardiac output versus Vo_2 is lower in patients with more severe disease.[3] This decrease in cardiac output is responsible for decreased perfusion of working skeletal muscle, resulting in early onset of fatigue. As mentioned above, although skeletal muscle can function anaerobically, most of the energy of working muscles is obtained through aerobic mechanisms.[1,2]

Although the slope of cardiac output versus Vo_2 in patients with chronic heart failure is an indicator of disease severity, the increase in pulmonary capillary wedge pressure (PCWP) with exercise has been reported to be a more sensitive indicator of cardiac dysfunction.[3,7] Mean PCWP in patients with chronic heart failure is increased in patients at rest and during exercise, although a significant number of patients have normal left ventricular filling pressures.[3]

It is clear that in patients with chronic heart disease, exercise capacity is not solely related to the degree of left ventricular systolic dysfunction. Peripheral changes in skeletal muscle, blood supply,[7] and in muscle metabolism, mass, and strength are often abnormal when compared with those in healthy subjects. An adequate muscle mass is required, and there must be normal function of intracellular contractile proteins, cell membranes, sarcoplasmic reticulum, mitochondria, and intracellular energy transport systems. In elderly people, disorders of the musculoskeletal system include muscle weakness and atrophy from disuse. However, healthy elderly people who show substantial decrease in muscle strength have a decrease in fat-free muscle mass without any alteration in muscle function.[8] Skeletal muscle atrophy, abnormalities of skeletal muscle blood flow, and abnormalities of skeletal muscle metabolism are all determinants of exercise intolerance.

Inadequate mobilization of energy resources can also be a factor in the ability to perform work. Fuel regulation depends on several variables, including the current state of training, the duration and intensity of exercise, and diet. Early in exercise, skeletal muscle fuel utilization relies primarily on carbohydrates. As exercise continues, working muscles derive an increasing amount of energy from circulating free fatty acids. With aerobic exercise training, exercising muscles rely more on fats and reduce their dependence on carbohydrates.[9] Additionally, new areas of research have shown that during exercise, there is a continual flux of amino acids between muscle and nonmuscular tissue, particularly the liver and kidney. This involves a continuous state of protein catabolism and anabolism to generate energy. Protein metabolism then also contributes to exercise endurance.[10]

How does all this relate to children? Exercise testing is difficult to perform in children under the age of 5 because of lack of cooperation. At the same time, it is more difficult to discriminate levels of fitness in children because they are generally more fit than adults. Healthy children can improve their performance in sports events without changes in their cardiovascular index capacities. Children with heart disease may show signs of reduced aerobic power, mainly because of inadequate training. Parental factors may also be involved, because children with congenital heart diseases typically perform above their parents' expectation. Supervised exercise training has been reported to improve cardiac indexes in children; for example, $V_{O_2 max}$ can be improved with endurance training during childhood. As with patients with chronic heart failure, children with chronic heart conditions may experience central hemodynamic dysfunction, which results in exercise intolerance. Although there are few relevant data, children with chronic illnesses, such as multisystem HIV disease and malnutrition, have similar reasons to be intolerant of exercise.

Changes in Exercise Physiology in the HIV-Positive Patient

Exercise testing in children infected with human immunodeficiency virus has not been formally reported, although there is anecdotal evidence of blunted blood pressure responses to exercise in this patient population (Table 15-1). However, older patients infected with HIV are known to experience exercise limitation independent of disease stage. A number of these patients experience a decline in their ability to perform mandatory physical training exercise.[7,11] Patients complaining of symptoms do not necessarily have evidence of exercise intolerance, and patients with evidence of exercise intolerance do not necessarily complain of daily fatigue or dyspnea on exertion. More puzzling is the fact that these limitations have a poor correlation with cardiac symptoms or disease stage. Contrary to observations in patients with chronic heart failure, limitations in exercise performance in patients with HIV infection may not have any predictive value

for cardiac decompensation. In the absence of opportunistic infections and in the presence of normal history and physical examination, Johnson and colleagues[11] concluded that this may reflect occult cardiac disease in the individual infected with HIV. These authors performed exercise testing in 32 patients with HIV infection but without acquired immunodeficiency syndrome. The patients complained of reduced capacity to perform activities of daily living, at a time when history, physical examination, and chest radiographs revealed no evidence of opportunistic infections. The authors excluded patients with history or symptoms suggestive of atherosclerotic heart disease or significant cardiac disease and those with asthma, other preexisting pulmonary disease, or significant complicating medical disorders. When compared with 22 healthy seronegative subjects, the HIV-positive patients achieved a significantly lower workload. They demonstrated mild tachypnea throughout exercise, compared with controls, and had a significant increase in the slope of the heart rate vs. $V_{O_2 max}$. There was no difference between the maximum expected heart rates of patients and those of controls. Nonetheless, 9 of the 32 patients had maximum heart rates lower than predicted. This subgroup of patients reached their $V_{O_2 max}$ at heart rates around 75% of predicted. The authors concluded that these findings were due mainly to a limitation of oxygen delivery to exercising muscles. Patients with HIV infection exercised to a significantly lower V_{O_2} maximum. The ventilatory anaerobic threshold was significantly lower in patients than

Table 15-1. Exercise Testing in HIV-Infected Children with Symptomatic HIV Infection (CDC Class P-2)

Age (yr)	Sex	Holter	ECG	Echo	Stress
11	F	Sinus tachycardia	Sinus tachycardia	SF = 35%	HR = 91–178 BP = 90/70–115/80
13	M	WAP RVCD	Sinus tachycardia Nonspecific ST-T	SF = 30%	HR = 95–202 BP = 108/80–140/80
9	F	Rare PAC	NSR, normal	SF = 33%	HR = 78–191 BP = 110/60–134/70
11	M	Sinus bradycardia Blocked PAC	Sinus bradycardia	SF = 33%	Normal; achieved 85% of maximum heart rate at stage V
7	M	NSR PAC	NSR PAC	SF = 44% ↑ contractility	HR = 97–170 BP = 106/50–118/58

BP, blood pressure; PAC, premature atrial contraction; HR, heart rate; NSR, normal sinus rhythm; SF, shortening fraction; WAP, wandering of atrial pacemaker; RVCD, right ventricular conduction delay.

in controls (1.44 ± 0.40 versus 1.83 ± 0.34 l/min of oxygen consumption; $P < .001$). The ventilatory anaerobic threshold expressed as a percentage of maximum predicted oxygen consumption was also considerably lower (49.2 ± 13.0 versus 61.9 ± 9.1%; $P < .001$). At maximum exercise, the patients' V_E was somewhat lower than that of the controls.

In a subsequent publication,[7] Johnson and collaborators studied nine HIV-positive patients who had symptoms of dyspnea on exertion. They had a VAT less than 46.2% of predicted VAT_{max}, a $V_{O2\,max}$ less than 80% of predicted, or both. These patients, together with 13 controls, underwent right heart catheterization during exercise. Patient and control groups had similar right atrial pressures and PCWP at rest. The nine HIV-positive patients had no signs or history of opportunistic infection. They had elevated exercise PCWP (14.6 ± 3.3 versus 9.9 ± 3.3 mmHg; $P < .005$) and elevated exercise right atrial pressure (10.1 ± 2.1 versus 4.7 ± 3.2 mmHg; $P < .001$). This increase in PCWP is a sensitive indicator of cardiac dysfunction.[3,4,7] There was no difference between patients and controls in cardiac index or stroke volume index at rest or with exercise. In the absence of valvular, pulmonary, and atherosclerotic disease, the authors concluded that otherwise occult cardiac impairment was responsible for these abnormal findings during exercise testing.

Another important aspect of exercise limitations described in the HIV-positive patient relates to abnormalities of the autonomic nervous system. Close to 40% of patients with AIDS present with clinical evidence of neurologic dysfunction.[12] They may present with multiple symptoms, including syncopal and near-syncopal episodes, dizziness, and orthostatic hypotension. Craddock and colleagues[13] reported rapid onset of bradycardia and hypotension in five patients who underwent fine-needle aspiration of the lung. One of the events was fatal, and the other four patients had formal autonomic function testing with Ewing's method meeting criteria for severe autonomic nerve damage. Lin-Greenberg and Taneja-Uppal[14] described low levels of norepinephrine in the supine position in a patient with AIDS who had severe orthostatic hypotension. Freeman and colleagues[15] performed formal autonomic function testing in 26 patients infected with HIV and 22 seronegative controls selected to match the age and sex distribution of the patients. The authors reported that autonomic dysfunction appeared to occur in a continuum from AIDS-related complex to AIDS. There was a significant difference between the AIDS patients and their controls, with patients with AIDS-related complex intermediate and manifesting a bimodal response.[15] These findings imply that the hemodynamic and autonomic responses gradually became compromised as HIV infection progressed. Although autonomic dysfunction occurred more frequently and with greater severity in patients with AIDS, dysautonomia in the HIV-infected patient may be present independent of disease stage.[13–18] If the autonomic nervous system is compromised, it may be difficult for an individual to mount an adequate tachycardia response to exercise; consequently, the individual will be unable to increase cardiac output as exercise intensifies, reaching exhaustion sooner than expected.

Resting tachycardia has also been noted, suggesting vagal neuropathy or unopposed cardiac sympathetic activity,[15] whereas rapid onset of bradycardia and orthostatic hypotension suggests vagal hyperreactivity.[13–15] All these may adversely affect exercise tolerance in HIV-positive patients. Other evidence of dysautonomia includes a lack of response to the Valsalva maneuver with no compensatory tachycardia and no overshoot of blood pressure,[14,15] a fall in mean arterial pressure with tilt testing, and an increase in diastolic blood pressure with isometric exercise.[15,18] Patients with AIDS-related complex may transiently show exaggerated normal responses, a phenomenon attributed to denervation supersensitivity.[15] These abnormalities place the patient at risk during invasive procedures.[13,14] Similarly, abnormal hemodynamic response to exercise can be expected.

Another factor that can limit exercise tolerance in patients with HIV infection relates to cardiac dysrhythmias.[12,19,20] Cardoso and associates[20] performed 24-hour Holter monitoring in 21 HIV-positive patients at different stages of the disease and found a high incidence of cardiac impulse conduction disturbances, such as supraventricular tachycardia, heart block, and premature atrial and ventricular contractions. Changes in the histology and anatomy of the conduction system in children with HIV have also been described. Histologic changes in children with HIV may include vascular, degenerative, and fibrotic changes of the pericardium, endocardium, and myocardium. These changes may affect the entire conduction system of the heart.[17]

Effects of Exercise on the Immune System

The effects of exercise on the immune system have long been a subject of controversy. Most current research, however, supports the conclusion that intense exercise, like trauma and sepsis, has negative effects on the immune system.[16,21] In animal models, electric shocks are well-proven means of inducing immunosuppression.[22] Intensive and exhaustive exercise, even of short duration, weakens nonspecific immunity.[23,24] Even well-conditioned athletes are advised to refrain from strenuous exercise if they have fever or other symptoms of infection, for exercise may reduce their resistance to infection.[1,16,21,23] However, there are conflicting reports over the short-term influence of exercise on the immune system. Circulating leukocyte numbers after acute exercise are increased, unchanged, or decreased, depending on the intensity of exercise, training status of the subjects, and timing of the blood sample.[21] The small transient changes observed acutely after exercise are often attributable to circadian rhythm or hemoconcentration. Those reports are often based on the observation that postexercise lymphocyte counts, proliferation rates, or helper:suppressor cell ratios remained lower than preexercise levels for many hours, returning to "normal" 24 hours later. For this reason, postexercise immunosuppression is often reported. Neutrophil counts are usually increased and neutrophil activity decreased, with a resultant decline in phagocytic defense against infections.[16] There are reports of lymphocytosis resulting in a greater increase in CD8+ lymphocytes than in CD4+ lymphocytes, causing a proportional decline of the CD4+:CD8+ ratio, similar to the effect of the HIV virus itself on the immune system. There are reports that B lymphocytes, although stable in number, may have decreased function as determined by mitogenic stimulation. Phytohemag-glutinin-stimulated proliferation of blood mononuclear cells is decreased after intensive exercise in healthy individuals.[25]

Exercise conditioning, nevertheless, has been reported to enhance immune parameters.[26] Lymphocytosis, granulocytosis, and increased serum immunoglobulin titers occur within minutes after completion of submaximal aerobic exercise.[26] The transient alterations return to normal values within an hour. Moderate exercise increases plasma interleukin-1 and interleukin-2 titers.[27,28] Moderate exercise also induces leukocytosis and increases monocyte and macrophage production of interferons.[29]

Is Exercise Beneficial to the HIV-Positive Patient?

What would be the advantages and disadvantages of exercise in the patient with HIV? The answer to this question is likely to remain controversial for some time. There is sufficient scientific evidence to suggest that HIV-positive patients should not exercise to exhaustion. In the presence of acute-phase HIV disease, opportunistic infections, or febrile illness, the HIV-infected individual should abstain from exercising. On the other hand, there may be more benefits than risks to exercising if the HIV-positive patient participates in controlled exercise programs. Exercise training can improve exercise capacity and potentially reduce symptoms, even subjects with impaired cardiac function. Improved cardiovascular fitness and skeletal muscle function may be observed after several weeks of sustained exercise training. Spencer and colleagues[30] report that muscle function can improve in patients with AIDS. MacArthur and colleagues[31] studied six subjects who completed a 24-week program of exercise training and concluded that all showed evidence of exercise training effect. They demonstrated improvement in ($Vo_{2 max}$), V_E, and their sense of well-being. All maintained stable subsets of T lymphocytes.

Nevertheless, there are reasons to believe that intense, vigorous exercise could have a negative effect on the already compromised immune system of HIV-infected patients. Although strenuous exercise acutely has a negative effect on the immune system, the effects of moderate supervised exercise training in the HIV-positive patient remain unknown. Moderate exercise training is thought to be beneficial for the cardiovascular, immunologic, and psychological system of the individual.[4,16,31] We conclude that HIV-infected patients with an already compromised immune system may benefit from regular, low-level training programs but should probably not exercise until exhaustion.

Exercise in patients with chronic heart failure may improve the quality of life. Fitter and stronger patients are more comfortable performing tasks of daily living, with greater independence and less depression.[4] Moderate exercise is relaxing and increases the sense of confidence and well-being, perhaps as a result of increased levels of endorphins, enkephalins, and natural opioids, which may have analgesic, euphoric effects. Exercise also relieves stress by decreasing cortisol release from the adrenal cortex.[32]. Exercise training as part of an integrated, multidisciplinary, rehabilitative program for the HIV-infected patient may soon find its place in the management of the patient. Considering the fact that children with HIV infection are surviving longer periods of time into school age and adolescence, supervised exercise training, together with other elements to encourage good nutrition and healthy lifestyle, may improve cardiovascular fitness, muscle strength, and quality of life.

Acknowledgments

We thank Dr. Alan Meyers, Dr. Sigmund Kharasch, Dr. Rounen Rubenoff, Dr. Barry Zuckerman, and Dr. Arnold W. Strauss for their helpful contributions.

References

1. Colan SD, MD. Exercise testing. In: Fyler DC (ed). *Nadas' Pediatric Cardiology*. Philadelphia: Hanley and Belfus, 1992:249–263.

2. Driscoll JD. Exercise testing. In: Emmanouilides GC, Allen HD, Riemenschneider TA, Gutgesell HP (eds). *Moss and Adams Heart Disease in Infants,* *Children, and Adolescents.* Baltimore: Williams & Wilkins, 1995:293–310.

3. Sullivan MJ, Hawthorn MH. Exercise intolerance in patients with chronic heart failure. *Prog Cardiovasc Dis* 1995;28:1–22.

4. McKelvie RS, Teo KK, McCartney N, et al. Effects of exercise training in patients with congestive heart failure: critical review. *J Am Coll Cardiol* 1995;25: 789–796.

5. Dell'Italia LJ. Exercise and exercise testing in congestive heart failure. In: McCall D, Rahimtoola SH (eds). *Heart Failure.* New York: Chapman and Hall, 1995;10:197–214.

6. Jones N, Campbell E. *Clinical Exercise Testing.* 2nd Ed. Philadelphia: WB Saunders, 1982.

7. Johnson JE, Slife DM, Anders GT, et al. Cardiac dysfunction in patients seropositive for the human immunodeficiency virus. *West J Med* 1991;155: 373–379.

8. Frontera WR, Hughes VA, Lutz KJ, et al. A cross-sectional study of muscle strength and mass in 45- to 78-yr-old men and women. *Am Physiol Soc* 1991;71:644–650.

9. Wahren J. Metabolic adaptation to physical exercise in man. In: Degroot LJ (ed). *Endocrinology.* Vol 3. New York: Grune and Stratton, 1979:1911–1926.

10. Evans WJ, Fisher EC, Hoerr RA, et al. Protein metabolism and endurance exercise. *J Phys Sports Med* 1983;11:63–72.

11. Johnson JE, Anders GT, Blanton HM, et al. Exercise dysfunction in patients seropositive for the human immunodeficiency virus. *Am Rev Respir Dis* 1990;141:618–622.

12. Villa A, Cruccu V, Foresti V, et al. HIV related functional involvement of autonomic nervous system. *Acta Neurol* 1990;12:14–18.

13. Craddock C, Bull R, Pasvol G, et al. Cardiorespiratory arrest and autonomic neuropathy in AIDS. *Lancet* 1987;2:16–18.

14. Lin-Greenberg A, Taneja-Uppal N. Dysautonomia and infection with the human immunodeficiency virus. *Arch Intern Med* 1987;196:167.

15. Freeman R, Roberts MS, Friedman LS, et al. Autonomic function and human immunodeficiency virus infection. *Neurology* 1990;40:575–580.

16. Lawless D, Jackson CGR, Greenleaf JE. Exercise and human immunodeficiency virus (HIV-1) infection. *Sports Med* 1995;19:235–239.

17. Bharati S, Joshi VV, Connor EM, et al. Conduction system in children with acquired immunodeficiency syndrome. *Chest* 1989;96:406–413.

18. Miller TL, Semple SJ. Autonomic neuropathy in AIDS. *Lancet* 1987;2:343–344.

19. Villa A, Foresti V, Cruccu V, et al. QT interval prolongation and HIV-related autonomic neropathy. [Abstract]. *Int Conf AIDS (Berlin)* 1993;9:414.

20. Cardoso J, Mota-Miranda A, Gomes NH, et al. Dysrhythmic profile of human immunodeficiency virus infected patients. *Int J Cardiol* 1995;49:249–255.

21. Cannon JG. Exercise and resistance to infection. *Am Physiol Soc* 1993;74:973–981.

22. Keller SE, Weiss JM, Schleifer SJ, et al. Suppression of immunity by stress: effect of a graded series of stressors on lymphocyte stimulation in the rat. *Science* 1981;213:1397–1400.

23. Lewicki R, Tchorzewski H, Denys A, et al. Effect of physical exercise on some parameters of immunity in conditioned sportsmen. *Int J Sports Med* 1987;8:309–314.

24. Tchorzewski H, Lewicki R, Majewska E. Changes in the helper and suppressor lymphocytes in human peripheral blood following maximal physical exercise. *Arch Immunol Ther Exp (Warsz)* 1987;35:307–312.

25. Pederson BK. Influence of physical activity on the cellular immune system: mechanisms of action. *Int J Sports Med* 1991;12(Suppl 1):S23-S29.

26. Nehlsen-Cannarella SL, Nieman DC, Balk-Lamberton AJ, et al. The effects of moderate exercise training on the immune response. *Med Sci Sports Exerc* 1991;23:64–70.

27. Carlson SL, Felten DL. Involvement of hypothalamic and limbic structures in neural-immune communication. In: Goetzl EJ, Spector NH (eds). *Neuroimmune Networks: Physiology and Diseases.* New York: Wiley-Liss, 1989:219–226.

28. Shechtman O, Elizondo R, Taylor M. Exercise augments interleukin–2 induction. [Abstract]. *Med Sci Sports Exerc* 1988;20:S18.

29. Shephard RJ, Verde TJ, Thomas SG, et al. Physical activity and the immune system. *Can J Sports Sci* 1991;16:163–185.

30. Spence DW, Galantino ML, Mosberg KA, et al. Progressive resistance exercise: effect on muscle function and anthropometry of a select AIDS population. *Arch Phys Med Rehabil* 1990;71:644–648.

31. McArthur RD, Levine SD, Birk TJ. Supervised exercise training improves cardiopulmonary fitness in HIV-infected persons. *Med Sci Sports Exerc* 1993;25:684–688.

32. Farrell PA, Gates WK, Maksud MG, et al. Increases in plasma B-endorphin/B-lipotropin immunoreactivity after treadmill running in humans. *J Appl Physiol* 1982;52:1245–1249.

Part 3
Pathogenesis

16

Pathologic Changes in the Hearts of Patients with AIDS

It is axiomatic to consider acquired immunodeficiency syndrome (AIDS) a global health crisis. The initial reports from Los Angeles described the occurrence of opportunistic infections (especially *Pneumocystis carinii* pneumonia) and unusual malignancies (particularly Kaposi's sarcoma) in previously healthy young homosexual men.[1,2] Since then, the prevalence of AIDS has grown to epidemic proportions. The intense domestic experience with AIDS over the past two decades was originally distributed among large metropolitan medical centers. Early in the epidemic, American patients consisted predominantly of homosexual males, intravenous drug abusers, blood transfusion recipients, and hemophiliacs treated with factor VIII concentrates.

Today, sexual partners and children of human immunodeficiency virus (HIV)-infected persons are increasing the number of patients with AIDS.[3] Typical presentations include opportunistic infections with *P. carinii*, *Toxoplasma gondii*, *Cryptosporidium*, cytomegalovirus, herpes simplex virus, *Candida* species, *Cryptococcus neoformans*, and *Mycobacterium avium-intracellulare*; malignancies, including Kaposi's sarcoma, non-Hodgkin's lymphomas, and oral and anorectal carcinomas; and the AIDS wasting syndrome.[4–7]

The impact of heart disease in AIDS may be increasing, since it is believed that cardiovascular problems may emerge more prominently.[8] Heart muscle diseases (including cardiomyopathy and myocarditis) have become the most important cardiac complications of AIDS in the Western world.[9,10] Additionally, it is generally accepted that myocardial dysfunction in AIDS may be overlooked because attention frequently is directed to urgent problems or symptoms attributed to pulmonary disease or other AIDS-related conditions.[11] Anderson and Virmani[12] estimated that more than 6% of HIV-infected patients may have symptomatic heart disease. They categorized AIDS heart disease into four headings: (1) endocardial disease, such as nonbacterial thrombotic endocarditis; (2) myocardial disease, including myocarditis and cardiomyopathy; (3) pericardial disease, including pericarditis and infections; and (4) neoplasms, including Kaposi's sarcoma.

Controversy remains regarding the prevalence and clinical impact of cardiac disease in AIDS. The role of HIV infection of the myocardium in the pathogenesis or natural history of some heart disease in persons with AIDS similarly remains controversial. We have described some of the pathologic findings in the heart of the adult with AIDS[13–17] and some findings from those studies and others[18–22] may be a useful background for review of cardiac changes in persons with AIDS. Virtually any organ

233

in a patient with AIDS, including the heart, may show pathologic changes due to opportunistic infection, to invasion by Kaposi's sarcoma or other malignancies, or to nonspecific compensatory or decompensatory effects. The lungs are frequently involved with *P. carinii* pneumonia. The brain is frequently affected by encephalitis due to *Toxoplasma* or *Cryptococcus*, HIV, or central nervous system lymphoma. Lesions from Kaposi's sarcoma affect the skin in particular but may also affect other organs. The upper and lower gastrointestinal tract may be the site of opportunistic infections from *Cryptosporidium* or other pathogens or of lesions from Kaposi's sarcoma. The adrenal glands may be infected with cytomegalovirus. The thymus may suffer from involution and the lymph nodes from hyperplasia or depletion.[23-25]

Cardiac Findings in Women with AIDS

This subgroup was classified separately because in previous pathologic studies women with AIDS were grouped with men. Previously, we reviewed nine cases of women with documented AIDS from more than 200 consecutive autopsies from the archives of the University of California at Los Angeles (UCLA) and the University of Cincinnati. The mean age for the women was 47.2 years compared to 39.1 years in the earlier study in which men comprised the vast majority of patients.[17] AIDS risk factors in women differed from those previously reported for the predominantly male group.[15,17] Of the nine cases, four were associated with transfusions, three with intravenous drug abuse, one with bisexual contact, and one with no known cause. Pathologic findings included cardiomegaly (400 g) with serous pericardial effusion (150 ml) as prominent findings. One case of a ring abscess of the tricuspid valve occurred in a patient with intravenous drug abuse. One *Candida* myocardial abscess was found. Nonbacterial thrombotic endocarditis was present in one case. Data suggest that clinically important cardiac lesions may be found in this growing segment of the AIDS population.[26]

Pathologic Changes in the Hearts of Patients with AIDS based on Anatomic Location

Pericardium

Pericardial involvement in AIDS is prevalent and includes serous pericardial effusion, or effusion with inflammation (pericarditis).[27-29] An extensive, clinically based study of HIV-infected gay men from the United Kingdom concluded that heart disease in AIDS was important and that pericardial effusion was the most commonly found cardiac change in patients with AIDS.[30] In a retrospective study from San Francisco, 7% of hospitalized patients with pericardial effusions were known to be HIV-positive at the time of echocardiography.[31] The mortality was 29%. Data from Tanzania suggested that pericardial effusion was strongly associated with HIV infection and may be a prevalent and early manifestation of the disease.[32]

Postmortem data from similar populations in Los Angeles (where, as in San Francisco, homosexuality is the most prevalent behavioral risk factor) show that pericardial effusions were common.[15,29] The most common were serous effusions (straw-colored clear effusions exceeding 75 ml volume, with or without pericarditis) (Figure 16-1), which accounted for nearly two-thirds of all cardiac lesions in the previous report[15] and appeared to be the most prevalent cardiac pathologic finding at autopsy.

In our studies, infectious etiologies of the effusions were not documented. However, postmortem studies showed that many of the patients with AIDS suffered from severe interstitial pulmonary diseases in life, were treated with ventilatory support, or had documented *P. carinii* pneumonia in the clinical history. A history of pulmonary disease (such as *P. carinii* pneumonia, or *Mycobacterium avium-intracellulare*) correlated with right ventricular hypertrophy in approximately two-thirds of the cases.

Other studies of infected pericardial effusions found that tuberculous pericardial effusions may be early manifestations of AIDS in patients where intravenous drug abuse was a risk behavior.[33-35] *Mycobacterium avium-intracellulare* was associ-

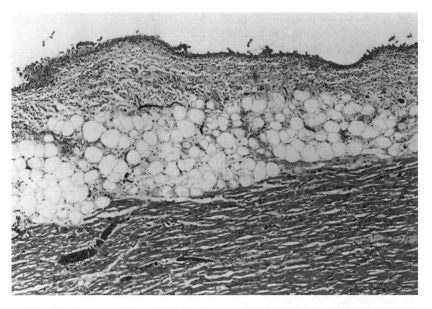

Figure 16-1. Fibrinous pericarditis. Focal inflammation of the pericardium was found fairly commonly at the University of California at Los Angeles. Mononuclear infiltrate (as shown here) was also present in some cases. (Hematoxylin and eosin; ×250.)

ated with pericarditis in AIDS[36] and is a cause of pericardial effusion in AIDS.[37] *T. gondii* also has been found as a cause of pericarditis in AIDS.[38]

Cardiac tamponade in the presence of HIV infection is common in patients from the inner city with AIDS.[39] *Streptococcus pneumoniae* is a rare and ominous etiologic agent found in this complication.[40] Tamponade also has been attributed to Kaposi's sarcoma involvement of the pericardium[41] and to other causes, including pericardial lymphoma.[42,43]

In a review of 45 children with AIDS, 21 had pericardial effusion at postmortem examination. Myocarditis or pericarditis was found in patients, three of whom had documented opportunistic infection with cytomegalovirus, *Candida* or *Staphylococcus aureus.*[44]

Myocardium

Controversy remains regarding the etiology, pathogenesis, clinical impact, and epidemiology of two commonly described diseases of the myocardium in AIDS: dilated cardiomyopathy, and myocarditis.

Cardiomyopathy in AIDS

AIDS cardiomyopathy was described in 1986.[45] Subsequent cases of AIDS cardiomyopathy have been reported.[46] The subcellular pathogenesis of cardiomyopathy in AIDS remains obscure, like that of myocarditis in AIDS (see below). In a one-year consecutive enrollment study of patients admitted to the intensive care unit in an urban center, 65 patients with confirmed HIV infection or AIDS-defining illness were identified from 1,550 admissions. Four such patients (6%) had echocardiographically documented cardiomyopathy. The mortality with cardiomyopathy in AIDS was 25%.[47] Some investigators believed that persistent echocardiographic abnormalities in AIDS were an ominous finding. Other changes were reversible and of less serious clinical consequence.[48] In one British study, myocardial dysfunction was prevalent in HIV-infected patients, and 13 of 173 patients had cardiomyopathy as a correlate of advanced HIV disease. The data suggested the myopathy was not caused by zidovudine, cytomegalovirus, or *T. gondii.*[49] In 27 hemophiliacs, 2 HIV-infected patients had echocardiographically documented cardiomyopathy.[50]

Nonetheless, the impact of unrelated illnesses on the cardiovascular health of patients with AIDS must be ascertained before describing AIDS as an etiologic factor in heart failure.[51]

Possible Etiologic and Pathogenetic Relationships in AIDS Cardiomyopathy

Some cases of dilated cardiomyopathy in patients with AIDS may have the same causes as dilated cardiomyopathy in patients with AIDS.[52] In one study of patients who underwent diagnostic endomyocardial biopsy for congestive heart failure, 5% of the patients were determined by serologic and pathologic methods to have a diagnosis of AIDS heart disease. The proposed causes of cardiomyopathy in AIDS include direct infection of the heart by HIV with or without myocarditis (see below), toxicity of AIDS therapeutics, effects of circulating or systemic toxins, infection of the heart by opportunistic pathogens, toxicity of illicit or self-prescribed pharmaceuticals or home remedies, and nutritional disorders. Additionally, more than one factor may be operative or present in a single patient. There is clinical and basic science evidence for some of these factors as causes of AIDS-related cardiomyopathy.[53-55] Some evidence is summarized below.

Toxicity of Antiretroviral Agents Including Zidovudine

We have proposed the mitochondrial DNA polymerase-γ hypothesis, based on work in our laboratories,[56-61] as a unifying explanation for some pathophysiologic events in zidovudine-induced cardiomyopathy, in cardiomyopathy induced by other antiviral nucleoside analogues, and in toxicity to mitochondria caused by antiviral nucleoside analogues in other tissues. It is reasonable to expect that alterations in mitochondrial DNA replication induced by antiviral nucleoside agents reflect the combined effects of (1) the subcellular availability and abundance of the antiviral nucleoside agent in the target tissue, (2) the ability of the antiviral nucleoside agent to serve as a substrate for cellular nucleoside kinases and to become phosphorylated intracellularly, (3) the ability of the antiviral nucleoside agent triphosphate to inhibit mitochondrial DNA polymerase-γ in the tissues, and (4) the metabolic requirements in the tissues for oxidative phosphorylation.

At this time, the hypothesis that toxicity to mitochondria caused by antiviral nucleoside agents is one of the causes of dilated cardiomyopathy in AIDS is supported anecdotally. Herskowitz and colleagues[62] described cases of patients with AIDS who received antiviral nucleoside agent s and subsequently developed cardiomyopathy. Removal of the toxic antiviral nucleoside agent resulted in reduction in zidovudine-associated left ventricular hypokinesis on echocardiographic examination. To reduce the possibility of cardiomyopathy caused by antiviral nucleoside agents, those authors suggested a "drug holiday" in which zidovudine therapy was alternated with other therapies or discontinued for some time.

We reported a single case of a 45-year-old, HIV-seropositive, homosexual man treated with high-dose zidovudine (1,200 mg/day) for 2 years before the development of AIDS. He manifested symptoms of congestive heart failure with left ventricular dilatation and a 20% ejection fraction. An endomyocardial biopsy showed no active myocarditis, but numerous intramyocytic vacuoles were present. Transmission electron microscopy revealed mitochondria cristae with distortion and myofibrillar loss. At autopsy, a 100-ml pericardial effusion with cardiomegaly and biventricular dilatation was found.[63]

Subsequently, four additional cases of cardiomyopathy associated with zidovudine treatment were referred to us for evaluation of pathologic changes of the heart. All shared documented HIV infection, long-term zidovudine therapy, and clinical features of cardiomyopathy. Pathologic and ultrastructural changes on endomyocardial biopsy correlated with clinical features and grossly resembled changes in cardiomyopathy of many other causes (Figure 16-2). Histologic findings included nonspecific changes consistent with cardiomyopathy. Myocarditis was absent. Mitochondrial degeneration, and swollen or enlarged mitochondria with vacuolization, fragmentation, and loss of cristae were present. Intramitochondrial paracrystals were not found. Despite the differences in behavioral risk factors for the development of AIDS, and the differences in patient age, the four cases shared pathologic

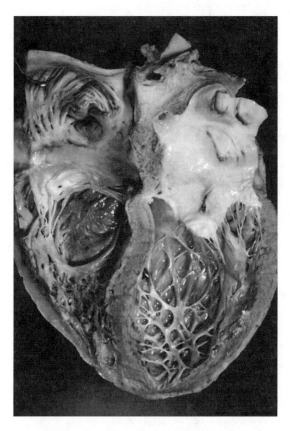

Figure 16-2. (See Color Plate 1 for image in full color.) Dilated cardiomyopathy in AIDS: Biventricular dilatation is seen. No evidence of endocarditis or inflammation. (Courtesy of Dr. Gallo and Dr. d'Amati, La Sapienza, Rome.)

changes involving cardiac mitochondria, a history of long-term zidovudine exposure, and the development of intractable heart failure. In one case, reversal of cardiac dysfunction followed discontinuation of zidovudine therapy[64] in ways that resembled those previously reported.[62]

Cardiomyopathy in Pediatric AIDS

Lipshultz and colleagues[65] reviewed cardiac dimensions and function in HIV-infected children and concluded that progressive left ventricular dilatation occurred irrespective of therapy with zidovudine. However, no myocardial biopsy was performed. One interpretation of these data based on evaluation of ejection performance supports the view that zidovudine exacerbated the development

of cardiomyopathy.[66] It should be noted that in children with AIDS, zidovudine-induced skeletal muscle myopathy is less frequently recognized and may be masked by coexistent AIDS encephalopathy.[67] By analogy to findings with zidovudine-induced skeletal muscle myopathy, zidovudine-induced cardiomyopathy may be rarer in children. A recent report suggests that zidovudine causes cardiomyopathy in HIV-infected children, but didanosine therapy does not.[68] In that report, no endomyocardial biopsy data were included.

Nutritional Deficiency

Evidence also exists that specific nutritional deficiencies (such as selenium and L-carnitine) have an effect on the pathophysiology of heart failure in AIDS and on the pathogenesis of AIDS cardiomyopathy. In experimental studies, carnitine administration reversed myopathic changes induced by zidovudine in vitro.[69,70]

Selenium deficiency has been suggested as a cause of cardiomyopathy in AIDS.[71] Analysis of autopsy samples showed that myocardial selenium content in AIDS was significantly reduced.[72] In one pediatric case, reversal of cardiomyopathy occurred after selenium supplementation.[73]

Global Left Ventricular Dysfunction in AIDS

A related entity described in the AIDS literature is acute global left ventricular dysfunction. Prospective evaluation of HIV-infected patients showed that this entity is not rare in the course of AIDS, is often fatal, and may be associated with active myocarditis.[74] Herskowitz and colleagues[75] showed a high rate of left ventricular dysfunction in HIV infection. A subgroup of those patients progressed to overt congestive heart failure. The pathologic findings were not completely described. Four of the seven patients used intravenous drugs which may itself cause left ventricular dysfunction. A study of 101 unselected HIV-infected patients (71 with AIDS) revealed a higher prevalence of echocardiographic abnormalities than in controls.[76]

Other Cardiotoxic Agents in AIDS That May Cause Cardiomyopathy

On an anecdotal basis, other therapeutic agents have been related to cardiomyopathy in AIDS, but the association has no experimental support. Foscarnet has caused reversible cardiac dysfunction in AIDS.[77] In three cases, interferon alfa therapy was associated with reversible cardiac dysfunction leading to cardiomyopathy.[78] Torsades de pointes ventricular tachycardia was a rare complication of pentamidine therapy for *P. carinii* pneumonia.[79,80]

Active Myocarditis in AIDS

Inflammatory heart disease in AIDS (myocarditis) receives continued attention,[81] but its pathogenesis and treatment remain speculative.[82] Myocarditis in AIDS was considered prevalent in some early reports, but this was not substantiated universally by all investigators who evaluated pathologic specimens. Variability in the reported prevalence of myocarditis in AIDS may have been due to inherent difficulties in separating AIDS risk behaviors in populations under review (particularly intravenous drug abusers) and the inherent prevalence of inflammatory lesions in the hearts irrespective of their AIDS status. Some investigators suggested that myocarditis in AIDS is multifactorial.[12] Myocarditis in AIDS may be related to "innocent bystander" destruction of cardiac myocytes, microvascular spasm with subsequent necrosis, or humorally mediated immune or autoimmune mechanisms of myocyte destruction with or without associated inflammation.

Prevalence of Myocarditis in AIDS

In a Scandinavian study of 60 consecutive autopsies of patients with AIDS, myocarditis was present in 42%, diffuse myocardial fibrosis in 67%, and dilatation and/or hypertrophy of the right ventricle in 38%. It was concluded that the prevalence of heart failure will increase in AIDS.[83] HIV-infected asymptomatic patients demonstrated cardiac abnormalities less commonly.[84] Investigators in southern California found a 74% prevalence of lymphocytic infiltrates of the myocardium.[85] Intravenous drug abuse was a prominent behavioral risk factor in that study population. In a recent review, 100 autopsies of patients with AIDS were reported from Puerto Rico. Almost all patients in that study had intravenous drug abuse as a behavioral risk factor, and pathologic changes in the heart were found in

32%. Histopathologically, myocarditis with mononuclear interstitial inflammation and necrosis was prominent. Opportunistic infections with *Histoplasma capsulatum*, *T. gondii*, *Mycobacterium tuberculosis*, cytomegalovirus, and *Cryptococcus* also were prominent.[86]

Interstitial inflammatory lesions are a prevalent and important histopathologic finding in the hearts of patients with AIDS. Reilly and colleagues[87] found that samples from 26 of 58 patients with AIDS satisfied the Dallas criteria for myocarditis and demonstrated clinical correlations of cardiac symptoms, including congestive heart failure and rhythm disturbances. A study that more closely resembled our previous one from Los Angeles[17] reported a prevalence of lymphocytic infiltrates of 34%.[88] In an autopsy series, the prevalence of myocardial inflammation was 52%.[89] Roldan and coworkers[90] found lymphocytic infiltrates and necrosis in 17 of 54 autopsies. In pediatric cases, Joshi and colleagues[91] demonstrated cardiomyopathy with small interstitial mononuclear infiltrates. It should be noted that benign small interstitial mononuclear infiltrates have been reported in cardiomyopathy of many causes[92] and their pathologic significance may be questioned.

Influence of Behavioral Risk

Since our initial studies were from a population consisting predominantly of gay men with AIDS who died of *P. carinii* pneumonia, *Mycobacterium avium-intracellulare*, or Kaposi's sarcoma, we found a lower prevalence of myocarditis in those samples. In the past, we suggested that different risk behaviors for the development of AIDS (such as intravenous drug abuse) may influence the pathologic changes found at autopsy.[13,15,17] Intravenous drug abuse is the second most common risk behavior associated with AIDS and accounts for 27% of reported AIDS cases (through 1989).[93] It is possible that such behavioral risk factors could also confound a casual relationship between AIDS and myocarditis per se. The relative contribution of AIDS and its inherent risk factors (such as intravenous drug abuse) must be addressed in studies that discriminate between multiple factors in the pathogenesis of AIDS myocarditis.[94] Other important elements (such as coronary artery disease or hypertension) can contribute to the development of heart failure in AIDS. The prevalence of idiopathic myocarditis and cardiomyopathy was higher in patients whose risk behavior was intravenous drug abuse.[51,95,96]

In a subsequent retrospective review of more than 500 histologic sections of myocardium,[17] focal microscopic interstitial mononuclear infiltrates were found in 16% of cases (from the UCLA archives). Although the inflammatory lesions were more commonly observed than was originally appreciated,[13] they were not widespread.[15] Generous sampling was required for their detection. Moreover, the inflammatory lesions observed in the UCLA series.[15] did not fit diagnostic criteria for active myocarditis.[97] It is possible that our adherence to strict criteria for diagnosing active myocarditis resulted in a lower prevalence. Repeated blinded review yielded essentially identical results.

Histopathological Changes of Inflammation in the Hearts of Patients With AIDS

Histopathologically, the interstitial inflammatory infiltrates were composed of mixtures of lymphocytes and plasma cells (Figure 16-3). Extensive scanning of microscopic fields was required to identify the small, usually isolated, and occasionally subendocardial lesions. Interstitial myocardial infiltrates did not correlate with the presence of other important gross pathologic findings that suggested myocardial disease in AIDS. Neither cardiomyopathy nor active myocarditis was diagnosed grossly at autopsy in cases where infiltrates were found subsequently on microscopic examination.

Cardiac Malignancies

Primary and metastatic tumors of the heart are relatively uncommon,[98] but the advent of AIDS changed both their prevalence and their appreciation in some ways.

Kaposi's Sarcoma Involving the Heart in AIDS

Kaposi's sarcoma involving the heart was relatively rare before the AIDS epidemic.[99] In a series of 565 autopsies of patients with AIDS, 1% had Kaposi's sarcoma involvement of the heart.[100] Early in the epidemic, we reported Kaposi's sarcoma involvement of the heart and epicardial blood vessels,[13] and Kaposi's sarcoma of the heart has been

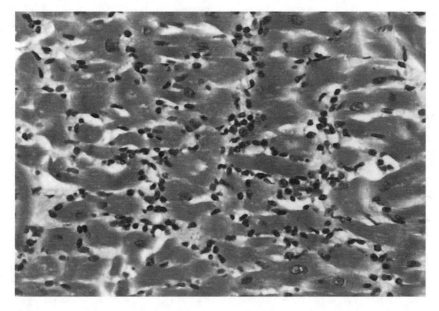

Figure 16-3. Mononuclear interstitial infiltrates. Zones of mononuclear inflammation were found in a number of cases, but not as frequently as described in other series. The infiltrates were frequently isolated and small. (Hematoxylin and eosin; ×1,000.)

reviewed editorially[101] and as part of a large series of Kaposi's sarcoma cases in which 2 of 47 autopsies of patients with Kaposi's sarcoma revealed cardiac involvement.[102] A relation between cardiac disease and AIDS was first suggested in the case of a Haitian woman with AIDS combined with cardiac Kaposi's sarcoma and Whipple's disease.[103] Since then, many investigators have examined cardiac involvement in AIDS-related Kaposi's sarcoma.[13,15,104–107]

The apparent prevalence of cardiac Kaposi's sarcoma has decreased in our autopsy population since the report of Cammarosano and Lewis.[13] In contrast to the earlier reported cases, none of the newer cases showed invasion of the epicardial coronary arteries by Kaposi's sarcoma. This latter point is concordant with the findings of Silver and colleagues.[105] It also is possible that this apparent change in the biology of cardiac Kaposi's sarcoma may relate to more effective use of antiretroviral therapy or other chemotherapeutic measures.

Treatment of Kaposi's sarcoma with daunorubicin, doxorubicin, or related anthracyclines may also affect the development of cardiomyopathy in AIDS and make the diagnosis of AIDS cardiomyopathy more difficult because of the known cardiotoxicity of anthracyclines. Liposomal encapsulated daunorubicin had an improved pharmacokinetic profile compared with free daunorubicin in patients with Kaposi's sarcoma and AIDS.[108,109] Other anthracycline regimens produced a less significant response.[110]

Cardiac Lymphoma

Malignant lymphoma of the heart is extremely rare but is found relatively frequently in patients with AIDS.[111–113] Two of 21 cases of diffuse large-cell cleaved lymphoma involved the myocardium.[18] Lymphoma should be considered in patients with AIDS whose cardiovascular symptoms progress rapidly.[114] Our previous autopsy experience suggested that cardiac lymphoma in AIDS is rare.[13,15,17] In one case, surgical resection of a right atrial lymphoma in AIDS was reported,[115] but the patient died of AIDS after 8 months. Primary lymphoma involving the heart alone is rare in AIDS.[116,117]

Endocardial Diseases

Endocarditis is the principal endocardial lesion identified pathologically in AIDS. Both infectious and noninfectious endocarditis have been described. At present, the prevalence of these lesions at autopsy appears lower than originally reported.[13] Nonetheless, they cause significant morbidity.

Noninfective Endocarditis (Nonbacterial Thrombotic Endocarditis)

An early case of nonbacterial thrombotic endocarditis appeared in 1983[118] and was described in autopsy series.[119] At UCLA, six cases were found in total (including cases described in our earlier studies).[13] One patient had lesions on all four valves, one had lesions on the tricuspid and pulmonary valves, and one had lesions only on the mitral valve. Systemic embolization (possibly from the valvular vegetations) was believed to contribute to morbidity and mortality. In one case, an isolated tricuspid valve vegetation was believed to be infected, but neither bacterial colonies nor tissue reaction could be identified histopathologically, and the case was included in the nonbacterial thrombotic endocarditis group.

Infective Endocarditis

In surgery for infective endocarditis in AIDS from intravenous drug abuse, lymphopenia from cardiopulmonary bypass was not associated with AIDS progression.[120,121] A poor prognosis was related to the factors in patients with intravenous drug abuse. As a precaution for all personnel involved in surgery, safe strategies and improved handling of instruments are stressed.[122]

A solitary case of documented infective endocarditis was found in one of our earlier studies[13] (Figure 16-4). In that case, heaped-up fibrinous vegetations were present on the mitral valve. Microscopic examination revealed clumps and chains of gram-positive cocci deep in the matrix of the fibrinous vegetations without destruction. The finding was consistent with clinical evidence of *Streptococcus viridans* bacteremia. The AIDS risk factors in that

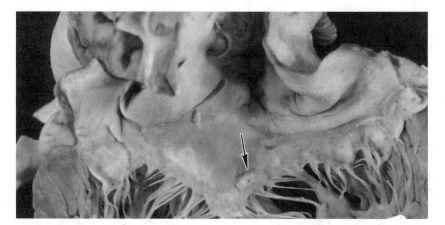

Figure 16-4.   Infective endocarditis in AIDS. Mitral valve vegetation showing platelet-fibrin mesh on endocardium (*arrow*). Gram-positive cocci in chains and clumps were present histopathologically.

case was homosexuality; there was no history of intravenous drug abuse.

Myocardial Abscess

Myocardial abscess is addressed separately because of a suggested pathogenetic relation to infective endocarditis, but no clear link between the lesions has been established. We have found two cases. In one case in our UCLA series, a large left ventricular abscess with myocardial liquefactive necrosis was found. Gram-positive cocci were present in clumps (consistent with *Staphylococcus* specifies) (Figure 16-5). A second case came from the University of Cincinnati. The pathogenesis of the

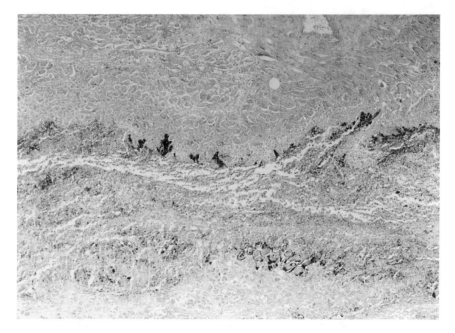

Figure 16-5.   Abscess of left ventricle. Zone of liquefactive necrosis of myocardium in the left ventricle. (Hematoxylin and eosin; ×100.)

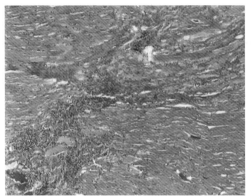

Figure 20-1, page 303

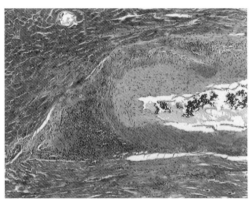

Figure 20-2, page 304

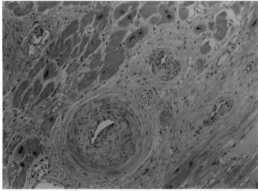

Figure 20-3, page 304

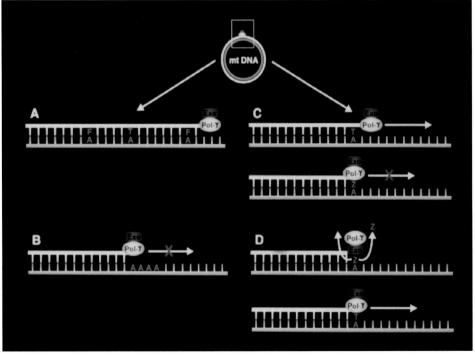

Figure 22-1, page 319

signal for HIV in medium-sized arterial endothelium from the myocardium of patients with AIDS (W. Lewis and W. W. Grody, unpublished observations). This finding served as an internal control, since endothelial cells are susceptible to infection by HIV. Our findings were independently confirmed or supported by other groups, using both in situ hybridization and other methods.[136–139] In one study of autopsies, in situ hybridization failed to show an HIV signal in the myocardium of patients with AIDS.[140]

Evidence of cardiac HIV infection was based on isolation and cultivation of HIV from an endomyocardial biopsy from a patient with AIDS and cardiomyopathy,[138] by detection of nucleic acid sequences of extracted DNA using the polymerase chain reaction and Southern blotting,[139] or by individually isolating cardiac myocytes by microdissection and polymerase chain reaction amplification of HIV sequences and Southern blotting.[137] Calabrese and colleagues[138] correctly raised the possibility that the positive culture results were caused by contamination of the heart biopsy specimen with HIV possibly from the patients' infected blood. Similarly, polymerase chain reaction amplification of a sample contaminated with as little as one HIV sequence (hypothetically) can yield artifacts that render interpretation of the data difficult.

As suggested previously, it is possible that the profoundly unbalanced immune function in AIDS[141] may give rise to clinical (or subclinical) myocarditis (see above). A viral cardiac infection in AIDS could account for the development of myocarditis and ultimately lead to the development of AIDS cardiomyopathy. If HIV were the etiologic infectious agent in the development of myocarditis in AIDS, various strains of HIV could exhibit different propensities of myocardial infectivity, but this had yet to be proven from clinical data. Different infectivities of HIV strains have been reported in studies on other tissues.[142] We determined that skeletal muscle samples from patients with AIDS revealed no diagnostic hybridization signals for HIV.

Cardiac Opportunistic Infections

Postmortem confirmation of the presence of a variety of opportunistic infections of the heart in patients with AIDS has been documented for the pericardium, myocardium, and endocardium. The infectious agents included *T. gondii* in the hearts of both adults and children,[23,143–145] *Cryptococcus* species,[14] cytomegalovirus,[119,146,147] *Candida* species,[15] disseminated *P. carinii* involving the myocardium,[17,148] atypical mycobacterium,[149] and others.

Fungal and Yeast Infections

Disseminated *Cryptococcus* and disseminated *Candida* were found in two cases each in our autopsy studies from UCLA (Figures 16-7 and 16-8).[13–15] Frequently, there was little gross evidence of myocardial involvement. In those cases, infection was widely disseminated, and finding focal myocyte necrosis was consistent with that illness. *Cryptococcus* infection is almost uniformly lethal in AIDS. Only *P. carinii* pneumonia, cytomegalovirus, and *Mycobacterium avium-intracellulare* cause higher mortality.[150]

Myocardial involvement with *Aspergillus* organisms in AIDS has been reported.[151,152] Five cases of pulmonary aspergillosis were reported, and no cardiac involvement occurred.[119] Aspergillosis was not documented at UCLA.[15,17] However, 5 of 37 cases of AIDS with invasive aspergillosis had documented cardiac involvement.[153] Pericarditis from *Nocardia asteroides* has been reported.[154,155] In one referred case, multiple small intramyocardial abscesses were found with irregular brown-black borders and necrotic yellow centers (Figure 16-9).

Myocbacterial Infection, Including *Mycobacterium Avium-Intracellulare* Infection of the Heart

Despite previous findings of disseminated *Mycobacterium avium-intracellulare* infection by other investigators,[149] and extensive histopathologic searches by us in the past, we were unable to document *M. avium-intracellulare* infection of the myocardium. *M. avium-intracellulare* has been shown to disseminate to the liver, spleen, and lymph nodes, and this is concordant with findings at UCLA (W. Lewis, unpublished observations). *M. tuberculosis*

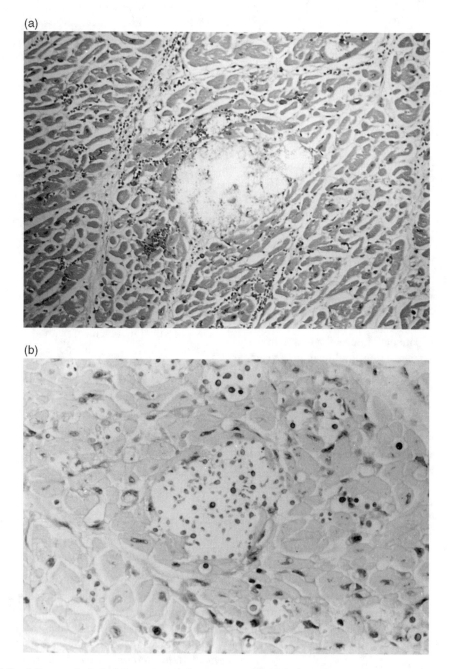

Figure 16-7. Microscopic foci of disseminated *Cryptococcus*. Multiple foci of necrotic myocytes are seen. Inflammation is minimal. Special stains reveal organisms (*arrow*) present within necrotic zones. **A**: Hematoxylin and eosin; ×400. **B**: Periodic acid-Schiff; ×1,000.

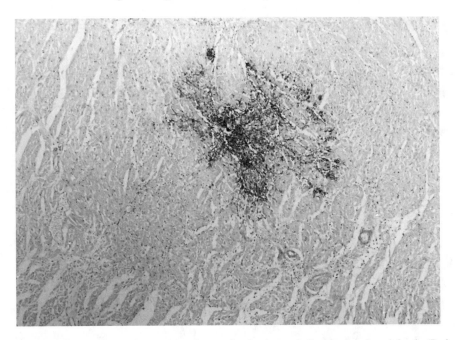

Figure 16-8. Microscopic focus of *Candida* abscess in the heart. Inflammation is minimal. (Periodic acid-Schiff; ×100.)

pericarditis in AIDS has been reported as well[113] and may become more prevalent.

Disseminated Infection With *Pneumocystis carinii*

Disseminated *P. carinii* has been reported to involve multiple organs.[156] We have found two cases of disseminated *P. carinii* infection (Figure 16-10). One showed intramyocardial lesions that consisted of multifocal microscopic zones of myocyte necrosis within dense matrix. Confirmation of authentic *P. carinii* was made both immunohistochemically and with modified Gomori methenamine silver stain. No inflammatory reaction or repair response was noted. Data from others support our previous findings[148,157] and help to emphasize the importance of *P. carinii* as a pathogen in the heart in AIDS.

Viral Opportunistic Pathogens

Evidence indirectly supported coninfection of the heart with *Herpesvirus viridiae* in AIDS. Early evidence suggested that serum antibodies against cytomegalovirus antigens were prominent in homosexual patients with AIDS.[158] Cytomegalovirus and herpes simplex virus were shown to be potentially important in the pathogenesis of Kaposi's sarcoma[159] and other vascular lesions. Herpes simplex virus was a pericardial pathogen in AIDS.[160] Cytomegalovirus inclusion bodies in cardiac myocytes have been reported. Investigators found the prevalence of cytomegalovirus infection in AIDS to be as high as 77% without clear definition of the anatomic site of the infection.[119] An autopsy case study of sudden death in an infant with AIDS documented disseminated cytomegalovirus and pancarditis.[161]

Using in situ DNA hybridization techniques, we examined 30 samples from 27 cases of AIDS with a cytomegalovirus-specific probe. Additionally, 16 samples (from 15 AIDS cases) were probed with a cDNA probe specific for herpes simplex virus. No positive hybridization signal was observed in either case. In our experience, and with the group of viruses examined, HIV was more easily identified in the heart by in situ hybridization than cyto-

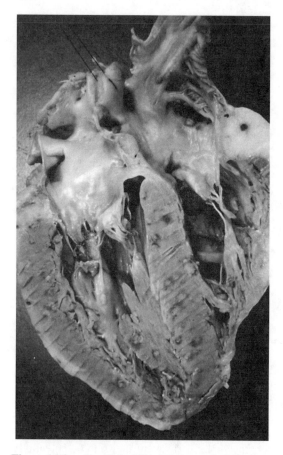

Figure 16-9. (See Color Plate 1 for image in full color.) Myocardial involvement by *Aspergillus*. Cut section reveals multiple irregular abscesses with pole centers and dark borders.

megalovirus or herpes simplex virus. By contrast, in one study, 6 of 12 biopsy samples demonstrated signal for the cytomegalovirus immediate early gene by in situ hybridization.[162]

Toxoplasmosis of the Heart

T. gondii myocarditis was described early in the AIDS epidemic. Cardiac involvement with *T. gondii* has been reported and demonstrated both by endomyocardial biopsy[163] and post mortem. In the latter study, the endemic risk may have been amplified, since the population involved was from Miami and Haitian immigrants were included. One case of toxoplasmosis involving the heart in a 44-year-old homosexual was reported in an autopsy series

from Los Angeles.[164] A review of 182 autopsies of patients with AIDS from France revealed cardiac toxoplasmosis diagnosed at autopsy in 12% of cases. It was associated with encephalitis in 10%.[165] Other studies suggested a lower prevalence.[166] Although *T. gondii* causes central nervous system lesions in AIDS, 15% to 91% of postmortem cases show cardiac involvement.[167,168] Pathologically, the encysted organisms are found in the myocardium. Generally, the inflammatory response is minimal if the cysts are intact (Figure 16-11).

Other Parasitic Infections

Acute Chagas myocarditis in AIDS has been reported.[169] Pathologic findings from 23 patients with AIDS and Chagas disease included myocarditis in 30% of cases.[170]

We documented a single case of *Microsporidium* infection in the myocardium of one patient with AIDS.[17] The patient had no clear cardiovascular symptoms, and the disease was diagnosed at autopsy. The organism was present diffusely on sections of the left ventricular myocardium. No mononuclear infiltrate or eosinophilic infiltrate was present. Myocytes demonstrated vacuolar clearing of cytoplasm with organisms within the sarcoplasm. In routine samples of other tissues, the organism could not be identified. There was no known risk factor for the pathogen.

Summary

Cardiac lesions in the adult heart that are prevalent in AIDS-infected patients frequently may relate to opportunistic infections, neoplasm, or inflammation, and may cause significant morbidity and mortality. Myocarditis prevalence varies in different studies and may reflect demographic or other factors of AIDS risk behavior. Heart failure in AIDS may relate to antecedent myocarditis or other factors in AIDS patients. Further detailed clinical and basic science studies may help clarify pathogenetic and pathophysiologic mechanisms of heart disease in AIDS.

(a)

(b)

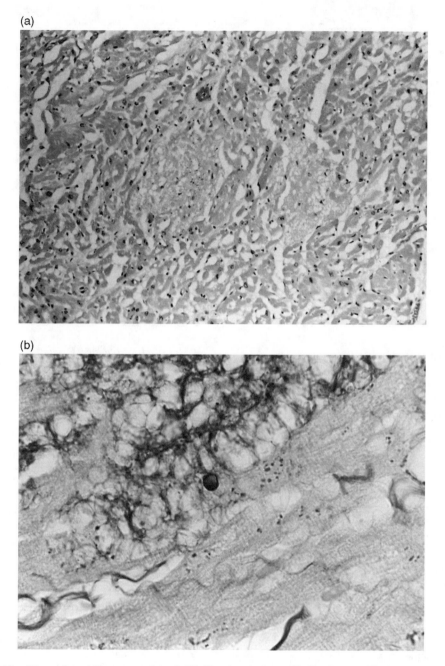

Figure 16-10.   Disseminated *Pneumocystis carinii* infiltrating the heart. Fluffy glycosaminoglycan matrix separates groups of myocytes. Organisms (*arrow*) are found within the fluffy material when stained with silver methenamine. The patient was found to have disseminated *P. carinii* in many organs sampled at autopsy. **A:** Hematoxylin and eosin; ×400. **B:** Silver methenamine; ×1000.

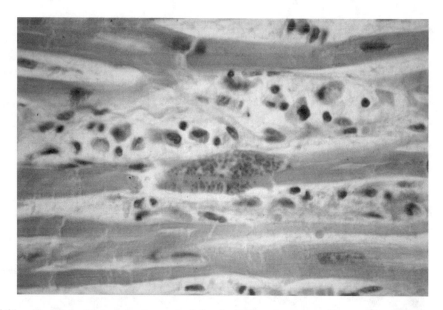

Figure 16-11. (See Color Plate 1 for image in full color.) *Toxoplasma gondii* cyst in myocardium. Interstitial inflammation with mononuclear cells is present. Encysted organisms are present with cardiac myocyte. (Hematoxylin and eosin; ×1,000.) (Courtesy of Dr. Gallo and Dr. d'Amati, LaSapienza, Rome.)

References

1. Centers for Disease Control . A cluster of Kaposi's sarcoma and *Pneumocystis carinii* pneumonia among homosexual male residents of Los Angeles and Orange counties, California. *MMWR* 1982; 31:305–307.

2. Gottlieb MS, Schroff R, Schanker HE, et al. *Pneumocystis carinii* pneumonia and mucosal candidiasis in previously healthy homosexual men. *N Engl J Med* 1981;305:1425–1431.

3. Rosenberg PS. Scope of the AIDS epidemic in the United States. *Science* 1995;270:1372–1375.

4. Masur H, Falloon J, Polis M, et al. Infectious complications of HIV. In: DeVita VT, Hellman S, Rosenberg SA. (eds). *AIDS: Etiology, Diagnosis, Treatment, and Prevention.* Philadelphia: JB Lippincott, 1992:157–209.

5. Safai B, Schwartz JJ. Kaposi's sarcoma and the acquired immunodeficiency syndrome. In: DeVita VT, Hellman S, Rosenberg SA (eds). *AIDS: Etiology, Diagnosis, Treatment, and Prevention.* Philadelphia: JB Lippincott, 1992:209–229.

6. Grunfeld C. What causes wasting in AIDS? *N Engl J Med* 1995;333:123–124.

7. Levine AM. Lymphoma and other miscellaneous cancer. In: DeVita VT, Hellman S, Rosenberg SA (eds). *AIDS: Etiology, Diagnosis, Treatment, and Prevention.* Philadelphia: JB Lippincott, 1992: 225–236.

8. Cotton P. AIDS giving rise to cardiac problems. *JAMA* 1990;263:2149.

9. Currie PF, Boon NA. Cardiac involvement in human immunodeficiency virus infection. *Q J Med* 1993;86:751–753.

10. Hsia JA, McQuinn LB. AIDS cardiomyopathy. *Res Staff Physician* 1993;39:21–24.

11. Jacob AJ, Boon NA. HIV cardiomyopathy: a dark cloud with a silver lining. *Br Heart J* 1991;66:1–2.

12. Anderson DW, Virmani R. Emerging patterns of heart disease in human immunodeficiency virus infection. *Hum Pathol* 1990;21:253–259.

13. Cammarosano C, Lewis W. Cardiac lesions in acquired immune deficiency syndrome (AIDS). *J Am Coll Cardiol* 1985;5:703–706.

14. Lewis W, Lipsick J, Cammarosano C. Cryptococcal myocarditis in acquired immune deficiency syndrome. *Am J Cardiol* 1985;55:1238–1239.

15. Lewis W. AIDS: cardiac findings from 115 autopsies. *Prog Cardiovasc Dis* 1989;32:207–215.

16. Grody WW, Cheng L, Lewis W. Infection of the heart by the human immunodeficiency virus. *Am J Cardiol* 1990;66:203–206.

17. Lewis W, Grody WW. AIDS and the heart: review and consideration of pathogenetic mechanisms. *Cardiovasc Pathol* 1992;1:53–64.

18. Hui AN, Koss MN, Meyer PR. Necropsy findings in acquired immunodeficiency syndrome: a comparison of premortem diagnoses with post-mortem findings. *Hum Pathol* 1984;15:670–676.

19. Welch K, Finkbeiner W, Alpers CE, et al. Autopsy findings in the acquired immune deficiency syndrome. *JAMA* 1984;252:1152–1159.

20. Acierno LJ. Cardiac complications in acquired immunodeficiency syndrome (AIDS): a review. *J Am Coll Cardiol* 1989;13:1144–1154.

21. Francis CK. Cardiac involvement in AIDS. In: O'Rourke RA, McCall D, Beller GA, et al. (eds). *Current Problems in Cardiology.* St. Louis: Mosby-Year Book, 1990:571–639.

22. Bestetti RB. Cardiac involvement in the acquired immune deficiency syndrome. *Int J Cardiol* 1989; 22:143–146.

23. Guarda LA, Luna MA, Smith LJ, et al. Acquired immune deficiency syndrome: postmortem findings. *Am J Clin Pathol* 1984;81:549–557.

24. Reichert CM, O'Leary TJ, Levens DL, et al. Autopsy pathology in the acquired immune deficiency syndrome. *Am J Pathol* 1983;112:357–382.

25. Grody WW, Fligiel S, Naiem F. Thymus involution in the acquired immunodeficiency syndrome. *Am J Clin Pathol* 1985;84:85–95.

26. Cusi MV, Lewis W. Cardiac changes in women with AIDS. *Mod Pathol* 1994;7:27A.

27. Dasco CC. Diseases of the pericardium. *Cardiol Clin* 1990;8:697–699.

28. Hsia J, Ross AM. Pericardial effusion and pericardiocentesis in human immunodeficiency virus infection. *Am J Cardiol* 1994;74:94–96.

29. Heidenreich PA, Eisenberg MJ, Kee L. Pericardial effusion in HIV positive patients: incidence and survival. [Abstract]. *J Am Soc Echocardiogr* 1993; 6:S19.

30. Akhras F, Dubrey S, Gazzard B, Noble MIM. Emerging patterns of heart disease in HIV infected homosexual subjects with and without opportunistic infections: a prospective colour flow Doppler echocardiographic study. *Eur Heart J* 1994; 15:68–75.

31. Eisenberg MJ, Gordon AS, Schiller NB. HIV associated pericardial effusions. *Chest* 1992;102: 956–958.

32. Cegielski JP, Ramaiya K, Lallinger GJ, et al. Pericardial disease and human immunodeficiency virus in Dar es Salaam, Tanzania. *Lancet* 1990; 335:209–212.

33. Serrano-Heranz R, Camino A, Vilacosta I, et al. Tuberculous cardiac tamponade and AIDS. *Eur Heart J* 1995;16:430–432.

34. Moskowitz LB, Kory P, Chan JC, et al. Unusual causes of death in Haitians residing in Miami. *JAMA* 1983;250:1187–1191.

35. Reynolds MM, Hecht SR, Berger M, et al. Large pericardial effusions in the acquired immnodeficiency syndrome. *Chest* 1992;102:1746–1747.

36. Woods GL, Goldsmith JC. Fatal pericarditis due to *Mycobacterium avium-intracellulare* in acquired immunodeficiency syndrome. *Mod Pathol* 1990; 3:625–630.

37. Choo PS, McCormack JG. *Mycobacterium avium:* a potentially treatable cause of pericardial effusions. *J Infect* 1995;30:55–58.

38. Guerot E, Aissa F, Kayal S, et al. Toxoplasma pericarditis in acquired immunodeficiency syndrome. *Intens Care Med* 1995;21:229–230.

39. Kwan T, Karve MM, Emerole O. Cardiac tamponade in patients infected with HIV: a report from an inner city hospital. *Chest* 1993;104:1059–1062.

40. Karve MM, Murali MR, Shah HM, Phelps KR. Rapid evoluation of cardiac tamponade due to bacterial pericarditis in two patients with HIV-1 infection. *Chest* 1992;101:1461–1463.

41. Stotka JL, Good CB, Downer WR, Kapoor WN. Pericardial effusion and tamponade due to Kaposi's sarcoma in acquired immunodeficiency syndrome. *Chest* 1989;951:1359–1361.

42. Turco M, Seneff M, McGrath BJ, Hsia J. Cardiac tamponade in the acquired immunodeficiency syndrome. *Am Heart J* 1990;120:1467–1468.

43. Aboulafia DM, Bush R, Picozzi VJ. Cardiac tamponade due to primary pericardial lymphoma in a patient with AIDS. *Chest* 1994;106:1295–1299.

44. Mast HL, Haller JO, Schiller MS, Anderson VM. Pericardial effusion and its relationship to cardiac disease in children with acquired immunodeficiency syndrome. *Pediatr Radiol* 1992;22:548–551.

45. Cohen IS, Anderson DW, Virmani R, et al. Congestive cardiomyopathy in association with the acquired immunodeficiency syndrome. *N Engl J Med* 1986;315:628–630.

46. Corboy JR, Fink L, Miller T. Congestive cardiomyopathy in association with AIDS. *Radiology* 1987;16:139–141.

47. De Palo VA, Millstein BH, Mayo PH, et al. Outcome of intensive care in patients with HIV infection. *Chest* 1995;107:506–510.

48. Blanchard DG, Hagenhoff C, Chow LC, et al. Reversibility of cardiac abnormalities in human immunodeficiency virus (HIV)-infected individuals: a serial echocardiographic study. *J Am Coll Cardiol* 1991;17:1270–1276.

49. Jacob AJ, Sutherland GR, Bird AG, et al. Myocardial dysfunction in patients infected with HIV: prevalence and risk factors. *Br Heart J* 1992; 68:549–553.

50. Jacob AJ, Sutherland GR, Boon NA, Ludian CA. Dilated cardiomyopathy in haemophiliacs infected with the human immunodeficiency virus. *Scott Med J* 1993;38:112–113.

51. van Hoeven KH, Segal B, Factor SM. AIDS cardiomyopathy: first rule out other myocardial risk factors. *Int J Cardiol* 1990;29:35–37.

52. Kasper EK, Agema WRP, Hutchins GM, et al. The causes of dilated cardiomyopathy: a clinicopathologic review of 673 consecutive patients. *J Am Coll Cardiol* 1994;23:586–590.

53. Kaminski HJ, Katzman M, Wiest PM, et al. Cardiomyopathy associated with the acquired immune deficiency syndrome. *J Acquir Immune Defic Syndr* 1988;1:105–110.

54. Leidig GA. Clinical, echocardiographic, and electrocardiographic resolution of HIV-related cardiomyopathy. *Mil Med* 1991;156:260–261.

55. Hecht SR, Berger M, Van Tosh A, Croxson S. Unsuspected cardiac abnormalities in the acquired immune deficiency syndrome: an echocardiographic study. *Chest* 1989;96:805–808.

56. Lewis W, Papoian T, Gonzalez B, et al. Mitochondrial ultrastructural and molecular changes induced by zidovudine in rat hearts. *Lab Invest* 1991; 65:228–236.

57. Lewis W, Gonzalez B, Chomyn A, Papoian T. Zidovudine induces molecular, biochemical, and ultrastructural changes in rat skeletal muscle mitochondira. *J Clin Invest* 1992;89:1354–1360.

58. Lewis W, Simpson JF, Meyer RR. Cardiac mitochondrial DNA polymerase-γ is inhibited competitively and noncompetitively by phosphorylated zidovudine. *Circ Res* 1994;74:344–348.

59. Lewis W, Meyer RR, Simpson JF, et al. Mammalian DNA polymerases, α, β, γ, δ, and ε incorporate fialuridine (FIAU) monophosphate into DNA

and are inhibited competitively by FIAU trisphosphate. *Biochemistry* 1994;33:14620–14624.

60. Lewis W, Levine ES, Griniuviene B, et al. Fialuridine and its metabolites inhibit DNA polymerase-γ at sites of multiple adjacent analog incorporation, decrease mtDNA abundance, and cause mitochondrial structural defects in cultured hepatoblasts. *Proc Natl Acad Sci USA* 1996;93:3592–3597.

61. Lewis W, Dalakas MC. Mitochondrial toxicity of antiviral drugs. *Nature Med* 1995;1:417–422.

62. Herskowitz A, Willoughby SB, Baughman KL, et al. Cardiomyopathy associated with antiretroviral therapy in patients with HIV infection: a report of six cases. *Ann Intern Med* 1992;116:311–313.

63. D'Amati G, Kwan W, Lewis W. Dilated cardiomyopathy in a zidovudine-treated AIDS patient. *Cardiovasc Pathol* 1992;1:317–320.

64. Koehler A, Lewis W. Mitochondrial cardiomyopathy in HIV patients with zidovudine. [Abstract]. *Lab Invest* 1995;72:33A.

65. Lipshultz SE, Orav EJ, Sanders SP, et al. Cardiac structure and function in children with human immunodeficiency virus infection treated with Zidovudine. *N Engl J Med* 1992;327:1260–1265.

66. Lewis W, Dorn G,II. Cardiac structure and function in HIV-infected children. *N Engl J Med* 1993;328:513–514.

67. Jay C, Dalakas MC. Myopathies and neuropathies in HIV-infected adults and children. In: Pizzo P, Wilfert CM (eds). *Pediatric AIDS*. Baltimore: Williams & Wilkins, 1994:559–573.

68. Domanski MJ, Sloas MM, Follmann DA, et al. Effect of zidovudine and didanosine treatment on heart function in children infected with human immunodeficiency virus. *J Pediatr* 1995;127: 137–146.

69. De Simone C, Tzantzoglou S, Jirillo E, et al. L-Carnitine deficiency in AIDS patients. *AIDS* 1992;6:203–205.

70. Semino-Mora MC, Leon-Monzon ME, Dalakas MC. The effect of L-carnitine on the AZT-induced destruction of human myotubes. Part II: treatment with L-carnitine improves the AZT-induced changes and prevents further destruction. *Lab Invest* 1994;71:773–781.

71. Dworkin BM. Selenium deficiency in HIV infection and the acquired immunodeficiency syndrome (AIDS). *Chem Biol Interact* 1994;181:186.

72. Dworkin BM, Antonecchia PP, Smith F, et al. Reduced cardiac selenium content in the acquired

immunodeficiency syndrome. *J Parenter Enter Nutr* 1989;13:644–647.

73. Kavanaugh-McHugh AL, Ruff A, Perlman E, et al. Selenium deficiency and cardiomyopathy in acquired immunodeficiency syndrome. *J Parenter Enter Nutr* 1991;15:347–349.

74. DeCastro S, D'Amati G, Gallo P, et al. Frequency of development of acute global left ventricular dysfunction in human immunodeficiency virus infection. *J Am Coll Cardiol* 1994;24:1018–1024.

75. Herskowitz A, Vlahov D, Willoughby S, et al. Prevalence and incidence of left ventricular dysfunction in patients with human immunodeficiency virus infection. *Am J Cardiol* 1993;71:955–958.

76. Fong IW, Howard R, Elzawi A, et al. Cardiac involvement in human immunodeficiency virus-infected patients. *J Acquir Immune Defic Syndr* 1993;6:380–385.

77. Brown DL, Sather S, Cheitlin MD. Reversible cardiac dysfunction associated with foscarnet therapy for cytomegalovirus esophagitis in an AIDS patients. *Am Heart J* 1993;125:1439–1440.

78. Deyton LR, Walker RE, Kovacs JA, et al. Reversible cardiac dysfunction associated with interferon alfa therapy in AIDS patients with Kaposi's sarcoma. *N Engl J Med* 1989;321:1246–1249.

79. Stein KM, Haronian H, Mensah GA, et al. Ventricular tachycardia and torsades de pointes complicating pentamidine therapy of *Pneumocystis carinii* pneumonia in the acquired immunodeficiency syndrome. *Am J Cardiol* 1990;66:888–890.

80. Wharton JM, Demopulos PA, Goldschlager N. Torsade de pointes during administration of pentamidine isethionate. *Am J Med* 1987;83:571–576.

81. Levy WS, Barghese PJ, Anderson DW, et al. Myocarditis diagnosed by endomyocardial biopsy in human immunodeficiency virus infection wtih cardiac dysfunction. *Am J Cardiol* 1988;62:658–659.

82. Fisher LL, Fisher EA. Myocarditis associated with human immunodeficiency virus infection. *Primary Cardiol* 1990;16:49–60.

83. Hansen BF. Pathology of the heart in AIDS: a study of 60 consecutive autopsies. *APMIS* 1992;100:273–279.

84. Thuesen L, Moller A, Kristensen BO, Black F. Cardiac function in patients with human immunodeficiency virus infection and with no other active infections. *Dan Med Bull* 1994;41:197–198.

85. Klatt EC, Meyer PR. Pathology of the heart in acquired immunodeficiency syndrome (AIDS). *Arch Pathol* 1988;112:114.

86. Altieri PI, Climent C, Lazala G, et al. Opportunistic invasion of the heart in Hispanic patients with acquired immunodeficiency syndrome. *Am J Trop Med Hyg* 1994;51:56–59.

87. Reilly JM, Cunnion RE, Anderson DW, et al. Frequency of myocarditis, left ventricular dysfunction and ventricular tachycardia in the acquired immune deficiency syndrome. *Am J Cardiol* 1988;62:789–793.

88. Baroldi G, Corallo S, Moroni M, et al. Focal lymphocytic myocarditis in acquired immunodeficiency syndrome (AIDS): a correlative morphologic and clinical study in 26 consecutive fatal cases. *J Am Coll Cardiol* 1988;12:463–469.

89. Anderson DW, Virmani R, Reilly JM, et al. Prevalent myocarditis at necropsy in the acquired immunodeficiency syndrome. *J Am Coll Cardiol* 1988;11:792–799.

90. Roldan EO, Moskowitz L, Hensley GT. Pathology of the heart in acquired immunodeficiency syndrome. *Arch Pathol* 1987;111:943–946.

91. Joshi VV, Gadol C, Connor E, et al. Dilated cardiomyopathy in children with acquired immunodeficiency syndrome: a pathologic study of five cases. *Hum Pathol* 1988;19:69–73.

92. Tazelaar HD, Billingham ME. Leukocytic infiltrates in idiopathic dilated cardiomyopathy: a source of confusion with active myocarditis. *Am J Surg Pathol* 1986;10:405–412.

93. Stein MD. Medical complications of intravenous drug use. *J Gen Intern Med* 1990;5:249–257.

94. Turnicky RP, Goodin J, Smialek JE, et al. Incidental myocarditis with intravenous drug abuse: the pathology, immunopathology, and potential implications for human immunodeficiency virus-associated myocarditis. *Hum Pathol* 1992;23:138–143.

95. Factor SM. Acquired immune deficiency syndrome: the heart of the matter. *J Am Coll Cardiol* 1989;13:1037–1038.

96. Segal BH, Factor SM. Myocardial risk factors other than human immunodeficiency virus infection may contribute to histologic cardiomyopathic changes in acquired immune deficiency syndrome. *Mod Pathol* 1993;6:769–773.

97. Aretz HT, Billingham M, Edwards WD, et al. Myocarditis: a histopathologic definition and classification. *Am J Cardiovasc Pathol* 1986;1:3–14.

98. McAllister HA. Tumors of the heart and pericardium. In: Silver MD (ed). *Cardiovascular Pathology.* New York: Churchill Livingston, 1991:1297–1134.

99. Levinson DA, Semple Pd'A. Primary cardiac Kaposi's sarcoma. *Thorax* 1976;31:595–600.

100. Klatt EC, Nichols L, Noguchi TT. Evolving trends revealed by autopsies of patients with the acquired immunodeficiency syndrome. *Arch Pathol* 1994; 118:884–890.

101. Stotka JL. Cardiac Kaposi's sarcoma in a patient with acquired immunodeficiency syndrome. *NY State J Med* 1992;92:332–333.

102. Ioachim HL, Adsay V, Giancotti FR, et al. Kaposi's sarcoma of internal organs: a multiparameter study of 86 cases. *Cancer* 1995;75:1376–1385.

103. Autran BR, Gorin I, Leibowitz M, et al. AIDS in a Haitian woman with cardiac Kaposi's sarcoma and Whipple's disease. *Lancet* 1983;1:767–768.

104. Moskowitz L, Hensley GT, Chan JC, Adams K. Immediate causes of death in acquired immunodeficiency syndrome. *Arch Pathol* 1985;109: 735–738.

105. Silver MA, Macher AM, Reichert CM, et al. Cardiac involvement by Kaposi's sarcoma in acquired immune deficiency syndrome (AIDS). *Am J Cardiol* 1984;53:983–985.

106. Fink L, Reichek N, St John Sutton MG. Cardiac abnormalties in acquired immune deficiency syndrome. *Am J Cardiol* 1984;54:1161–1163.

107. Steigman CK, Anderson DW, Macher AM, et al. Fatal cardiac tamponade in acquired immunodeficiency syndrome with epicardial Kaposi's sarcoma. *Am Heart J* 1988;116:1105–1106.

108. Gill P, Espina BM, Muggia R, et al. Phase I/II clinical and pharmacokinetic evaluation of liposomal daunorubicin. *J Clin Oncol* 1995;13:996–1003.

109. Harrison M, Tomlinson D, Stewart S. Liposomal-entrapped doxorubicin: an active agent in AIDS-related Kaposi's sarcoma. *J Clin Oncol* 1995; 13:914–920.

110. Fischl MA, Krown SE, O'Boyle KP, et al. Weekly doxorubicin in the treatment of patients with AIDS-related Kaposi's sarcoma. *J Acquir Immune Defic Syndr* 1993;6:259–264.

111. Balasubramanyam A, Waxman M, Kazal HL, Lee MH. Malignant lymphoma of the heart in acquired immune deficiency syndrome. *Chest* 1986;90: 243–246.

112. Guarner J, Brynes RK, Chan WC, et al. Primary non-Hodgkin's lymphoma of the heart in two patients with the acquired immunodeficiency syndrome. *Arch Pathol* 1987;111:254–256.

113. D'Cruz IA, Sengupta EE, Abrahams C, et al. Cardiac involvement, including tuberculous pericardial effusion, complicating acquired immune deficiency syndrome. *Am Heart J* 1986;112: 1100–1102.

114. Holladay AO, Siegel RJ, Schwartz DA. Cardiac malignant lymphoma in acquired immune deficiency syndrome. *Cancer* 1992;70:2203–2207.

115. Horowitz MD, Cox MM, Neibart RM, et al. Resection of right atrial lymphoma in a patient with AIDS. *Int J Cardiol* 1992;34:139–142.

116. Constantino A, West TE, Gupta M, Loghmanee F. Primary cardiac lymphoma in a patient with acquired immune deficiency syndrome. *Cancer* 1987;60:2801–2805.

117. Goldfarb A, King CL, Rosenzweig BP, et al. Cardiac lymphoma in the acquired immunodeficiency syndrome. *Am Heart J* 1989;118:1340–1344.

118. Garcia I, Fainstein V, Rios A, et al. Nonbacterial thrombotic endocarditis in a male homosexual with Kaposi's sarcoma. *Arch Intern Med* 1983;143:1243–1244.

119. Niedt GW, Schinella RA. Acquired immunodeficiency syndrome: clinicopathologic study of 56 autopsies. *Arch Pathol* 1985;109:727–734.

120. Lemma M, Vanelli P, Botta BM, et al. Cardiac surgery in HIV-positive intravenous drug addicts: influence of cardiopulmonary bypass on the progression to AIDS. *Thorac Cardiovasc Surg* 1992; 40:279–282.

121. Cegielski JP, Lwakatare J, Dukes CS, et al. Tuberculous pericarditis in Tanzanian patients with and without HIV infection. *Tuber Lung Dis* 1994;75: 429–434.

122. Royle JP. AIDS and the vascular surgeon. *J Cardiovasc Surg* 1992;33:139–142.

123. Egan TM, Maitland A, Sinave C, et al. Myocardial abscess in a patient with AIDS-related complex: pericardial patch repair. *Ann Thorac Surg* 1990; 49:481–482.

124. Koenig S, Gendelman HE, Orenstein JM. Detection of AIDS virus in macrophages in brain tissues from AIDS patients with encephalopathy. *Science* 1986;233:1089–1093.

125. Feremans WW, Huygen K, Menu R, et al. Fifty cases of human immunodeficiency virus (HIV) infection: immunoultrastructural study of circulating lymphocytes. *J Clin Pathol* 1988;41:62–71.

126. Salahuddin SZ, Palestine A, Heck E, Ablashi D. Isolation of the human T-cell leukemia/lymphotropic virus type III from the cornea. *Am J Ophthalmol* 1986;101:149–152.

127. Wiley CA, Schrier RD, Nelson JA, et al. Cellular localization of human immunodeficiency virus infection within the brains of acquired immune deficiency syndrome patients. *Proc Natl Acad Sci USA* 1986;83:7089–7093.

128. Rabeneck L, Popovic M, Gartner S, et al. Acute HIV infection presenting with painful swallowing and esophageal ulcers. *JAMA* 1990;263:2318–2322.

129. Bailey RO, Baltch AL, Venkatesh R, et al. Sensor motor neuropathy associated with AIDS. *Neurology* 1988;38:886–891.

130. Da Silva M, Shevchuk MM, Cronin WJ, et al. Detection of HIV-related protein in testes and prostates of patients with AIDS. *Am J Clin Pathol* 1990;93:196–201.

131. Hoda SA, Gerber MA. Immunohistochemical studies of human immunodeficiency virus type 1 (HIV 1) in liver tissues of patients with AIDS. [Abstract]. *Am J Clin Pathol* 1990;93:452.

132. Karlsson-Parra A, Dimeny E, Fellstom B, Klareskog L. HIV receptors (CD4 antigen) in normal human glomerular cells. *N Engl J Med* 1989;320:741.

133. Coudray N, De Zuttere D, Force G, et al. Left ventricular diastolic function in asymptomatic and symptomatic human immunodeficiency virus carriers: an echocardiographic study. *Eur Heart J* 1995;16:61–76.

134. Hsi D, Manders WT, Shannon RP. SIV in nonhuman primates causes myocardial injury and cardiomyopathy following chronic but not acute infection. [Abstract]. *Circulation* 1995;92:I471–1471.

135. Dittrich H, Chow L, Denaro F, Spector S. Human immunodeficiency virus, coxsackievirus, and cardiomyopathy. *Ann Intern Med* 1988;108:308–309.

136. Lipshultz S, Fox CH, Perez-Atayde AR, et al. Identification of human immunodeficiency virus–1 RNA and DNA in the heart of a child with cardiovascular abnormalities and congenital acquired immune deficiency syndrome. *Am J Cardiol* 1990;66:246–250.

137. Wu AY, Forouhar F, Cartan RW, et al. Identification of human immunodeficiency virus in the heart of a patient with acquired immunodeficiency syndrome. *Mod Pathol* 1990;3:625–630.

138. Calabrese LH, Proffitt M, Yen-Lieberman B, et al. Congestive cardiomyopathy and illness related to the acquired immunodeficiency syndrome (AIDS) associated with isolation of retrovirus from myocardium. *Ann Intern Med* 1987; 107: 691–692.

139. Flomenbaum M, Soeiro R, Udem SA, et al. Proliferative membranopathy and human immunodeficiency virus in AIDS hearts. *J Acquir Immune Defic Syndr* 1989;2:129–135.

140. Beschorner WE, Baughman K, Turnicky RP, et al. HIV-associated myocarditis: pathology and immunopathology. *Am J Pathol* 1990;137:1365–1371.

141. Pantaleo G, Graziosi C, Fauci SA. The immunopathogenesis of human immunodeficiency virus infection. *N Engl J Med* 1993;328:327–335.

142. Cheng–Mayer C, Seto D, Tateno M, Levy JA. Biologic features of HIV-1 that correlate with virulence in the host. *Science* 1988;240:80–82.

143. Medlock MD, Tilleli JT, Pearl GS. Congenital cardiac toxoplasmosis in a newborn with acquired immunodeficiency syndrome. *Pediatr Infect Dis J* 1990;9:129–132.

144. Adair OV, Randive N, Krashow N. Isolated toxoplasma myocarditis in acquired immune deficiency syndrome. *Am Heart J* 1989;118:856–857.

145. Tolat D, Kim HS. Toxoplasmosis of the brain and heart: autopsy report of a patient with AIDS. *Tex Med* 1989;85:40–42.

146. Schindler JM, Neftkel KA. Simultaneous primary infection with HIV and CMV leading to severe pancytopenia, hepatitis, nephritis, perimyocarditis, myositis and alopecia totalis. *Klin Wochenschr* 1990;15:237–240.

147. Scott PJ, Conway SP, Da Costa P. Cardiac tamponade complicating cytomegalovirus pericarditis in a patient with AIDS. *J Infect* 1990;20:92–93.

148. Ravalli S, Garcia RL, Vincent RA, Schein R. Disseminated *Pneumocystis carinii* infection in the acquired immunodeficiency syndrome. *NY State J Med* 1990;90:155–157.

149. Cantwell AR. Necroscopic findings of variably acid-fast bacteria in a fatal case of acquired immunodeficiency and Kaposi's sarcoma. *Growth* 1983; 47:129–134.

150. Zuger A, Louis E, Holzman RS, et al. Cryptococcal disease in patients with the acquired immunodeficiency syndrome. *Ann Intern Med* 1986;104:234–240.

151. Henochowicz S, Mustafa M, Lawinson WE, et al. Cardiac aspergillosis in acquired immune deficiency syndrome. *Am J Cardiol* 1985;55:1239–1240.

152. Cox JN, diDio F, Pizzolato GP, et al. Aspergillus endocarditis and myocarditis in a patient with the acquired immunodeficiency syndrome (AIDS): a review of the literature. *Virchows Arch* 1990;417:255–259.

153. Minamoto GY, Barlam TF, Vander Els NJ. Invasive aspergillosis in patients with AIDS. *Clin Infect Dis* 1992;14:66–74.

154. Joshi N. Nocardia asteroides pericarditis. *Mayo Clin Proc* 1990;6:1276.

155. Holtz MA, Lavery DP, Kapila R. Actinomycetes infection in the acquired immunodeficiency syndrome. *Ann Intern Med* 1985;102:203–205.

156. Cote RJ, Rosenblum M, Telzak EE, et al. Disseminated *Pneumocystis carinii* infection causing extrapulmonary organ failure: clinical, pathologic, and immunohistochemical analysis. *Mod Pathol* 1990;3:25–30.

157. Grimes MM, La Pook J, Bar M, et al. Disseminated *Pneumocystis carinii* infection in a patient with acquired immune deficiency syndrome. *Hum Pathol* 1987;17:307–308.

158. Drew WL, Conant MA, Miner RC, et al. Cytomegalovirus and Kaposi's sarcoma in young homosexual men. *Lancet* 1982;II:125–127.

159. Giraldo G, Beth E, Huang ES. Kaposi's sarcoma and its relationship to cytomegalovirus (CMV) III. CMV DNA and CMV early antigens in Kaposi's sarcoma. *Int J Cancer* 1980;26:23–29.

160. Freedberg RS, Gindea AJ, Dieterich DT, Greene JB. Herpes simplex pericarditis in AIDS. *NY State J Med* 1987;87:304–306.

161. Brady MT, Reiner CB, Singley C, et al. Unexpected death in an infant with AIDS: disseminated cytomegalovirus infection wtih pancarditis. *Pediatr Pathol* 1988;8:205–214.

162. Wu TC, Pizzorno MC, Hayward GS, et al. In situ detection of human cytomegalovirus immediate-early gene transcripts within cardiac myocytes of patients with HIV-associated cardiomyopathy. *AIDS* 1992;6:777–785.

163. Mullins RJ, Bastian B, Sutherland DC. AIDS and the heart. *NZ J Med* 1988;18:809–811.

164. Tschirhart D, Klatt EC. Disseminated toxoplasmosis in acquired immunodeficiency syndrome. *Arch Pathol Lab Med* 1988;112:1237–1241.

165. Hofman P, Bernard E, Michiels JF, et al. Extracerebral toxoplamosis in the acquired immunodeficiency syndrome (AIDS). *Pathol Res Pract* 1993;189:894–901.

166. Rabaud C, May T, Amiel C, et al. Extracerebral toxoplasmosis in patients infected with HIV. *Medicine* 1994;73:306–314.

167. Hofman P, Drici MD, Gibelin P, et al. Prevalence of toxoplasma myocarditis in patients with the acquired immunodeficiency syndrome. *Br Heart J* 1993;70:376–381.

168. Jautzke G, Sell M, Thalmann U, et al. Extracerebral toxoplasmosis in AIDS: histological and immunohistological findings based on 80 autopsy cases. *Pathol Res Pract* 1993;189:428–436.

169. Oddo D, Casanova M, Acuna G, et al. Acute Chagas disease (trypanosomiasis americana) in acquired immunodeficiency syndrome. *Hum Pathol* 1992;23:41–44.

170. Rocha A, DeMeneses ACO, DaSilva AM, et al. Pathology of patients with Chagas' disease and acquired immunodeficiency syndrome. *Am J Trop Med Hyg* 1994;50:261–268.

17

Cardiac Cancers in HIV-Infected Patients

Hal B. Jenson, M.D., and Brad H. Pollock, M.P.H., Ph.D.

Malignant tumors of the heart, defined as those involving the heart or the pericardium, are very infrequent and rarely diagnosed antemortem. Primary neoplasms of the heart are found in only 0.0017% to 0.28% of autopsies in the general population.[1,2] The most common primary cancers of the heart are soft-tissue sarcomas.[3] Nearly all neoplasms involving the heart are metastasic. The prevalence of metastatic cardiac involvement ranges from 1% to 26% for all cases of cancer and is largely dependent on the histology of the primary neoplasm. Cardiac metastases are most commonly associated with primary cancers of the lung and breast, lymphomas, and malignant melanomas.[4-7] The majority of patients with metastatic involvement of the heart lack cardiac symptoms; cardiac involvement is usually diagnosed only at autopsy.

More than 40% of patients with the acquired immunodeficiency syndrome (AIDS) develop cancer.[8] The development of tumors is a relatively late manifestation of human immunodeficiency virus (HIV) infection and likely reflects the multifactorial pathogenesis of these tumors. The incidence of three types of tumors has greatly increased in patients with HIV infection: Kaposi's sarcoma, non-Hodgkin's lymphoma (especially primary central nervous system lymphoma), and

leiomyosarcoma. The majority of cardiac cancers in patients with AIDS have been metastatic Kaposi's sarcoma, followed by metastatic lymphoma (Table 17-1). A few cases of primary cardiac Kaposi's sarcoma and primary cardiac lymphoma have been reported. These and the less common malignant tumors (e.g., germinal testicular tumors, cervical carcinomas, lung cancers, colorectal cancers, acute lymphoblastic leukemia, and chronic lymphocytic leukemia) of patients with AIDS are characterized by the relatively young age of the affected patients.[9]

Primary rhabdomyosarcoma of cardiac muscle tissue, the second most common primary sarcoma after angiosarcoma of the heart in non-HIV-infected patients, has not been reported in HIV-infected patients to date. The potential for primary tumors of muscle cell origin in patients with AIDS is indicated by the intriguingly high incidence of (noncardiac) leiomyosarcomas in young people with AIDS.[10–19] Leiomyosarcomas are rare malignant tumors of smooth muscle origin that occur at a rate of less than 2/10,000,000 in the normal population.[20] Muscle tumor cells have been demonstrated to harbor Epstein-Barr virus in leiomyosarcomas from HIV-infected patients[17,18] and in patients receiving immunosuppressive therapy for transplantation[21] or cancer treatment.[22] The finding of an increased number

Cardiology in AIDS

Table 17-1. Comparison of Cardiac Kaposi's Sarcoma and Cardiac Lymphoma in HIV-Infected Patients

Attribute	Kaposi's Sarcoma	Lymphoma
Incidence	Rare (400–500 times increased incidence in AIDS)	Rare (60–100 times increased incidence in AIDS)
Virus association		
Epstein-Barr virus	None	30%–40% of small noncleaved (Burkitt or Burkitt-like) lymphomas 75%–80% of large cell immunoblastic lymphomas Almost all central nervous system lymphomas
Human herpesvirus-8	100%	100% of body cavity-based lymphomas (e.g., of the pericardial, pleural, or abdominal cavities)
Pathogenesis	Usually metastatic, occasionally primary	Usually metastatic, occasionally primary
Anatomic location of cardiac involvement	Visceral subepicardial adipose tissue	Patchy nodules of the epicardium
Myocardial infiltration	Uncommon	Common; may result in progressive heart block
Associated pericardial effusion	Occasional	Usual
Malignant cells in pericardial fluid	No	Usual
Clinical symptoms		
Cardiac symptoms	Usually asymptomatic	Common
Conduction defects	No	Common
Overall prognosis	Poor	Poor

of Epstein-Barr virus receptors on smooth muscle cells in benign leiomyomas in patients with AIDS, together with the association of Epstein-Barr virus only with leiomyosarcoma, but not with leiomyoma, strongly suggests a direct role for Epstein-Barr virus in the development of these tumors.[17] There is no evidence that HIV is directly involved in the development of leiomyosarcoma in patients with AIDS, beyond the associated immunologic abnormalities related to impaired immune surveillance of cells that have undergone malignant transformation. Profound immunosuppression, including the immunosuppression associated with AIDS, may predispose smooth muscle cells to Epstein-Barr virus infection and development of these rare tumors. The possibility of Epstein-Barr virus and human herpesvirus-8 acting together as cofactors for the development of muscle tumors is suggested by the finding of concomitant infection in cell lines of Kaposi's sarcoma,[23,24] but human herpesvirus-8 has not been found in leiomyosarcomas in children with AIDS.[25]

Cardiac Kaposi's Sarcoma in AIDS

Various terms have been used as synonyms for Kaposi's sarcoma, including angiosarcoma.[26] Kaposi's sarcoma has been distinguished from angiosarcoma by the presence of cutaneous involvement with Kaposi's sarcoma.[27] Primary angiosarcoma and Kaposi's sarcoma involving the heart are extremely rare tumors.[3] A very few cases of primary Kaposi's sarcoma of the heart in patients without HIV infection have been reported.[26,28–32] Many cases termed angiosarcoma of the heart were characterized by localization to the atria, especially the right atrium.[32]

Numerous cases of Kaposi's sarcoma involving the heart have been reported in HIV-infected patients, which is not unexpected, since Kaposi's sarcoma is the most common cancer associated with AIDS.

Association With Human Herpesvirus-8

Human herpesvirus-8 was first identified in tissues from AIDS-associated cutaneous Kaposi's sarcoma.[33] Human herpesvirus-8 has been found by polymerase chain reaction amplification in more than 90% of Kaposi's sarcoma tissues from patients with AIDS[34–37] as well as in classical Kaposi's sarcoma occurring in otherwise healthy persons[34–36,38,39] and in non-Kaposi's sarcoma skin lesions of organ transplant recipients.[40] Seroconversion to human herpesvirus-8 seropositivity precedes the clinical appearance of Kaposi's sarcoma.[41] Human herpesvirus-8 has also been found in AIDS-associated[42] and non-AIDS-associated[43] body cavity-based lymphomas, also called primary effusion lymphoma, and in tissues from patients with Castleman's disease, a multicentric lymphoproliferative disease.[37] The role of human herpesvirus-8 in AIDS-associated cardiac tumors is linked to its role in the etiology of Kaposi's sarcoma and body cavity-based lymphoma, including lymphoma of the pericardium, rather than to isolated involvement of the heart specifically.

Pathology

Kaposi's sarcoma appears to have a predilection for subepicardial adipose tissue adjacent to a major coronary artery, with or without involvement of the adventitia of the ascending aorta or pulmonary trunk.[27,44–47] The tumor may encase the outflow tracts, usually without compression. The metastatic sarcomatous plaques and nodules are typically small and localized on the epicardial surface, and typically do not involve either the underlying myocardium or the overlying parietal pericardium, although concomitant myocardial involvement has been reported in one patient.[45] At autopsy the epicardial nodules appear violaceous. The histologic appearance of cardiac Kaposi's sarcoma is typical and is similar to that of Kaposi's sarcoma found in other anatomic sites.

Clinical Features

Kaposi's sarcoma of the heart in HIV-infected patients is usually an incidental finding at autopsy, with cardiac metastases in conjunction with widespread visceral, mucocutaneous, and gastrointestinal Kaposi's sarcoma.[27,44,45,48,49] Most cases of disseminated Kaposi's sarcoma do not involve the heart; Silver and colleagues[27] found cardiac involvement in only 5 of 18 (28%) HIV-infected patients with widespread Kaposi's sarcoma. A few primary cases of cardiac Kaposi's sarcoma (without involvement of other sites) have been reported.[46,48]

Specific clinical symptoms or signs of cardiac dysfunction are almost always lacking in patients with cardiac Kaposi's sarcoma. Symptoms are usually attributed to concomitant infection or respiratory involvement, with the diagnosis of cardiac Kaposi's sarcoma made only postmortem. Cardiac symptoms are more common if there is concomitant pericardial effusion. The electrocardiogram and chest radiograph are usually normal.[27]

Pericardial effusion with Kaposi's sarcoma usually reflects epicardial involvement, although most large pericardial effusions in patients with HIV infection are secondary to infection, frequently due to mycobacterial disease.[50] The pericardial effusion associated with Kaposi's sarcoma typically is of serosanguineous fluid with unremarkable chemistry results, yields negative culture results for infectious pathogens, lacks fibrosis or fibrin deposition, and does not demonstrate malignant cells by cytologic examination.[47,51,52] Antemortem diagnosis of cardiac Kaposi's sarcoma is infrequent but has been reported with pericardial effusion that may progress to cardiac tamponade.[47] Two-dimensional echocardiography is useful in delineating pericardial effusions and can also identify focal masses that may suggest the possibility of Kaposi's sarcoma.[53]

Treatment

There is little information on the specific therapy of cardiac Kaposi's sarcoma. Radiation therapy has been used, because the tumor is susceptible to this modality. Most patients with Kaposi's sarcoma involving the heart do not succumb directly to the cardiac tumor but to the opportunistic infections associated with advanced stages of AIDS.

Lymphoma

Primary lymphoma of the heart is extremely rare in otherwise healthy persons and constitutes only approximately 1.3% of primary cardiac neoplasms.[1] Fewer than 50 cases have been reported.[54–56] Metastatic involvement of the heart with lymphoma is up to 40 times more common than primary lymphoma of the heart but constitutes only 9% of all metastatic tumors of the heart.[1] Metastatic cardiac involvement occurs in up to 8% to 24% of non-HIV-infected patients with Hodgkin's or non-Hodgkin's lymphoma, with few demonstrating gross myocardial or endocardial involvement.[7,57,58] In most patients, the cardiac involvement is clinically silent and is found only at autopsy.

Lymphomas occur with greatly increased frequency in patients with primary immunodeficiency disorders and in patients with acquired immunodeficiency resulting from immunosuppression associated with HIV infection[59] or solid organ transplantation.[60] These tumors are characterized by aggressive growth, rapid progression, extranodal involvement, and poor response to therapy, with poor patient survival.

Association with Epstein-Barr Virus

Approximately 90% of lymphomas associated with HIV infection are high-grade B-lymphocyte lymphomas of small, noncleaved cell type (Burkitt or Burkitt-like) or of large-cell immunoblastic cell type.[61] Low-grade B-lymphocyte lymphomas, T-lymphocyte lymphomas, and Hodgkin's disease occur in patients with AIDS, but these tumors do not have increased incidence in patients with AIDS and are not considered AIDS-defining conditions.

Burkitt-like lymphomas characteristically appear early in the course of AIDS before severe impairment of immune function.[61,62] These lymphomas have reciprocal translocations characteristic of all Burkitt lymphomas at or near the site of the c-*myc* locus and have Epstein-Barr virus present

in approximately 30% to 40% of cases. They resemble classic Burkitt lymphomas histologically but have anatomic sites of presentation similar to the sporadic pattern, more frequently involving the abdomen rather than the jaw or orbit.

Immunoblastic lymphomas typically appear in the later stages of AIDS. These tumors are characterized by profound immunosuppression[62] and have many features in common with posttransplantation lymphoproliferative disorders.[60] Non-Hodgkin's lymphomas in patients with AIDS are highly aggressive compared with those in non-HIV-infected patients, and are characterized by multifocal distribution of disease, with metastatic invasion of organs that are not commonly associated with lymphoma. They have a poor response to chemotherapeutic or irradiation regimens used for lymphoma. Extranodal involvement at the time of presentation is found in approximately 80% to 90% of cases of lymphoma in patients with AIDS, compared with only approximately 40% of non-AIDS-related cases. The tumors histologically have a heterogeneous morphologic appearance, and some demonstrate immunophenotypic or genotypic evidence of oligoclonality or polyclonality.[63] Presentation in the central nervous system is common and is usually associated with Epstein-Barr virus. Approximately 75% of immunoblastic lymphomas presenting outside the central nervous system harbor Epstein-Barr virus.[64]

Epstein-Barr virus infection has not been associated with primary cardiac lymphomas in otherwise healthy persons. Ito and colleagues[65] report not finding Epstein-Barr virus using in situ hybridization and immunostaining of two primary cardiac lymphomas and five secondary cardiac B-lymphocyte lymphomas in immunocompetent patients.[65]

Pathology

Cardiac lymphomatous involvement in patients with AIDS is characterized by various pathologic patterns. The infiltration of either primary or secondary lymphoma of the heart appears most commonly as focal, circumscribed, whitish homogeneous nodules predominantly involving the pericardium, often extending into the myocardium, and occasionally involving the endocardium.[66-68] The myocardial lymphomatous infiltrates may be solitary or multiple discrete lesions, or may be diffuse with patchy lymphocytic cellular infiltrates. The myocardial and subendocardial extension of AIDS-associated cardiac lymphoma is distinctly unusual compared with cardiac lymphomas in non-AIDS patients.[7,57,58] The lymphomatous infiltration histologically demonstrates a coarse chromatin pattern, numerous typical and atypical mitotic figures, prominent, enlarged nucleoli, prominent nuclear membranes, and cellular polymorphism.[69] Extensive diffuse infiltration of the myocardium results in cardiomegaly and a pale-appearing heart.[70] Cardiac lymphoma has also been reported as a solitary tumor mass, sometimes characterized as multilobulated, that arises from the atrial or ventricular wall harboring lymphomatous tumor.[71-73] Valvular or arteriopathic lesions are not typical. The pericardium may be obliterated by fibrosis and fibrinous organization.[69]

The AIDS-associated body cavity-based lymphomas, also called primary effusion lymphomas, occur much less frequently than non-Hodgkin's lymphomas, and are distinguished by their growth in a body cavity (e.g., pleural, pericardial, or peritoneal cavity), without an identifiable solid tumor mass, and regular association with human herpesvirus-8,[42] even in non-HIV-infected patients.[43] Two of the eight body cavity-based lymphomas reported by Cesarman and coworkers[42] were of the pericardium. It is probable that many of the previously reported AIDS-associated lymphomas involving the pericardium also harbored human herpesvirus-8.

Clinical Features

Lymphoma in patients with AIDS is characterized by a higher frequency of involvement of the heart,[67,68,70,73-76] especially at the time of initial diagnosis.[67] Extranodal lymphoma can occur in virtually any body site as an isolated focus, although disseminated nodal and extranodal disease is much more common. Extranodal involvement is typically found in the gastrointestinal tract, with extensive involvement of the liver, kidney, and adrenal glands. In one large series of AIDS-related lymphoma, cardiac involvement occurred in only 1 of 90 patients.[66] Very few cases of cardiac lymphoma judged to be primary on the basis of the absence of lymphoma outside the heart have been reported in patients with AIDS.[68,69] Extracardiac sites, if present, may be more amenable to biopsy, although transvenous endocardial biopsy has been used for antemortem diagnosis of cardiac lymphoma.[72,73]

Patients with AIDS and cardiac lymphoma typically have no specific clinical symptoms of cardiac involvement. Early symptoms and findings may include gastrointestinal symptoms (e.g., nausea and abdominal pain), myocardial infarction (e.g., chest pain),[67] congestive heart failure, progressive or complete heart block, cardiac tamponade,[72,75,77] or superior vena cava syndrome.[67] Rapid progression of cardiac dysfunction to cardiac failure is common. The classic constitutional ("B") symptoms of lymphoma are present in approximately half of such patients and may be the only presenting symptoms.[67]

The electrocardiogram is usually abnormal and variably demonstrates ST- and T-wave changes, low voltage, and conduction abnormalities,[67,78,79] including complete atrioventricular block.[76] The two-dimensional echocardiogram is the most sensitive test for cardiac involvement. The most common finding is pericardial effusion, found to some extent in almost all patients, and thickened myocardium or luminal tumor masses, found in 50% to 75% of patients. The myocardium may appear speckled, with disseminated nodular areas, producing heterogeneous echogenicity.[73,80] Intravenous gadolinium injection can improve the contrast between tumor infiltration and normal myocardium.[79] Hypokinesia, akinesia/dyskinesia, and right ventricular hypertrophy are also occasionally found. Intense infiltration of the myocardium may be evident by two-dimensional echocardiography.[80] The pericardial effusion typically harbors malignant cells, facilitating definitive diagnosis,[73,75] but may be histologically normal.[72] Pleural effusions are frequently found in patients with pericardial effusions and may also contain malignant cells.[78] Cardiac tamponade with AIDS-related cardiac lymphoma has been reported in several cases.[67,72,75,77,79] Large hemodynamically significant lymphomatous masses have also been observed, often originating in the right atrium.[71,73]

Treatment

Treatment regimens for AIDS-associated cardiac lymphoma have primarily involved multiagent chemotherapy, with or without local radiation,[67,78] and surgery for large, hemodynamically significant masses.[71] The ultimate prognosis for patients with AIDS and lymphomas involving the heart is very poor, with median survival of a few months, although survival for 6 to 12 months has been reported.[78,79] Primary lymphoma of the heart in non-HIV-infected patients is similarly characterized by acute onset and rapid clinical deterioration.[55] These are characteristically aggressive tumors that respond poorly to cancer chemotherapy[70] and that infiltrate the myocardium and affect the conducting system, leading to progressive conduction abnormalities, myocardial dysfunction, and death. The underlying immune deficiency associated with HIV infection, the difficulty of diagnosing cardiac involvement, the generally widespread lymphomatous involvement, and the high tumor burden at the time of diagnosis are contributing factors to the poor prognosis in HIV-infected patients.

References

1. McAllister HA Jr, Fenoglio JJ Jr. Tumors of the cardiovascular system. In: *Atlas of Tumor Pathology,* 2nd series. Washington, DC: Armed Forces Institute of Pathology, 1978:Fasicicle 15:99–100.

2. Dapper F, Gorlach G, Hoffman C, et al. Primary cardiac tumors: clinical experiences and late results in 48 patients. *Thorac Cardiovasc Surg* 1988;36: 80–85.

3. Raaf HN, Raaf JH. Sarcomas related to the heart and vasculature. *Semin Surg Oncol* 1994;10:374–382.

4. Bisel HF, Wroblewski F, LaDue JS. Incidence and clinical manifestations of cardiac metastases. *JAMA* 1953;153:712–715.

5. Young JM, Goldman JR. Tumor metastasis to the heart. *Circulation* 1954;9:220–229.

6. Hanfling SM. Metastatic cancer of the heart. *Circulation* 1960;22:474–483.

7. Roberts WC, Glancy DL, DeVita VT Jr. Heart in malignant lymphoma (Hodgkin's disease, lymphosarcoma, reticulum cell sarcoma and mycosis fungoides): a study of 196 autopsy cases. *Am J Cardiol* 1968;22:85–107.

8. Peters BS, Beck EJ, Coleman DG, et al. Changing disease patterns in patients with AIDS in a referral centre in the United Kingdom: the changing face of AIDS. *BMJ* 1991;302:203–207.

9. Monfardini S, Vaccher E, Pizzocaro G, et al. Unusual malignant tumors in 49 patients with HIV infection. *AIDS* 1989;3:449–452.

10. Chadwick EG, Conner EJ, Hanson GC, et al. Tumors of smooth muscle origin in HIV-infected children. *JAMA* 1990;263:3182–3184.

11. McLoughlin LC, Nord KS, Joshi VV, et al. Disseminated leiomyosarcoma in a child with acquired immune deficiency syndrome. *Cancer* 1991;67: 2618–2621.

12. Orlow SJ, Kamund H, Lawrence RL. Multiple subcutaneous leiomyosarcomas in an adolescent with AIDS. *Am J Pediatr Hematol Oncol* 1992;14: 365–368.

13. Ross JS, Del Rosario A, Bui HX, et al. Primary hepatic leiomyosarcoma in a child with acquired immunodeficiency syndrome. *Hum Pathol* 1992; 23:69–72.

14. Smith MB, Silverman JF, Raab S, et al. Fine-needle aspiration cytology of hepatic leiomyosarcoma. *Diagn Cytopathol* 1994;11:321–327.

15. Prevot S, Neris J, de Sain Maur P. Detection of Epstein-Barr virus in an hepatic leiomyomatous neoplasm in an adult human immunodeficiency virus 1-infected patient. *Virchows Arch* 1994;425: 321–325.

16. Radin R, Kiyabu M. Multiple smooth muscle tumors of the colon and adrenal gland in an adult with AIDS. *Am J Radiol* 1992;159:545–546.

17. McClain KL, Leach CT, Jenson HB, et al. Association of Epstein-Barr virus with leiomyosarcomas in children with AIDS. *N Engl J Med* 1995;332: 12–18.

18. Jenson HB, McClain KL, Leach CT, et al. Benign and malignant smooth muscle tumors containing Epstein-Barr virus in children with AIDS. *Leuk Lymphoma* 1997;27:303–314.

19. Zetler PJ, Filipenko D, Bilbey JH, Schmidt N. Primary adrenal leiomyosarcoma in a man with acquired immunodeficiency syndrome (AIDS): fur-

ther evidence for an increase in smooth muscle tumors related to Epstein-Barr infection with AIDS. *Arch Pathol* 1995;119:1164–1167.

20. Lack EE. Leiomyosarcomas in childhood: a clinical and pathologic study of 10 cases. *Pediatr Pathol* 1986;6:181–197.

21. Lee ES, Locker J, Nalesnik M, et al. The association of Epstein-Barr virus with smooth-muscle tumors occurring after organ transplantation. *N Engl J Med* 1995;332:19–25.

22. Yunis EJ. Role of Epstein-Barr virus in tumor development. *J Pediatr* 1996;128:438.

23. Cesarman E, Moore PS, Rao PH, et al. In vitro establishment and characterization of two acquired immunodeficiency syndrome-related lymphoma cell lines (BC-1 and BC-2) containing Kaposi's sarcoma-associated herpesvirus-like (KSHV) DNA sequences. *Blood* 1995;86:2708–2714.

24. Renne R, Zhong W, Herndier B, et al. Lytic growth of Kaposi's sarcoma-associated herpesvirus (human herpesvirus 8) in culture. *Nature Med* 1996; 2:342–346.

25. Jenson HB, Leach CT, Montalvo EA, et al. Absence of herpesvirus in AIDS-associated smooth-muscle tumors (letter). *N Engl J Med* 1996;335:1690.

26. Glancy DL, Morales JB Jr, Roberts WC. Angiosarcoma of the heart. *Am J Cardiol* 1968;21:413–419.

27. Silver MA, Macher AM, Reichert CM, et al. Cardiac involvement by Kaposi's sarcoma in acquired immune deficiency syndrome (AIDS). *Am J Cardiol* 1984;53:983–985.

28. Levison DA, Semple PD. Primary cardiac Kaposi's sarcoma. *Thorax* 1976;31:595–600.

29. Lothe F, Murray JF. Kaposi's sarcoma: autopsy findings in the African. *Acta Unio Int Contra Cancrum* 1962;18:429–452.

30. Ayer JP, Paul O, Capps RB. Clinical pathologic conference. *Am Heart J* 1962;63:566–572.

31. Gelfand M. Kaposi's hemangiosarcoma of the heart. *Br Heart J* 1957;19:290–292.

32. Janigan DT, Husain A, Robinson NA. Cardiac angiosarcomas: a review and a case report. *Cancer* 1986;57:852–859.

33. Chang Y, Cesarman E, Pessin MS, et al. Identification of herpesvirus-like DNA sequences in AIDS-associated Kaposi's sarcoma. *Science* 1994;266: 1865–1869.

34. Moore PS, Chang Y. Detection of herpesvirus-like DNA sequences in Kaposi's sarcoma in patients

with and without HIV infection. *N Engl J Med* 1995;332:1181–1185.

35. Ambroziak JA, Blackbourn DJ, Herndier BG, et al. Herpes-like sequences in HIV-infected and uninfected Kaposi's sarcoma patients. *Science* 1995; 268:582–583.

36. Su I-J, Chang Y-C, Wang I-W. Herpesvirus-like DNA sequence in Kaposi's sarcoma from AIDS and non-AIDS patients in Taiwan. *Lancet* 1995; 35:722–723.

37. Dupin N, Gorin I, Deleuze J, et al. Herpes-like DNA sequences, AIDS-related tumors, and Castleman's disease. *N Engl J Med* 1995;333:798–799.

38. Gyulai R, Kemeny L, Kiss M, et al. Herpesvirus-like DNA sequence in angiosarcoma in a patient without HIV infection. *N Engl J Med* 1996;334: 540–541.

39. Dupin N, Grandadam M, Calvez V, et al. Herpesvirus-like DNA sequences in patients with Mediterranean Kaposi's sarcoma. *Lancet* 1995;345: 761–762.

40. Rady PL, Yen A, Rollefson JL, et al. Herpesvirus-like DNA sequences in non-Kaposi's sarcoma skin lesions of transplant patients. *Lancet* 1995;345: 1339–1340.

41. Gao S-J, Kingsley L, Hoover DR, et al. Seroconversion to antibodies against Kaposi's sarcoma-associated herpesvirus-related latent nuclear antigens before the development of Kaposi's sarcoma. *N Engl J Med* 1996;335:233–241.

42. Cesarman E, Chang Y, Moore PS, et al. Kaposi's sarcoma-associated herpesvirus-like DNA sequences in AIDS-related body-cavity-based lymphomas. *N Engl J Med* 1995;332:1186–1191.

43. Nador RG, Cesarman E, Knowles DM, Said JW. Herpes-like DNA sequences in a body-cavity-based lymphoma in an HIV-negative patient. *N Engl J Med* 1995;333:943.

44. Welch K, Finkbeiner W, Alpers CE, et al. Autopsy findings in the acquired immunodeficiency syndrome. *JAMA* 1984;252:1152–1159.

45. Cammarosano C, Lewis W. Cardiac lesions in acquired immune deficiency syndrome (AIDS). *J Am Coll Cardiol* 1985;5:703–706.

46. Reichert CM, O'Leary TJ, Levens DL, et al. Autopsy pathology in the acquired immune deficiency syndrome. *Am J Pathol* 1983;112:357–382.

47. Remick SC, Hoisington SA, Migliozzi A. Epidemic Kaposi sarcoma presenting with pleuropericarditis. *NY State J Med* 1992;92:359–360.

48. Autran B, Gorin I, Leibowitch M, et al. AIDS in a Haitian woman with cardiac Kaposi's sarcoma and Whipple's disease. *Lancet* 1983;1:767–768.

49. Anderson DW, Virmani R, Reilly JM, et al. Prevalent myocarditis at necropsy in the acquired immunodeficiency syndrome. *J Am Coll Cardiol* 1988; 11:792–799.

50. Reynolds M, Hecht S, Berger M, et al. Large pericardial effusions in the acquired immune deficiency syndrome. *Chest* 1992;102:1746–1747.

51. Stotka JL, Good CB, Downer WR, Kapoor WN. Pericardial effusion and tamponade due to Kaposi's sarcoma in acquired immunodeficiency syndrome. *Chest* 1989;95:1359–1361.

52. Steigman CK, Anderson DW, Macher AM, et al. Fatal cardiac tamponade in acquired immunodeficiency syndrome with epicardial Kaposi's sarcoma. *Am Heart J* 1988;116:1105–1107.

53. Corallo S, Mutinelli MR, Moroni M, et al. Echocardiography detects myocardial damage in AIDS: prospective study in 102 patients. *Eur Heart J* 1988; 9:887–892.

54. Somers K, Lothe F. Primary lymphosarcoma of the heart: review of the literature and report of 3 cases. *Cancer* 1960;13:449–457.

55. Chou ST, Arkles LB, Gill GD, et al. Primary lymphoma of the heart: a case report. *Cancer* 1983;52: 744–747.

56. Curtsinger CR, Wilson MJ, Yoneda K. Primary cardiac lymphoma. *Cancer* 1989;64:521–525.

57. McDonnell PJ, Mann RB, Bulkley BH. Involvement of the heart by malignant lymphoma: a clinicopathologic study. *Cancer* 1982;49:944–951.

58. Petersen CD, Robinson WA, Kurnick JE. Involvement of the heart and pericardium in the malignant lymphomas. *Am J Med Sci* 1976;272:161–165.

59. Biggar RJ, Rabkin CS. The epidemiology of acquired immunodeficiency syndrome-related lymphomas. *Curr Opin Oncol* 1992;4:883–893.

60. Craig FE, Gulley ML, Banks PM. Post-transplantation lymphoproliferative disorders. *Am J Clin Pathol* 1993;99:265–276.

61. Hamilton-Dutoit SJ, Pallesen G, Franzmann MB, et al. AIDS-related lymphoma: histopathology, immunophenotype, and association with Epstein-Barr virus as demonstrated by in situ nucleic acid hybridization. *Am J Pathol* 1991;138:149–163.

62. Pedersen C, Gerstoft J, Lundgren JD, et al. HIV-associated lymphoma: histopathology and association with Epstein-Barr virus genome related to clinical, immunological and prognostic features. *Eur J Cancer* 1991;27:1416–1423.

63. Meeker TC, Shiramizu B, Kaplan L, et al. Evidence for molecular subtypes of HIV-associated lymphoma: division into peripheral monoclonal, polyclonal and central nervous system lymphoma. *AIDS* 1991;5:669–674.

64. Hamilton-Dutoit SJ, Raphael M, Audouin J, et al. In situ demonstration of Epstein-Barr virus small RNAs (EBER 1) in acquired immunodeficiency syndrome-related lymphomas: correlation with tumor morphology and primary site. *Blood* 1993; 82:619–624.

65. Ito M, Nakagawa A, Tsuzuki T, et al. Primary cardiac lymphoma: no evidence for an etiologic association with Epstein-Barr virus. *Arch Pathol* 1996;120:555–559.

66. Ziegler JL, Beckstead JA, Volberding PA, et al. Non-Hodgkin's lymphoma in 90 homosexual men: relation to generalized lymphadenopathy and the acquired immunodeficiency syndrome. *N Engl J Med* 1989;311:565–570.

67. Gill PS, Chandraratna PA, Meyer PR, Levine AM. Malignant lymphoma: cardiac involvement at initial presentation. *J Clin Oncol* 1987;5:216–224.

68. Guarner J, Brynes RK, Chan WC, et al. Primary non-Hodgkin's lymphoma of the heart in two patients with the acquired immunodeficiency syndrome. *Arch Pathol* 1987;111:254–256.

69. Constantino A, West TE, Gupta M, Loghmanee F. Primary cardiac lymphoma in a patient with acquired immune deficiency syndrome. *Cancer* 1987; 60:2801–2805.

70. Ioachim HL, Cooper MC, Hellman GC. Lymphomas in men at high risk for acquired immune deficiency syndrome (AIDS): a study of 21 cases. *Cancer* 1985;56:2831–2842.

71. Horowitz MD, Cox MM, Neibart RM, et al. Resection of right atrial lymphoma in a patient with AIDS. *Int J Cardiol* 1992;34:139–142.

72. Andress JD, Polish LB, Clark DM, Hossack KF. Transvenous biopsy diagnosis of cardiac lymphoma in an AIDS patient. *Am Heart J* 1989;118:421–423.

73. Goldfarb A, King CL, Rosenzweig BP, et al. Cardiac lymphoma in the acquired immunodeficiency syndrome. *Am Heart J* 1989;118:1340–1344.

74. Balasubramanyam A, Waxman M, Kazal HL, Lee MH. Malignant lymphoma of the heart in acquired immune deficiency syndrome. *Chest* 1986;90: 243–246.

75. Abdoulafia DM, Bush R, Picozzi VJ. Cardiac tamponade due to primary pericardial lymphoma in a patient with AIDS. *Chest* 1994;106:1295–1299.

76. Holladay AO, Seigal RJ, Schwartz D. Cardiac malignant lymphoma in acquired immunodeficiency syndrome. *Cancer* 1992;70:2203–2207.

77. Helfand J. Cardiac tamponade as a result of American Burkitt's lymphoma of the heart and pericardium. *Conn Med* 1990;54:186–189.

78. Kelsey RC, Saker A, Morgan M. Cardiac lymphoma in a patient with AIDS. *Ann Intern Med* 1991;115:370–371.

79. Pousset F, Le Heuzey JY, Pialoux G, et al. Cardiac lymphoma presenting as atrial flutter in an AIDS patient. *Eur Heart J* 1994;15:862–864.

80. Dalli E, Quesada A, Paya R. Cardiac involvement by non-Hodgkin's lymphoma in acquired immune deficiency syndrome. *Int J Cardiol* 1990;26: 223–225.

18

Molecular Mechanisms of HIV Cardiovascular Disease

Carol Kasten-Sportès, M.D., and Constance Weinstein, Ph.D.

Human immunodeficiency virus (HIV) infection can result in damage to many organs, including the heart. Very little is known about factors that determine the target organ and the extent of dysfunction or disease. Such factors might include the viral mutant, coinfections, genetic susceptibility, age, hormonal status, and prescribed medications, as well as the interactions among these possible factors. The amount of fundamental research that needs to be done is formidable. Although progress has been made in understanding the disease process in some organs, notably the brain, similar understanding of the effects of HIV on the cardiovascular system has been much slower to develop. In fact, there is very little to summarize. Our intent in this chapter, then, is to present data from diverse areas of research to provide the basis for the generation of hypotheses and the initiation of research regarding the pathogenesis of HIV cardiovascular disease.

There are several reasons for the paucity of knowledge of the etiology of HIV cardiovascular disease. First, in the early years of the acquired immunodeficiency syndrome (AIDS) epidemic, most patients died of infectious complications before the cardiovascular manifestations were apparent. Second, because cardiomyocytes do not have CD4 receptors, the heart was thought to be unaffected by HIV infection. It has only recently been

documented that HIV can infect non-CD4+ tissues by fusion of viral and host cell membranes or by contact between an infected and an uninfected cell, principally in lymph nodes and the central nervous system.[1] However, these processes have not been shown to occur in the cardiovascular system in any widespread, uniform fashion. An additional factor that makes it difficult to study HIV cardiovascular disease in humans is the presence of risk factors that may cause heart disease in the absence of HIV infection. Such factors may include poor nutrition, smoking, and alcohol and drug abuse. Finally, cardiac dysfunction can be detected in many HIV-positive pediatric[2] and adult patients[3] who are not symptomatic. Symptomatic cardiac involvement appears to be more frequent in the more advanced stages of infection and in patients with lower CD4+ lymphocyte counts.[4]

In a consideration of mechanisms that may underlie HIV cardiovascular disease, it is important to bear in mind the integrated physiology of the cardiovascular system and the hemodynamic, neural, and hormonal factors that are intrinsic to the maintenance of normal cardiac output and compensation for a failing myocardium. Among these are the autonomic nervous system, the renin–angiotensin–aldosterone system, endothelins, atrial natriuretic factor (ANF), prostaglandins, arginine vasopressin, and other peptides, such as bradykinin (and the kallikrein–kinin system), neuropeptide Y, and substance P.

There is no doubt that dysregulation of factors such as these has a role in HIV cardiovascular disease. For example, renal complications are known to occur in HIV and may cause occult changes in fluid balance leading to volume overload and congestive heart failure. Total peripheral resistance may also be affected and cause hemodynamic changes. HIV-positive patients with congestive heart failure may have elevated levels of circulating norepinephrine, as do HIV-negative patients with congestive heart failure. Knowledge of the levels of ANF and prostaglandins, for example, in patients with HIV cardiovascular disease may be important in determining which hypotheses to pursue in seeking the underlying causes of cardiac disease and dysfunction in HIV-positive patients.

What Is HIV Cardiovascular Disease?

This book describes all aspects of HIV cardiovascular disease. However, most clinical studies reported in the literature have dealt largely with disease and dysfunction of the myocardium. Therefore the focus of this chapter is on HIV cardiovascular disease and altered functions of the endothelium, autonomic nerves, and immune cells as they may affect the heart. In particular, it deals with mechanisms that might account for the signs or symptoms of cardiac dysfunction in HIV-positive adults and children, including dilated or hypertrophic cardiomyopathy, myocarditis, arrhythmias, and coronary arteriopathy. The chapter also speculates about mechanisms that might account for the fact that seronegative infants born to seropositive mothers may also present with the signs and symptoms of disturbances in cardiac function.

Is HIV Cardiomyopathy Primary?

The most commonly reported cardiovascular complication of HIV infection is cardiomyopathy. If this were the result of infection of the myocardium (myocytes, fibroblasts, or endothelium) by HIV, it could be considered a primary cardiomyop-

athy. Much has been written about infection of the cardiomyocyte by HIV.[5–7] Some authors have detected an occasional focus of HIV-1 RNA in the myocardium by in situ hybridization[5,6]; however, its presence seems unrelated to the occurrence of symptomatic cardiovascular disease.[8] Because HIV, with rare exceptions, infects only cells that express the CD4 antigen, which has not been found to be expressed on myocytes, it seems unlikely that HIV cardiomyopathy is a direct result of infection of the mycocytes by HIV. Widespread infection of the myocardium by HIV, which might be expected given the global contractile dysfunction in affected patients, has never been documented.

This conclusion parallels that regarding HIV-associated skeletal muscle dysfunction and disease. In patients with polyomyositis, Leon-Monzon and colleagues[9] found evidence of HIV only in sparse lymphoid cells but not within muscle fibers. Lange[10] noted similar findings in both noninflammatory and inflammatory myopathies associated with HIV infection. Biopsies of muscles of patients taking zidovudine typically show ragged red fibers and loss of mitochondrial DNA. Since the condition is reversible on cessation of zidovudine treatment, it is not considered to be a response to HIV. It is, therefore, reasonable to postulate that cardiac and skeletal muscle dysfunction and disease do not occur as a direct result of infection of the cardiomyocyte or myocyte by HIV.

One must consider, however, other mechanisms of a possible primary effect of HIV on the myocardium. Peptides and transactivating factors produced by the virion itself for self-replication might have direct effects on components of the myocardium. The extraordinary effects of gp120 on the astrocyte are the result of processes that are unknown with any other infectious disease.[11,12] Similar phenomena may be contributing factors to HIV cardiovascular disease.

Is HIV Cardiomyopathy Secondary?

According to Werdan and coworkers,[13] a secondary cardiomyopathy occurs as "myocardial damage within the scope of a systemic disease." Such a cardiomyopathy would not include myocardial changes induced by essential hypertension, aortic stenosis, or other diseases whose effects are purely secondary to alterations in hemodynamics. Cytokines are agents that are known to induce a secondary cardiomyopathy via their negative inotropic effects, particularly during sepsis.[13] For the most part, cytokines secreted by leukocytes function locally in a manner similar to neurotransmitters.[14] Hence, macrophages or lymphocytes present in the myocardium or cardiac vessels may secrete cytokines that affect the subjacent myocytes, endothelium, or fibroblasts. In the case of the cardiac vasculature, this could have a global impact on the heart (see the section Endothelial Dysfunction below).

During sepsis and a few other conditions (such as congestive heart failure), circulating levels of various cytokines may be present. Accurate measurement of these cytokines in blood (serum or plasma), however, has been difficult until just a few years ago. Recent studies using more reproducible assays have provided reassuring confirmation of most earlier reports. Hence studies indicating systemic concentrations of cytokines in primary HIV infection presumably reflect the clinical state.[15] There appear, as well, to be several perturbations of cytokine production associated with progressive HIV infection in adults and children.[16] Interleukin-1α (IL-1α), tumor necrosis factor-α (TNF-α) and interferon gamma (IFN-γ) have been reported most recently to be present in the systemic circulation, with older reports also indicating interleukin-6 (IL-6) may be measurable in the circulation at more advanced stages of HIV infection.[16,17] Some have correlated these systemic levels of cytokines with concurrent infections, although for the most part these elevations appear to be unrelated to a specific pathogen.

Extensive recent research has revealed the basis for the negative inotropic effects of these cytokines. A fascinating network of interactions between the myocardium, the endothelium, and the immune system has been discovered of a complexity that was virtually unknown 10 years ago and that may be involved in HIV cardiomyopathy. These studies indicate that acute myocardial depression often occurs in such diverse conditions as major trauma, extensive burns, and severe bacterial or viral infections. The contractile failure seen in each instance appears to be the end result of a final common

pathway produced by the systemic immune response syndrome (SIRS).[18] In the case of sepsis, lipopolysaccharide (endotoxin) stimulates release of several mediators, including TNF-α and IL-1, which then produce myocardial depression. Other cytokines, such as IFN-γ and interleukin-2, (IL-2),[19–21] have also been implicated. This process of contractile dysfunction in SIRS, often in the setting of peripheral vasodilatation, does not appear to be the result of myocardial ischemia.[18,22–25] Rather, one or more soluble factors present in plasma have been shown to be capable of inducing these changes.

Perturbation of Cardiomyocyte Function

The most cogent framework for understanding the effects of cytokines, nitric oxide, and bacterial or viral toxins on the cardiomyocyte is presented in the comprehensive review of Werdan and associates,[25] which the reader is advised to consult. This framework proposes that there are four basic mechanisms, or negative inotropic cascades, by which substances may affect cardiomyocyte function in sepsis:

1. Dysfunction of the β_1-adrenoceptor–G protein–adenylyl cyclase axis
2. Inhibition of protein synthesis
3. Impairment of cellular Ca^{2+} homeostasis
4. Cytotoxicity mediated by polymorphonuclear leukocytes
5. Possibly, unknown routes of interference with the function of myocytes

Mechanisms 1 to 4 would also be operative in noninfectious causes of cardiomyopathy and congestive heart failure. We also propose one additional mechanism of secondary cardiomyopathies: induction of apoptosis. These mechanisms are discussed below.

Nitric Oxide

Originally identified as endothelial-derived relaxing factor, nitric oxide is now known to play a complex role in the function of many organs and cells. Physiologically, it is involved in signal transduction, neurotransmission, and mediation of tumoricidal and bactericidal actions of macrophages. Pathologically, it can cause cellular dysfunction and death.[26–28]

Nitric oxide is produced by nitric oxide synthases. The constitutive isoform present in endothelial cells produces small amounts of nitric oxide to regulate vascular tone, platelet aggregation, and neutrophil adhesion to vascular walls. The inducible isoform, which produces nitric oxide in larger quantities over a longer period of time, is generally thought to be the source of the toxic effects of nitric oxide.

Nitric oxide can be produced by inducible nitric oxide synthase both in activated macrophages infiltrating into the myocardium and in cardiac myocytes. Pinsky and associates[27] have shown increased expression of both inducible nitric oxide synthase message and protein in cardiac myocytes treated with TNF-α, IL-1β, and IFN-γ. Increased myocyte death in culture paralleled increased nitric oxide synthesis. This group showed that cardiac myocyte death could occur as a result of nitric oxide produced by macrophages or by nitric oxide produced within the myocyte. The latter mechanism is implicated in cytotoxicity induced by infusions of a variety of agents (TNF-α, IFN-α, IL-2).[27] These observations must be borne in mind when considering the mechanism of action of the immune system on the cardiovascular system.

Interference With the β_1-Adrenoceptor–G Protein–Adenylyl Cyclase Axis

Although cytokines do not appear to cause myocyte malfunction or necrosis directly, there is evidence that they can alter the function of the myocytes by several mechanisms, one of which is through effects on the β_1-adrenoceptor–G protein–adenylyl cyclase axis.[25,29,30] Interference with this axis has been studied by in vitro experiments. Long-term treatment of cardiomyocytes with immune cell supernatants (found to contain IL-1 and TNF-α) reduced contractility and cyclic adenosine monophosphate (cAMP) accumulation by inhibition of β-adrenergic responsiveness.[31]

TNF-α is the cytokine whose myocardial depressant effects have been most studied. In addition to its effects on cardiomyocytes in culture, its infusion in dogs has been shown to cause left ventricular dysfunction.[32] Myocardial dysfunction during sepsis has been reduced by anti-TNF-α antibodies.[33] TNF-α has been found to be elevated in congestive heart failure and non-HIV cardiomyopathy. Although the cause is unclear, it is reasonable to speculate that its effect may be similar to that described for in vitro and in vivo animal experiments.[34,35]

IL-1β has a suppressive effect on β-adrenergic agonist mediated increases in cAMP in neonatal rat cardiomyocytes.[25,31] In animal models, reversible myocardial depressant effects have been reported with infusions of IL-2[20] and IL-6.[36] These effects appear to be mediated by nitric oxide.[37] In humans, Kawamura and colleagues[38] have identified IL-6 as a chemical mediator of myocardial injury, and Finkel and colleagues[36] have reported on IL-6 as a mediator of stunned myocardium.

Further research correlating in vitro with in vivo myocardial contractile abnormalities is needed. This is particularly true in light of recent evidence for nitric oxide as the probable mediator for some, if not all, of these effects. Moreover, the relevance of these phenomena to HIV cardiovascular disease should be investigated.

Alterations in Cell Proteins

One of the more common bacterial infections in severely compromised patients with AIDS is *Pseudomonas aeruginosa*, which, with sepsis, can cause myocardial dysfunction. This infection becomes a significant risk in patients with CD4+ lymphocyte counts <100.[39] *Pseudomonas* exotoxin A, one of the main virulence factors of this organism, inhibits total protein synthesis by interfering with elongation factor-2 (EF-2).[25] EF-2 is required for translation of polyadenylated mRNA. Werdan and colleagues[25] found that this exotoxin suppressed protein synthesis in neonatal rat cardiomyocytes in a concentration- and time-dependent fashion. This inhibition was reversible with neutralization of the exotoxin by *Pseudomonas* hyperimmunoglobulin G. Although a short-term reduction of protein synthesis by as much as 20% does not impair the function of cardiac myocytes in vitro,[13] chronic reduction impairs function because of impaired protein turnover. On the other hand, some infections may cause increases in selected proteins. For example, TNF-α can induce expression of a 30-kDa stress protein.[25] The full range of altered induction, synthesis, and degradation of cell proteins under these conditions has yet to be studied.

Impairment of Cellular Ca²⁺ Homeostasis

Another pathway for cytokines to affect the cardiomyocyte has been identified by Thaik.[40] When neonatal rat cardiac myocytes were exposed to IL-1β, in addition to the induction of cardiac myocyte hypertrophy and fetal genes expressing ANF and β-myosin heavy-chain mRNA expression of three central calcium regulatory genes was found to be decreased: sarcoplasmic reticulum Ca²⁺ ATPase (SERCA2), calcium release channel (CRC), and voltage-dependent Ca channel (VDCC). The addition of a nitric oxide antagonist, *N*-monomethyl-L-arginine (NMMA), had no effect on this reduction in mRNA, which suggests that the IL-1β effect is independent of nitric oxide. Similar reductions in cardiomyocyte calcium regulatory gene expression were found in studies of rat left ventricular myocardium following intraperitoneal lipopolysaccharide treatment.[40] Reports of alterations in calcium regulatory gene expression in human heart disease indicate that there may be a decrease in mRNA for some or all of these genes.[40] Further research is necessary to ascertain the potential significance of these findings for the disruption of excitation-contraction coupling in negative inotropic cascades.

Fixler and colleagues[41] have discussed the possibility that the elevated levels of cytosolic Ca²⁺ observed during incubation of cardiac myocytes with lymphocytes may be responsible for physiologic changes but may not be an essential prelytic condition for ultimate cell death. Their experiments demonstrated changes in the amplitude of contraction, impairment of relaxation, prolongation of the action potential and of contraction, and the appearance of cell oscillations after cardiac myocytes were incubated with lymphocytes. These changes were reversible on washout or on application of vera-

pamil if it was applied early. Such observations demonstrate an important distinction between immune mechanisms resulting in reversible impaired function and those that result in irreversible cell death.

Cytotoxicity

Bacterial toxins, such as streptolysin O and staphylococcal α toxin, have in vitro and in vivo deleterious effects on myocyte function.[25] Both perturb membrane integrity, although different mechanisms have been proposed. They have not been found to have protein-inhibiting effects; rather, their deleterious effects appear to be cytotoxic. Seko and coworkers[42] demonstrated the infiltration of perforin-expressing killer cells and enhanced expression of human leukocyte antigen (HLA) and intracellular adhesion molecule-1 (ICAM-1) in myocardial tissue of patients with cardiomyopathy and myocarditis. Furthermore, they showed that T-lymphocyte receptor V-alpha and V-beta usage by infiltrating cells was restricted. This indicates that the infiltrating cells specifically recognized and damaged myocardial cells.[42]

Another possible cause of myocardial dysfunction and/or cytotoxicity is the adhesion of neutrophils to cardiac myocytes[43] and the intracellular generation of oxygen free radicals resulting in myocyte contracture. Ikeda and coworkers[44] reported on the increase in ICAM-1 expression after exposure of cultured cardiac myocytes to TNF-α. ICAM-1 interacts with CD11/CD18 integrins expressed on the surface of neutrophils and subsequently causes production of toxic oxygen species. The resulting oxidative injury is intracellular and cannot be prevented by extracellular free-radical scavengers. Monoclonal antibodies to ICAM-1, CD11b, or CD18 can inhibit the injury.[45]

Apoptosis

Another possibility is that HIV may lead by indirect means to apoptosis, that is, cell death without an inflammatory response. Ameisen[46] has based this theory on the finding that the occurrence of HIV-infected cells in the immune system and brain is very low. This suggests that direct pathogenic effects of the virus cannot account for cell dysfunction and loss. Although myocyte death has generally been thought to occur by necrosis, several studies have shown that apoptosis can occur. Gottleib and colleagues[47] showed that, under their experimental conditions, apoptosis occurred in reperfused ischemic myocardium, but not in ischemic myocardium.[47] Tanaka and colleagues[48] demonstrated apoptosis in hypoxic neonatal rat cardiomyocytes. More importantly, Liu and colleagues[49] demonstrated apoptosis in dogs with congestive myopathy due to prolonged rapid ventricular pacing. They were able to observe DNA fragmentation characteristic of apoptosis in cardiac myocytes, and they calculated that 3,700 cells per million myocytes were undergoing apoptosis in their experiment. Additionally, Kajstura and colleagues[50] showed that apoptosis occurred postnatally during cardiac maturation. Apoptotic death was shown to be largely responsible for the smaller number of myocytes in the right ventricle than in the left ventricle. Thus, if the normal processes of apoptosis are perturbed by the in utero environment, one might speculate that developmental abnormalities of the myocardium in infants of seropositive mothers could occur (see below).

Other Routes for Interference With Myocyte Function

Most of the studies discussed in the previous section have recorded the inotropic effects of cytokines; still other studies have recorded chronotropic effects. Oddis and coworkers[51] observed that treatment of rat cardiomyocytes in vitro with IL-1, IL-6, TNF, and L-NMMA significantly enhanced beating rates. Only IL-1 significantly raised nitrite levels in the culture media; however, other experiments suggested that the chronotropic effect was independent of nitric oxide for all the cytokines tested. On the other hand, Roberts and coworkers[52] reported that IL-1 suppressed the beating rate of mycocytes and that transforming growth factor-β (TGF-β) antagonized this effect. Both these factors had antagonistic effects on the secretion of nitric oxide, by these myocytes. Their effects on nitric oxide production correlate inversely with their effects on beating rates. Furthermore, L-arginine, a source of

nitric oxide, suppressed the beating rate, but the inhibitor of nitric oxide, L-NMMA, enhanced the beating rate. One explanation of the differences in findings between the two groups is that the in vitro culture conditions were quite different. It must also be emphasized that neither condition may reflect conditions in vivo.

Increased Myocardial Mass

The previous discussion has dealt with mechanisms of negative inotropic cascades and cardiomyocyte toxicity. Some of these mechanisms induce cell death, which could perhaps lead to a dilated cardiomyopathy in humans. For other mechanisms, however, the corresponding in vivo expression is speculative. This uncertainty is pertinent because one of the key features of HIV cardiovascular disease is increased myocardial mass. This hypertrophy is found even in the face of severe cachexia and muscle wasting. A possible correlate of this has also been reported in fetuses of HIV-positive mothers. These fetuses have increased left and right ventricular end-diastolic wall thickness, irrespective of whether the fetus is actually infected at birth or not.[53] Lipshultz and colleagues[2] have speculated that infected patients may have a chronic catecholamine excess. This could be a potent stimulator of myocyte hypertrophy (and possibly hyperplasia).

Another possibility for the increased myocardial mass seen in HIV cardiovascular disease is suggested by recent in vitro research on IL-6, cardiotrophin-1 (CT-1), and the gp130 portion of the putative receptor of CT-1. CT-1, a recently identified cytokine, is a member of the IL-6 cytokine family, which includes leukemia inhibitory factor, ciliary neurotrophic factor, and oncostatin M. CT-1 and some other members of this family have been found to induce cardiomyocyte hypertrophy in vitro.[54,55] The receptors for this family of cytokines have a transmembrane signaling subunit, gp130, in common.[55] The binding of CT-1 to its receptor leads to tyrosine phosphorylation and signal transduction via the Jak-STAT pathway. These recently discovered protein tyrosine kinase (Jak) and transcription factor (STAT) families are critical parts of the post-receptor signaling machinery of the cytokine receptor superfamily that may contribute to mitogenic responses. All the tissues that express CT-1 receptors are not known; however, it is clear that the cardiomyocyte does express these receptors.[55]

Further insight into a possible role for CT-1 and IL-6 in cytokine-induced myocardial hypertrophy comes from recent research using transgenic mice. A transgenic mouse line that overexpressed Il-6 and had no discernible phenotype was crossed with another transgenic mouse line that overexpressed the IL-6 receptor (IL-6R) and was also without phenotype.[56] The net effect of mating these two lines was a line of mice with a chronically activated IL-6R and its gp130 transmembrane subunit. These IL-6/IL-6R mice now had a phenotype, ventricular hypertrophy.[56] This suggests that one cause of the increased myocardial mass seen in HIV cardiovascular disease may be secondary to binding of IL-6 to its receptors on the myocardium.

The wide array of agents that may impair the function or cause the death of cardiomyocytes is daunting. Moreover, each has been discussed as if it acted in isolation from other agents. Clearly, multiple interactions may be operative. Nevertheless, certain themes emerge, for example, that IL-1, IL-6, and TNF are key players in the interactions that result in myocardial dysfunction and damage under conditions of infection or inflammation. Investigations both in vitro and in vivo will be needed to understand the cellular and molecular pathogenesis of the cardiovascular disease that is associated with HIV.

Could a Coinfection Cause or Contribute to Cardiac Dysfunction?

A wide variety of fungal, protozoan, bacterial, and viral infections have been described in HIV-infected patients,[57] and many of these are myocardial pathogens.[58] Furthermore, as with the nervous system, the cardiovascular system exhibits a spectrum of pathologies that complicate any attempt to construct a coherent pathogenetic scheme. Valvular endocarditis, pericardial disease, dilated cardiomyopathy, rhythm disorders, right ventricular dilatation and left ventricular dysfunction have all been reported.

Luginbuhl and coworkers[59] observed that coinfection with Epstein-Barr virus was the strongest correlate of chronic congestive heart failure in HIV-positive children; their analytical techniques did not yield a significant association between cytomegalovirus and adverse cardiac outcomes. However, Herskowitz and coworkers[8] found a diffuse pattern of cytomegalovirus *IE-2* gene expression within myocytes and endothelial cells from biopsy specimens of adult patients with myocarditis and congestive heart failure. These findings suggest that the response of immature and growing myocardium to the sequelae of infections may be different from those of mature myocardium.

The relationship between a cardiotropic infection and cardiac disease is only partially understood, notwithstanding considerable investigative efforts. One possibility is that there may be a direct immune attack on cardiac muscle cells, as suggested by studies of Lawson and colleagues,[60] who have shown that autoantibodies to cardiac myosin are produced in mice following infection with mouse cytomegalovirus and that anti-cardiac myosin antibodies cross-react with mouse cytomegalovirus protein(s) and cause myocardial inflammation and necrosis.

Studies with coxsackievirus B3, the most common cause of myocarditis in non-HIV-infected patients, have shown that TNF-α, IL-1β, IL-6, and IFN are released by monocytes after exposure to the virus, a similar response to that noted for HIV. Furthermore, these monocytes exhibit increased spreading, development of pseudopodia, and enhanced adherence when compared to control cells.[61] In these studies, which used a cardiac myocyte cell line (Girardi), TNF-α was found to have considerable toxicity. However, these experiments need to be repeated by using a primary culture of heart cells.

In summary, infection with a second pathogen may play a key role in HIV cardiovascular disease. Studies on viral myocarditides may provide insight into this process. Finally, examination of bacterial pathogens, particularly those that produce superantigens (*Staphylococcus* and *Streptococcus*), should also be considered. The association of superantigens with Kawasaki disease in children and its effective treatment with intravenous immunoglobulin suggests that further research in this area may be fruitful for patients with HIV-associated cardiovascular disease.

Endothelial Dysfunction

HIV, circulating factors produced by HIV, or coinfections and the factors they produce, may cause perturbation of normal structure and function of the endothelium, which plays an essential role in the regulation of myocardial function and in the protection of the myocardium from infiltrating cells. Since infection of endothelial cells by HIV is considered to happen rarely, if ever, it is necessary to consider other mechanisms that may affect the endothelium.

Hofman and associates[62] have shown that tat protein can activate endothelial cells to express leukocyte adhesion molecules and IL-6. IL-6 enhances endothelial permeability, thus permitting transmigration of leukocytes and HIV-infected cells, such as macrophages, into tissue. Dhawan and associates[63] reported that HIV infection of monocytes resulted in a twofold increase in the cell adhesion molecules, lymphocyte function-associated antigens 1 and 3 (LFA-1 and LFA-3), and a marked increase in monocyte adherence to human capillary endothelial cells from brain, lung, and skin. Cocultivation of HIV-infected monocytes with endothelial cell monolayers resulted in disruption of the monolayer and increased monocyte expression of gelatinase B and 1 and 2 (TIMP-1 and TIMP-2), tissue inhibitors of metalloproteases, indicating an effect on endothelial–extracellular matrix interactions. Birdsall and collaborators[64] noted increased quantities of adhesion molecules CD11a and CD11b, and very late antigen-4 (VLA-4), which facilitated transendothelial migration of HIV-infected leukocytes. They also noted that gp120 participates with LFA-1 to mediate monocyte–neural cell interactions. Whether such reactions occur in the cardiovascular system remains to be examined.

That the status of the endothelium can affect cardiac function is, however, well established. Endothelin-1 (ET-1), a product of endothelial cells

and a potent vasoconstrictor, also causes inotropic and chronotropic effects by directly affecting both the myocardium and the nodal tissues.[65] TNF-α, which is increased in HIV infection, was shown to cause an increase in circulating levels of ET-1 in rats.[66] Moreover, macrophages and mast cells, among other cell types, have also been shown to produce endothelins, which are a family of peptides with a molecular weight of about 2.5 kDa. Those most studied are endothelin-1 (ET-1), endothelin-2 (ET-2), and endothelin-3 (ET-3). Rolinski and associates[67] observed elevated ET-1 immunoreactivity in HIV-infected patients with retinal microangiopathic syndrome. They related this finding to the enhanced penetration of macrophages into the perivascular tissue and to the ischemia produced by the potent vasoconstrictor activity of ET-1 secreted by the infected macrophages. Ehrenreich and colleagues[68] have shown that the HIV envelope glycoprotein, gp120, stimulates the secretion of endothelin as well as TNF-α from macrophages. In humans, circulating levels of endothelin were found to be elevated in cardiogenic shock, acute myocardial infarction, ischemic heart disease, and heart failure.[65] Under these conditions it is likely that tissues such as heart and endothelium also release ET-1. Receptors for ET-1 were found in higher density in the atria than in the ventricles of human hearts.[69] It was also noted that the cardiac nerves were richest in binding sites, followed by the atria, ventricles, and coronary arteries. Clearly, elevated levels of endothelin could affect the function of the cardiovascular system in HIV-positive patients.

The loss of integrity of the endothelium permits infiltrating cells to have a direct effect on organ tissue. Plata[70] has summarized the evidence that the production of HIV-specific cytotoxic T lymphocytes could result in local inflammatory reactions in the lungs, central nervous system, and lymph nodes. Presumably, similar reactions could result in injury to the cardiovascular system. This view is consistent with the finding at autopsy of accumulated lymphocytes in the heart, as well as in the lungs, nervous system, and lymph nodes. The "restrained myocarditis" that has been reported in many AIDS patients at autopsy is consistent with a possible role for leukocytes (lymphocytes and monocytes) in HIV cardiovascular disease.

Current knowledge of the immune mechanisms whereby endothelial cells could be activated have been summarized by Barry,[29] mainly in the context of cardiac transplant rejection. However, many of the molecules participating in that process are present in increased amounts in the HIV-positive patient. For example, TNF-α and IL-1 stimulate the expression of adhesion molecules such as ICAM-1 on the surface of endothelial cells, which then interact with receptors such as LFA-1 on the surface of circulating monocytes and neutrophils. The resulting injury to the endothelium could result in decreased endothelial-dependent vasodilatation and in interstitial edema, a cause of decreased ventricular compliance. Of immune cells migrating into the myocardium, CD8+ cells comprise a considerable fraction in grafts undergoing rejection. These cells are known to be present in an increased percentage in HIV-infected patients. Since cardiac myocytes express class I major histocompatibility complex molecules, they can presumably be lysed by CD8+ cells.

Alterations in Autonomic Nervous System Regulation

Overview of Neurologic Complications of HIV

Although this section specifically addresses abnormalities of the autonomic nervous system, this system is integrated with the central and peripheral nervous systems which are well known to be seriously affected by HIV infection. In retrospective studies, HIV neurologic disease may be found in 10% of patients at presentation, in 40% during the course of the disease, and in 75% at autopsy.[12,71] Multiple different clinical syndromes have been reported, which vary with the severity of the disease. During the asymptomatic period, HIV meningitis, peripheral neuropathy, or an inflammatory demyelinating polyneuropathy may occur. As the disease progresses, patients may go on to develop a myelopathy or encephalopathy.[10,72] A mononeuropathy or mononeuropathy multiplex can occur at any stage of the disease and may be caused by cytomegalovirus.[10]

Autonomic nervous system disturbances have also been reported in asymptomatic patients. They appear, however, to be more common as HIV symptomatology progresses.[71,73–76] Several have reported the cardiovascular consequences of HIV autonomic dysfunction.[71,73–78] (See Chapter 10.)

Two HIV-specific pathologic findings are HIV encephalitis and HIV leukoencephalopathy. The former consists of multiple small gray and white matter foci of microglia and macrophages which show intensive staining for HIV.[79,80] The latter is characterized by a reduction in myelin, reactive astrogliosis, and multinucleated HIV-infected microglia or macrophages in the deep white matter of the cerebral hemispheres.[79,80] Other neuropathologic findings that are associated with HIV but that may be secondary to infections are multifocal vacuolar leukoencephalopathy, vacuolar myelopathy, and diffuse gray matter disease with astrogliosis and occasional nerve cell loss.[79,80] The most consistent feature of peripheral neuropathies is a mononuclear cell infiltration around the vessels of the nerve sheaths (epineurial and endoneurial vessels). Demyelination and axonal degeneration are also common.[81] In the cardiac conduction system of children with vertically transmitted AIDS, Bharati et al.[82] found vascular changes in the sinoatrial and atrioventricular nodes, including thrombosis. One child with a left anterior hemiblock was found to have fibrosis and vacuolization of the left bundle branch.

Anatomy of the Autonomic Nervous System

One of the key regulators of cardiac function is the autonomic nervous system, whose nerve fibers are widely distributed in the heart, blood vessels, smooth muscle, visceral organs, glands, and skin. The hypothalamus is the center for integration of information, with higher cortical input significantly affecting this process. Three areas of the brainstem active in autonomic cardiovascular regulation that are known to receive hypothalamic input are the excitatory or pressor center (rostrolateral medulla), the inhibitory or depressor center (mediocaudal medulla), and the dorsal motor nucleus of the vagus, which is inhibitory.[83]

The inotropic state of the myocardium is primarily regulated by catecholamines produced by the autonomic nervous system, although circulating catecholamines may play a role under conditions such as chronic stress and heart failure. Sympathetic nerve stimulation produced by fibers lying close to the myocardium releases norepinephrine which binds to β_1 and β_2 receptors found in both the atria and ventricles and the sinoatrial and atrioventricular nodes. Parasympathetic vagal stimulation acts predominantly on the atria and the sinotrial and atrioventricular nodes by releasing acetylcholine. A few vagal fibers have also been shown to innervate the ventricles, causing a decrease in myocardial contractility when stimulated.[84]

The systemic vasculature, peripheral vascular resistance, and venous return are reflexly regulated by the autonomic nervous system. Input for this regulation comes from the carotid sinus and aortic stretch receptors, the carotid body chemoreceptors, and the stretch receptors of the low-pressure areas of the intrathoracic vascular bed.

This input is affected by a balance of sympathetic and parasympathetic activity produced by the release of norepinephrine and acetylcholine.[83] Other autonomic neurotransmitters are also important for the regulation of vascular tone. It now appears that most neurons in the central and peripheral nervous systems store and release more than one neurotransmitter. These compounds include purines, autocoids (eicosanoids and leukotrienes), and peptides (enkephalins, substance P, vasoactive intestinal peptide, and neuropeptide).[85] Although at this time there is no clinical or experiemental data, one could speculate that HIV infection may affect the release of some of these compounds.

Multiple neurotransmitters have been reported in the hypothalamus, where autonomic nervous system integration occurs. The primary neurotransmitter responsible for most, if not all, excitatory hypothalamic synaptic activity is the amino acid glutamate.[86] There are two principal postsynaptic glutamate receptors: those that are coupled to G proteins and those that contain an integral ion channel. The latter group of receptors includes two types, N-methyl-D-aspartate (NMDA) and α-amino-3-hydroxy-5-methyl-4-isoxazole propionic acid (AMPA). Both have been shown to be affected by portions of the HIV virion itself or by cytokines that are dysregulated by HIV.[87]

In summary, systemic HIV infection causes damage to the central, peripheral, and autonomic nervous systems. Cardiovascular regulation and the autonomic nervous system are fundamentally interconnected. Thus, there is every reason to expect that regulation of the cardiovascular system by the autonomic nervous system could be significantly hampered by HIV infection, contributing to alterations of contractility, blood pressure, and heart rate.

Potential Mechanisms of Damage to the Nervous System By HIV and Their Possible Role in HIV Cardiovascular Disease

A great deal of research has been directed toward understanding the mechanism(s) of HIV neurologic disease. Analogous to HIV cardiovascular disease, direct infection of neural tissue by HIV has never been documented, despite widespread dysfunction.[80,88–90] Yet extraordinary damage to both the central and peripheral nervous systems is obvious, both antemortem from the manifestation of debilitating symptoms, and postmortem at autopsy.

At this time, there appear to be several possible routes for HIV neurotoxicity. The HIV envelope glycoprotein gp120 has multiple toxic effects.[87,90,91] It stimulates the release of neurotoxins from microglia and macrophages[92] and binds to NMDA receptors, leading to an increase in the local concentration of nitric oxide.[11,92] Lastly, gp120 has been reported to activate Na^+-H^+ exchange in astrocytes, which could lead to neuronal dysfunction or death.[12]

Autoimmunity, a more familiar pathologic phenomenon than some of the other mechanisms noted above, has also been proposed as a cause for some HIV neuropathic changes. An aute, Guillain-Barré-like, inflammatory demyelinating polyneuropathy,[10,93] as well as a chronic form, have been reported with HIV. Both may result from an autoimmune process. Interestingly, signs of an acute demyelinating polyneuropathy have been reported to disappear as HIV infection progresses and immunoglobulin levels fall.

In conclusion, HIV neurologic disease has many similarities to and may be the genesis of significant aspects of HIV cardiovascular disease pathology. Mechanisms for this neurologic damage are under active investigation and may be similar to those responsible for HIV cardiovascular disease. Careful consideration of these processes may facilitate research on and treatment of HIV cardiovascular disease.

Does Vertical Transmission of HIV Affect the Expression of Cardiovascular Disease in Children?

It is even more difficult to unravel how the cardiovascular system becomes affected in some children born to HIV-positive mothers than it is to unravel the cardiovascular effects in adults infected with HIV. First, much remains to be understood about the manner in which vertical transmission occurs, whether in utero or peripartum. It is not known why some, but not all, children born to HIV-positive mothers are infected; however, the same is true for other teratogenic infections. It is known that not all fetuses exposed to rubella or toxoplasmosis via maternal infection become infected. Second, it is not clear whether the cardiovascular effects on fetuses of seropositive mothers are due to HIV, to coinfections such as cytomegalovirus, or to more complex mechanisms such as those described in the preceding paragraphs. Third, there is considerable evidence (see Chapter 6) that children's cardiovascular systems may be affected even if they themselves are not infected with HIV, suggesting that the maternal environment is a significant factor. It is a well-recognized fact that a variety of bacterial, protozoal, and viral infections of the mother can affect the developing fetus without actually infecting the fetus or the placenta. Bacterial, protozoal, and viral infections may affect the fetus indirectly, resulting in abortion, stillbirth, or premature delivery. A well-studied example is the association of maternal urinary infection with premature delivery and low birth weight. Treatment with antibiotics reduced the incidence of pyelonephritis but did not affect the rate of premature delivery and low birthweight. The basis for this effect is unknown, but it has been suggested that it relates to fetal lymphocytes exposed and sensitized to antigen in utero.[94] However, this is controversial. Others have suggested that this may be a chance association, given the frequency of urinary tract infections in pregnancy.

The pathogenetic mechanisms whereby infectious agents can cause fetal anomalies also remain obscure, although histologic studies have suggested that infectious agents may cause cell death, alterations in growth, and chromosomal damage.[94] It is significant that cardiac anomalies can occur in both HIV-positive and HIV-negative children of HIV-positive mothers. This suggests that maternal factors and not direct HIV infection are responsible for both fetal and postnatal cardiac changes.[2]

If vertical transmission of HIV occurs in utero, the placenta, the fetus, or both may be infected, and infection may occur at any time during gestation. HIV is not thought to infect sperm or oocytes, but the developing embryo might be infected via HIV-infected white blood cells in semen. For most congenital cardiovascular malformations to occur, infection must presumably have its effects during the first trimester, while morphogenesis is occurring. The viral antigen p24 has been detected in macrophages and occasionally in trophoblasts and endothelial cells of HIV-infected placentas as early as the eighth week of gestation.[95] Several reports have documented infection of the placenta with HIV and concomitant placental abnormalities. Kesson and colleagues[96] have demonstrated the expression of CD4 on the surface of placental macrophages and have shown that these cells are permissive for HIV-1 replication. Cells reported to stain positive for gp41 antigen and HIV nucleic acid include maternal decidual leukocytes, villous macrophages, and endothelial cells. David and colleagues[97] have shown that trophoblasts from human placenta can be infected with HIV-1. Using cell lines derived from the trophoblast, they were able to show the presence of CD4 molecules on the surface of these cells and to show that the level of infection depends on both the cell line and the virus strain. However, the relevance of this finding to the situation in vivo is not clear. Lairmore and colleagues[98] were unable to identify CD4 RNA in immunoaffinity-purified cytotrophoblasts and more mature syncytiotrophoblast cultures, and they suggested that transmission of HIV-1 across syncytioblasts may occur by mechanisms other than by binding the CD4 receptor.

The effects of HIV transmission in utero involve the timing of fetal infection in terms of developmental stage of the organs affected and the immune system. The development of the immune system, the effects of HIV, as far as they are known, and the differences between the immature and the adult systems have been described in detail.[16] In general, it would appear that HIV infection in infants brings about broad functional abnormalities in immune cells, most of which are uninfected. This may account for the infants' susceptibility to infections. Additionally, in infected immune cells the virus assumes control of the genetic and biochemical machinery, which then synthesizes and releases large amounts of cytokines. These include factors that act on B lymphocytes, which in turn produce large amounts of immunoglobulins. These immunoglobulins have cross-reactive autoantibody function, which may account for cardiac disease as well as hematologic disease and diseases of other organs.[99]

Cytomegalovirus and toxoplasmosis are common congenital, perinatal, and postnatal infections that do not have direct effects on the cardiovascular system. They may, however, have cardiovascular sequelae. It seems likely that the alterations in cytokine production caused by these infections may mediate cardiac dysfunction via the pathways described earlier in this chapter, but this question has not yet been investigated.

Some have argued that the cardiac dysfunction and disease seen in adult HIV-positive patients may be the result of lifestyles that include risk factors affecting the cardiovascular system, but this cannot be true for HIV-positive infants. These patients provide convincing evidence for an effect that is related to HIV infection and that warrants further investigation. Clearly, the amount of information that can be obtained from studies of infants is limited, and research must be pursued with cells, tissues, and animal models.

Future Directions

One approach to understanding some of the mechanisms of dysfunction and disease of various organs and tissues seen in patients with AIDS is to examine the role of various gene products by constructing transgenic mice, possibly with cardiotropic promoters. Several attempts at developing transgenic models have been successful for organs and tissues other than heart, using various strains of mice, including severe combined immunodeficient (SCID) mice. The latter model may be useful in studying the role of immunodeficiency in the development of cardiac dysfunction and as an approach to cardiac disease in pediatric patients with HIV infection.[100,101] However, it must be emphasized that most of the experiments to be conducted in mice will require careful analysis of physiology as well as pathology. Because of recent advances in technology, such experiments are feasible in animals as small as mice.[102–106]

Transgenic mice containing the complete HIV coding sequences fused to the mouse mammary tumor virus long terminal repeat have been generated. These mice produce gag and env HIV proteins in organs such as mammary gland, spleen, and liver. In some transgenic lines, low levels of HIV proteins could also be detected in serum.[107] The report states that animals sacrificed at 17 months of age were indistinguishable from nontransgenic mice on macroscopic and histologic examination. Thus, it would appear that cells from various tissues in the mouse are capable of replicating retroviruses and producing HIV proteins without causing disease. However, the heart was not among the tissues examined.

Transgenic mice expressing the entire HIV genome under the control of the promoter for the human neurofilament *NF-L* gene exhibited neuropathologic changes 7 to 12 months after birth.[91] HIV was expressed in the neurons of these mice, in contrast to humans, where neurons are only rarely found to be infected with HIV. However, there were parallels between the hypoactivity of these mice and the psychomotor slowing and apathy seen in the early stages of AIDS dementia. These experiments are somewhat inconclusive as far as human neurologic disease is concerned. It is conceivable that postmitotic neurons might be infected but express the viral genome at very low levels, that surrounding infected cells might secrete neurotoxins, and that metabolic disturbances without morphologic disease might contribute to AIDS dementia. Such mechanisms might be considered when speculating about possible causes of cardiovascular disease in HIV-infected patients.

Of more specific relevance is the transgenic

mouse constructed to investigate the pathogenesis of HIV-associated nephropathy, which occurs in about 10% of HIV-infected patients. The mice were made transgenic for a subgenomic proviral HIV construct, pNL4-3:d1443, which lacks the *gag* and *pol* genes and is therefore noninfectious. Abnormal renal histology was noted beginning at about 35 to 45 days of age.[108] About 20% of these animals developed cardiac lesions at the base of the aortic valve, an adventitial process with macrophage and neutrophil infiltrates. Vasculitis involving the coronary arteries was also observed. The interesting aspect of this proviral construct is that its expression in heart tissue could not be detected by Northern analysis (T. B. Kopp and P. E. Klotman, personal communication), although low-level expression would only be detected by more sensitive methods. However, there was increased expression of ANF, a molecular marker of myocyte hypertrophy, in the ventricles of these mice.

One line of these transgenic mice carrying a subgenomic HIV proviral construct lacking the *gag* and *pol* genes was found to develop proliferative epidermal lesions with some similarities to those seen in HIV-infected patients. Dermal lesions similar to Kaposi's sarcoma were not seen in this model, in contrast to those seen in an HIV *LTR-tat* transgenic mouse. Thus, the proteins expressed by the genes appear to play an important but specific role in the pathogenesis of skin disorders in HIV-infected patients[109] and could possibly be involved in the effects of HIV on the cardiovascular system.

As mentioned earlier, there have been a few reports of the detection of HIV transcripts in endomyocardial biopsies of HIV-infected patients, but the significance of these findings is unclear, since the transcripts have been detected in cardiac tissues of patients with and without known cardiac dysfunction.[8] This adds to the speculation that it is not the virus itself, but immune mechanisms and cytokine and growth factor dysregulation, that are involved in the pathogenesis of cardiac dysfunction in HIV-positive patients.[30] It is possible that host genetic susceptibility may also play a role, since it has been shown that, in mice infected with CVB3, macrophage inflammatory protein (MIP-l-alpha) is an absolute requirement for the development of myocarditis.[110] It is also possible that the constant,

repeated cycles of viral replications lead to mutations with differential pathogenic effects, which result in neurologic, kidney, or heart disease or cancer.

It should be noted that recent studies of peripheral blood monocytes during HIV infection show phenotypic and functional changes as the disease progresses. Although in the early stages, the ability of monocytes to phagocytose bacteria and migrate across endothelium is normal or enhanced, in later stages their ability to mount a host defense declines. These findings undoubtedly complicate the picture of the role of macrophages described above, but they may account for the complex expression of the sequelae of HIV infection in vivo.[111] They should also be kept in mind in designing in vitro experiments.

Summary

We have described multiple different mechanisms by which HIV may affect normal functioning of the cardiovascular system. Although some have reported direct infection of the myocardium by HIV, this would not explain the global myocardial failure seen in many AIDS patients. Primary effects of the virus on the heart via a peptide such as gp120 are possible, although there is no evidence to support this at present. Research on the SIRS and the effects of cytokines, leukocytes, and nitric oxide on the myocardium provide a solid framework. Testable hypotheses regarding the pathogenesis of HIV cardiovascular disease may now be generated by using these data. Consideration should be given to the role that HIV central nervous system disease plays in HIV cardiovascular disease as well as the mechanisms by which HIV produces these diseases. They may share many pathogenetic processes. Endothelial dysfunction induced by HIV infection is in the background of all of the above phenomena. It is a source of, and is affected by, cytokines and nitric oxide, ubiquitous agents in infection. Lastly, the extraordinary effects of HIV extend even to fetuses and infants who are not infected. The cardiovascular alterations observed in these children should also be borne in mind as research plans are designed.

Acknowledgments

We thank Dr. Mason Barr, Dr. Pat Fast, and Dr. Steven Leber for their constructive advice, Dr. Lan-Hsiang Wang for her invaluable contributions to the section on autonomic nervous system regulation, and Dr. Rani Rao for reviewing the manuscript.

References

1. Zeichner SL. The molecular biology of HIV. *Clin Perinatol* 1994;21:39–73.

2. Lipshultz SE, Bancroft EA, Boller AM. Cardiovascular manifestations of HIV infection in children. In: Bricker, JT (ed). *The Science and Practice of Pediatric Cardiology,* 2nd Ed. Baltimore: Williams & Wilkins, 1997.

3. Coudray N, Zuttere DD, Force G, et al. Left ventricular diastolic function in asymptomatic and symptomatic human immunodeficiency virus carriers: an echocardiographic study. *Eur Heart J* 1995;16:61–67.

4. Cardoso JS, Miranda AM, Moura B, et al. Cardiac morbidity in human immunodeficiency virus infection. *Rev Port Cardiol* 1994;13:901–911.

5. Lipshultz SE, Fox CH, Perez-Atayde AR, et al. Identification of human immunodeficiency virus-1 RNA and DNA in the heart of a child with cardiovascular abnormalities and congenital acquired immune deficiency syndrome. *Am J Cardiol* 1990; 66:246–250.

6. Grody WW, Cheng L, Lewis W. Infection of the heart by human immunodeficiency virus. *Am J Cardiol* 1990;60:203–206.

7. Lewis W, Grody W. AIDS and the heart: review and consideration of pathogenetic mechanisms. *Cardiovasc Pathol* 1992;1:53–64.

8. Herskowitz A, Wu T, Willoughby SB, et al. Myocarditis and cardiotropic viral infection associated with severe left ventricular dysfunction in late-stage infection with human immunodeficiency virus. *J Am Coll Cardiol* 1994;24:1025–1032.

9. Leon-Monzon M, Lamperth L, Dalakas MC. Search for HIV proviral DNA and amplified sequences in the muscle biopsies of patients with HIV polymyositis. *Muscle Nerve* 1993;16: 408–413.

10. Lange DJ. Neuromuscular diseases associated with HIV-1 infection. *Muscle Nerve* [AAEM minimonograph no.41] 1994;17:16–30.

11. Mollace V, Colasanti M, Persichini T, et al. HIV gp120 glycoprotein stimulates the inducible isoform of NO synthase in human cultured astrocytoma cells. *Biochem Biophys Commun* 1993;194: 439–444.

12. Benos D, McPherson S, Hahn BH, et al. Cytokines and HIV envelope glycoprotein gp120 stimulate Na^+H^+ exchange in astrocytes. *J Biol Chem* 1994; 269:13811–13816.

13. Werdan K, Muller U, Reithmann C, et al. Mechanisms of acute septic cardiomyopathy: evidence from isolated myocytes. *Basic Res Cardiol* 1991; 86:411–421.

14. Durum SK, Oppenheim JJ. Macrophage-derived mediators: interleukin 1, tumor necrosis factor, interleukin 6, interferon and related cytokines. In: Paul WE (ed). *Fundamental Immunology,* 2nd Ed. New York: Lippincott-Raven, 1989:639–661.

15. Tindall B, Carr A, Cooper DA. Primary HIV infection: clinical, immunologic and serologic aspects. In: Dande MA, Volberding PA (eds). *The Medical Management of AIDS,* 4th Ed. Philadelphia: WB Saunders, 1995:105–129.

16. Koup RA, Wilson CB. Clinical Immunology of HIV-infected Children. In: Pizzo PA, Wilfert CM (eds). *Pediatric AIDS: The Challenge of HIV Infection in Infants, Children, and Adolescents,* 2nd Ed. Baltimore: Williams & Wilkins, 1994: 129–157.

17. Senaldi G, Peakman M, Natoli C, et al. Relationship between the tumor-associated antigen 90k and cytokines in the circulation of persons infected with human immunodeficiency virus. *J Infect* 1994;28:31–39.

18. Ungureanu-Longrois D, Balligand JL, Kelly RA, et al. Myocardial contractile dysfunction in the systemic inflammatory response syndrome: role of cytokine-inducible nitric oxide synthase in cardiac myocytes. *J Mol Cell Cardiol* 1995;27:155–167.

19. Natanson C, Eichenholz PW, Danner RL, et al. Endotoxin and tumor necrosis factor challenges in dogs stimulate the cardiovascular profile of human septic shock. *J Exp Med* 1989;169:823–832.

20. Ognibene FP, Rosenberg SA, Lotze M, et al. Interleukin-2 administration causes reversible hemodynamic changes and left ventricular dysfunction similar to those seen in septic shock. *Chest* 1988; 94:750–754.

21. Deyton LR, Walker RE, Kovacs JA, et al. Reversible cardiac dysfunction associated with interferon alpha therapy in AIDS patients with Kaposi's sarcoma. *N Engl J Med* 1989;321:1246–1249.

22. Cunnion RE, Schaer GL, Parker MM, et al. The coronary circulation in human septic shock. *Circulation* 1986;73:637–644.

23. Dhainault JF, Huyghebacrt MF, Monsallier JF, et al. Coronary hemodynamics and myocardial metabolism of lactate, free fatty acids, glucose, and ketones in patients with septic shock. *Circulation* 1987;75:533–541.

24. Papadakis EJ, Abel FL. Left ventricular performance in canine endotoxin shock. *Circ Shock* 1988;24:123–131.

25. Werdan K, Muller U, Reithman C. Negative inotropic cascades in cardiomyocytes triggered by substances relevant to sepsis. In: Schlag G, Redl H (eds). *Pathophysiology of Shock, Sepsis and Organ Failure.* Berlin: Springer-Verlag, 1993: 787–834.

26. Rand MJ, Li CG. Nitric oxide as a neurotransmitter in peripheral nerves: nature of transmitter and mechanism of transmission. *Annu Rev Physiol* 1995;57:659–682.

27. Pinsky DJ, Cai B, Ynag X, et al. The lethal effects of cytokine-induced nitric oxide on cardiac myocytes are blocked by nitric oxide synthase antagonism or transforming growth factor beta. *J Clin Invest* 1995;95:677–685.

28. Vladutiu AO. Short analytical review: role of nitric oxide in autoimmunity. *Clin Immunol Immunopathol* 1995;76:1–11.

29. Barry WH. Mechanisms of immune-mediated myocyte injury. *Circulation* 1994;89:2422–2432.

30. Lange LG, Schreiner GF. Immune mechanisms of cardiac disease. *N Engl J Med* 1994;330:1129–1135.

31. Gulick TS, Chung MK, Pieper SJ, et al. Interleukin-1 and tumor necrosis factor inhibit cardiac myocyte beta-adrenergic responsiveness. *Proc Natl Acad Sci USA* 1989;86:6753–6757.

32. Pagani FD, Baker LS, Hsi C, et al. Left ventricular systolic and diastolic dysfunction after infusion of tumor necrosis factor-alpha in conscious dogs. *J Clin Invest* 1992;90:389–398.

33. Vincent JL, Bakker J, Marecaux G, et al. Administration of anti-TNF antibody improves left ventricular function in septic shock patients. *Chest* 1992;101:810–815.

34. Weidermann CJ, Beimpold H, Herold M, et al. Increased levels of serum nonprotein and decreased production of neutrophil superoxide anions in chronic heart failure with elevated levels of tumor necrosis factor-alpha. *J Am Coll Cardiol* 1993;22:1897–1901.

35. Matumori A, Yamada T, Suzuki H, et al. Increasing circulating cytokines in patients with myocarditis and cardiomyopathy. *Br Heart J* 1994;72: 561–566.

36. Finkel MS, Hoffman RA, Shen L, et al. Interleukin-6 (IL-6) as a mediator of stunned myocardium. *Am J Cardiol* 1993;71:1231–1232.

37. Finkel MS, Oddis CV, Jacob TD, et al. Negative inotropic effects of cytokines on the heart mediated by nitric oxide. *Science* 1992;257:387–389.

38. Kawamura T, Inada K, Okada H, et al. Methylprednisolone inhibits increase of interleukin 8 and 6 during open heart surgery. *Can J Anaesthesiol* 1995;42:399–403.

39. Jacobson MA. Disseminated and other bacterial infections In: Sande MA, Volberding PA (eds). *The Medical Management of AIDS,* 4th Ed. Philadelphia: WB Saunders, 1995:402–415.

40. Thaik CM, Calderone A, Takahashi N, et al. Interleukin-1beta modulates the growth and phenotype of neonatal rat cardiac myocytes. *J Clin Invest* 1995;96:1093–1099.

41. Fixler R, Shimoni Y, Hassin D, et al. Physiological changes induced in cardiac myocytes by cytotoxic lymphocytes: an autoimmune model. *J Mol Cell Cardiol* 1994;26:351–360.

42. Seko Y, Ishiyama S, Nishikawa T, et al. Restricted use of T cell receptor $v\alpha$-$v\beta$ genes in infiltrating cells in the hearts patients with acute myocarditis and dilated cardiomyopathy. *J Clin Invest* 1995; 96:1035–1041.

43. Entman ML, Youker K, Shappel SB, et al. Neutrophil adherence to isolated adult canine myocytes. *J Clin Invest* 1990;85:1497–1506.

44. Ikeda U, Ikeda M, Kano S, et al. Neutrophil adherence to rat cardiac myocyte by proinflammatory cytokines. *J Cardiovasc Pharmacol* 1994; 23:647–652.

45. Entman ML, Youker K, Shoji T, et al. Neutrophil induced oxidative injury of cardiac myocytes. *J Clin Invest* 1992;90:1335–1345.

46. Ameisen JC. The programmed cell death theory of AIDS pathogenesis: implications, testable pre-

dictions, and confrontation with experimental findings. *Immunodefic Rev* 1992;3:237–246.

47. Gottlieb RA, Burleson KO, Kloner RA, et al. Reperfusion injury induces apoptosis in rabbit cardiomyocytes. *J Clin Invest* 1994;94:1621–1623.

48. Tanaka M, Ito H, Adachi S, et al. Hypoxia induces apoptosis with enhanced expression of FAS antigen messenger RNA in cultured neonatal rat cardiomyocytes. *Circ Res* 1994;75:426–433.

49. Liu Y, Cigola E, Cheng W, et al. Myocyte nuclear mitotic division and programmed myocyte cell death characterize the cardiac myopathy induced by rapid ventricular pacing in dogs. *Lab Invest* 1995;73:771–787.

50. Kajstura J, Mansukhani M, Cheng W, et al. Programmed cell death and the expression of the protoncogene *bcl-2* in myocytes during postnatal maturation of the heart. *Exp Cell Res* 1995;219:110–121.

51. Oddis CV, Simmons RL, Hattler BG, et al. Chronotropic effects of cytokines and the nitric oxide synthase inhibitor, L-NMMA, on cardiac myocytes. *Biochem Biophy Res Commun* 1994;205:992–997.

52. Roberts AB, Vodovtz Y, Roche NS, et al. Role of nitric oxide in antagonistic effects of transforming growth factor-beta and interleukin-1 beta on the beating rate of cultured cardiac myocytes. *Mol Endocrinol* 1992;11:1921–1930.

53. Hornberger LK, Lipshultz SE, Easley KA, et al. for the P^2C^2 Study Group Cardiac structure and function in fetuses of human immunodeficiency virus-infected mothers: the prospective P^2C^2 multicenter study. (Submitted).

54. Pennica D, Shaw KJ, Swanson TA, et al. Cardiotrophin-1. *J Biol Chem* 1995;270:10915–10922.

55. Pennica D, King KL, Shaw KJ, et al., Expression cloning of cardiotrophin-1, a cytokine that induces cardiac myocyte hypertrophy. *Proc Natl Acad Sci USA* 1995;92:1142–1146.

56. Hirota H, Yoshida K, Kishimoto T, Taga T. Continuous activation of gp130, a signal-transducing receptor component for IL-6 related cytokines, causes myocardial hypertrophy in mice. *Proc Natl Acad Sci USA* 1995;92:4862–4866.

57. Mueller BU, Pizzo PA. Acquired immunodeficiency syndrome in the infant. In: Remington JS, Klien JO (eds). *Infectious Diseases of the Fetus and Newborn Infant,* 4th Ed. Philadelphia: WP Saunders, 1995:377–403.

58. De Castro S, d'Amati G, Gallo P, et al. Frequency of development of acute global left ventricular dysfunction in human immunodeficiency virus infection. *J Am Coll Cardiol* 1994;24:1018–1024.

59. Luginbuhl LM, Orav EJ, McIntosh K, et al. Cardiac morbidity and related mortality in children with HIV infection. *JAMA* 1993;269:2869–2875.

60. Lawson CM, O'Donoghue HL, Reed WD. Mouse cytomegalovirus infection induces antibodies which cross-react with virus and cardiac myosin: a model for the study of molecular mimicry in the pathogenesis of viral myocarditis. *Immunology* 1992;75:513–519.

61. Henke A, Mohr C, Sprenger H, et al. Coxsackievirus B3-induced production of tumor necrosis factor-α, IL-1β, and IL-6 in human monocytes. *J Immunol* 1992;148:2270–2277.

62. Hofman FM, Wright AD, Dohadwala MM, et al. Exogenous tat protein activates human endothelial cells. *Blood* 1993;82:2774–2780.

63. Dhawan S, Weeks BS, Soderland C, et al. HIV-1 infection alters monocyte interactions with human microvascular endothelial cells. *J Immunol* 1995;154:422–432.

64. Birdsall HH, Trial J, Jennifer AH, et al. Phenotypic and functional activation of monocytes in HIV-1 infection: interactions with neural cells. *J Leukocyte Biol* 1994;56:310–317.

65. Golfman LS, Hata T, Beamish RE, et al. Role of endothelin in heart function in health and disease. *Can J Cardiol* 1993;9:635–653.

66. Klemm P, Warner TD, Hohlfeld T, et al. Endothelin-1 mediates ex vivo coronary vasoconstriction caused by exogenous and endogenous cytokines. *Proc Natl Acad Sci USA* 1995;92:2691–2695.

67. Rolinski B, Geier SA, Sadri I, et al. Endothelin-1 immunoreactivity in plasma is elevated in HIV-1 infected patients with retinal microangiopathic syndrome. *Clin Invest* 1994;72:288–293.

68. Ehrenreich H, Rieckmann P, Sinowatz F, et al. Potent stimulation of monocytic endothelin-1 production by HIV-1 glycoprotein 120. *J Immunol* 1993;150:4601–4609.

69. Davenport AP, Nune DJ, Hall JA, et al. Autoradiographical localisation of binding sites for porcine-^{125}I endothelin-1 in humans, pigs and rats: functional relevance in humans. *J Cardiovasc Pharmacol* 1989;13:166–170.

70. Plata F. Implications of HIV-specific cytotoxic T lymphocytes in AIDS. *Biotherapy* 1992;5:31–45.

71. Freeman R, Roberts MS, Friedman LS, et al. Autonomic function and human immunodeficiency virus infection. *Neurology* 1990;40:575–580.

72. Harrison MJG. Neurological complications of HIV infection: clinical aspects. In: Scaravelli F (ed). *The Neuropathology of HIV Infection.* London: Springer-Verlag, 1993:21–33.

73. Craddock C, Pasvol G, Bull R, et al. Cardiorespiratory arrest and autonomic neuropathy in AIDS. *Lancet* 1987;4:16–18.

74. Miller RF, Semple SJG. Autonomic neuropathy in AIDS. *Lancet* 1987;2:343–344.

75. Ruttimann S, Hilti P, Spinas GA, et al. High Frequency of HIV-associated autonomic neuropathy and more severe involvement in advanced stages of human immunodeficiency virus disease. *Arch Intern Med* 1991;151:2441–2443.

76. Villa A, Crucci V, Foresti V, et al. Confalonieri F. HIV-related functional involvement of autonomic nervous system. *Acta Neurol* 1990;12:14–18.

77. Villa A, Foresti V, Confalonieri F. Autonomic neuropathy and prolongation of QT interval in human immunodeficiency virus infection. *Clin Auton Res* 1995;5:48–52.

78. Walsh CA, Better D, Adam HM, et al. Holter monitor and ECG abnormalities in children with HIV. [Abstract]. *Am J Dis Child* 1990;144:434.

79. Budka H. HIV-related dementia: pathology and possible pathogenesis. In: Scaravelli F (ed). *The Neuropathology of HIV Infection.* London: Springer-Verlag, 1993:141–185.

80. Dickson DW, Lee SC, Lattiace LA, et al. Microglia and cytokines in neurological disease, with special reference to AIDS and Alzheimer's disease. *Glia* 1993;7:75–83.

81. Fuller GN, Jacobs JM. Peripheral nerve and muscle disease in HIV infection. In: Scaravelli F (ed). *The Neuropathology of HIV Infection.* London: Springer-Verlag, 1993:215–233.

82. Bharati S, Joshi VV, Connor EM, et al. Conduction system in children with acquired immunodeficiency syndrome. *Chest* 1989;96:406–413.

83. Lefkowitz RJ, Hoffman BB, Taylor P. Neurohumoral transmission: the autonomic and somatic nervous systems. In: Gilman AG, Rall TW, Nies AS, Taylor P (eds). *Goodman and Gilman's The Pharmacological Basis of Therapeutics,* 8th Ed. New York: Pergamon Press, 1990:84–121.

84. Schlant RC, Sonnenblick EH. Normal physiology of the cardiovascular system In: Schland RC, Alexander RW (eds). *Hurst's The Heart,* 8th Ed. New York: McGraw-Hill, 1994:113–151.

85. Campbell WB. Lipid-derived autocoids: eicosanoids and platelet-activating factor In: Gilman AAG, Rall TW, Nies As, Taylor P (eds). *Goodman and Gilman's The Pharmacological Basis of Therapeutics,* 8th Ed. Elmsford, NY: McGraw-Hill, 1990:600–617.

86. Van der Pol AN, Trombley PQ. Glutamate neurons in hypothalamus regulate excitatory transmission. *J Neurosci* 1993;13:2829–2836.

87. Magnuson DSK, Knudsen BE, Geiger JD, et al. Human immunodeficiency virus type 1 *tat* activates non-*N*-methyl-D-aspartate excitatory amino acid receptors and causes neurotoxicity. *Ann Neurol* 1995;37:373–380.

88. Scaravelli F, Gray F, Mikol J, et al. Pathology of the nervous system. In: Scaravelli F (ed). *The Neuropathology of HIV Infection.* London: Springer-Verlag, 1993:99–169.

89. Everall IP, Hudson L, Al-Sarraj S, et al. Decreased expression of AMPA receptor messenger RNA and protein in AIDS: a model for HIV-asociated neurotoxicity. *Nature Med* 1995;1:1174–1178.

90. Toggas SM, Masliah E, Rockenstein EM, et al. Central nervous system damage produced by expression of HIV-1 coat protein gp120 in transgenic mice. *Nature* 1994;367:188–193.

91. Thomas FP, Chalk C, Lalonde R, et al. Expression of human immunodeficiency virus type 1 in the nervous system of transgenic mice leads to neurologic disease. *J Virol* 1994;68:7099–7107.

92. Giulian D, Wendt E, Vaca K, et al. The envelope glycoprotein of human immunodeficiency virus type 1 stimulates release of neurotoxins from monocytes. *Proc Natl Acad Sci USA* 1993;90: 2769–2773.

93. Rostami AM. Pathogenesis of immune-mediated neuropathies. *Pediatr Res* 1992;33:S90-S94.

94. Klein JO, Remington JS. Current concepts of infections of the fetus and newborn infant. In: Remington JS, Klein Jo (eds). *Infectious Diseases of the Fetus and Newborn Infant,* 4th Ed. Philadelphia: WB Saunders, 1995:1–19.

95. Kaplan C. The placenta and viral infections. *Semin Diagn Pathol* 1993;10:232–250.

96. Kesson AM, Fear WR, Williams L, et al. HIV infection of placental macrophages: their potential role in vertical transmission. *J Leukocyte Biol* 1994;56:241–246.

97. David FJ, Tran HC, Serpente N, et al. HIV infection of choriocarcinoma cell lines derived from human placenta: the role of membrane CD4 and Fc-Rs into HIV entry. *Virology* 1995;208: 784–788.

98. Lairmore MD, Cuthbert PS, Utley LL, et al. Cellular localisation of CD4 in the human placenta. *J Immunol* 1993;151:1673–1681.

99. Frenkel LD, Gaur S. Perinatal HIV infection and AIDS. *Clin Perinatol* 1994;21:95–107.

100. Reinhardt B, Torbett BE, Gulizia RJ, et al. Human immunodeficiency virus type 1 infection of neonatal severe combined immunodeficient mice xenografted with human cord blood cells. *AIDS Res Hum Retrov* 1994;10:131–141.

101. Aldrovandi GM, Feuer G, Gao L, et al. The SCID-hu mouse as a model for HIV-1 infection. *Nature* 1993;363:732–736.

102. Chien KR. Molecular advances in cardiovascular biology. *Science* 1993;269:916–917.

103. Rockman HA, Ono S, Ross RS, et al. Molecular and physiological alterations in murine ventricular dysfunction. *Proc Natl Acad Sci USA* 1994; 91:2694–2698.

104. Bond RA, Leff P, Johnson TD, et al. Physiological effects of inverse agonists in transgenic mice with myocardial overexpression of the beta 2-adreno-ceptor. *Nature* 1995;374:272–276.

105. Milano CA, Allen LF, Rockman HA, et al. Enhanced myocardial function in transgenic mice overexpressing the beta 2-adrenergic receptor. *Science* 1994;264:582–586.

106. Luo W, Grupp IL, Harrer J, et al. Targeted ablation of the phospholamban gene is associated with markedly enhanced myocardial contractility and loss of beta-agonist stimulation. *Circ Res* 1994; 75:401–409.

107. Jolicoeur P, Laperriere A, Beaulieu N. Efficient production of human immunodeficiency virus proteins in transgenic mice. *J Virol* 1992;66:3904–3908.

108. Kopp JB, Ray PE, Adler SH, et al. Nephropathy in HIV-transgenic mice. *Contrib Nephrol* 1994; 107:194–204.

109. Kopp JB, Rooney JF, Wohlenberg C, et al. Cutaneous disorders and viral gene expression in HIV-1 transgenic mice. *AIDS Res Hum Retrov* 1993; 9:267–275.

110. Cook DN, Beck MA, Coffman TM, et al. Requirement of MIP-1 for an inflammatory response to viral infection. *Science* 1995;269:1583–1585.

111. Trial JA, Birdsall HH, Hallum JA, et al. Phenotypic and functional changes in peripheral blood monocytes during progression of human immunodeficiency virus infection. *J Clin Invest* 1995; 95:1690–1701.

19

Immunopathogenesis of Cardiovascular Complications of HIV Infection

Alistair I. Fyfe, M.D., Ph.D

At a superficial level, it would seem paradoxical that an immunodeficiency virus such as human immunodeficiency virus-1 (HIV) might lead to cardiovascular complications that are immunologically mediated. This would not be the first paradox associated with the acquired immunodeficiency syndrome (AIDS), as the disease has provided many new and complicated insights into the human immune repertoire, which transcend the classic responses characterized historically with more traditional bacterial and viral agents. The following are some of the paradoxes that may be explored in order to understand the potential mechanisms of the immunopathogenesis of cardiovascular disease in HIV infection:

1. Consideration of immunity in its broadest sense, rather than being restricted to the traditional lymphocyte-based concepts. Elements of the so-called nonspecific immune system, including antigen-presenting cells, such as dendritic cells and macrophages, represent major cellular targets involved in HIV pathogenesis.

2. Imbalance within the immune system created by the deletion of specific cell subsets by HIV infection leads to unopposed effects of the remaining or uninfected cells, which produce pathophysiologic consequences.

3. It has been assumed for many years that the immune system is destructively involved in many classic immune diseases and some degenerative diseases, such as atherosclerosis. However, withdrawal of various elements of the immune system can lead to enhanced disease, suggesting a protective role of the immune system in these diseases.

4. Many of the cytokines that have traditionally been within the repertoire of immune system effectors have been demonstrated to be produced and secreted by a number of nonimmune cells, such as endothelial cells and smooth muscle cells. These cytokines are pathologic in the absence of a sustained immune response.

5. There have been new insights into the pathophysiologic consequences of antibodies targeting functional proteins within the myocardium and vasculature.

6. Factors classically thought to be immune-related in the induction of apoptosis in both immune and nonimmune cells have been assessed as effector mechanisms in HIV infection.

One common feature of HIV cardiomyopathy is the general association with low CD3+ or CD4+ lymphocyte counts in peripheral blood.[1] Explanations for this include the following: (1) The achievement of a critical level of immunosuppression either

283

results in the appearance of other pathogenic organisms or represents a critical level of depletion of a protective cell type.[2] (2) Because CD3+ and CD4+ lymphocyte counts inversely parallel virus load, a critical mass of viral replication has occurred not only in immunologic tissues but also in cardiac tissues. In many cases, a direct and causal relationship among HIV, immunity, and cardiovascular disease has not been conclusively proved, and the role of the immune response to HIV in these complications can only be inferred from related cardiovascular diseases. The resistance of cardiac myocytes to productive infection with HIV, and the lack of data supporting active viral infection and proliferation in vitro and in vivo, suggest that mechanisms other than HIV infection play a role in the pathogenesis of the cardiac complications of HIV.[3] Further complicating our understanding in infants with HIV is the possibility that maternal cytokines and antibodies are transferred to the fetus and are active in utero. In the first 6 months of life, some of the immunologic damage, particularly humoral immune-mediated damage, may result from the prenatal transfer of maternal antibodies. There are no comparative data on cardiac function using simultaneous assessments in mothers and fetuses to provide information on this question.

Immunologic Consequences of and Responses to HIV Infection

In an effort to provide some insights into the immunologic effects of and responses to HIV infection and how these might translate into cardiovascular pathogenesis, the natural history of HIV will first be reviewed. HIV infection occurs in two distinct phases. First, there is a latent phase of infection of T lymphocytes and other antigen-presenting cells, which lasts from weeks to years. HIV infection propagates at both local and systemic levels by migration of infected cells within and between tissues, as well as by transfer of HIV from infected to uninfected cells via cell-to-cell communication. Propagation of infection by these mechanisms is more common than propagation by release of free virions. For example, it has been shown that myocardial interstitial cells, including dendritic cells,

are not only susceptible to HIV infection but efficiently transmit HIV-1 to CD4+ T lymphocytes through cell-to-cell syncytia.[3]

The development of the full AIDS syndrome usually follows a stimulus that activates HIV replication and gene expression. Many of these stimuli result from independent or interrelated immunologic or inflammatory events causing the release of soluble factors and cytokines, such as tumor necrosis factor (TNF), lymphotoxin, interleukin (IL)-1, IL-3, IL-6, interferon (IFN), and granulocyte-macrophage colony-stimulating factor (GM-CSF). One common pathway by which these various factors switch on HIV transcription is nuclear factor kappa B (NF-kB)-mediated transcription of the viral long terminal repeat sequences. The production of these cytokines and other soluble HIV gene products not only serves to amplify further production of cytokines but may enhance the ability of HIV to infect nearby cells or to switch on HIV proliferation in nearby cells. This will be a common theme in HIV infection in general and cardiovascular complications in particular. It has been shown that HIV-1 infection of T lymphocytes induces the expression of TNF but not IL-1 and IL-6 in the infected cells via the *tat* gene product,[4] and that TNF can induce the expression of IL-1 and IL-6 in an autocrine fashion in nearby cells. These cytokines then act to increase the expression of HIV in other infected cells, completing the positive feedback loop.[5] The stimuli for the specific production of cytokines in nonimmune tissues are largely unknown, but the functional consequences for HIV replication and T-lymphocytes apoptosis are the same.[6] In this local environment massive HIV-1 production can occur. If such production occurs in the presence of IFN-γ and IL-10, apoptosis of the infected or activated T-helper lymphocytes occurs.[7] Thus, the local cytokine milieu can determine the balance between productive infection and immunosuppression due to cell death.

The preferential infection of CD4+ lymphocytes by HIV, leading via a number of pathways to selective CD4+ lymphocyte depletion, produces local and systemic immunologic imbalance. The resulting overabundance of CD8+ cells changes both local and systemic cytokines. It subsequently became apparent that HIV infection showed a predilection for the T-helper 2 (T_H2) subset (producers of IL-4, IL-5, IL-6, and IL-10) rather than the T_H1 subset (secreting IFN-γ, IL-2, and IL-12) The relationship between these two subsets in the pathogenesis of cardiomyopathy is poorly understood, although specific disease states are associated with similar imbalances. The T_H1 subset is active more acutely and attempts to destroy foreign antigen present on grafts and infectious agents. T_H2 cells appear to be more active chronically in accommodating antigenic stimuli and are often seen in chronic infectious or inflammatory processes, such as atherosclerosis and leprosy.[8] In the chronic immunologic conditions, T_H2 cells appear to limit both the damage done by the infectious or inflammatory agent and the damage from the immune response to the agent. One can therefore imagine that deletion of this accommodating cell population leads to more briskly aberrant immune responses than a balanced depletion.

Initial data seemed to indicated that the preferential loss of CD4+ T_H1 cell function in HIV-infected persons was related to an imbalance or switch from T_H1 to T_H2 cytokine production. Others have suggested that the loss of CD4+ lymphocytes results from inadequate renewal of T-helper cells.[9] More recent evidence suggests that infection of CD4+ lymphocytes leads to activation-induced death via T-lymphocyte receptor or fas-mediated apoptosis[10] and depletion of this cell population. Even within the T-helper cell subset, there is a further level of complexity, as imbalance exists between the infectivity of T_H1 and T_H2 cells, with T_H2 cells able to prevent the apoptotic death of infected T_H1 cells. T_H2 cytokines such as IL-12 appear to prevent the apoptosis of infected T_H1 cells. The absence of T_H2 cells allows apoptosis to occur, with further imbalance of the immune system. The $T_H2:T_H1$ ratio then changes the balance of the immune system by affecting CD8+ lymphocytes. Treatment of CD8+ lymphocytes with a prototypical T_H1 cytokine, IL-2, enhances anti-HIV viral activity, but the T_H2-type cytokines IL-4 and IL-10 reduce the ability of CD8+ lymphocytes to suppress HIV replication and to produce IL-2. HIV disease progression may result from a shift in cytokine production from a T_H1 to a T_H2 pattern.[11] The imbalance between T_H1 and T_H2 lymphocyte subpopulations not only affects

other cellular elements of the immune response, it also directly affects HIV replication. In prestimulated peripheral blood mononuclear cells, the typical T_H1 cytokines IL-12, IL-4, and IL-2 induced production of HIV p24 antigen, which was not due to induction of IL-1, IL-2, (TNF)-α, or TNF-β. T_H1 and T_H2 cytokines may be produced by a number of nonclassical immune cells, such as macrophages, endothelial cells, and dendritic cells.

The cardiac significance of imbalances created by these two cell subsets will be discussed in greater detail later. Evidence for significant imbalances within the myocardium in human cardiac disease is provided by studies on coronary sinus cytokine concentrations.[12]

There are both classical and nonclassical responses to HIV infection by the immune system. The reponses vary with time depending on the number of CD4+ lymphocytes depleted. The predilection of HIV for CD4+ lymphocytes is a mechanism to prevent immunosurveillance and detection. Normally, viral infection of a nucleated cell leads to the formation of complexes between viral peptides and major histocompatibility complex (MHC) molecules on the surface of the cell. These are typically class I MHC molecules for viral and other intracellular proteins and class II MHC molecules for extracellular proteins. The consequences of viral peptide presentation by a class I MHC molecule to a CD8+ lymphocyte are both the amplification of an immune response and the death of the infected cell. After it is injected into mice, HIV tat protein (which may circulate) can be found associated with cardiac vascular cells, such as endothelium,[13] where it may incite an independent immune response when presented as expected in the context of class I MHC.[14] The normal sequence of immune activation in response to viral infection is aberrant in HIV infection as CD4+ lymphocytes, which by definition are class II MHC-restricted, cannot process and present antigens via class I MHC molecules to CD8+ lymphocytes. Even if they were able, the resulting death of the presenting cells would further augment the loss of CD4+ lymphocytes. CD8+ lymphocytes also detect and are activated by HIV peptides on alternative antigen-presenting cells, such as endothelial cells or macrophages.[15] There is evidence from the cellular immune responses to HIV that antigen presentation of HIV proteins occurs in the context of class I MHC molecules.[14] HIV may have associated on its surface a human leukocyte antigen (HLA)-DR molecule which can act as a super-antigen to cause T-lymphocyte proliferation and IL-2 production. Such HLA-DR-bearing HIV strains can under appropriate conditions induce T-lymphocyte apoptosis.[16] HIV soluble glycoprotein gp120 bears structural similarities to MHC class I and class II molecules and is able to stimulate the T-lymphocyte receptor aberrantly, producing immune activation, anergy, and apoptosis, depending on the context of antigen recognition.[17]

CD8+ lymphocyte-derived cytokines, normally used to signal CD4+ helper lymphocytes and amplify the immune response, produce aberrant consequences in the presence of HIV infection, with activation and amplification of HIV replication in CD4+ lymphocytes and apoptosis in HIV-infected cells. Further problems occur because CD8+ lymphocytes therefore cannot eradicate HIV-infected CD4+ lymphocytes, as they have no ability to detect that they are infected; and because CD8+ lymphocytes do not necessarily have access to body compartments such as the testis and the central nervous system where HIV-infected cells may exist. There is therefore a chronic class I MHC-dependent stimulus to CD8+ lymphocytes, together with an inherent lack of ability to control CD8+ lymphocytes because of the selective depletion of T_H2 lymphocytes. Chronic activation of specific elements of the immune system contributes to cytokine imbalances, particularly the production of TNF-α, which is a direct myocardial toxin.

The productive infection of cells by HIV leads to production of several viral proteins that circulate, such as tat, gp120, p24, and vpr. These proteins themselves play pathophysiologic roles and stimulate antibody responses which may also play a pathophysiologic role in HIV manifestations. This will be discussed in detail later. It is apparent, then, that HIV infection or the immunologic responses to infection may play a role in the development of cardiomyopathy and vascular disease by the following mechanisms:

- Infection of myocardial and vascular cells
- Depletion of protective immunity

- Production of HIV proteins that may directly or indirectly affect cardiovascular structure and function
- Production of immune responses to HIV that may directly (cytokines) or indirectly (antibodies) affect cardiovascular structure and function

The role of each of these factors will be discussed in relation to the development of cardiomyopathy[18] (for which there are more data) and then for the development of vascular disease (for which there are few data except for Kaposi's sarcoma).

HIV Myocarditis: Virus versus Immunity

There is evidence of myocarditis from necropsy of HIV-infected adults with global left ventricular dysfunction.[19] In a larger series of adults, 51% of patients with global left ventricular dysfunction and CD4+ lymphocyte counts <100 cells/mm³, showed evidence of myocarditis, including infiltrating CD8+ lymphocytes.[14] It is not clear from the published literature, either in HIV infection or in the more common myocarditis, whether myocardial damage leading to cardiomyopathy results from the direct action of the virus itself, from a vigorous immune response directed at infected cardiomyocytes, or from an attack on cardiomyocytes as innocent bystanders. There is conflicting evidence about the direct infection of myocytes by HIV in myocarditis that relates in part to the techniques of detection used. In one report, both HIV and cytomegalovirus (CMV) viral sequences were found; however, detection of viral DNA does not prove productive infection.[20] In fact, there is only one report that conclusively documents the presence of productive HIV infection in human cardiomyocytes.[21] In the myocarditis associated with the dilated cardiomyopathy of Chagas' disease in *Trypanosoma cruzi* infection, nonparasitized myocytes are damaged as a result of the immune response to infection.[22] The interstitial lymphocytes and macrophages form contacts with myocytes that lead to focal loss of the myocyte basement membrane. As in HIV infection, contacts are formed between lymphocytes and endothelial cells.[22] Transforming growth factor (TGF) is a general inhibitor of acute immune responses but is associated with longer-term chronic inflammatory responses, such as scarring. Mice lacking TGFβ$_1$ (knockout mice) die by 3 to 4 weeks of age from a multifocal inflammatory disease, which includes myocarditis involving primarily macrophages.[23]

Endothelium, Immunity, and Cardiomyopathy

A number of observations suggest a role for vascular endothelium in the pathogenesis of myocarditis and idiopathic dilated cardiomyopathy. The proximity of endothelial cells to cardiac myocytes at a microscopic level suggests that cardiomyopathy might arise as a direct result of endothelial damage, or result from endothelial activation and the production of proinflammatory cytokines that are directly toxic to myocardial structure and function. One potential link between the microvasculature and cardiomyopathy is through the production of ischemia. There is evidence in both human tissue[24] and animal models[25] that ischemia may play a role in the pathogenesis of idiopathic dilated cardiomyopathy. Risk factors for the development of cardiomyopathy, such as hypertension and coronary artery disease, are also present in adults with HIV infection[26] but are unlikely to be present in children; they might support a role for endothelium in cardiomyopathy. There is evidence for a primary role of viral infection of the endothelium in myocarditis that ultimately develops into cardiomyopathy. In a large-animal model of cardiomyopathy induced by encephalomyocarditis virus, viral particles were detected in the cytoplasm of many endothelial cells, but not in cardiac myocytes.[27] An alternative interaction between endothelium and myocytes in the pathogenesis of myocarditis, and HIV myocarditis in particular, is mediated by nitric oxide produced by the endothelium in response to viral infection.[28] Nitric oxide is also produced by endothelium in response to TNF and is believed to be the primary mediator of endotoxic shock.[29] Nitric oxide production associated with myocardial macrophages has also been shown to reduce viral replication in a murine model of myocarditis.[30]

There is evidence for a larger role of the vascular endothelium in the pathogenesis of HIV myocarditis and cardiomyopathy than is apparent for other more traditional viruses, such as coxsackievirus. Vascular endothelium is a major reservoir for HIV. HIV infects human endothelial cells independent of CD4,[31] and endothelial cells participate in the spread of HIV in a complex manner involving interactions with monocytes. As a barrier between the circulation and the tissues, the vascular endothelium is able to transmit HIV to monocytes transmigrating between endothelial cells directly by cell-to-cell communication and indirectly via secreted HIV-related protein interactions with vascular endothelial cells. A positive feedback appears to exist, as HIV infection of monocytes increases CD11/CD18 integrin-dependent monocyte–monocyte and monocyte–endothelial interactions.[20] HIV-infected monocytes in turn markedly disrupt the endothelial monolayer by producing gelatinases and metalloproteinases, which degrade extracellular matrix.[32] Monoclonal antibodies to integrins, but not the ligands lymphocyte function antigen-1 and platelet endothelial cell adhesion molecule-1, increase HIV infection of human endothelial cells by enhancing HIV absorption.[33] Vascular endothelial cells appear selectively and specifically to upregulate HIV replication in macrophages when cultured in close proximity. This process depends on cell-to-cell contact and appears to be mediated through the same CD11/CD18 integrin pathway.[34] HIV infection changes the ability of infected monocytes to interact with extracellular matrix, and that matrix in turn affects viral replication in infected cells.[35] Endothelial cells and monocytes appear to act synergetically in the production of inflammatory cytokines as well as in viral infection, transmission, and replication. HIV-infected endothelial cells produce cytokines such as IL-6 and IL-1 in significant amounts,[36] but not TNF, IFN-α, or IFN-γ.[37] The production of cytokines such as IL-6, IL-1β, and GM-CSF by endothelial cells augments HIV replication in infected monocytes.[38] HIV gene products in turn stimulate the transmigration of more monocytes by activating the expression of endothelial cell adhesion molecules and the production of growth factors and cytokines. HIV tat stimulates endothelial cells to express E-selectin and to increase synthesis of IL-6, particularly in the presence of low levels of TNF.[39]

The HIV gene product tat adheres to and promotes the growth of vascular endothelial cells, which may differentiate into Kaposi's sarcoma cells via an integrin receptor.[28] Again a complex interplay is noted, with upregulation of the integrin receptor for tat by inflammatory cytokines.[40]

Cell-Mediated Immunity and Dilated Cardiomyopathy

Given the paucity of data supporting the ability of HIV to infect cardiac myocytes directly and cause myocarditis, it is useful to explore the role of the immune system in the development of idiopathic dilated cardiomyopathy. There are certainly many animal and human data that link the development of dilated cardiomyopathy to prior episodes of myocarditis. There is evidence for the coexistence of these two processes in the same patient. In 176 patients with suspected dilated cardiomyopathy, strict criteria for myocarditis were met in only 14 cases (8%). However, a further 67 cases (38%) showed pathologic lymphocytic infiltrates with activated lymphocytes, macrophages, and vascular endothelium.[41] One piece of evidence against systemic cell-mediated immune responses in the development of HIV cardiomyopathy is the temporal relationship to the fall in CD4+ lymphocyte counts in both adults[42] and children,[43] although this is not related to the local immune events that are occurring. Data for the relationship between immunity and cardiomyopathy have derived from human mechanistic and genetic studies as well as animal models. Observations in humans have focused on local and systemic markers of immune activation, as well as genetic studies looking for associations between immune response genes and cardiomyopathy.

The data from genetic studies are conflicting. Early studies suggested a relationship between HLA types and dilated cardiomyopathy, particularly at the class II loci DR, DP, and DQ, although systematic genetic linkage analysis has failed to confirm this.[44,45] More detailed analysis of the particular peptides corresponding to the fine detail of the MHC molecules continues to show enrichment for particular class II molecules such as DRB1*1401, DQB1*0503, and the combination of

DRB1*1401 and DQB1*0503 in certain populations.[46] An independent association study comparing 44 normal controls with 34 patients with idiopathic dilated cardiomyopathy also found an increased frequency of two different DQA1-DQB1 haplotypes (*0102-*0604 and *0102-*0501).[47] In other large pedigrees, however, detailed genetic mapping over the human HLA region on chromosome 6 in 12 families with idiopathic dilated cardiomyopathy failed to identify significant loci.[48] No evidence for genetic linkage was found from more exhaustive linkage maps that included markers linked to the genes for HLA antigens; immunoglobulin heavy and light chains; immunoglobulin Fc and T-cell receptor; CD3, CD4, CD8, and CD45 antigens; interleukins IL-1, IL-3, IL-4, IL-5, IL-6, IL-9, and IL-11, the IL-1 and IL-2 receptors; and the genes coding for the β_1 adrenoreceptor, the adenine nucleotide translocator-1, and the cardiac α and β myosin heavy chains.[49] There are two important caveats in genetic association studies. The first is that the combined effects of multiple genes (which are individually small but synergize to activate the immune system to target cardiac myocytes) are hard to determine in small populations, as it is likely that different combinations of genes are responsible in each population studied. The second is that genetic studies only reflect the static structural determinants of DNA and do not provide information on the activation of any particular gene or series of genes.

A few studies have looked specifically at immune activation markers in HIV cardiomyopathy, although the development of cardiomyopathy as a terminal manifestation of HIV infection at the same time as other infectious complications makes interpretation of the data difficult. In this regard, data from non-HIV-mediated cardiomyopathy are more instructive. Elevated soluble IL-2 receptor levels, representing generalized[49] and nonspecific activation of T lymphocytes, have been demonstrated in patients with dilated cardiomyopathy,[50] although in a small series of patients the opposite is noted; cutaneous anergy associated with decreased T-lymphocyte responsiveness has been reported.[51] In patients with dilated cardiomyopathy, there was a significant positive correlation between soluble CD4+ lymphocyte levels in serum and the clinical and immunohistologic findings, including the endomyocardial CD4+:CD8+ lymphocyte ratio,[52] consistent with a major role for CD4+ lymphocytes in the pathogenesis of this disease. This paradox can be resolved when one considers that the CD4+ lymphocytes present in the myocardium of HIV-infected patients are likely targets and that activation of these targets as a result of infection might produce a similar pathophysiologic process. Soluble CD4+ lymphocyte levels have not been measured in HIV cardiomyopathy. In non-HIV-infected patients with IDCM, there is an enrichment of infiltrating cells with CD8+ T lymphocytes and macrophages in the myocardium. The majority of T lymphocytes also express either activation markers, such as IL-2 receptors, or memory markers, such as CD45RO.[53] Infiltrates containing perforin-expressing killer CD8+ T lymphocytes and enhanced expression of HLA class I and intercellular adhesion molecule-1 (ICAM-1) are noted in myocardial tissue of patients with dilated cardiomyopathy. The repertoires of T-lymphocyte receptor V alpha genes as well as V beta gene transcripts were restricted, indicating a highly specific immune response to a cardiac antigen.[54]

Cytokines and Dilated Cardiomyopathy

Myocarditis and dilated cardiomyopathy are associated with local production of cytokines, which may be markedly elevated over circulating levels, making peripheral cytokine levels uninformative.[12] As discussed previously, the local cytokine milieu may determine the ateome of viral infection, which might either resolve spontaneously or develop into myocarditis or cardiomyopathy.[55] The local production of cytokines has been demonstrated to markedly enhance the cardiotoxicity of viral infection and myocardial damage in strains of mice. Viral infection in the context of a nonspecific stimulator of monokines such as IL-1 and TNF was much more likely to lead to myocarditis and myocyte damage than viral infection alone,[56] and antagonists of IL-1 were able to ameliorate the severity of myocarditis in susceptible mice.[57]

A number of studies have looked at the profile of cytokines produced in myocarditis, cardiomyopathy, and heart failure, as well as the sites of production, with varied results. In a study of 13 patients with acute myocarditis, elevated plasma TNF levels were found in 46% of patients, with a mean concentration of 61 ± 31 pg/ml.[52] In 8 of 23 patients who developed dilated cardiomyopathy, TNF levels were elevated to an average concentration of 402 pg/ml, suggesting a pathophysiologic role in the progression of the disease.[58] In a series of patients developing mild or moderate heart failure from dilated cardiomyopathy, no increases in circulating levels of IL-1α, soluble IL-2 receptor, or TNF-α were noted, but IL-6 levels were elevated.[59] Vascular endothelial cells and monocytes/macrophages are rich sources for these cytokines, although data from endomyocardial biopsies have not conclusively proven which cell type is predominant. GM-CSF was also elevated at 2.5 ± 1.8 ng/ml.

Many of the factors leading to the production of cytokines in infected cells have been discussed above. HIV-1 envelope glycoprotein gp120 can directly induce TNF-α production in monocytes/macrophages.[60] The site of cytokine production in cardiomyopathy has been elucidated in animals and myocardial biopsies.

Messenger RNA for leukocyte chemotactic cytokines IL-8 and monocyte chemotactic protein-1 is produced in all cases of idiopathic dilated cardiomyopathy.[61] Endomyocardial biopsies have demonstrated local expression of the genes for IL-1β, IL-6, IL-8, and TNF in 100% of myocarditis patients, and the TNF gene continues to be expressed in 57% of patients whose disease progresses to cardiomyopathy.[62]

Antibody and Humoral Immune Responses in Cardiomyopathy

Despite the cellular immunodeficiency and lack of T-lymphocyte help to B lymphocytes created by depletion of CD4+ lymphocytes in HIV infection, enhanced and aberrant antibody responses, including an expanded repertoire of autoantibodies, occur in HIV-infected patients. This may represent a change in the balance between protective antibodies such as IgA and the complement-fixing antibodies IgG and IgM. Lipshultz and coworkers[63] were the first to show an association between abnormal serum immunoglobulins and abnormalities in left ventricular structure and function. In part, the immunologic responses responsible for the cardiomyopathy in HIV infection might result from the immune responses to CMV immediate early gene sequences in cardiac myocytes that are seen in HIV[64] as well as in non-HIV myocarditis. Antibodies to cholinergic receptors have been demonstrated in HIV infection and may explain conducting system disease, QT prolongation,[65] and sudden death that accompany HIV cardiac disease. In a separate series of studies, IgA and IgG antibodies from HIV-infected patients inhibited tension development in cardiac muscle cells by their activities on the cholinergic receptor. Autoantibodies to acetylcholine receptors have been demonstrated in non-HIV idiopathic dilated cardiomyopathy, and immunization of rabbits with the antigenic epitope of the acetylcholine receptor leads to changes in both the sarcolemma and the mitochondria of cardiac myocytes.[66] Antibodies to other cardiac structural components, such as cardiolipin, have been demonstrated in as many as 47% of HIV-seropositive individuals. As in other diseases, anticardiolipin antibodies may coexist with antibodies to endothelial cells.[67] Antibodies to other myocardial structural proteins, including myosin light and heavy chains, tropomyosin, and actin, have been demonstrated in approximately 50% of patients with dilated cardiomyopathy.[68] The presence of β-receptor adrenergic autoantibodies and their relationship to restriction fragment length polymorphisms of the HLA class II genes were studied in 42 affected and unaffected members of a family with a heritable disorder of the conduction system and cardiac muscle. Antibodies were detected in 34% of all members (59% of affected and 22% of unaffected; $P < .01$). Significant differences between affected and unaffected individuals and between individuals who were positive and negative for anti-β-receptor antibodies were noted in the prevalence of polymorphisms obtained with Taq I for the HLA-DR beta and HLA-DQ alpha genes. In affected individuals, there was a strong positive correlation between these polymorphisms and the presence of anti-β-receptor antibodies.[69] There is also evidence for restricted immunoglobulin subclass usage in dilated cardiomyopathy, and this appears to be associated with the presence of both cardiac-specific antibodies and generalized autoantibodies.[70] This restricted immunoglobulin response was also associated with a higher incidence of HLA-DR4 than in normal people, suggesting that particular HLA molecules present cardiac-specific proteins, as well as other tissue peptides in a manner that facilitates the production of autoantibody. There is also a correlation between the presence of antibodies to the β₁-adrenergic receptor that inhibit isoproterenol-stimulated Ca^{2+} uptake in cardiomyocytes, antibodies that inhibit sarcoplasmic calcium transport, and the HLA-DR4 antigen.[71]

In animal models of myocarditis, coxsackievirus infection is associated with the development of antibodies to cardiac structural proteins, such as myosin,[72] and myocarditis may also be produced by specific immunization using cardiac myosin as the antigen. Antibodies to other cardiac structural proteins, such as vimentin, have also been demonstrated in mouse models of myocarditis, although it is difficult to know whether such antibodies occur as a result of the interstitial injury produced by the virus.[73] These data support a close link between virus infection and cellular and humoral immune responses in the production of the final myocarditis/cardiomyopathy phenotype.

HIV Apoptosis and Cardiomyopathy

Although immune-mediated cytotoxicity and apoptosis are not normally thought to coexist, since apoptosis is defined as cell death that occurs in the absence of an inflammatory or immune response, there is accumulating evidence for the participation of apoptosis in the pathogenesis of HIV infection. One of the common pathways for apoptosis is through ligation of the combination of the TNF receptor and the fas ligand with the fas receptor. The role of TNF in the pathgenesis of HIV disease and also in the development of cardiovascular complications has already been alluded to. There is evidence from DNA fragmentation assays that circulating lymphocytes in HIV-infected children are undergoing apoptosis in vivo. These were preferentially of the CD8+ phenotype and were strongly correlated with evidence of active Epstein-Barr virus replication. Infected peripheral blood mononuclear cells rapidly induce apoptosis in uninfected cells. Infected cells themselves appear to be protected from programmed cell death in a gp120-CD4-dependent pathway.[74] Thus, in HIV-infected patients, infected lymphocytes may cause the depletion of the much larger population of uninfected CD4+ cells without actually infecting them, by triggering apoptosis.[75] These findings, together with others, suggest that triggering of T lymphocytes by foreign antigen or by other viruses may lead to HIV replication, apoptosis, or both.[76] A number of studies have documented the ability of HIV-related proteins, particularly vpr, gp120, and tat, to induce apoptosis in immune cell subtypes. HIV-1 tat protein induces apoptosis of lymphocytes from healthy donors.[77] Plasma from four patients with acute HIV-related thrombotic thrombocytopenic purpura (TTP) induced apoptosis in cultured microvascular endothelial cells via a fas-dependent pathway.[78] Conversely, there is evidence that extracellular tat can suppress apoptosis in a Bcl-2-dependent manner, which may contribute to immune system dysregulation and hyperplastic or neoplastic disorders.[79] An oxidative stress state that occurs in HIV infection is sensed through the NF-κB pathway,[80] a pathway used to induce apoptosis in response to stimulation via the TNF/fas pathway.[81] Again there appears to be a complex interplay between factors that induce productive infection of HIV in infected cells and activation of programmed cell death via the same pathway.

There is an accumulating body for evidence of apoptosis of cardiac myocytes in the genesis of cardiac development,[82] idiopathic dilated cardiomyopathy,[83] and arrhythmogenic right ventricular hypoplasia.[84] In animal models of dilated cardiomyopathy induced by rapid ventricular pacing, activation of myocyte apoptosis is associated with the induction of the TNF/fas pathway.[85] The more common causes of human heart failure secondary to hypertrophic responses to hypertensive heart disease are also associated with apoptosis.[86] There is no direct evidence for HIV-induced apoptosis of cardiac myocytes.

Immunity and Cardiovascular Developmental Defects and Delays

Given the role of HIV infection and the resulting cytokine production in the induction of apoptosis, and the role of apoptosis in development, it is somewhat surprising that there is little evidence that the immune system plays a major role in cardiovascular development. There is no evidence that the cardiovascular developmental delays noted in HIV infection might be immunologically mediated. The only relevant evidence is the recent observation that homozygous defective mice lacking TGFs show early arrested cardiac development,[87] which can be reversed by maternally produced TGF-β.

HIV, Immunity, and Atherogenesis

There are few studies looking at the role of HIV and immunosuppression in the development of coronary artery disease. Recent autopsy studies have shown that advanced 80% to 90% stenotic eccentric atherosclerotic plaques occur in young adults (average age: 27 years) with HIV infection.[88] In a small series of indigenous Africans with HIV infection, atypical vascular lesions were reported, including focal necrotizing vasculitis with aneurysm formation and rupture and slow, progressive development of granulomatous vasculitis with fibroproliferative aortic occlusion.[89] In a small postmortem series of eight HIV-seropositive patients, both proximal and distal coronary arterial lesions were demonstrated. Characteristic pathologic findings included eccentric typical atherosclerotic plaques, but also fibrosis and thickening of the tunica media with sclerohyalinosis of the smaller arteries.[90]

HIV infection causes lesions not only in the arterial and microvascular circulations, but also in the pulmonary arterial and venous circulatory beds.[91] In macaque monkeys infected with simian immunodeficiency virus, the arterial disease primarily affected the pulmonary vasculature, with marked intimal thickening and pulmonary thromboses in all 19 animals. The endothelial cells showed evidence of activation, injury, and denudation. Macrophages were more prominent in the adventitia than in the intima and media.[92]

Endothelial activation in HIV-infected patients is measured by markers such as von Willebrand factor, tissue plasminogen activator, plasminogen activator inhibitor and protein S. Von Willebrand factor, tissue-type plasminogen activator, and plasminogen activator inhibitor, are increased in AIDS patients.[93] Such changes might result from endothelial injury or activation and produce a hypercoagulable state, as seen in venoocclusive disease. A particularly common and lethal cardiovascular complication of HIV is Kaposi's sarcoma. Although the lineage of the sarcoma cells continues to be uncertain, an accumulating body of evidence suggests Epstein-Barr transformation of vascular endothelial cells. Other putative transforming agents, including oxidant stress responses, have also been proposed.[94]

Initial studies suggested a proinflammatory role of both nonspecific and specific immunity in atherogenesis, although recent studies have suggested that elements of the specific immune system play a role in suppressing the nonspecific immunity that targets the oxidized low-density lipoprotein modifications in the artery wall. It important to note that many of the early events in atherogenesis are mediated through the same oxidant stress response systems that play a major role in HIV pathogenesis, including NF-κB.[95] The immunodeficiency secondary to HIV allows dominance of CD8+ cellular immune events that are proatherogenic.[96]

A number of studies demonstrate both direct and indirect endothelial injury in HIV infection. These forms of injury might be more closely related to atherogenesis than the endothelium–myocyte interactions described above, which are believed to be important in the pathogenesis of cardiomyopathy. The forms of injury, like spontaneous atherosclerosis, involve both functional activation and structural damage. Endothelial cells, although CD4– can bind HIV-1, especially in the presence of IL-1 and TNF, and viral replication is enhanced in the presence of the same cytokines.[97] In bone marrow, microvascular endothelial cells are the predominant cells infected by HIV (5% to 20%) and show impaired release of IL-6 and GM-CSF after stimulation by IL-1.[98] HIV-tat secreted by HIV-infected cells promotes endothelium–monocyte interactions, that favor extravasation into underlying tissues.[99] Monocyte adhesion molecules on endothelial cells, such as β₂ integrins, are up-regulated with increased adhesion to and disruption of an endothelial monolayer. Treatment of monocytes with tat upregulates the protease MMP-9, which is associated with de-

tachment of endothelial cells and the basement membrane.[100] HIV-tat promotes vascular cell proliferation and migration, basement membrane degradation, and angiogenesis.[101] Conditioned media from activated T lymphocytes induce endothelial cells to proliferate in response to basis fibroblast growth factor and HIV-1 tat.[102] Other viruses, such as CMV, that have been implicated in atherogenesis might also be more common after HIV infection. Infection of vascular endothelial cells causes vasculitis and ischemia.[103] The incidence and potential reactivation of *Chlamydia pneumoniae* in HIV infection has not been studied. There is an accumulating body of evidence to link this infectious agent with spontaneous atherogenesis.

Summary

The role of the immune system in the pathogenesis of cardiovascular complications in HIV infection has been reviewed. Several distinct pathophysiologic links emerge. HIV infection of vascular endothelium is an early and central event in the pathogenesis of AIDS in general and cardiovascular complications in particular. Infection of the vascular endothelium contributes to spread of infection as the virus is transferred to nearby cells, including monocytes, with potential spread to cardiac myocytes. Infection of endothelium also leads to production of HIV proteins and cytokines that affect neighboring cells, such as cardiac myocytes. The change in the local and systemic immunologic milieu caused by HIV further enhances cytokine production, induces autoantibody formation, activates HIV replication in latently infected neighboring cells, and induces programmed cell death in specific cell subsets. All these changes produce an environment that favors HIV replication, which, together with the production of viral and immunologic cytotoxic factors, causes cardiovascular damage.

References

1. Herskowitz A, Vlahov D, Willoughby S, et al. Prevalence and incidence of left ventricular dys-

function in patients with human immunodeficiency virus infection. *Am J Cardiol* 1993;71:955–958.

2. Currie PF, Jacob AJ, Foreman AR, et al. Heart muscle disease related to HIV infection: prognostic implications. *BMJ* 1994;309:1605–1607.

3. Herskowitz A, Wu TC, Willoughby SB, et al. Myocarditis and cardiotropic viral infection associated with severe left ventricular dusfunction in late-stage infection with human immunodeficiency virus. *J Am Coll Cardiol* 1994;24:1025–1032.

4. Sharma V, Knobloch TJ, Benjamin D. Differential expression of cytokine genes in HIV-1 tat transfected T and B cell lines. *Biochem Biophys Res Commun* 1995;208:704–713.

5. Buonaguro L, Barillari G, Chang HK, et al. Effects of the human immunodeficiency virus type I tat protein on the expression of inflammatory cytokines. *J Virol* 1992;66:7159–7167.

6. Cleric M, Shearer GM. The Th1-Th2 hypothesis of HIV infection: new insights. *Immunol Today* 1994;15:575–581.

7. Ludewig B, Gelderblom HR, Becker Y, et al. Transmission of HIV-1 from productively infected mature Langerhans cells to primary CD4+ T lymphocytes results in altered T cell responses with enhanced production of IFN-gamma and IL-10. *Virology* 1996;215:51–60.

8. Uyemura K, Demer LL, Castle SC, et al. Cross-regulatory roles of interleukin (IL)-12 and IL-10 in atherosclerosis. *J Clin Invest* 1996;97:2130–2138.

9. Heeney JL. AIDS: a disease of impaired Th-cell renewal? *Immunol Today* 1995;16:515–520.

10. Estaquier J, Idziorek T, Zou W, et al. T helper type 1/T helper type 2 cytokines and T cell death: preventive effect of interleukin 12 on activation-induced and CD95 (FAS/APO-1)-mediated apoptosis of CD4+ T cells from human immunodeficiency virus-infected persons. *J Exp Med* 1995;182:1759–1767.

11. Barker E, Mackewicz CE, Levy JA. Effects of TH1 and TH2 cytokines on CD8+ cell response against human immunodeficiency virus: implications for long-term survival. *Proc Natl Acad Sci USA* 1995;92:11135–11139.

12. Fyfe AI, Daly PA, Galligan L, et al. Coronary sinus sampling of cytokines after cardiac transplantation: evidence for macrophage activation and interleukin 4 production within the graft. *J Am Coll Cardiol* 1993;21:171–176.

13. Fawell S, Seery J, Daikh Y, et al. Tat-mediated delivery of heterologous proteins into cells. *Proc Natl Acad Sci USA* 1994;91:664–668.

14. Matsui M, Warburton RJ, Cogswell PC, et al. Effects of HIV-1 Tat on expression of HLA class I molecules. *J Acquir Immun Defic Synd Hum Retrov* 1996;11:233–240.

15. Itescu S, Dalton J, Zhang HZ, Winchester R. Tissue infiltration in a CD8 lymphocytosis syndrome associated with human immunodeficiency virus-1 infection has the phenotypic appearance of an antigenically driven response. *J Clin Invest* 1993;91:2216–2225.

16. Rossio JL, Bess J Jr, Henderson LE, et al. HLA class II on HIV particles is functional in superantigen presentation to human T cells: implications for HIV pathogenesis. *AIDS Res Hum Retrov* 1995;11:1433–1439.

17. Sheikh MJ, Ongradi J, Austen BM, et al. The gp 120 envelope of HIV-1 binds peptides in a similar manner to human leukocyte antigens. *AIDS* 1995;9:1229–1235.

18. Barry WH. Mechanisms of immune-mediated myocyte injury. *Circulation* 1994;89:2421–2432.

19. De Castro S, d'Amati G, Gallo P, et al. Frequency of development of acute global left ventricular dysfunction in human immunodeficiency virus infection. *J Am Coll Cardiol* 1994;24:1018–1024.

20. Herskowitz A, Wu TC, Willoughby SB, et al. Myocarditis and cardiotropic viral infection associated with severe left ventricular dysfunction in late-stage infection with human immunodeficiency virus. *J Am Coll Cardiol* 1994;24:1025–1032.

21. Kovacs A, Hinton DR, Wright D, et al. Human immunodeficiency virus type I infection of the heart in three infants with acquired immunodeficiency syndrome and sudden death. *Pediatr Infect Dis J* 1996;15:819–824.

22. Andrade ZA, Andrade SG, Correa R, et al. Myocardial changes in acute *Trypanosoma cruzi* infection: ultrastructural evidence of immune damage and the role of microangiopathy. *Am J Pathol* 1994;144:1403–1411.

23. Kulkarni AB, Ward JM, Yaswen L, et al. Transforming growth factor-beta 1 null mice: an animal model for inflammatory disorders. *Am J Pathol* 1995;146:264–275.

24. Hammond EH, Menlove RL, Yowell RL, Anderson JL. Vascular HLA-DR expression correlates

with pathologic changes suggestive of ischemia in idiopathic dilated cardiomyopathy. *Clin Immunol Immunopathol* 1993;68:197–203.

25. Dong R, Liu P, Wee L, et al. Verapamil ameliorates the clinical and pathological course of murine myocarditis. *J Clin Invest* 1992;90:2022–2030.

26. Segal BH, Factor SM. Myocardial risk factors other than human immunodeficiency virus infection may contribute to histologic cardiomyopathic changes in acquired immune deficiency syndrome. *Mod Pathol* 1993;6:560–564.

27. Marcato PS, Sarli G, Della Salda L, et al. Ultrastructural study of experimental myocarditis induced by cardiovirus (EMCV-M) in swine. *J Submicrosc Cytol Pathol* 1992;24:371–379.

28. Hiraoka Y, Kishimoto C, Takada H, et al. Nitric oxide and murine coxsackievirus B3 myocarditis: aggravation of myocarditis by inhibition of nitric oxide synthase. *J Am Coll Cardiol* 1996;28:1610–1615.

29. Finkel MS, Oddis CV, Jacob TD, et al. Negative inotropic effects of cytokines on the heart mediated by nitric oxide. *Science* 1992;257:387–389.

30. Lowenstein CJ, Hill SL, Lafond-Walker A, et al. Nitric oxide inhibits viral replication in murine myocarditis. *J Clin Invest* 1996;97:1837–1843.

31. Cenacchi G, Re MC, Preda P, et al. Human immunodeficiency virus type-1 (HIV-1) infection of endothelial cells in vitro: a virological, ultrastructural and immuno-cytochemical approach. *J Submicrosc Cytol Pathol* 1992;24:155–161.

32. Dhawan S, Weeks BS, Soderland C, et al. HIV-1 infection alters monocyte interactions with human microvascular endothelial cells. *J Immunol* 1995;154:422–432.

33. Scheglovitova O, Scanio V, Fais S, et al. Antibody to ICAM-1 mediates enhancement of HIV-1 infection of human endothelial cells. *Arch Virol* 1995;140:951–958.

34. Gilles PN, Lathey JL, Spector SA. Replication of macrophage-tropic and T-cell-tropic strains of human immunodeficiency virus type 1 is augmented by macrophage-endothelial cell contact. *J Virol* 1995;69:2133–2139.

35. Dhawan S, Vargo M, Meltzer MS. Interactions between HIV-infected monocytes and the extracellular matrix: increased capacity of HIV-infected monocytes to adhere to and spread on extracellular matrix associated with changes in extent of virus replication and cytopathic effects in infected cells. *J Leukocyte Biol* 1992;52:62–69.

36. Tanowitz HB, Gumprecht JP, Spurr D, et al. Cytokine gene expression of endothelial cells infected with *Trypanosoma cruzi*. *J Infect Dis* 1992;166:598–603.

37. Corbeil J, Evans LA, McQueen PW, et al. Productive in vitro infection of human umbilical vein endothelial cells and three colon carcinoma cell lines with HIV-1. *Immunol Cell Biol* 1995;73:140–145.

38. Fan ST, Hsia K, Edgington TS. Upregulation of human immunodeficiency virus-1 in chronically infected monocytic cell line by both contact with endothelial cells and cytokines. *Blood* 1994;84:1567–1572.

39. Hofman FM, Wright AD, Dohadwala MM, et al. Exogenous tat protein activates human endothelial cells. *Blood* 1993;82:2774–2780.

40. Barillari G, Gendelman R, Gallo RC, Ensoli B. The Tat protein of human immunodeficiency virus type 1, a growth factor for AIDS Kaposi sarcoma and cytokine-activated vascular cells, induces adhesion of the same cell types by using integrin receptors recognizing the RGD amino acid sequence. *Proc Natl Acad Sci USA* 1993;90:7941–7945.

41. Kuhl U, Noutsias M, Schultheiss HP. Immunohistochemistry in dilated cardiomyopathy. *Eur Heart J* 1995;16:100–106.

42. Currie PF, Jacob AJ, Foreman AR, et al. Heart muscle disease related to HIV infection: prognostic implications. *BMJ* 1994;309:1605–1607.

43. Domanski MJ, Sloas MM, Follman DA, et al. Effect of zidovudine and didanosine treatment on heart function in children infected with human immunodeficiency virus. *J Pediatr* 1995;127:137–146.

44. Carlquist JF, Ward RH, Husebye D, et al. Major histocompatibility complex class II gene frequencies by serologic and deoxyribonucleic acid genomic typing in idiopathic dilated cardiomyopathy. *Am J Cardiol* 1994;74:918–920.

45. Olson TM, Thibodeau SN, Lundquist PA, et al. Exclusion of a primary gene defect at the HLA locus in familial idiopathic dilated cardiomyopathy. *J Med Genet* 1995;32:876–880.

46. Nishi H, Koga Y, Koyanagi T, et al. DNA typing of HLA class II genes in Japanese patients with dilated cardiomyopathy. *J Mol Cell Cardiol* 1995;27:2385–2392.

47. Limas CJ, Limas C, Goldenberg IF, Blair R. Possible involvement of the HLA-DQB1 gene in sus-

ceptibility and resistance to human dilated cardio-myopathy. *Am Heart J* 1995;129:1141–1144.

48. Olson TM, Thibodeau SN, Lundquist PA, et al. Exclusion of a primary gene defect at the HLA locus in familial idiopathic dilated cardiomyopa-thy. *J Med Genet* 1995;32:876–880.

49. Krajinovic M, Mestroni L, Severini GM. Absence of linkage between idiopathic dilated cardiomyop-athy and candidate genes involved in the immune function in a large Italian pedigree. *J Med Genet* 1994;31:766–771.

50. Limas CJ, Goldenberg IF, Limas C. Soluble inter-leukin-2 receptor levels in patients with dilated cardiomyopathy: correlation with disease severity and cardiac autoantibodies. *Circulation* 1995;91: 631–634.

51. Maisel AS. Beneficial effects of metoprolol treat-ment in congestive heart failure: reversal of sym-pathetic-induced alterations of immunologic func-tion. *Circulation* 1994;90:1774–1780.

52. Klappacher G, Mehrabi M, Plesch K, et al. Serum-soluble CD4 as a clinical and immunological marker in patients with dilated cardiomyopathy. *Immunol Lett* 1993;38:103–109.

53. Holzinger C, Schollhammer A, Imhof M, et al. Phenotypic patterns of mononuclear cells in di-lated cardiomyopathy. *Circulation* 1995;92:2876–2885.

54. Seko Y, Ishiyama S, Nishikawa T, et al. Restricted usage of T cell receptor V alpha-V beta genes in infiltrating cells in the hearts of patients with acute myocarditis and dilated cardiomyopathy. *J Clin Invest* 1995;96:1035–1041.

55. Lane JR, Neumann DA, Lafond-Walker A, et al. Role of IL-1 and tumor necrosis factor in Cox-sackie virus-induced autoimmune myocarditis. *J Immunol* 1993;151:1682–1690.

56. Lane JR, Neumann DA, Lafond-Walker A, et al. Interleukin 1 or tumor necrosis factor can promote Coxsackie B3-induced myocarditis in resistant B10.A mice. *J Exp Med* 1992;175:1123–1129.

57. Neumann DA, Lane JR, Allen GS, et al. Viral myocarditis leading to cardiomyopathy: do cyto-kines contribute to pathogenesis? *Clin Immunol Immunopathol* 1993;68:181–190.

58. Matsumori A, Yamada T, Suzuki H, et al. In-creased circulating cytokines in patients with myo-carditis and cardiomyopathy. *Br Heart J* 1994; 72:561–566.

59. Munger MA, Johnson B, Amber IJ, et al. Circulat-ing concentrations of proinflammatory cytokines in mild or moderate heart failure secondary to ischemic or idiopathic dilated cardiomyopathy. *Am J Cardiol* 1996;77:723–727.

60. Karsten V, Gordon S, Kirn A, Herbein G. HIV-1 envelope glycoprotein gp120 down-regulates CD4 expression in primary human macrophages through induction of endogenous tumour necrosis factor-alpha. *Immunology* 1996;88:55–60.

61. Seino Y, Ikeda U, Sekiguchi H, et al. Expression of leukocyte chemotactic cytokines in myocardial tissue. *Cytokine* 1995;7:301–304.

62. Satoh M, Tamura G, Segawa I, et al. Expression of cytokine genes and presence of enteroviral ge-nomic RNA in endomyocardial biopsy tissues of myocarditis and dilated cardiomyopathy. *Vir-chows Arch* 1996;427:503–509.

63. Lipshultz SE, Orav EJ, Sanders SP, Colan SD. Immunoglobulins and left ventricular structure and function in pediatric HIV infection. *Circula-tion* 1995;92:2220–2225.

64. Wu TC, Pizzorno MC, Hayward GS, et al. In situ detection of human cytomegalovirus immediate-early gene transcripts within cardiac myocytes of patients with HIV-associated cardiomyopathy. *AIDS* 1992;6:777–785.

65. Villa A, Foresti V, Confalonieri F. Autonomic neuropathy and prolongation of QT interval in human immunodeficiency virus infection. *Clin Auton Res* 1995;5:48–52.

66. Fu ML, Schulze W, Wallukat G, et al. A synthetic peptide corresponding to the second extracellular loop of the human M2 acetylcholine receptor in-duces pharmacological and morphological changes in cardiomyocytes by active immuniza-tion after 6 months in rabbits. *Clin Immunol Immu-nopathol* 1996;78:203–207.

67. Weiss L, You JF, Giral P, et al. Anti-cardiolipin antibodies are associated with anti-endothelial cell antibodies but not with anti-beta 2 glycoprotein I antibodies in HIV infection. *Clin Immunol Immu-nopathol* 1995;77:69–74.

68. Latif N, Baker CS, Dunn MJ, et al. Frequency and specificity of antiheart antibodies in patients with dilated cardiomyopathy detected using SDS-PAGE and Western blotting. [See comments]. *J Am Coll Cardiol* 1993;22:1378–1384.

69. Limas C, Limas CJ, Boudoulas H, et al. Anti-beta-receptor antibodies in familial cardiomyopathy:

correlation with HLA-DR and HLA-DQ gene polymorphisms. *Am Heart J* 1994;127:382–386.

70. Martinetti M, Dugoujon JM, Caforio AL, et al. HLA and immunoglobulin polymorphisms in idiopathic dilated cardiomyopathy. *Hum Immunol* 1992;35:193–199.

71. Limas CJ, Limas C. Immune-mediated modulation of sarcoplasmic reticulum function in human dilated cardiomyopathy. *Basic Res Cardiol* 1992; 87(Suppl 1):269–276.

72. Neumann DA, Rose NR, Ansari AA, Herskowitz A. Induction of multiple heart autoantibodies in mice with Coxsackie virus B3- and cardiac myosin-induced autoimmune myocarditis. *J Immunol* 1994;152:343–350.

73. Sato Y, Matsumori A, Sasayama S. Autoantibodies against vimentin in a murine model of myocarditis. *Autoimmunity* 1994;18:145–148.

74. Maldarelli F, Sato H, Berthold E, et al. Rapid induction of apoptosis by cell-to-cell transmission of human immunodeficiency virus type 1. *J Virol* 1995;69:6457–6465.

75. Nardelli B, Gonzalez CJ, Schechter M, Valentine FT. CD4+ blood lymphocytes are rapidly killed in vitro by contact with autologous human immunodeficiency virus-infected cells. *Proc Natl Acad Sci USA* 1995;92:7312–7316.

76. Lauener RP, Huttner S, Buisson M, et al. T-cell death by apoptosis in vertically human immunodeficiency virus-infected children coincides with expansion of CD8+/interleukin-2 receptor-/HLA-DR+ T cells: sign of a possible role for herpes viruses as cofactors? *Blood* 1995;86:1400–1407.

77. Patti AH, Lederman MM. HIV-1 Tat protein and its inhibitor Ro 24-7429 inhibit lymphocyte proliferation and induce apoptosis in peripheral blood mononuclear cells from healthy donors. *Cell Immunol* 1996;169:40–46.

78. Laurence J, Mitra D, Steiner M, et al. Plasma from patients with idiopathic and human immunodeficiency virus-associated thrombotic thrombocytopenic purpura induces apoptosis in microvascular endothelial cells. *Blood* 1996;87:3245–3254.

79. Zauli G, Gibellini D, Caputo A, et al. The human immunodeficiency virus type-1 Tat protein upregulates Bcl-2 gene expression in Jurkat T-cell lines and primary peripheral blood mononuclear cells. *Blood* 1995;86:3823–3834.

80. Pace GW, Leaf CD. The role of oxidative stress in HIV disease. *Free Radical Biol Med* 1995;19: 523–528.

81. Rensing-Ehl A, Hess S, Ziegler-Heitbrock HW, et al. Fas/Apo-1 activates nuclear factor kappa B and induces interleukin-6 production. *J Inflammat* 1995;45:161–174.

82. James TN. Normal and abnormal consequences of apoptosis in the human heart: from postnatal morphogenesis to paroxysmal arrhythmias. *Circulation* 1994;90:556–573.

83. Narula J, Haider N, Virmani R, et al. Apoptosis in myocytes in end-stage heart failure. *N Engl J Med* 1996;335:1182–1189.

84. Mallat Z, Tedgui A, Fontaliran F, et al. Evidence of apoptosis in arrhythmogenic right ventricular dysplasia. *N Engl J Med* 1996;335:1190–1196.

85. Liu Y, Cigola E, Cheng W, et al. Myocyte nuclear mitotic division and programmed myocyte cell death characterize the cardiac myopathy induced by rapid ventricular pacing in dogs. *Lab Invest* 1995;73:771–787.

86. Katz AM. Cell death in the failing heart: role of an unnatural growth response to overload. *Clin Cardiol* 1995;9:IV36–44.

87. Letterio JJ, Geiser AG, Kulkarni AB, et al. Maternal rescue of transforming growth factor-beta 1 null mice. *Science* 1994;264:1936–1938.

88. Paton P, Tabib A, Loire R, Tete R. Coronary artery lesions and human immunodeficiency virus infection. *Res Virol* 1993;144:225–231.

89. Marks C, Kuskov S. Pattern of arterial aneurysms in acquired immunodeficiency disease. *World J Surg* 1995;19:127–132.

90. Paton P, Tabib A, Loire R, Tete R. Coronary artery lesions and human immunodeficiency virus infection. *Res Virol* 1993;144:225–231.

91. Ruchelli ED, Nojadera G, Rutstein RM, Rudy B. Pulmonary veno-occlusive disease: another vascular disorder associated with human immunodeficiency virus infection? *Arch Pathol* 1994;118: 664–666.

92. Chalifoux LV, Simon MA, Pauley DR, et al. Arteriopathy in macaques infected with simian immunodeficiency virus. *Lab Invest* 1992;67:338–349.

93. Lafeuillade A, Alessi MC, Poizot-Martin I, et al. Endothelial cell dysfunction in HIV infection. *J AIDS* 1992;5:127–131.

94. Mallery SR, Bailer RT, Hohl CM, et al. Cultured AIDS-related Kaposi's sarcoma (AIDS-KS) cells demonstrate impaired bioenergetic adaptation to oxidant challenge: implication for oxidant stress in

AIDS-KS pathogenesis. *J Cell Biochem* 1995;59: 317–328.

95. Berliner JA, Navab M, Fogelman AM, et al. Atherosclerosis: basic mechanisms: oxidation, inflammation, and genetics. *Circulation* 1995;91: 2488–2496.

96. Fyfe AI, Qiao JH, Lusis AJ. Immune-deficient mice develop typical atherosclerotic fatty streaks when fed an atherogenic diet. *J Clin Invest* 1994; 94:2516–2520.

97. Conaldi PG, Serra C, Dolei A, et al. Productive HIV-1 infection of human vascular endothelial cells requires cell proliferation and is stimulated by combined treatment with interleukin-1 beta plus tumor necrosis factor-alpha. *J Med Virol* 1995;47:355–363.

98. Moses AV, Williams S, Heneveld ML, et al. Human immunodeficiency virus infection of bone marrow endothelium reduces induction of stromal hematopoietic growth factors. *Blood* 1996;87: 919–925.

99. Lafrenie RM, Wahl LM, Epstein JS, et al. HIV-1-Tat modulates the function of monocytes and alters their interactions with microvessel endothelial cells: a mechanism of HIV pathogenesis. *J Immunol* 1996;156:1638–1645.

100. Albini A, Benelli R, Presta M, et al. HIV-tat protein is a heparin-binding angiogenic growth factor. *Oncogene* 1996;12:289–297.

101. Albini A, Barillari G, Benelli R, et al. Angiogenic properties of human immunodeficiency virus type 1 Tat protein. *Proc Natl Acad Sci USA* 1995;92: 4838–4842.

102. Fiorelli V, Gendelman R, Samaniego F, et al. Cytokines from activated T cells induce normal endothelial cells to acquire the phenotypic and functional features of AIDS-Kaposi's sarcoma spindle cells. *J Clin Invest* 1995;95:1723–1734.

103. Golden MP, Hammer SM, Wanke CA, Albrecht MA. Cytomegalovirus vasculitis: case reports and review of the literature. *Medicine* 1994;73: 246–255.

20

Simian Immunodeficiency Virus-Associated Cardiomyopathy in Nonhuman Primates

Richard P. Shannon, M.D.

Cardiomyopathy is being recognized with increasing frequency as an important clinical sequela of chronic infection with human immunodeficiency virus (HIV). Current estimates suggest that 6% of all acquired immunodeficiency syndrome (AIDS)-related deaths are due to HIV cardiomyopathy, and it is estimated that 10% to 18% of HIV-seropositive patients will have subclinical evidence of left ventricular dysfunction. It is estimated that there will be between 21,000 and 40,000 new cases of heart failure attributable to HIV cardiomyopathy by the year 2000. Despite the increase in recognition of this clinical syndrome, there has been little understanding of the pathogenesis of retroviral infection and its consequences for cardiac function. In this regard, it seems unlikely that substantial information about the chronic pathogenesis of HIV cardiomyopathy can be obtained exclusively from clinical studies, for both technical and ethical reasons. The availability of a relevant experimental model that manifests signs and symptoms of human AIDS, including cardiovascular involvement, seems most appropriate for the study of basic mechanisms of the pathogenesis of AIDS-related cardiomyopathy. In this review, we discuss the immunodeficiency syndrome that develops after experimental infec-

tion with simian immunodeficiency virus (SIV) in nonhuman primates. We review the relationship of this lentivirus to other retroviruses and review the clinical, immunologic, and pathologic abnormalities that have been identified within this syndrome in nonhuman primates. Finally, we present, in preliminary form, recent findings with respect to cardiovascular involvement in nonhuman primates infected with SIV.

Simian AIDS

SIV is a class of lentiviruses that are found in African nonhuman primates and are closely related to HIV. These viruses were isolated from rhesus macaque monkeys, but they have also been identified from healthy African green monkeys and from healthy sooty mangabeys. These viruses appear to occur as exogenous nonpathogens in these nonhuman primates, in which viral specific antibody responses are quite robust.[1,2] However, when SIV isolated from West African macaques is experimentally introduced into Asian macaques, an immunodeficiency syndrome develops. The clinical syndrome following experimental infection with SIV

299

is referred to as simian AIDS. The general features include the development of an transient maculopapillary rash over the trunk, face, and extremities of infected animals. Visceral and axillary adenopathy develops within 6 to 8 weeks after infection. Chronic manifestations include the development of weight loss and a wasting syndrome, the superimposition of opportunistic infections, and end-organ involvement, principally in the brain, lung, kidney, intestine, and lymph nodes. By contrast, most earlier pathologic studies of simian AIDS suggested that the heart is generally spared as a direct target of SIV infection or its sequelae. To our knowledge, there has been no earlier report of functional cardiovascular impairment in this model.

Simian Immunodeficiency Virus

SIV shares with its human retroviral counterpart a specific tropism for bone marrow-derived cells, which include cells bearing the CD4 surface molecule present on specific subsets of T lymphocytes, monocytes, and macrophages. Considerable controversy exists with respect to whether SIV infects cells not bearing the CD4 receptor. The immunologic manifestations of SIV infection are numerous and considerable. Animals that succumb rapidly to SIV infection within the first 6 months are generally conspicuous for the absence of significant titers of anti-SIV antibody, little or no detectable viral-specific T-lymphocyte effector function, and significant nonspecific qualitative and quantitative T-lymphocyte functional abnormalities. By contrast, animals chronically infected with SIV usually live for 1 or 2 years after the onset of infection. These animals manifest a prolonged clinical latency not unlike that observed in HIV infection. Nonetheless, the course tends to be truncated with fully 70% of SIV-infected animals demonstrating immunodeficiency within 1 year. The immunologic characteristics of those animals in which the disease has a more chronic course include the development of high-titer antibody responses specific to SIV derived from macrophages (SIVmac), as well as early-detected, viral-specific T-lymphocyte effector responses. Notably, there is limited experimental

evidence that suggests that the ability to generate a SIVmac gag-specific cytotoxic T-lymphocyte response is associated with lower viral loads and a chronic as opposed to an acute course. Animals with a more chronic course also develop qualitative and quantitative nonspecific T-lymphocyte abnormalities remote from the initiation of infection. Nonetheless, as is the case with humans, monitoring the peripheral blood CD4+ lymphocyte count provides the most useful immunologic marker with respect to disease progression.

Opportunistic Infections

Like humans with AIDS, nonhuman primates, specifically rhesus macaques, infected with SIV develop a wide range of opportunistic infections. The most common infections include *Pneumocystis carinii* pneumonia, cytomegalovirus infections, and cryptosporidiosis. Cytomegalovirus infection tends to be disseminated, with involvement of multiple organ systems, including lymph nodes, liver, lungs, spleen, heart, and large and small intestine. The lesions usually consist of focal necrosis and neutrophilic inflammation, with the cytomegalovirus-infected cells containing intranuclear inclusions. Other viral pathogens in simian AIDS include adenoviral infections, which most commonly involve the pancreas but are occasionally more diffuse. Papovavirus infections, particularly SV40, frequently result in lesions involving the brain, the kidney, and, less frequently, the lung. The bacterial infection seen most commonly in simian AIDS is *Myobacterium avium-intracellulare*. This tends to be disseminated, with the most intense findings in the intestine. Histologically, these lesions consist of macrophages with foamy cytoplasm, principally located in the lamina propria.

P. carinii pneumonia is the major life-threatening opportunistic infection in SIV-infected macaques. It is found in the lungs of 52% of terminally ill SIV-infected animals. The lesions associated with *P. carinii* pneumonia include eosinophilic infiltrates of the alveoli, hyperplasia of type 2 pneumocytes, and a variable degree of interstitial fibrosis and edema, with minimal inflammatory cell infiltrates. It is rare that *Pneumocystsis carinii* infection extends beyond the thorax. *Cryptosporidium* is also a common protozoan that is generally associated with gastrointestinal distress, watery diarrhea, and dehydration. *Cryptosporidium* is most commonly isolated from the small intestine, the gallbladder, and the biliary and pancreatic ducts of SIV-infected animals. In the small intestine, crytosporidiosis is associated with blunting and fusion of the villi, while the response in the biliary tree is characterized by a hyperplastic reaction.

Pathologic Findings

We will discuss those lesions known to be due directly to SIV infection. These include principal involvement of the lymph nodes, in which the SIV-mac p27 core protein can be identified in paracortical and medullary zones of lymph nodes within the first 3 to 9 weeks after experimental infection. Lymphadenopathy is usually seen within 6 to 8 weeks following inoculation, and is associated with proliferation of large follicular cell centers that are particularly rich in B lymphocytes. One theory suggests that the follicular hyperplasia observed soon after SIV infection is due to trapping of SIV antigens by follicular dendritic cells, with subsequent presentation of these antigens to cells within the germinal center, resulting in their proliferation. Even at this early stage, the paracortical region of the lymph nodes is characterized by depletion of CD4+ T lymphocytes and a corresponding increase in CD8+ lymphocytes. After follicular hyperplasia, the chronic phase of SIV infection is characterized by follicular involution and expansion of CD8+ lymphocytes and macrophages in the paracortex. This is frequently associated with severe depletion of both cortical and paracortical lymphocytes within peripheral and visceral lymph nodes. Variations on these peripheral manifestations include massive infiltration of peripheral lymph nodes by histiocytes and multinucleated giant cells. This enlargement of peripheral lymph nodes is distinct from the follicular hyperplastic response and is seen soon after SIV inoculation. Importantly, the histiocytes and multinucleate giant cells frequently stain positive for SIV mac p27 core protein, and furthermore, the RNA of the SIV virus can frequently be identified in these cells by in situ hybridization. Finally, a small subset of animals develop lymphoproliferative syndromes again, distinct from the follicular hyperplastic response seen commonly in SIV-infected monkeys. In this case, lymphadenopathy is due to proliferation of large plasmacytoidlike cells that replace the normal architecture of the node, obliterating the subcapsular and medullary sinuses. In general, the proliferative response is contained in the capsule of the lymph node, although occasionally aggregates of lymphoid cells can be found in salivary glands, lung, liver, bone marrow, and thymus.

SIV Infection Involving the Nervous System

Approximately 50% of rhesus macaques experimentally infected with SIV develop meningoencephalitis. Inflammatory lesions have been identified in both the gray and the white matter of the brain and the spinal cord, with some predilection for white matter. The lesions themselves are multifocal perivascular infiltrates comprised of histiocytes and multinucleated giant cells. SIV core proteins can be found within the histiocytes and macrophages by electron microscopy.

SIV Infection Involving the Respiratory System

Distinct from the opportunistic infections described above, the lung can also be a primary target for SIV infection. SIV-induced giant cell pneumonia is characterized by infiltration of the parenchyma and alveolar spaces by foamy macrophages and multinucleated giant cells. This is usually associated with thickening of the alveolar wall as a consequence of inflammatory cell infiltration and proliferation of type II pneumocytes lining the alveolar spaces. This can be seen distinct from, but also in association with, parabronchial lymphoid hyperplastic responses.

SIV Infection Involving the Kidney

The renal glomerulus is a frequent target of SIV infection. The glomeruli themselves are associated with hyperplasia of visceral epithelial cells and with thickening and redundancy of the basement membrane. There is also proliferation of the mesangial matrix and occasional focal areas of tubular atrophy frequently associated with replacement fibrosis.

SIV Infections Involving the Gastrointestinal Tract

SIV infection can be seen in association with a nonspecific enteropathy that appears to be independent of opportunistic infection. This is associated with blunting and atrophy of the intestinal villi, with varying degrees of crypt hyperplasia. There is usually an associated hyperplastic response within the lymphoid tissues, although in the advanced stage, one may see actual depletion of lymph tissue, as described above. These lesions are frequently identified as the proximate cause of the acute diarrheal syndromes in the absence of an identifiable opportunistic infection, and they contribute significantly to the subsequent morbidity of these animals.

Cardiovascular Involvement with SIV Infection

There has been relatively little systematic examination of the cardiovascular pathology and functional consequences in rhesus macaques chronically infected with SIV. We recently had the opportunity to examine the functional cardiovascular consequences of chronic SIV infection in rhesus macaques using noninvasive echocardiographic techniques. A cohort of rhesus macaques that had been infected with mutated nonpathogenic SIV strains were used as controls. These initial data revealed that 5 of the 6 animals chronically infected with pathogenic SIV had an average depressed left ventricular ejection fraction of 43%. This is in contrast to the animals that had been infected chronically with nonpathogenic SIV strains, in which the resting left ventricular ejection fraction averaged 63%. Only two of 9 animals chronically infected with nonpathogenic strains of SIV had ejection fractions less than 50%. Importantly, there was evidence of significant ventricular remodeling in those rhesus macaques with simian AIDS and depressed left ventricular ejection fractions. Specifically, there was evidence of left ventricular dilatation and an increase in left ventricular end-systolic volumes, even when normalized for body mass. Furthermore, the finding of depressed left ventricular ejection fraction and associated ventricular dilatation is evident only in rhesus monkeys chronically infected with SIV. A cohort of rhesus monkeys acutely infected with pathogenic SIV revealed no evidence of left ventricular dysfunction. Taken together, these retrospective data suggest that there are significant functional cardiovascular sequelae associated with chronic SIV infection.

We have subsequently reviewed the pathologic findings from 24 consecutive rhesus macaques chronically infected with pathogenic SIV that had died of simian AIDS. Fifteen rhesus macaques had pathologic evidence of cardiac involvement. There was no difference in age between the monkeys with manifest cardiac pathology (5.9 years) and those without (5.8 years.) Similarly, the duration of infection with SIV was comparable in the two groups, with those manifesting cardiac pathology being infected for an average of 23 months and those with no evidence of cardiac pathology being infected for 22 months. The rhesus macaques with simian AIDS that manifested cardiac pathology were more emaciated than those without cardiac involvement. Most importantly, the rhesus macaques with simian AIDS and no cardiac involvement had a greater frequency of opportunistic infections (7 of 9 animals) than those in which cardiac involvement was identified (6 of 15). The cardiac pathology evident in the 15 of the 24 animals chronically infected with pathogenic HIV included 9 animals with evidence of myocarditis (Figure 20-1). Myocarditis itself was associated with extensive inflammatory infiltrates with associated myocyte necrosis, which in most cases was mild, but which in some cases was associated with extensive myocyte loss and replacement fibrosis. In the other six animals, the

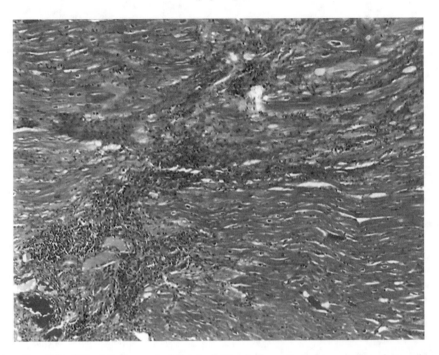

Figure 20-1. (See Color Plate 2 for image in full color.) Histologic section of myocardium from a rhesus macaque chronically infected with SIV. There is an extensive area of cellular infiltration associated with myocyte necrosis.

most common lesion observed was coronary arteriopathy, involving both large epicardial coronary arteries and intramyocardial coronary arterioles. The lesions were characterized by perivascular inflammation and associated intimal and endothelial hyperplastic responses (Figure 20-2), culminating in many cases in the development of extensive intimal hyperplasia (Figure 20-3) with resultant encroachment upon the lumen. In two rhesus macaques, there was actually evidence of in situ thrombosis and associated myocardial injury close to areas subtended by the involved vessels. It should be noted that of the 15 animals with cardiac involvement, two actually died in apparent cardiogenic pulmonary edema. In these animals, the dominant pathology was that of coronary arteriopathy, with evidence of in situ thrombosis and actual luminal occlusion leading to myocardial ischemic injury.

Summary

Chronic infection with SIV in nonhuman primates results in a clinical syndrome of simian AIDS that is akin to that observed in humans. In animals with a particularly prolonged and protracted course, there appears to be a high incidence of pathologic cardiac involvement. The most common cardiac lesion is inflammatory myocarditis. However, we also observed an extensive coronary arteriopathy not unlike that reported in pediatric populations with human AIDS. It should be noted that the rhesus macaques used in these experimental studies were both juvenile and naive. In contrast to what has been reported in humans, the animals with cardiac involvement tended to have relative preservation of immunologic responses, with a tendency to higher circulating antibody levels against SIV and greater preservation of their CD4+ lymphocytes. In addition, the animals with cardiac involvement appeared to have fewer opportunistic infections. Taken together, these data suggest the possibility that some degree of immunocompetency is required to have cardiac inflammatory involvement following SIV. However, many fundamental cellular and physiologic questions remain to be answered. These include the relative role of SIV itself in the direct pathogenesis of cardiomyopathy and coronary arte-

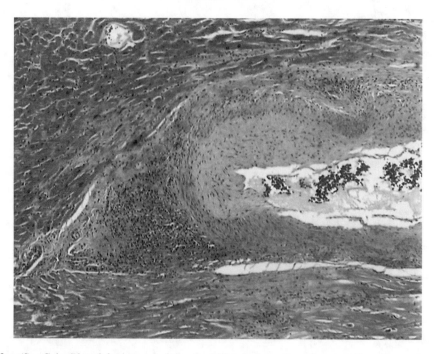

Figure 20-2. (See Color Plate 2 for image in full color.) Histologic section of myocardium from a rhesus macaque chronically infected with SIV. There is evidence of perivascular inflammatory infiltrate involving an epicardial coronary artery with associated intimal hyperplastic response.

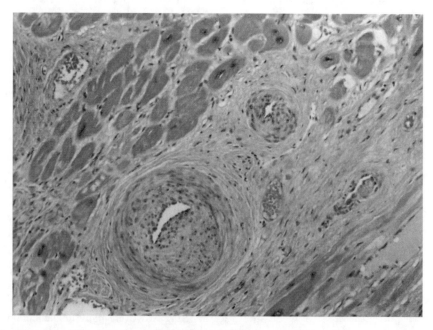

Figure 20-3. (See Color Plate 2 for image in full color.) Histologic section of myocardium from a rhesus macaque chronically infected with SIV. There is a symmetric intimal hyperplastic response involving an intramyocardial arteriole with resultant encroachment upon the luminal diameter.

riopathy. It is also possible that these findings are due to associated opportunistic infections in the more immunocompetent chronically SIV-infected animals. More studies will be required to determine the role of SIV directly using colocalization techniques, as well as to characterize the nature and extent of the inflammatory infiltrate in those animals, both the infiltrates in the myocardial lesions and the infiltrates associated with development of coronary arteriopathy. Finally, the relationships between commonly observed cardiac pathologic involvement and the findings of functional cardiac impairment remain to be established prospectively. Nonetheless, this model promises to be an exciting source of new information, specifically with respect to the pathogenesis of cardiac involvement in human AIDS.

Acknowledgment

This work was supported in part by U.S. Public Health Service grant RR-0016B.

References

1. Lackner AA. Pathology of simian immunodeficiency virus induced disease. *Curr Top Microbiol Immunol* 1994;188:35–64.

2. Letvin NL, King NW. Immunologic and pathologic manifestations of the infection of rhesus monkeys with simian immunodeficiency virus of macaques. *J Acquir Immune Defic Syndr* 1990;3:1023–1040.

21

Malnutrition and Cardiovascular Disease in Patients Infected With HIV

Tracie L. Miller, M.D.

The nutritional problems of human immunodeficiency virus (HIV)-infected patients contribute significantly to the morbidity and mortality from this disease. Statistics generated from the Centers for Disease Control and Prevention[1] have shown that nutritional- and gastrointestinal-related conditions in HIV-infected children are among the leading causes of pediatric acquired immunodeficiency syndrome (AIDS). Malnutrition can influence many organ systems. Although there was initial widespread belief that the heart is resistant to change with malnutrition,[2] more recent scientific data have shown that the nutritional status of a patient can affect cardiac mass and function in diverse ways and across a variety of disease states. Heart mass, one component of the lean body compartment of the individual, changes with other lean body compartments, yet is subject to the influence of chemical mediators, such as those derived from the sympathetic nervous system. Fluctuations in cardiac mass, as a result of nutritional status, can also lead to changes in cardiac function. Malnutrition can lead to micronutrient deficiencies with resulting cardiac disease. Specific micronutrients known to influence cardiac function include carnitine,[3] selenium,[4] and thiamine.[5] As strong as the influence of nutrition on cardiac mass and function is, the opposite relationship is equally as strong. Chronic cardiac compromise can also produce an entity known as "cardiac cachexia," in which chronic congestive heart failure, as the primary process, influences nutritional status. Although there are few reports linking cardiac disease with the nutritional condition of the HIV-infected person, it is logical to expect that there is an interaction between these two highly prevalent conditions in patients infected with HIV. This chapter provides current background information on nutrition in HIV infection and the associations between nutrition and cardiac disease, with a focus on the effects of changing lean body mass, micronutrient deficiencies, and chemical mediators that may produce changes in both nutritional and cardiac parameters.

Nutrition and HIV Infection

Nutritional problems are common in patients infected with HIV, and the wasting syndrome is considered one of the major AIDS-defining illnesses.[1] Most, if not all, children with HIV infection will experience nutritional deficits during the course of their illness, and a large number of adults will have problems with the wasting condition associated with HIV.[6,7] For many drug-treatment protocols, nutritional parameters are important entry and failure criteria. Data are now emerging that show a direct correlation of these nutritional abnormalities with morbidity and survival.[6,8,9] Weight loss and gastrointestinal symptoms are among the most common presenting symptoms of HIV disease in developing countries. In a Tanzanian study, 200 children with severe malnutrition and controls who were matched for age, sex, and area of residence were screened for evidence of HIV infection.[10] Of the malnourished group, 25% were HIV-positive, compared with 1.5% of the control group. Based on the high prevalence of HIV in the malnourished group, the authors recommended routine screening for HIV infection in malnourished children in developing countries.

Malnutrition is measured in many ways, depending on the population that is being studied (children versus adults) and the time frame that is being considered (acute versus chronic). For children, acute malnutrition is manifested by a decline in weight before a decline in height, with lower weight-for-height percentiles. Chronic nutritional deprivation will result in below-standard weight and height, with nearly normal weight-for-height. This is a growing child's adaptation to undernutrition. Children with this condition are often referred to as nutritional dwarfs. For adults, since height is preserved, malnutrition is based on weight changes that can reflect either changes in the percentage of normal weight or changes in the percentage of ideal weight based on height and sex.

Children with HIV infection have similar birthweights and are at no higher risk of prematurity compared with children who are not HIV-infected but who are born to HIV-infected women.[11] Thus, growth abnormalities begin postnatally and can occur rapidly even in asymptomatic children. Patterns of growth are not always predictable, since the clinical course of HIV is variable. In some studies, growth patterns are found that suggest acute undernutrition, with low weight-for-height percentiles,[11,12] and other studies have shown symmetric changes in weight and height, with nearly normal weight-for-height.[13,14] Factors such as variability of HIV disease and other potential confounders could account for conflicting results, and therefore these variable factors should be experimentally controlled.

Although data are emerging on growth disturbances in HIV-infected children, more studies have been conducted on HIV-infected adults. There appear to be characteristic patterns of weight loss in adults with HIV infection. Macallan[15] evaluated the weight changes in 30 men with an AIDS-defining illness over a 9- to 49-month period. He found that episodes of acute weight loss (greater than 4 kg in <4 months) were associated primarily with nongastrointestinal systemic infections such as *Pneumocystis carinii* pneumonia. Chronic weight loss events of greater than 4 kg for >4 months were most often associated with gastrointestinal symptoms. There were significant periods of weight stability in 43% of patients, and episodes of weight gain were recorded in most of the patients, coincident with recovery from an acute infection. The patients usually did not fully regain all of the lost weight. Thus, weight loss in adults with HIV infection occurs over defined intervals with intervening periods of weight stability.

Weight loss and decrease in growth velocity are simple markers to diagnose malnutrition of HIV-infected patients. However, using weight as the only marker of nutritional status can be misleading, since vomiting, diarrhea, or hydration therapy can dramatically change body weight without changing nutritional status. A more accurate measure of nutritional status is body composition, the compartments of fat mass and fat-free mass (roughly equivalent to lean body mass). With typical malnutrition, the body's first response to starvation (inadequate food intake) is the preferential loss of body fat. When fat stores have been depleted, then wasting of lean body mass occurs. By contrast, cachexia or wasting disorder refers to the preferential and inappropriate loss of lean body mass over fat mass, with or without concomitant weight loss. Cachexia has been described previously in patients with cancer but most recently has been found in patients with HIV infection. Cachexia may be mediated by chemical intermediates such as cytokines.

There are few studies measuring the body composition of HIV-infected children. We have reported body composition measurements of 89 children born to HIV-infected women, 52 of whom were HIV-infected. By 2 years of age, lean body mass, as measured by arm muscle circumference, was significantly less in the HIV-infected children than in those who were not infected. There were no differences in fat mass between the two groups of children.[11] These findings are suggestive of cachexia rather than starvation. Another study[16] also supported the cachexia model in pediatric HIV infection in a group of nine children who were beginning 2′,3′-dideoxycytidine (ddC) therapy. Lean body mass was significantly diminished in these children as well.

As in the pediatric population, early body composition changes have been noted in adults with HIV infection,[17,18] with loss of lean body mass evident in people with asymptomatic infection. Kotler and colleagues[19] found that the presence of active cytomegalovirus infection in patients with AIDS significantly affected weight gain and lean body mass. There was a repletion of lean body mass in those patients who received appropriate antiviral therapy.[20]

Since early and pervasive changes in muscle mass are found in HIV-infected patients, similar changes may be apparent in the hearts of these patients as well.

Influence of Malnutrition on Cardiac Mass

Initially, there was widespread belief that the heart was unaltered with a change in nutritional status, so that with significant weight loss, cardiac muscle mass was preserved. Voit's[2] study of 1866 compared two cats, one of which was starved for 13 days, while the other was normally nourished. The hearts of the cats were compared at autopsy and he found that the starved cat's heart was only slightly smaller. Thus, he concluded that the heart is spared in malnutrition. Although it is attractive to consider that the most vital organs, such as the brain and the heart, are preserved with malnutrition, this has not been supported by subsequent studies. A landmark study by Keyes and colleagues[21] during World War II showed that heart size was markedly reduced with severe caloric restriction. Keyes and colleagues placed conscientious objectors on a European famine diet. After 6 months on a low-energy, low-protein diet, the volunteers lost 25% of their body weight. Radiographs showed that heart size was markedly reduced in all dimensions, and the decrease in calculated cardiac volume was 70% of the decrease in total body weight. This was the first study showing a decrease in heart size and myocardial atrophy with malnutrition. Since then, this concept has been widely documented in malnourished patients by different methods.

Bloom and Smith[22] determined heart size and plasma volume of 21 patients before and after a fast. Heart size was determined by standard six-foot x-rays of the chest, and plasma volume was measured by the apparent volume of distribution of albumin tagged with ^{131}I in seven of the patients. They found that heart size decreased in all patients studied, and there was a significant decrease in plasma volume as well. They did not find any correlation between change in heart size or blood volume and amount of weight loss or duration of fasting. The heart weights of children with kwashiorkor are generally diminished.[23,24] In addition, obese patients undergoing rapid weight loss can also show a loss in heart mass at autopsy.[25] In echocardiograms of women with anorexia nervosa, there is a marked thinning of the walls of the ventricle, with no evidence of sparing of cardiac mass.[26]

When cachexia is due to chronic disease rather than pure caloric restriction, there seems to be some sparing of ventricular mass.[27] However, the metabolic demand that exists at the time of starvation may be an important determinant of the severity of cardiac muscle loss. In conditions where there is a demand for increased cardiac output, such as the hypermetabolism of chronic diseases, there may be some preservation of cardiac mass at the expense of skeletal muscle and visceral mass. These findings may be relevant in patients with HIV infection and are similar to our recent findings in HIV-infected children.

We recently reported on 36 children with symptomatic HIV infection who underwent simultaneous anthropometric and echocardiographic evaluations over an 8-year period.[28] These measurements were performed before the children had received antiretroviral therapy or supplemental feedings, to assess the effect of HIV infection on nutritional and cardiac parameters. Children infected with HIV were significantly below age-adjusted standards for height, weight, triceps skinfold thickness, and arm muscle circumference. Left ventricular mass normalized to body surface area was below standard, and contractility was normal. Correlation analyses found an inverse relationship between left ventricular mass and weight z score, height z score, and arm muscle circumference percentile. An inverse relationship was also found between heart rate and weight z score and arm muscle circumference percentile. We concluded that in malnourished children with HIV infection, a paradoxical relation exists between nutritional status and cardiac muscle mass, so that there is relative cardiac sparing. The inverse relationship between heart rate and nutritional status may suggest increased metabolic rates mediated through increased sympathetic tone.

Microscopy

Studies by Rossi and Zucoloto[29] showed the ultrastructural features of nutritional cardiomyopathy in protein-calorie-malnourished rats. Protein-calorie malnutrition was induced in young rats by feeding them a low-protein diet for 6 weeks. Control animals were fed a high-protein diet. The deficient rats showed severe weight loss, fatty liver, and hypoproteinemia. The morphologic changes of the rat heart on light microscopy showed hyalinization and vacuolization of muscle fibers, loss of cross-striations and myofibrils, small foci of necrosis, interstitial fibrosis, and mononuclear cell infiltration. The ultrastructural lesions were characterized by myofibrillar degeneration, contraction band formation, dilatation of sarcoplasmic reticulum, mitochondrial swelling, dehiscence of intercalated disks, and widened interstitial spaces, especially around vessels. These findings were due to edema and cellular infiltration by mononuclear cells and activated fibroblasts within collagen fibers and myofibrils. In humans it appears macroscopically that the musculature in all chambers of the heart wastes proportionately. Microscopically the starved heart initially shows reduction in the size of the fibers, but as the person becomes more malnourished, the signs of degeneration multiply, so that there may be fatty degeneration and brown atrophy. Cytologi-

cally, cloudy swelling and loss of striation and vacuolization occur.

Cardiac Function with Malnutrition

The chief function of the heart is to deliver blood containing oxygen and nutrients to tissues, and carry away carbon dioxide and waste products. As less energy is supplied to the tissues during starvation, a number of normal physiologic adaptations occur in the context of a progressively hypometabolic state. As myocardial mass decreases with starvation, stroke volume and cardiac output can fall proportionately. However, because of the decrease in body size, the stroke volume index and the cardiac index may remain normal or rise slightly. In addition, systolic ejection phase indices of left ventricular function, such as the ejection fraction and the mean rate of shortening of left ventricular circumferential fibers, remain normal or increase slightly. Therefore, despite the decrease in muscle mass, the needs of the circulation are met by these compensatory mechanisms. Thus, although significant changes occur in the cardiovascular system, congestive heart failure is rare, because these compensatory mechanisms mask the effect of myocardial atrophy.

There are several human and animal studies that define cardiovascular function in individuals with malnutrition. A study of 43 infection-free African children with marasmic kwashiorkor used simultaneous measurements of body weight, plasma albumin, intravascular volumes, cardiac index, and intravascular and related hemodynamic parameters to determine the effect of malnutrition on cardiac function in children.[30] These measurements were compared with similar measurements in 24 convalescent children. The malnourished children showed a prolonged circulatory time, with a tendency to bradycardia and hypotension. Cardiac index, stroke index, and heart work were significantly reduced in these malnourished children, as were the intravascular volumes. Hemodynamic data correlated with either body weight or plasma albumin and cardiac index bore a direct relation to cell volume. In the most severely malnourished patients, ventricle filling pressures were low and vascular resistances were high. It can be inferred that most patients were in an adaptive hypocirculatory state, comparable to hypothyroidism, while the most severely malnourished children showed frank peripheral circulatory failure, comparable to hypovolemic shock. Circulatory failure on admission was associated with a high death rate during treatment, but the relation between cause and effect could not be clearly demonstrated.

Although these findings were significant and obvious, most patients with malnutrition are relatively well compensated cardiovascularly. In the absence of any other disturbance, bradycardia is the most common hemodynamic abnormality in the malnourished heart. Even after periods of prolonged exercise, there may be a relative bradycardia, with resting heart rates in adults of <50 beats per minute. Bradycardia with malnutrition has been best described in patients with anorexia nervosa.[31] This cardiovascular change is an adaptive response to starvation in the context of a progressively hypometabolic state, where there are diminished demands of tissue perfusion. The mechanism of bradycardia is unclear, but it may be caused by an autonomic imbalance, with low sympathetic tone.[32]

The importance of catecholamines in the regulation of metabolic processes has been recognized for decades now.[33] Catecholamines influence metabolism in two ways: (1) they increase the rate of cellular metabolism, and (2) they stimulate the conversion of complex fuels into regularly used substrates by stimulating glycogenolysis, lipolysis, and gluconeogenesis. The increased rate of cellular metabolism induced by catecholamines is manifested by elevations in heat production and in fuel and oxygen consumption; however, the cellular mechanisms involved have not been established. Fasting and feeding induce changes in sympathetic nervous activity: fasting suppresses and overfeeding stimulates the sympathetic nervous.[34,35] These observations are consistent with the hypothesis that during fasting, suppression of sympathetic activity conserves calories by diminishing metabolism and heat production; during overfeeding, stimulation of sympathetic activity expends calories by accelerating metabolism and producing heat. Catecholamine effects on thyroid function may also lead to hypometabolism, where decreased adrenergic stimuli promote the deiodination of thyroxine to produce reverse triiodothyronine instead of triiodothyronine. With lowered catecholamine levels in the malnourished state, a relative hypothyroidism results, with a further decrease in metabolism and resulting heart rate.

Attempts to assess sympathetic activity during fasting have included measurement of urine and plasma catecholamines or metabolites, which yielded inconsistent results. The action of the sympathetic nervous system on the heart can be assessed in a more direct manner by evaluating tritiated norepinephrine turnover in the hearts of fasting rats.[36] In one study, the turnover of endogenous norepinephrine was 23.1 ng per heart per hour in a fed group of rats and 3.1 ng per heart per hour in a fasting group, a significant difference. In patients with pheochromocytoma, in which myocardial epinephrine is elevated, cardiomyopathy manifested by various pathologic changes, including myofibrillar degeneration, edema, round cell infiltration, interstitial fibrosis, and myocardial hypertrophy, has been reported.

Resting oxygen consumption is reduced in starvation and, in particular, has been shown in patients with anorexia nervosa by indirect calorimetry, which measures the respiratory quotient (oxygen consumption as it relates to carbon dioxide production). Additionally, obese patients studied by right heart catheterization before and after a 30% weight loss showed a 17.5% fall in oxygen consumption.[37] In these patients with obesity and weight loss, lower cardiac output and blood volume were also noted, which were thought to be secondary to lowered metabolic demands due to tissue mass loss.

Our recent study on nutrition and cardiac changes in children with HIV infection suggests that these metabolic adaptations may not be in effect for HIV-infected patients.[28] Our finding of an inverse relationship between heart rate and nutritional status is not consistent with other malnutrition states, such as anorexia nervosa or pure starvation. Our findings, coupled with the findings of others[38] showing that basal metabolic rates are increased, even in early, asymptomatic phases of HIV infection in adults, suggest that there is modulation of the normal response to malnutrition by chemical intermediates (such as catecholamines) that can alter heart rate and metabolism and may be, in part, responsible for the nutritional wasting that is so common in people infected with HIV.

In summary, most of the data from both human and animal studies indicate that there is a fall in cardiac output and systolic performance that is consistent with metabolic adaptation of the organism to starvation. This is most clearly seen by the clinician, who observes bradycardia, hypotension, and delayed circulation time on examination. The depression of systolic performance is mild and of little functional consequence in the unstressed, malnourished state. In patients with HIV infection, it is currently unclear how common these adaptations are. It is likely that catecholamine levels, which are usually depressed in pure starvation, are increased because of the stress of infections and chronic disease. Thus, the usual adaptive mechanisms are not apparent. As a result, the association of increased heart rate and increased metabolism would put the individual at risk for progressive wasting.

Electrophysiology

A recognized problem of malnourished patients undergoing rehabilitation is sudden death, thought to be due primarily to arrhythmias. Specific changes in electrocardiographic (EKG) readings are common with malnutrition, and some of these changes are clearly secondary to depletion of total body potassium stores. Other changes reflect loss of muscle mass. Keyes and coworkers[21] described changes in ECG readings with malnutrition and subsequent rehabilitation in a group of starved volunteers. ECG findings in that study revealed a pronounced slowing of the heart rate and low voltage of the P wave, QRS complex, and T wave in all leads. There was an increase in the QT interval, but this was consistent with the observed slowing of the heart rate. Smythe and colleagues[23] studied ECG patterns of hospitalized South African children with kwashiorkor. Children with broad concave ST- and T-wave depression with prolonged QT intervals, and children with low voltage and flat T waves, had a combined mortality of 59%, compared with a mortality of 17.5% in children with less severe ST-segment and T-wave abnormalities. Some of these

abnormalities were corrected with orally administered potassium. The axis of the EKG has also been found to be useful in predicting recovery from kwashiorkor.[39] A rightward axis shift and failure to shift to the left with refeeding correlated with a poor prognosis in patients with severely edematous malnutrition. The rightward axis shift most likely resulted from elevated pulmonary artery pressures due to electrolyte imbalance and consequent fluid retention.

In summary, there is widespread evidence of abnormal electrophysiologic findings in malnutrition and refeeding. It is difficult to discern how much of the observed change is due to electrolyte imbalance and how much is due to primary myocardial dysfunction.

Vitamin and Mineral Deficiencies

Malnutrition of HIV-infected patients may be due, in part, to suboptimal or inadequate dietary intake. As much as diminished or inadequate intake results in weight loss or suboptimal growth, specific deficiencies of vitamins and trace minerals can also occur, which may relate to inadequate intake of micronutrients or altered processing of these micronutrients (abnormal intestinal absorption or metabolic pathways). The HIV-infected patient may have one or many micronutrient deficiencies. Deficiencies of vitamin A, vitamin E, vitamin B_{12}, thiamine, carnitine, zinc, selenium, and iron, to name a few, have been described. Deficiencies of these micronutrients can have multiple effects on the individual, including altered immune function, effects on the central nervous system, hematologic effects, and changes in the cardiovascular system. In particular, deficiencies of selenium, carnitine, and thiamine can affect the cardiovascular system in all diseases, including HIV infection.

Thiamine deficiency has been established as an etiologic factor in altered cardiac metabolism, electrophysiologic changes, and myocardial hypertrophy. There were early descriptions of the human syndrome of cardiac beriberi with right ventricular failure and peripheral vasodilatation. This peripheral vasodilatation can result in high output cardiac failure. Upon the appearance of neurologic signs after an average of 53 days of a thiamine-deficient diet, left ventricular muscle preparations from thiamine-deficient rats showed a decrease in performance associated with a decrease in the duration of contraction and the rate of tension development.[5]

Carnitine (3-hydroxy-4-*n*-trimethoaminobutyric acid) is a cofactor for transport of long-chain fatty acids across the inner mitochondrial membrane. It is present in the diet, notably in meat. Carnitine of dietary or endogenous origin is released from the liver and kidneys into the plasma and is taken up by the peripheral tissues. Deficiency of carnitine blocks the mitochondrial oxidation of fatty acids to carbon dioxide in all tissues and leads to lipid accumulation in the cytosol. The skeletal muscle, in particular cardiac muscle, depends on oxidation of fat for most of its energy, and muscle is the tissue most severely affected by carnitine deficiency. Carnitine deficiency in humans is found in two forms, myopathic and systemic, on the basis of tissue carnitine contents. In myopathic carnitine deficiency, carnitine levels are reduced only in muscle, but in systemic carnitine deficiency, carnitine levels are reduced in several tissues, including the muscle, plasma, and liver. Cardiac disease has been described in both forms of carnitine deficiency. A hypertrophic cardiomyopathy with a decreased ejection fraction, resembling a dilated cardiomyopathy, results.

A cardiomyopathy was described in China 100 years ago that was responsive to selenium supplementation. This cardiomyopathy, called Keshan disease, is geographically distributed from the northwest to the southwest of China and targets children and women in the childbearing years. The susceptible population includes peasants consuming crops grown in soils with low selenium content. In the United States, selenium deficiency has been described in patients receiving long-term parenteral hyperalimentation.[40] Selenium is a cofactor required for the activity of the enzyme glutathione peroxidase, which catalyzes the removal of reactive oxygen molecules. Glutathione peroxidase activity may be important under ischemic conditions, where there is an increased production of oxygen radicals, and may protect the heart against cardiotoxic effects of these elements. With selenium deficiency, lipid peroxide accumulates in the myocardium, espe-

cially under ischemic conditions. Lipid peroxides in the heart may damage the cell membrane and may lead to impaired calcium transport, with uncontrolled calcium accumulation in the cell, leading to cardiomyopathy. Histologically, there is multifocal necrosis and replacement fibrosis. Selenium has a protective effect against drugs that are cardiotoxic, such as doxorubicin, has protective effects against viral infections that affect the heart (coxsackievirus), and may increase the resistance of the heart to hypoxia.

Selenium levels can be low and can affect cardiac function and have an impact on nonspecific immunity in HIV-infected patients. Kavanaugh-McHugh[41] published a case report of a 5-year-old boy with HIV infection and selenium deficiency. Cardiac dysfunction was associated with selenium deficiency, and cardiac function improved on selenium supplementation. In a cohort of patients studied at Children's Hospital, Boston,[42] 61% of the patients had low serum selenium levels. Selenium levels significantly correlated with weight z score, albumin levels, and CD4+ lymphocyte counts, suggesting a strong relationship with nutrition and immunity. There was no correlation between low selenium levels and cardiac function in this small study. Dworkin[43] compared 12 adult patients with AIDS and 27 healthy controls, and found a significant decrease in whole blood selenium and red blood cell selenium levels in the patients with AIDS. He also found that myocardial biopsies in AIDS patients demonstrate significant selenium deficits.[44] These data may provide a link between selenium deficiency in cardiomyopathy and AIDS.

The Refeeding Syndrome

Although congestive heart failure is rare in malnutrition, it can occur when the malnourished patient is refed. Starvation is associated with a fall in heart rate, blood pressure, and blood volume, whereas refeeding is associated with a sudden reversal of these compensatory factors. Furthermore, since severe malnutrition can result in interstitial myocardial edema, cardiac compliance can decrease. With refeeding, the malnourished patient must cope metabolically with increased salt, water, and energy loads. Carbohydrate and fat are potent stimuli for the release of catecholamines and activation of the renin–angiotensin–aldosterone axis, with a further increase in blood volume and blood pressure. Furthermore, catecholamines augment the shift of potassium, magnesium, and phosphorus into cells, with potential deleterious effects on cardiac function and rhythm.

Refeeding causes a change from the hypometabolism of starvation to the hypermetabolism of refeeding. Increasing energy intake leads to a corresponding increase in oxygen consumption to meet this demand. Cardiac output must increase. Increased carbon dioxide production requires increased respiratory ventilation and an increased work of breathing. Heat production and heart rate progressively rise with increasing energy intake. Reversal of cardiac atrophy and the ability to generate cardiac output may not keep pace with these rapidly increasing demands. Cardiac failure is a concern in nutritionally supplemented patients, even when the sodium and water load is kept low. It is important to begin with low energy loads in patients who are at risk for cardiac decompensation. It may be useful in these patients to give a higher proportion of energy as fat rather than carbohydrate. The lower respiratory quotient of fat oxidation results in less carbon dioxide production, thereby decreasing the work of breathing and facilitating ventilator weaning in patients with respiratory failure.

Although congestive heart failure is a well-recognized complication of refeeding therapy in underweight patients, few data exist that describe cardiac function during the refeeding period. Heymsfield and coworkers[27] evaluated cardiac parameters of 12 patients with severe protein-calorie undernutrition and subsequent refeeding. In this study, five patients were selected for hyperalimentation. With nutritional repletion, there was progressive improvement in body weight and lean body mass during therapy. Body weight increased by 0.3 kg/day, with increasing positive metabolic balances. The cardiovascular status of these patients also changed during the hyperalimentation phase. During the first 5 to 15 days of therapy, intracardiac volume expanded, the left ventricular mass enlarging by 15%. The absolute stroke volume and cardiac output also

increased during this period by 21% and 31%, respectively. The cardiac index increased, and in some patients, exceeded the normal range. During the next 3 weeks, ventricular volume, cardiac output, and stroke volume continued to increase gradually. By contrast, left ventricular mass increased by only 10% of the initial phase per week. The ejection fraction remained within the normal range throughout. Heart rate remained unchanged or slightly increased during hyperalimentation. During hyperalimentation, two of the five patients developed physical signs and symptoms of congestive heart failure, one at approximately 20 and the other at approximately 30 days of hyperalimentation. A pericardial effusion developed in two patients on day 20. Heymsfield and colleagues advocate the use of low-salt regimens, a slower rate of hyperalimentation, and serial monitoring of cardiac dimensions and function by clinical examination and echocardiography to prevent cardiac decompensation during refeeding. Although little has been written on refeeding the HIV-infected patients similar principles must also apply.

Conclusion

Nutritional status, including body composition, micronutrients, and response to refeeding, can impact significantly on cardiac mass, function, and rhythm in non-HIV human and animal models. Because malnutrition is common in people infected with HIV, nutritional effects on cardiac mass and function must be common, although not currently fully studied. Little scientific data exists on the relationship between nutrition and cardiac disease in HIV-infected patients, yet preliminary studies suggest that nutritional status can impact on cardiac mass and function. Alternatively, altered cardiac function, as a presumed response to intrinsic and abnormal metabolic function can impact, in a primary way, on the nutritional status of HIV-infected patients. Future studies are needed to determine metabolic factors that can alter both cardiac and nutritional parameters simultaneously. In addition, the effects of nutritional rehabilitation with dietary components, including micronutrient supplementation on cardiac outcomes should be studied.

References

1. Centers for Disease Control. Revised classification system for human immunodeficiency virus infection in children less than 13 years of age. *MMWR* 1994;43:1–10.

2. Voit C. Über die Verchiedenheiten der Erweissersetzung beim Hunger. *Z Biol* 1866;2.

3. Waber LJ, Valle D, Neill C, DiMauro S, Shug A. Carnitine deficiency presenting as familial cardiomyopathy: a treatable defect in carnitine transport. *J Pediatr* 1982;101:700–705.

4. Oster O, Prellwitz W. Selenium and cardiovascular disease. *Biol Trace Element Res* 1990;24:91–103.

5. Cohen EM, Abelmann WH, Messer JV, Bing OHL. Mechanical properties of rat cardiac muscle during experimental thiamine deficiency. *Am J Physiol* 1976;231:1390–1394.

6. Kotler DP, Tierney AR, Wang J, Pierson RN. Magnitude of body-cell-mass depletion and the timing of death from wasting in AIDS. *Am J Clin Nutr* 1989;50:444–447.

7. Grunfeld C, Kotler DP. Wasting in the acquired immunodeficiency syndrome. *Semin Liver Dis* 1992;12:175–187.

8. Guenter P, Muurahainen N, Simons G, et al. Relationships among nutritional status, disease progression, and survival in HIV infection. *J Acquir Immune Defic Syndr* 1993;6:1130–1138.

9. Miller TL, Awnetwant EL, Evans SE, et al. Gastrostomy tube supplementation for HIV-infected children. *Pediatrics* 1995;96:696–702.

10. Mgone CS, Mhalu FS, Shao JF, et al. Prevalence of HIV-1 infection and symptomatology of AIDS in severely malnourished children in Dar Es Salaam, Tanzania. *J Acquir Immune Defic Syndr* 1991;4:910–913.

11. Miller TL, Evans SJ, Orav EJ, et al. Growth and body composition in children with human immunodeficiency virus–1 infection. *Am J Clin Nutr* 1993;57:588–592.

12. Moye J Jr, Rich KC, Kalish LA, et al. for the Women and Infants Transmission Study Group. Natural history of somatic growth in infants born to women infected by human immunodeficiency virus. *J Pediatr* 1996;128:58–69.

13. McKinney RE Jr, Robertson JW, and the Duke Pediatric AIDS Clinical Trials Unit. Effect of human immunodeficiency virus infection on the growth of young children. *J Pediatr* 1993;123:579–582.

14. Saavedra JM, Henderson RA, Perman JA, et al. Longitudinal assessment of growth in children born to mothers with human immunodeficiency virus infection. *Arch Pediatr Adolesc Med* 1995;149:497–502.

15. Macallan DC, Noble C, Baldwin C, et al. Prospective analysis of patterns of weight change in stage IV human immunodeficiency virus infection. *Am J Clin Nutr* 1993;58:417–424.

16. Danker WM, Nyhan WL, Spector SA. Effect of salvage dideoxycytidine (ddC) on growth, nutritional parameters, and metabolic rates of children with advanced HIV disease. [Abstract No. 272]. *Proc Natl Conf Hum Retrov Relat Infect.* 1995;Jan 29–Feb 2.

17. Ott M, Lembcke B, Fischer H, et al. Early changes of body composition in human immunodeficiency virus-infected patients: tetrapolar body impedance analysis indicates significant malnutrition. *Am J Clin Nutr* 1993;57:15–19.

18. Kotler DP, Wang J, Pierson RN. Body composition studies in patients with the acquired immunodeficiency syndrome. *Am J Clin Nutr* 1985;42:1255–1265.

19. Kotler DP. Cytomegalovirus colitis and wasting. *J Acquir Immune Defic Syndr* 1991;4(Suppl 1):S36–S41.

20. Kotler DP, Tierney AR, Altilio D, et al. Body mass repletion during ganciclovir treatment of cytomegalovirus infections in patients with acquired immunodeficiency syndrome. *Arch Intern Med* 1989;149:901–905.

21. Keys A, Henschel A, Taylor HL. The size and function of the human heart at rest in semistarvation and in subsequent rehabilitation. *Am J Physiol* 1947;150:153–169.

22. Bloom WL, Azar G, Smith EG Jr. Changes in heart size and plasma volume during fasting. *Metab Clin Exp* 1966;15:409–413.

23. Smythe PM, Swanepoel A, Campbell JAH. The heart in kwashiorkor. *BMJ* 1962:67–75.

24. Wharton B. *Q. J Med News* 1969.

25. Isner JM, Roberts WC, Heymsfield SB, Yager J. Anorexia nervosa and sudden death. *Ann Intern Med* 1985;102:49–52.

26. Gottdiener JS, Gross HA, Henry WL, et al. Effects of self-induced starvation on cardiac size and function in anorexia nervosa. *Circulation* 1978;58: 425–433.

27. Heymsfield SB, Bethel RA, Ansley JD, et al. Cardiac abnormalities in cachectic patients before and during nutrition repletion. *Am Heart J* 1978; 95:584–594.

28. Miller TL, Orav EJ, Colan S, Lipshultz SE. Nutritional status and cardiac mass and function in children infected with the human immunodeficiency virus. *Am J Clin Nutr* 1997;66:660–664.

29. Rossi MA, Zuccoloto S. Ultrastructural changes in nutritional cardiomyopathy of protein-calorie malnourished rats. *Br J Exp Pathol* 1982;63:242–247.

30. Viart P. Hemodynamic findings in severe protein-calorie malnutrition. *Am J Clin Nutr* 1977;30: 334–348.

31. Kalager T, Brubakk O, Bassoe HH. Cardiac performance in patients with anorexia nervosa. *Cardiology* 1978;63:1–4.

32. Kreipe RE, Harris JP. Myocardial impairment resulting from eating disorders. *Pediatr Ann* 1992; 21:760–768.

33. Landsberg L, Young JB. Fasting, feeding and regulation of the sympathetic nervous system. *N Engl J Med* 1978;298:1295–1300.

34. Young JB, Landsberg L. Suppression of the sympathetic nervous system during fasting. *Science* 1977; 196:1473–1475.

35. Young JB, Landsberg L. Stimulation of the sympathetic nervous system during sucrose feeding. *Nature* 1977;269:615–617.

36. Pissaia O, Rossi MA, Oliveira JSM. The heart in protein-calorie malnutrition in rats: morphological, electrophysiological and biochemical changes. *J Nutr* 1980;110:2035–2044.

37. Alexander JK, Peterson KL. Cardiovascular effects of weight reduction. *Circulation* 1972;45:310–318.

38. Grunfeld C, Feingold KR. Metabolic disturbances and wasting in the acquired immunodeficiency syndrome. *N Engl J Med* 1992;327:329–337.

39. Stephens AJH. ECG as a prognostic instrument in kwashiorkor. *Ann Trop Med Parasitol* 1978;69:85.

40. Fleming CR, Lie JT, McCall JT, et al. Selenium deficiency and fatal cardiomyopathy in a patient on home parenteral nutrition. *Gastroenterology* 1982; 83:689–693.

41. Kavanaugh-McHugh AL, Ruff A, Perlman E, et al. Selenium deficiency and cardiomyopathy in acquired immunodeficiency syndrome. *J Parenter Enteral Nutr* 1991;15:347–349.

42. Miller TL, Orav EJ, McIntosh K, Lipshultz SE. Is selenium deficiency clinically significant in pediatric HIV infection? *Gastroenterology* 1993;104: A746

43. Dworkin BM, Rosenthal WS, Wormser GP, Weiss L. Selenium deficiency in the acquired immunodeficiency syndrome. *J Parenter Enteral Nutr* 1986;10:405–407.

44. Dworkin BM, Antonecchia PP, Smith F, et al. Reduced cardiac selenium content in the acquired immunodeficiency syndrome. *J Parenter Enteral Nutr* 1989;13:644–647.

22

Mitochondrial Toxicity of Antiviral Nucleosides Used in AIDS: Insights Derived From Toxic Changes Observed in Tissues Rich in Mitochondria

William Lewis, M.D.

Evidence is mounting to link alterations in mitochondrial DNA replication in various tissues to toxicity of antiviral nucleoside agents[1] used as therapy in acquired immunodeficiency syndrome (AIDS) and other viral infections. However, some controversy exists regarding the prevalence and overall clinical impact of such toxicities in AIDS patients. Clinically useful agents such as zidovudine (3'-azido-2',3'-deoxythymidine), zalcitibine (2',3'-dideoxycytidine), didanosine (2',3'-dideoxyinosine), and stavudine (2',3'-didehydro-3'-dideoxythymidine) serve as tools in models of inhibition of mitochondrial DNA polymerase-γ . Other agents that showed promise for treating AIDS-related viral infections, such as fialuridine (1-[2-deoxy-2-fluoro-β-D-arabinofuranosyl]-5-iodouracil) for chronic hepatitis B infection, were extremely toxic to liver, skeletal and cardiac muscle, and peripheral nerve tissues in clinical trials resulting in early termination of the studies. On the basis of clinical evidence and data extrapolated from preclinical studies, it seems reasonable to consider mitochondrial toxicity of antiviral nucleoside agents as an organelle-specific toxicity affecting many tissues. Table 22-1 shows the extent of clinical involvement of mitochondrial toxicity of antiviral nucleoside agents.

Biological Basis of Antiviral Nucleoside Agent Toxicity: the DNA Polymerase-γ Hypothesis

Recently, we suggested the mitochondrial DNA polymerase-γ hypothesis to explain some events of the newly described antiviral nucleoside agent mitochondrial toxicity. The hypothesis relates mitochondrial toxicity to inhibition of eukaryotic DNA polymerase-γ by the antiviral nucleoside agent and its incorporation into DNA.[2] The DNA polymerase-γ hypothesis states that alterations in mitochondrial DNA replication induced by antiviral nucleoside agents are a result of the following:

1. Subcellular availability and abundance of the antiviral nucleoside agent in the target tissue

317

Table 22-1. Mitochondrial Toxicity of Antiviral Agents

Antiviral Agent	Anatomic or Tissue Target	Clinical Evidence for Mitochondrial Toxicity [Refs.]	Experimental Evidence for Mitochondrial Toxicity [Refs.]
Zidovudine	Skeletal muscle	Features of mitochondrial myopathy includng ragged red fibers; decreased muscle mitochondrial DNA, paracrystals; phosphocreatine depletion in exercised patients [2,49,52,55]	Decreased mitochondrial DNA in vitro; decreased mitochondrial DNA, mitochondrial RNA, mitochondrial polypeptides, and ultrastructural damage to mitochondria in vivo; low K_i for zidovudine triphosphate with mammalian DNA polymerase-γ; failure of exonulcleolytic excision of terminally incorporated zidovudine [5,11,22,24,25,26,35]
	Heart muscle	Cardiomyopathy with cardiac dilatation and failure; mitochondrial cristae dissolution [61,62,63]	Decreased mitochondrial RNA; altered mitochondria on transmission electron microscopy; mixed (competitive and noncompetitive) K_i with cardiac DNA polymerase-γ [10,34,35,36]
	Lactic acidosis with anaerobic metabolism in many tissues	Markedly elevated serum lactate; Reyes syndromelike findings [67,68]	After 7 days, lactate in HepG2 cells is 200% of control levels at 250 µM zidovudine [29]
	Liver	Hepatomegaly with fatty change (steatosis) [26]	Intracytoplasmic lipid droplet accumulation in HepG2 cells with disrupted mitochondrial cristae [29]
Zalcitibine	Peripheral nerve	Painful peripheral neuropathy in 50% to 100% of patients [43,71,72,73]	Inhibition of mitochondrial DNA replication in MOLT cells; lactate accumulation in HTB11 neuronal cells; mitochondrial structural changes and lipid accumulation in nerves of zalcitibine-treated rabbits [25,27,31,40,41,88]
Didanosine	Peripheral nerve	Painful peripheral neuropathy in 3% to 22% of patients [89,70]	Distorted cristae and decreased mitochondrial DNA in cultured cells; lactate accumulates in HTB11 neuronal cells [32]
Stavudine	Peripheral nerve	Painful peripheral neuropathy in 55% of patients [70,89]	Distorted cristae and decreased mitochondrial DNA in CEM [32]
Fialuridine	Liver, skeletal and cardiac muscle, peripheral nerve	Lactic acidosis; hepatic failure and steatosis; renal failure; skeletal and cardiac myopathy; peripheral neuropathy [77,90]	fialuridine incorporation into mitochondrial DNA in vivo and in vitro; mitochondrial structural defects and intracellular fat accumulation in vitro and in vivo. Competitive K_i of fialuridine triphosphate with DNA polymerase-γ (0.02 µM) [10,12,14,23,30,38,39]

2. Ability of the antiviral nucleoside agent to serve as a substrate for cellular nucleoside kinases and to become phosphorylated intracellularly

3. Ability of the antiviral nucleoside triphosphate to serve as an inhibitor of mitochondrial DNA polymerase-γ (possibly reflected in its K_i in vitro)

4. Metabolic requirements of the tissues for oxidative phosphorylation

Parts of the DNA polymerase-γ hypothesis serve as corollaries to the oxidative phosphorylation paradigm of Wallace.[3,4] Furthermore, antiviral nucleoside agents may serve as tools to create animal models of genetic illnesses of mitochondria in which disturbances in mitochondrial DNA replication are integral features. Treatment with agents like zidovudine yields phenotypically similar mitochondrial disease, with alterations in mitochondrial DNA, mitochondrial RNA, mitochondrial polypeptide synthesis, and mitochondrial ultrastructure.[5] At present, animal models of genetic mitochondrial illnesses are not readily available,[6] but mitochondrial toxicity caused by nucleoside analogues is considered an acquired model of mitochondrial DNA depletion. Other investigators[7,8] suggested that the antiviral nucleoside agents can be divided into two classes of mitochondrial DNA replication inhibitors according to the relative importance of

DNA chain termination, or internalization of the analogue into nascent mitochondrial DNA and its substitution for the natural base.

One class of compound inhibits mitochondrial DNA replication in ways that resemble the action of fialuridine (Figure 22-1A). The toxic mechanism with such agents involves the incorporation of antiviral nucleoside monophosphate into mitochondrial DNA. To that extent, FIAC (1-[2-deoxy-2-fluoro-*b*-D-arabinofuranosyl]-5-iodocytosine), fialuridine, FMAU (1-[2-deoxy-2-fluoro-*b*-D-arabinofurano-syl]-5-methyluracil), and FEAU (1-[2-deoxy-2-fluoro-*b*-D-arabinofuranosyl]-5-ethyluracil) each

demonstrated efficacy in viral disease models.[9] However, many of their triphosphates inhibit mammalian DNA polymerase-γ in vitro.[10]

The second type of compound is represented by some anti-AIDS dideoxynucleosides such as zidovudine, zalcitibine, and stavudine. With agents that resemble zidovudine structurally, the 5′-triphosphates serve as substrates for mitochondrial DNA synthesis by DNA polymerase-γ and compete with the natural nucleotides. Such agents terminate nascent mitochondrial DNA chains once incorporated into the chain because they lack 3′-hydroxyl groups (3′-OH), which are necessary for continued poly-

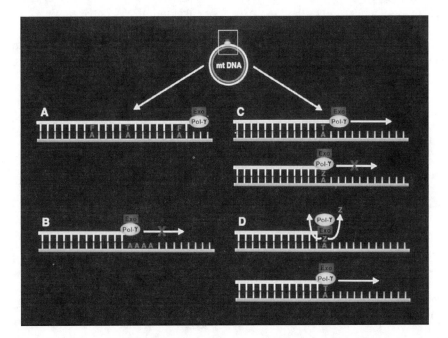

Figure 22-1. (See Color Plate 2 for image in full color.) Mechanism of toxicity of antiviral nucleoside agent to mitochondrial DNA replication (small double circle), with attached DNA polymerase-γ (in block) in which antiviral nucleoside triphosphates serve as inhibitors of mitochondrial DNA replication. **A,B**: Enlarged view of interaction of mitochondrial DNA with DNA polymerase-γ. Incorporation of antiviral nucleoside agents into mitochondrial DNA as an alternate substrate for DNA polymerase-γ. Fialuridine triphosphate serves as an alternate substrate for thymidine triphosphate with DNA polymerase-γ and is incorporated (inserted into mitochondrial DNA as **F**) into the nascent chain because it possesses a 3′-OH group (**A**). The nascent mitochondrial DNA can be extended beyond the inserted fialuridine. If there is a run of adenine in the template (signaling insertion of thymine), then fialuridine monophosphate cannot be inserted into the run, perhaps relating to changes of interaction between the polymerase and the template (**B**). By contrast, antiviral nucleoside triphosphates (such as zidovudine triphosphate) that lack a 3′-OH group also compete with thymidine triphosphate as substrates of DNA polymerase-γ. **C**: The latter antiviral nucleoside agents terminate mitochondrial DNA synthesis (inserted into DNA as **Z**) because bases cannot be added to the nascent chain after zidovudine is inserted. **D**: If the exonuclease recognizes the misinserted **Z**, it has the potential for removing it as shown.

merization of DNA. This results in inhibition of mitochondrial DNA synthesis (Figure 22-1C). The inhibition of mitochondrial DNA replication and manifestations of antiviral nucleoside agent toxicity may be reversible because the 3'→5' exonuclease of DNA polymerase-γ may excise the inserted zidovudine (Figure 22-1D), but only at the point of its insertion into the nascent mitochondrial DNA. If the antiviral nucleoside agent (such as zidovudine) is not recognized as an erroneous insertion, it will remain in the nascent chain and mitochondrial DNA synthesis of that chain of mitochondrial DNA will cease (Figure 22-1C). A recent biochemical study found that terminally incorporated zidovudine monophosphate was not removed by the 3→5' exonuclease of *Saccharomyces cerevisiae* DNA polymerase-γ[11] and the investigators suggested this was a mechanism operative in the mitochondrial toxicity of DNA polymerase-γ.

There is no reported postreplicational repair mechanism to remove the internally incorporated antiviral nucleoside monophosphate (see below), and the damage to mitochondrial DNA is more likely to be permanent or more difficult to reverse. Incorporated fialuridine (as fialuridine monophosphate) or fialuridine metabolites could be released from degraded DNA. Evidence also supports a role of template-related "hot spots," analogous to those found in some heritable mitochondrial diseases,[3,4] in the altering of mitochondrial DNA synthesis by antiviral nucleoside agents. "Adenosine tracts" in DNA templates appear to inhibit the incorporation of fialuridine monophosphate into DNA in vitro (Figure 22-1B).[12]

Pharmacology and Biochemistry of Antiviral Nucleoside Agent Toxicity

Metabolism of Antiviral Nucleoside Agents in Tissues

Nucleoside kinases are enzymes responsible for activating antiviral nucleoside agents intracellularly. Activation is accomplished by 5'-phosphorylation of the antiviral nucleoside agent using the same system that phosphorylates ribonucleosides and 2'-deoxynucleosides.[13] Antiviral nucleoside agents including zidovudine, fialuridine and stavudine are phosphorylated by thymidine kinase.[14,15] Tissue-specific forms of mammalian thymidine kinase exist: thymidine kinase 1 (cytosolic, with low activity in skeletal muscle) and thymidine kinase 2 (mitochondrial, with higher activity in skeletal muscle). The tissue distribution of thymidine kinase isoforms and their ability to phosphorylate an antiviral nucleoside agent may relate to the selective toxicity of some antiviral nucleoside agents at specific tissue sites. After 5'-monophosphorylation, antiviral nucleoside agents ultimately are phosphorylated by other cellular enzymes to antiviral nucleoside triphosphates that function as inhibitors of viral or eukaryotic DNA polymerases.

Antiviral Nucleoside Agent Interactions With DNA Polymerases

On a structural basis, antiviral nucleoside triphosphates could inhibit mammalian nuclear DNA polymerases (DNA polymerase-α, DNA polymerase-β, DNA polymerase-δ, and DNA polymerase-ε) and DNA polymerase-γ (for mitochondrial DNA replication). Both the mechanisms for DNA polymerization and the choice of nucleotide substrates are similar among eukaryotic DNA polymerases. Some antiviral nucleoside triphosphates inhibit nuclear DNA polymerases in vitro.[16] However, there is no evidence that the inhibition of nuclear DNA polymerases by antiviral nucleoside triphosphates is as important as inhibition of DNA polymerase-γ in the clinical toxicity.[1] By contrast, the data suggest that antiviral nucleoside triphosphates inhibit DNA polymerase-γ relatively effectively. The resultant mitochondrial structural and functional changes in target tissues have been demonstrated. These facts suggest that the mitochondria are targets for antiviral nucleoside agent toxicity regardless of the tissue and may help explain some of the diverse clinical manifestations of the mitochondrial toxicity of antiviral nucleosides.

Biochemical Features of DNA Polymerase-γ That Affect the Mitochondrial Toxicity

One important clinical and experimental observation in some forms of antiviral nucleoside toxicity is a decreased steady-state abundance of mitochondrial DNA. This may relate to the functions of DNA polymerase-γ, a nuclear-encoded DNA polymerase for mitochondrial DNA replication.[17] The *polymerase* function of DNA polymerase-γ is fundamental to antiviral nucleoside agent toxicity. However, a $3' \rightarrow 5'$ *exonuclease* is present.[18,19] The exonuclease is inhibited by nucleoside 5'-monophosphates.[20] DNA polymerase-γ is processive. *Processivity* allows each DNA polymerase-γ molecule to replicate mitochondrial DNA completely after one initiation event.

The processivity of DNA polymerase-γ also may relate to *heteroplasmy* (an intracellular mix of normal and mutant mitochondrial DNA molecules[3,4]). Because of the processivity of DNA polymerase-γ, deletion mutants (shortened mitochondrial DNA) may be replicated more quickly and efficiently than native mitochondrial DNA counterparts.[4,6] As a result, the abundance of mitochondrial DNA mutants may increase, with associated functional changes at a threshold of mutant mitochondrial DNA. Similarities exist between antiviral nucleoside agent toxicity (as is zidovudine myopathy) and with mitochondrial DNA depletion seen in some forms of heritable mitochondrial illnesses.[21]

Experimental Models that Support Mitochondrial Toxicity of Antiviral Nucleoside Agents

Biochemical Evidence for Mitochondrial Toxicity of Antiviral Nucleoside Agent

Incubation of zidovudine triphosphate with DNA polymerase-γ in vitro resulted in mixed kinetics with a competitive K_i of 1.8 ± 0.2 μM and a noncompetitive K_i' of 6.8 ± 1.7 μM.[22] A similar mixed inhibition pattern was determined for inhibition of cardiac DNA polymerase-γ by stavudine triphosphate, but with a much lower K_i.[23] In studies by other investigators, zidovudine triphosphate inhibited DNA polymerase-γ activity approximately 30% at 4 μM, compared with 80% inhibition of reverse transcriptase activity at the same concentration in vitro.[24]

We showed that fialuridine triphosphate inhibited DNA polymerase-γ competitively with a nano-

molar K_i and that fialuridine monophosphate was incorporated into DNA.[10,12] Fialuridine triphosphate and FMAU triphosphate demonstrated nanomolar, competitive K_i values. By contrast, the K_i for fialuridine 1-(2-deoxy-2-fluoro-β-*d*-arabinofuranosyl)-5-metgyluracil) triphosphate was micromolar.

Cell Biologic Evidence for Antiviral Nucleoside Agent Mitochondrial Toxicity

Cell biologic data on the effects antiviral nucleoside agents support the hypothesis that these agents have selective mitochondrial toxicity. Zidovudine decreased the abundance of mitochondrial DNA in human lymphoblastoid cells.[25] In vitro, 25 μM zidovudine inhibited the incorporation of [³H]thymidine by 90% and 1 μM zidovudine inhibited it by 25% to 38%.[26] Selective loss of mitochondrial DNA occurred in MOLT-4F lymphoblasts exposed to zalcitibine, zidovudine, and other dideoxynucleosides in vitro.[25,27,28] In various human and rodent muscle cell lines, exposure to zidovudine causes abnormal mitochondria with extensive lipid accumulation.

Treatment of HepG2 cells with fialuridine and FMAU caused both antiviral nucleoside agents to be found in nuclear and mitochondrial DNA. Ultrastructural defects were found in mitochondria.[14] We determined that mitochondrial DNA decreased in abundance in HepG2 cells after 14 days' exposure to fialuridine and FMAU,[12] and that fialuridine and FMAU but *not* FAU caused mitochondrial structural defects in vitro after at least 2 weeks' treatment. Changes in HepG2 cells were easily visible using rapid, sensitive, and simple Oil-red-O staining of cells and were correlated with increased lactate in the medium.[29] In U937 or MOLT-4 cells treated with fialuridine, a higher IC_{50} was found with 1% to 2% replacement of cellular thymidine by fialuridine.[30]

Zalcitibine decreased the abundance of mitochondrial DNA in PC12 mouse neuronal cell lines in vitro[31] and in cultured cells cells treated with zalcitibine, stavudine, or didanosine.[32] We found decreased abundance of mitochondrial DNA in HTB11 neuroblastoma cells treated with zalcitibine, didanosine, or stavudine. In vitro, Dalakas and colleagues[33] showed that zidovudine increased the abundance of lactate in the culture medium and caused the development of abnormal mitochondria in the cytoplasm of myotubes with accumulation of neutral fat. These changes, in contrast to those with zidovudine, were irreversible and consistent with the incorporation of fialuridine monophosphate and its internalization into mitochondrial DNA as noted earlier.

In Vivo Evidence for Mitochondrial Toxicity

Oral zidovudine decreased rat cardiac mitochondrial RNA and altered mitochondrial ultrastructure.[5,34–36] In similarly treated rats, zidovudine administration decreased mitochondrial DNA, mitochondrial RNA, and mitochondrial polypeptide expression, and altered mitochondrial ultrastructure in skeletal muscle.[5] Other data suggest that the mitochondrial changes we observed in the zidovudine-treated rat heart and muscle are found in striated muscle of hamsters treated with zidovudine intraperitoneally.[37] Rats treated with zidovudine developed ultrastructural abnormalities in their skeletal and cardiac muscle mitochondria associated with depression of muscle mitochondrial DNA and mitochondrial polypeptide synthesis, impaired cytochrome c reductase, and an uncoupling effect.[33,35]

Woodchucks developed severe hepatic steatosis after 8 weeks' treatment with fialuridine (B. Tennant, personal communication), and rodents, primates, and canines incorporated fialuridine monophosphate into DNA in vivo.[38]

Oil-red-O-stained heart samples from fialuridine-treated woodchucks revealed lipid droplets in cardiac myocytes but not in other cardiac cells (such as smooth muscle cells[39]). This was associated with ultrastructural evidence of mitochondrial destruction. The steady-state abundance of mitochondrial DNA in the liver, myocardium, skeletal muscle, and kidney decreased in fialuridine-treated woodchucks compared with controls, but the amount of the decrease mitochondrial DNA varied among the tissues. This point suggests further similarities to genetic diseases of mitochondrial DNA in which the abundance of mitochondrial DNA varies from tissue to tissue[21] and supports the oxidative phosphorylation paradigm of Wallace[3,4] in a pharmacologic model.

Although zalcitibine and didanosine have not caused cardiac lesions similar to those caused by treating rodents with zidovudine (W. Lewis, unpublished observations), administration of zalcitibine to rabbits caused dose-related structural damage to the Schwann cells of the peripheral nerves.[40,41] This so-called "schwannopathy" involved mitochondrial changes with some similarities to those found with zidovudine myopathy.

Clinical Mitochondrial Toxicity of Antiviral Nucleoside Agents and Anatomic Targets

Hematologic Toxicity

Hematologic toxicity is the most common side effect of zidovudine, occurring in up to 21% of patients.[42,43] The manifestations include anemia (usually macrocytic), leukopenia, thrombocytopenia, and bone marrow suppression. Pancytopenia and marrow aplasia are rare. Zidovudine produces significant loss of hematopoietic precursors in the peripheral blood before affecting the bone marrow itself. The hematopoietic toxicity of zidovudine is attributed to the inhibition of cellular DNA polymerases,[44] possibly including DNA polymerase-γ, or to the depletion of thymidine pools.[45] The effects of zidovudine on bone marrow cultures include time- and dose-dependent inhibition of marrow erythroid and granulocyte/macrophage precursors. Burst and colony-forming units for erythroid cells are five- to eightfold more sensitive to zidovudine than colony-forming units for granulocytes and macrophages and mixed colonies. Analogies between zidovudine myelotoxicity and at least one heritable illness of mitochondrial DNA may be made. Mitochondrial deletions and associated bone marrow failure are important components of Pearson's marrow-pancreas syndrome.[46] It also should be noted that one important manifestation of didanosine toxicity is acute pancreatitis; pancreatitis also is a feature of Pearson syndrome.

Zidovudine-Induced Skeletal Muscle Myopathy

All evidence to date suggests that zidovudine causes a mitochondrial skeletal myopathy in adult

AIDS patients receiving long-term zidovudine treatment. The literature on AIDS therapy now includes zidovudine-induced skeletal muscle myopathy as a complication of zidovudine therapy,[6,47] but some controversy persists.[48]

Dalakas and colleagues[49] reported zidovudine-induced mitochondrial myopathy with microscopic "ragged red fibers" and ultrastructural paracrystalline inclusions in the mitochondria. Ragged red fibers are characteristic histopathologic features that result from subsarcolemmal accumulation of mitochondria in the skeletal muscle of patients with mitochondrial myopathies.[50] By transmission electron microscopy, the mitochondria are enlarged and swollen, and contain disrupted cristae and occasional paracrystalline inclusions; analogous changes have occurred in experimental treatment.[2,34,35,51] Further studies of extracts of muscle biopsy specimens of zidovudine-treated patients with AIDS revealed decreased skeletal muscle mitochondrial DNA from crude extracts. Pathologic changes were absent in samples from nonmyopathic control patients with AIDS.[52] The absence of viral particles was noted ultrastructurally.[53]

Clinically, the myopathy presents with fatigue, myalgia, muscle weakness, wasting, and elevation of serum creatine kinase,[49,52] but elevated lactate dehydrogenase, creatine kinase and serum glutamic-oxaloacetic transaminase serum levels after 6.5 to 17 months of zidovudine were reported.[54] Exercise decreased muscle phosphocreatine (detected by ^{31}P nuclear magnetic resonance) in zidovudine-treated patients.[55] Assays of muscle homogenates revealed abnormal mitochondrial respiratory function. Enzyme histochemical analysis of muscle biopsy specimens from patients showed partial deficiency of cytochrome c oxidase activity.[56,57] A high lactate/pyruvate ratio (consistent with abnormal mitochondrial function) is seen in the blood of patients with zidovudine myopathy.[58] Assessment of muscle metabolism in vivo using magnetic resonance spectroscopy showed marked phosphocreatine depletion with slow recovery only in zidovudine-treated, HIV-positive patients.[55]

Because of mitochondrial dysfunction in zidovudine-induced myopathy, long-chain fatty acids may not be mobilized effectively for β-oxidation. Consequently, fat accumulates within the muscle fiber and is visualized histopathologically as lipid droplets.[56] Extracts of muscle biopsy specimens from patients with zidovudine myopathy contained decreased mitochondrial DNA compared to nuclear DNA.[52] This correlates with decreased mitochondrial DNA, decreased mitochondrial RNA, decreased mitochondrial polypeptide synthesis, altered mitochondrial histochemistry, and ultrastructural changes in mitochondria in animal systems.[5,34,35] Similarly, morphologic, functional, and molecular changes were absent in zidovudine. The pathologic changes in zidovudine-induced myopathy are reversible following discontinuation of zidovudine-naive, myopathic AIDS patients' muscle samples. Clinical improvement accompanies histologic improvement and reversal of zidovudine-induced mitochondrial DNA changes.[49,52] The pathologic and clinical reversibility of zidovudine myopathy is consistent with the mechanism of inhibition of DNA polymerase-γ by zidovudine triphosphate that includes termination of mitochondrial DNA.[2]

Zidovudine myopathy develops slowly after at least 6 months of therapy and occurs in up to 17% of the zidovudine-treated patients.[59] Dalakas and his colleagues showed that it occurs not only with the high-dose therapy used early in the epidemic but also with current low-dose regimens. In pediatric populations with AIDS, zidovudine myopathy is less frequently recognized and may be masked by coexisting encephalopathy.[60]

Zidovudine Cardiac Mitochondrial Toxicity

Dilated cardiomyopathy related to zidovudine or other antiretroviral therapy has been reported in AIDS patients. Cessation of therapy with the presumed toxic antiviral nucleoside agent resulted in improvement of left ventricular function on echocardiographic examination.[61] The clinical features of zidovudine-dilated cardiomyopathy occur after prolonged (at least 2 years) treatment and include congestive heart failure, left ventricle dilatation, and 7% to 26% reduced ejection fractions. Endomyocardial biopsies showed intramyocytic vacuoles, myofibrillar loss, dilated sarcoplasmic reticulum, and disruption of mitochondrial cristae.[62]

Four patients with antiviral nucleoside agent di-

Table 22-2. Cardiomyopathy Related to Antiviral Nucleoside Agent Treatment

Patient No.	Sex	Age (years)	Risk Factor	Ejection Fraction (%)	Therapy	Duration (years)
1	M	9.7	HE	7	Zidovudine/didanosine	3 .
2	M	36	IVDA	25	Zidovudine	2
3	M	36	HO	NA	Zidovudine	NA
4	M	36	HO	15	Zidovudine	1.6

HE, hemophiliac; IVDA, intravenous drug abuse; HO, homosexual; NA, not available.

lated cardiomyopathy were referred to us for evaluation of pathologic changes of the hearts. All shared documented HIV infection, long-term zidovudine therapy, and clinical features of dilated cardiomyopathy. All were males. Pathologic and ultrastructural changes on endomyocardial biopsies correlated with clinical features and grossly resembled changes in dilated cardiomyopathy of many causes (Table 22-2).

Nonspecific histologic changes consistent with dilated cardiomyopathy were seen. Myocarditis was absent. Mitochondrial degeneration and swollen or enlarged mitochondria with vacuolization, fragmentation, and loss of cristae were present. Intramitochondrial paracrystals were not found. Despite differences in behavioral risk factors for AIDS and in age, the four patients shared pathologic changes involving cardiac mitochondria, a history of long-term zidovudine exposure, and development of intractable heart failure. In one case, reversal of cardiac dysfunction followed discontinuation of zidovudine therapy.[63]

In pediatric patients with AIDS who were treated with zidovudine, Lipshultz and colleagues[64] reported that impaired cardiac function was not attributed to zidovudine. However, no myocardial biopsy findings were reported. zidovudine-skeletal myopathy is also uncommon in children with AIDS.[60] There is contrasting evidence in other reports that zidovudine dilated cardiomyopathy in pediatric patients may be more prevalent than previously reported.[65]

Hepatic Mitochondrial Toxicity of Nucleoside Analogs

Hepatic toxicity from zidovudine treatment (and treatment with other antiviral nucleoside agents including didanosine and zalcitibine) was reported recently[66–68] and was believed to relate to toxic effects of antiviral nucleoside agents on mitochondria. Fatal hepatomegaly with severe steatosis,[66] severe lactic acidosis,[67] and adult Reye syndrome[68] in zidovudine-treated HIV-seropositive patients were all pathogenetically linked to zidovudine-induced hepatotoxicity. The clinical features resembled some of those seen in fialuridine toxicity and in some uncommon metabolic conditions in which neutral fat accumulates in the liver, but the pathophysiologic basis for this unusual accumulation of intracellular fat is poorly understood.

Peripheral Neuropathy From Antiviral Nucleoside Analogs

Although it is important to identifying other causes of neuropathy in AIDS,[69] it is established that many antiviral nucleoside agents have associated peripheral neuropathies as major limiting side effects.[2,70] Dose-related, painful peripheral neuropathies occurred in up to 100% of patients with zalcitibine doses of 0.03 to 0.09 mg /kg^{-1}/day^{-1}.[43,71–73] Peripheral neuropathy with didanosine was unexpected on the basis of preclinical studies (see below)[40] but it occurred in 3% to 22% of patient's in early clinical studies[74,75] after at least 8 weeks of therapy. With stavudine, peripheral neuropathy occurred in 55% of patients between 5 and 46 weeks after initiation of therapy. This neuropathy is characterized clinically by painful dysesthesias in the feet and toes, areflexia, distal sensory loss, and mild muscle weakness. Electrophysiologic studies confirm axonal involvement. Sural nerve biopsies of patients with zalcitibine-induced neuropathy showed axonal degeneration. Dalakas and colleagues observed mitochondria with disrupted cristae in some axons in sural nerve biopsies of treated patients (M. C. Dalakas, personal communication). These findings resembled mitochondrial Schwann-opathy induced in the peripheral nerves of rabbits fed zalcitibine.[40] The dideoxynucleoside-related neuropathy can be reversible when zalcitibine or didanosine is discontinued. However, clinical evidence suggests that these agents can aggravate pre-existing neuropathy related to HIV (M. C. Dalakas, personal communication).

One common finding is a relatively slow onset of neuropathic changes. To some extent, the clinical manifestations resembled those of the unexpected but clinically important findings of zidovudine-induced mitochondrial myopathy[76] and fialuridine toxicity to liver mitochondria,[77] in which delayed onset of toxicity was a common feature.[2]

Multisystem Mitochondrial Toxicity of Fialuridine

The documented antihepatitis virus activity of fialuridine was the basis for a clinical trial in patients with chronic active hepatitis B virus. Serious fialuridine toxicity occurred (including in some patients liver failure, necessitating liver transplantation, and death) in the National Institutes of Health clinical trial.[1,78–80] The clinical manifestations of toxicity were profound lactic acidosis, hepatic failure, skeletal and cardiac myopathy, pancreatitis, and neuropathy. Micro- and macrovesicular steatosis was found in some livers from autopsies and explants from patients who survived liver transplant. In the fialuridine clinical trial, we extracted liver DNA for enzymatic hydrolysis. The hydrolysates of liver DNA were analyzed radioimmunochemically with a polyclonal antibody specific for fialuridine. fialuridine was detected in DNA hydrolysates from fialuridine-treated patients, but not in the hydrolysates from an untreated patient.

Neuropathy also occurred with fialuridine treatment. However, fialuridine-induced neuropathy had a later onset and persisted longer than the neuropathy of zalcitibine or didanosine. Fialuridine neuropathy may be pathogenetically linked to inhibition of DNA polymerase-γ by fialuridine triphosphate and its incorporation of fialuridine monophosphate into mitochondrial DNA in the affected nerves,

which explains the persistence of the toxicity over time.

Other Cardiotoxins in AIDS Therapy

On an anecdotal basis, other therapeutic agents have been related to dilated cardiomyopathy in AIDS, but the association has no experimental support. Foscarnet has caused reversible cardiac dysfunction in AIDS.[81] In three cases, interferon alfa therapy was associated with reversible cardiac dysfunction leading to dilated cardiomyopathy.[82]

Pentamidine therapy for *P. carinii* pneumonia had side effects that have an impact on therapy. About 29% of patients experienced major adverse effects including cardiac arrest, hypoglycemia, and pancreatitis.[83,84] Foscarnet therapy for cytomegalovirus also has been associated with electrophysiologic abnormalities.[81] Effects of foscarnet on DNA polymerases were not considered likely. In a prospective nonrandomized study of HIV-1, 3 of 14 patients developed torsades de pointes.[85] Torsades de pointes ventricular tachycardia was a rare complication of pentamidine therapy for *P. carinii* pneumonia.[86,87]

Summary

It is clear that a variety of therapeutic agents in AIDS may have cardiotoxicity as an important side effect. Mitochondrial toxicity of antiviral nucleoside agents may represent a significant limitation on the usefulness of such agents. The toxicity of antiviral nucleoside agents is directed not against a tissue target (such as cardiac or skeletal muscle or liver) but against a subcellular *organelle* (the mitochondrion). The observation of mitochondrial toxicity, as shown most dramatically with zidovudine skeletal myopathy and fialuridine toxicity, has brought to light the mitochondrial toxicity of antiviral drugs as a new class of adverse drug effects.[1]

Despite the DNA polymerase-γ hypothesis, which suggests a common subcellular target, the tissue target varies with each antiviral nucleoside agent. For example, zidovudine does not cause a neuropathy, and didanosine and zalcitibine do not exacerbate zidovudine myopathy. Myopathy improves when zidovudine is discontinued and with didanosine or zalcitibine is continued. Such tissue selectivity may be related to differential phosphorylation of antiviral nucleoside agents in specifc tissues, to antiviral nucleoside agent and nucleotide subcellular pools, or to isoform distribution and substrate specificity of thymidine kinase in different tissues. Through detailed basic studies and creation of authentic models, the mechanisms of toxicity of antiviral nucleoside agents to mitochondria can be understood, and the toxicities can be treated and prevented.

References

1. Swartz MN. Mitochondrial toxicity: new adverse drug effects. *N Engl J Med* 1995;333:1146–1148.

2. Lewis W, Dalakas MC. Delayed mitochondrial toxicity of antiviral nucleoside analogs. *Nature Med* 1995;1:417–422.

3. Wallace DC. Mitochondrial genetics: a paradigm for aging and degenerative diseases? *Science* 1992; 256:628–632.

4. Wallace DC. Diseases of the mitochondrial DNA. *Annu Rev Biochem* 1992;61:1175–1212.

5. Lewis W, Chomyn A, Gonzalez B, Papoian T. Zidovudine induces molecular, biochemical and ultrastructural changes in rat skeletal muscle mitochondria. *J Clin Invest* 1992;89:1354–1360.

6. Johns DR. Mitochondrial DNA and disease. *N Engl J Med* 1995;333:638–644.

7. Parker WB, Cheng YC. Mitochondrial toxicity of antiviral nucleoside analogs. *J NIH Res* 1994;6: 57–61.

8. Wright GE, Brown NC. Deoxyribonucleotide analogs as inhibitors and substrates of DNA polymerases. *Pharmacol Ther* 1990;47:447–497.

9. Fourel I, Hantz O, Wantanabe KA, et al. Inhibitory effects of 2′-fluorinated arabinosylpyrimidine nucleosides on woodchuck hepatitis virus replication in chronically infected woodchucks. *Antimicrob Agents Chemother* 1990;34:473–475.

10. Lewis W, Simpson JF, Colacino JM, et al. Fialuridine (fialuridine) triphosphate competitively inhibits mitochondrial DNA polymerase-γ. *Biochemistry* 1994;33:14620–14624.

11. Eriksson S, Xu B, Clayton DA. Efficient incorporation of anti-HIV deoxynucleotides by recombinant yeast mitochondrial DNA polymerase. *J Biol Chem* 1995;270:18929–18934.

12. Lewis W, Levine ES, Griniuviene B, Tankersley KO, et al. Fialuridine and its metabolites inhibit DNA polymerase-γ, substitute for thymidine DNA, decrease mitochondrial DNA abundance, and cause mitochondrial structural defects in cultured hepatoblasts. *Proc Natl Acad Sci USA* 1996;93:3592–3597.

13. Reichard P. Interactions between deoxyribonucleotide and DNA synthesis. *Annu Rev Biochem* 1988; 57:349–374.

14. Cui L, Yoon S, Schinazi RF, Sommadossi J-P. Cellular and molecular events leading to mitochondrial toxicity of 1-[2′-deoxy-2′-fluoro-β-D-arabinofuranosyl]-5-iodouracil in human liver cells. *J Clin Invest* 1995;95:555–563.

15. Munch-Petersen B, Bloos L, Trysted G, Eriksson S. Diverging substrate specificity of pure human thymidine kinase 1 and 2 against antiviral dideoxynucleosides. *J Biol Chem* 1991;266:9032–9038.

16. Fry M, Loeb LA. *Animal Cell DNA Polymerases.* Boca Raton, FL: CRC Press, 1986:221.

17. Wang TSF. Eukaryotic DNA polymerases. *Annu Rev Biochem* 1991;60:513–552.

18. Kunkel TA, Mosbaugh DW. Exonucleolytic proofreading by a mammalian DNA polymerase γ. *Biochemistry* 1989;28:988–995.

19. Kunkel TA, Soni A. Exonucleolytic proofreading enhances fidelity of DNA synthesis by chick embryo DNA polymerase γ. *J Biol Chem* 1988;263: 4450–4459.

20. Kaguni LS, Wernette CM, Conway MC, Yang-Cashman P. Structural and catalytic features of the mitochondrial DNA polymerase from *Drosophila melanogaster* embryos. Cold Spring Harbor Symp Quant Biol 1988;6:425–432.

21. Moraes CT, Shanske S, Fritschler H-J, et al. mitochondrial DNA depletion with variable tissue expression: a novel genetic abnormality in mitochondrial diseases. *Am J Hum Genet* 1991;48:492–501.

22. Lewis W, Simpson JF, Meyer, RR. Cardiac mitochondrial DNA polymerase-γ is inhibited competitively and non-competitively by phosphorylated zidovudine. *Circ Res* 1994;74:344–348.

23. Lewis W, Tankersley KO. Triphosphorylated fialuridine (fialuridine) and metabolites inhibit cardiac mitochondrial DNA polymerase-γ (DNA polymer-

ase-γ): alternative substrates for thymidine triphosphate (dTTP). [Abstract]. *Circulation* 1995; 92:I186.

24. König H, Behr E, Lower J, Kurth R. Azidothymidine triphosphate is an inhibitor of both human immunodeficiency virus type 1 reverse transcriptase and DNA polymerase g. *Antimicrob Agents Chemother* 1989;33:2109–2114.

25. Chen C-H, Vazquez-Padua M, Cheng Y-C. Effect of anti-human immunodeficiency virus nucleoside analogs on mitochondrial DNA and its implications for delayed toxicity. *Molec Pharmacol* 1991;39: 625–628.

26. Simpson MV, Chin CD, Keilbaugh SA, et al. Studies on the inhibition of mitochondrial DNA replication by 3′-azido–3′-deoxythymidine. *Biochem Pharmacol* 1989;38:1033–1036.

27. Chen C-H, Cheng Y-C. Delayed cytotoxicity and selective loss of mitochondrial DNA in cells treated with the anti-human immunodeficiency virus compound 2′,3′-dideoxycytidine. *J Biol Chem* 1989; 264:11934–11937.

28. d'Amati G, Lewis W. Zidovudine causes early increases in mitochondrial ribonucleic acid abundance and induces ultrastructural changes in cultured mouse muscle cells. *Lab Invest* 1994;71: 879–884.

29. Levine ES, Lewis W. The thymidine analogs fialuridine and zidovudine inhibit mitochondrial energy metabolism in cultured hepatoblasts. [Abstract]. *FASEB J* 1995;9:A1398.

30. Klecker RW, Kai AG, Collins JM. Toxicity, metabolism, DNA incorporation with lack of repair and lactate production for 1-(2′-deoxy-2′-fluoro-β-D-arabinofuranosyl)-5-iodouracil in U-937 and MOLT-4 cells. *Mol Pharmacol* 1994;46:1204–1209.

31. Keilbaugh SA, Hobbs GA, Simpson MV. Anti-human immunodeficiency virus type 1 therapy and peripheral neuropathy: prevention of 2′,3′-dideoxy-cytidine toxicity in PC 12 cells, a neuronal model, by uridine and pyruvate. *Mol Pharmacol* 1993; 44:702–706.

32. Medina DJ, Tsai C-H, Hsiung GD, Cheng Y-C. Comparison of mitochondrial morphology, mitochondrial DNA content and cell viability in cultured cells treated with three anti-human immunodeficiency virus dideoxynucleosides. *Antimicrob Agents Chemother* 1994;38:1824–1828.

33. Semino-Mora MC, Leon-Monzon ME, Dalakas MC. The effect of L-carnitine on the zidovudine-induced destruction of human myotubes. Part 1: L-Carnitine prevents the myotoxicity of zidovudine in vitro. *Lab Invest* 1994;70:102–112.

34. Lewis W, Papoian T, Gonzalez B, et al. Mitochondrial ultrastructural and molecular changes induced by zidovudine in rat hearts. *Lab Invest* 1991;65: 228–236.

35. Lamperth L, Dalakas DC, Dagani F, et al. Abnormal skeletal and cardiac mitochondria induced by zidovudine (azidothymidine) in human muscle in vitro and in an animal model. *Lab Invest* 1991;65: 742–751.

36. Cocuera Pindado MT, Lopez Bravo A, Martinez-Rodriguez R, et al. Histochemical and ultrastructural changes induced by zidovudine in mitochondria of rat cardiac muscle. *Eur J Histochem* 1994; 38:311–318.

37. Reyes MG, Casanova J, Varricchio F, et al. Zidovudine mitochondriopathy of hamster quadriceps muscle. [Abstract]. *Lab Invest* 1991;64:89A.

38. Richardson FC, Engelhardt JA, Bowsher RR. Fialuridine accumulates in DNA of dogs, monkeys, and rats following long-term oral administration. *Proc Natl Acad Sci USA* 1994;91:12003–12007.

39. Lewis W, Levine ES, Tennant BC. Fialuridine (fialuridine) treatment causes microvesicular fat to accumulate in myocardium in vivo. [Abstract]. *FASEB J* 1995;9:A628.

40. Anderson TD, Davidovich A, Feldman D, et al. Mitochondrial schwannopathy and peripheral myelinopathy in a rabbit model of dideoxycytidine neurotoxicity. *Lab Invest* 1994;70:724–739.

41. Anderson TD, Davidovich A, Arceo R, et al. Peripheral neuropathy induced by 2′,3′-dideoxycytidine: a rabbit model of 2′,3′-dideoxycytidine neurotoxicity. *Lab Invest* 1992;66:63–74.

42. Richman, DD, et al. The toxicity of zidovudine in the treatment of patients with AIDS and AIDS-related complex. *N Engl J Med* 1987;317:192–197.

43. Yarchoan R, Thomas RV, Allain J-P, et al. Phase 1 studies of 2′,3′-dideoxycytidine in severe human immunodeficiency virus infection as a single agent and alternating with zidovudine (azidothymidine). *Lancet* 1988;1:76–80.

44. Nickel W, Austermann S, Bailek G, Grosse F. Interactions of azidothymidine triphosphate with the cellular DNA polymerases α, δ, and ε and with DNA primase. *J Biol Chem* 1992;267:848–854.

45. Falcone A, Darnowski JW, Ruprecht RM, et al. Different effect of benzylacyclouridine on the toxic

and therapeutic effects of azidothymidine in mice. *Blood* 1990;76:2216–2221.

46. Rötig A, et al. Pearson's marrow-pancreas syndrome. *J Clin Invest* 1990;86:1601–1608.

47. Groopman JE. Zidovudine intolerance. *Rev Infect Dis* 1990;12:S500-S506.

48. Till M, MacDonell KB. Myopathy with human immunodeficiency virus type 1 (HIV-1) infection: HIV-1 or zidovudine? *Ann Intern Med* 1990;113:492–494.

49. Dalakas MC, Illa I, Pezeshkpour G, et al. Mitochondrial myopathy caused by long term zidovudine therapy. *N Engl J Med* 1990;322:1098–1105.

50. Shoubridge EA. Mitochondrial DNA diseases: histological and cellular studies. *J Bioenerg Biomemb* 1994;26:301–310.

51. Pezeshkpour G, Illa I, Dalakas MC. Ultrastructural characteristics and DNA immunocytochemistry in human immunodeficiency virus and zidovudine-associated myopathies. *Hum Pathol* 1991;22:1281–1288.

52. Arnaudo E, Dalakas M, Shanske S, et al. Depletion of muscle mitochondrial DNA in AIDS patients with zidovudine-induced myopathy. *Lancet* 1991;337:508–510.

53. Gertner E, Thurn J, Williams D, et al. Zidovudine associated myopathy. *Am J Med* 1989;86:814–818.

54. Bessen LJ, Greene JB, Louie E, et al. Severe polymyositis-like syndrome associated with zidovudine therapy of AIDS and ARC. *N Engl J Med* 1988;318:708. [Letter].

55. Sinnwell TM, Sivakumar K, Soueidan S, et al. Metabolic abnormalities in skeletal muscle of patients receiving zidovudine therapy observed by ³¹P in vivo magnetic resonance spectroscopy. *J Clin Invest* 1995;96:126–131.

56. Dalakas MC. Carnitine loss and zidovudine-myopathy. *Ann Neurol* 1994;36:680–681.

57. Chariot P, Gherardi R. Partial cytochrome c oxidase deficiency and cytoplasmic bodies in patients with zidovudine myopathy. *Neuromusc Dis* 1991;5:357–363.

58. Chariot P, et al. Blood lactate/pyruvate ratio is a noninvasive test for the diagnosis of zidovudine myopathy. *Arthritis Rheum* 1994;37:583–586.

59. Peters RS, Winer J, Landon DN, et al. Mitochondrial myopathy associated with chronic zidovudine therapy in AIDS. *Q J Med* 1993;86:5–15.

60. Jay C, Dalakas MC. Myopathies and neuropathies in HIV-infected adults and children. In: Pizzo P, Wilfert CM (eds). *Pediatric AIDS,* 2nd Ed. Baltimore: Williams & Wilkins, 1994:559–573.

61. Herskowitz A, Willoughby SB, Baughman KL, et al. Cardiomyopathy associated with antiretroviral therapy in patients with HIV infection: a report of 6 cases. *Ann Intern Med* 1992;116:311–313.

62. d'Amati G, Kwan W, Lewis W. Dilated cardiomyopathy in a zidovudine-treated AIDS patient. *Cardiovasc Pathol* 1992;1:317–320.

63. Koehler A, Lewis W. Mitochondrial cardiomyopathy in HIV patients treated with zidovudine. [Abstract]. *Lab Invest* 1995;72:33A.

64. Lipshultz SE, Oray J, Sanders SP, et al. Cardiac structure and function in children with human immunodeficiency virus infection treated with zidovudine. *N Engl J Med* 1992;327:1260–1265.

65. Domanski MJ, Sloas MM, Follmann DA, et al. Effect of zidovudine and didanosine treatment on heart function in children infected with human immunodeficiency virus. *J Pediatr* 1995;127:137–146.

66. Freiman JP, Helfert KE, Hamrell MR, Stein DS. Hepatomegaly with severe steatosis in HIV-seropositive patients. *AIDS* 1993;7:379–385.

67. Chattha G, Arieff AI, Cummings C, Tierney LM. Lactic acidosis complicating the acquired immunodeficiency syndrome. *Ann Intern Med* 1993;118:37–39.

68. Jolliet P, Widmann JJ. Reye's syndrome in adult with AIDS. *Lancet* 1990;335:1457.

69. Simpson DM, Tagliati M. Nucleoside analogue-associated peripheral neuropathy in human immunodeficiency virus infection. *J AIDS Hum Retrovir* 1995;9:153–161.

70. Cohen PT, Sande MA, Volberding PA. *The AIDS Knowledge Base,* 2nd Ed. Boston: Little, Brown, 1994:12–14.

71. Dubinsky RM, Yarchoan R, Dalakas M, Broder S. Reversible axonal neuropathy from the treatment of AIDS and related disorders with 2′,3′-dideoxycytidine (zalcitibine). *Muscle Nerve* 1989;12:856–860.

72. Merigan TC, Skowron G, Bozzette SA, et al. Circulating p24 antigen levels and responses to dideoxycytidine in human immunodeficiency virus (HIV) infections: a phase I and II study. *Ann Intern Med* 1989;110:189–194.

73. Berger AR, Arezzo JC, Schaumburg HH, et al. 2′,3′-Dideoxycytidine (zalcitabine) toxic neuropathy. *Neurology* 1993;43:358–362.

74. Lambert JS, Seidlin M, Reichman RC, et al. 2′,3′-Dideoxyinosine (didanosine) in patients with the acquired immunodeficiency syndrome or AIDS-related complex. *N Engl J Med* 1990;322:1332–1340.

75. Cooley TP, Kunches LM, Saunders CA, et al. Once-daily administration of 2′,3′-dideoxyinosine (didanosine) in patients with acquired immunodeficiency syndrome or AIDS-related complex. *N Engl J Med* 1990;1340–1345.

76. Dalakas MC, Lamperth L, Dagani F. Abnormal muscle mitochondria induced by zidovudine in vitro and in an animal model: morphological, enzymatic and oxygen consumption studies. *Neurology* 1991;41:375.

77. Manning FJ, Schwartz M. *Institute of Medicine Review of the Fialuridine (fialuridine) Clinical Trials.* Washington, DC: National Academy Press, 1995:1219–1221.

78. Brahams D. Deaths in US fialuridine trial. *Lancet* 1994;343:1494–1495.

79. Marshall E. Drug trial deaths deemed unavoidable. *Science* 1994;264:1530.

80. Macilwain C. US health agencies at odds over trial deaths. *Nature* 1994;369:433.

81. Brown DL, Sather S, Cheitlin MD. Reversible cardiac dysfunction associated with foscarnet therapy for cytomegalovirus esophagitis in an AIDS patient. *Am Heart J* 1993;125:1439–1441.

82. Deyton LR, Walker RE, Kovacs JA, et al. Reversible cardiac dysfunction associated with interferon alpha therapy in AIDS patients with Kaposi's sarcoma. *N Engl J Med* 1989;321:1246–1249.

83. Balslev U, Nielsen TL. Adverse effects associated with intravenous pentamidine isethionate as treatment of *Pneumocystis carinii* pneumonia in AIDS patients. *Dan Med Bull* 1992;39:366–368.

84. Cortese LM, Gasser RA, Bjornson DC, et al. Prolonged recurrence of pentamidine-induced torsades de pointes. *Ann Pharmacother* 1992;26:1365–1369.

85. Eisenhauer MD, Eliasson AH, Taylor AJ, et al. Incidence of cardiac arrhythmias during intravenous pentamidine therapy in HIV-infected patients. *Chest* 1994;105:389–394.

86. Stein KM, Haronian H, Mensah GA, et al. Ventricular tachycardia and torsades de pointes complicating pentamidine therapy of *Pneumocystis carinii* pneumonia in the acquired immunodeficiency syndrome. *Am J Cardiol* 1990;66:888–889.

87. Wharton JM, Demopulos PA, Goldschlager N. Torsades de pointes during administration of pentamidine isethionate. *Am J Med* 1987;83:571–576.

88. Feldman D, Brosnan C, Anderson TD. Ultrastructure of peripheral neuropathy in rabbits induced by 2′,3′-dideoxycytidine (zalcitibine). *Lab Invest* 1992; 66:75–85.

89. Browne MJ, Mayer KH, Chafee SBD, et al. 2′,3′-Didehydro-3′-deoxythymidine (stavudine) in patients with AIDS or AIDS-related complex: phase 1 trial. *J Infect Dis* 1993;167:21–29.

90. Stevenson W, Gaffey M, Ishitani M, et al. Clinical course of four patients receiving the experimental antiviral agent fialuridine for the treatment of chronic hepatitis B infection. *Transplant Proc* 1995; 27:1219–1221.

23

Cardiovascular Complications of Pharmacotherapeutic Agents (Excluding the Antiretrovirals) in HIV-Infected Patients

Julia C. L. Wong, M.B.B.S., M.Med., and Steven E. Lipshultz, M.D.

Human immunodeficiency virus (HIV)-infected patients frequently receive multiple medical therapies in addition to antiretroviral pharmacotherapy. Each of these medications has known side effects or toxicities, some of which may affect the cardiovascular system. Some cardiovascular side effects or toxicities have not been previously recognized in patients without HIV have become apparent in treating HIV-infected patients. This chapter reviews some of the medications that may be used to treat HIV-infected patients who have been shown to have cardiovascular side effects or toxicities that would be of clinical interest to their care providers. This chapter is not intended as a comprehensive look at all therapies a HIV-infected patient might receive, but is selectively focused on those that appear to be either most significant or most frequent in their association with cardiovascular abnormalities. The variety of new experimental therapies that are being used in an expanded way in HIV-infected patients and their cardiovascular toxicities and side effects are largely uncharacterized. Nevertheless, it is important for the care provider to understand that new unexpected toxicities are associated with well-studied therapies that were not known to be cardiotoxic in the HIV-uninfected population.

Interferon

Interferon alfa (IFN-α) is used to treat acquired immunodeficiency syndrome (AIDS)-associated Kaposi's sarcoma and other non-AIDS-related malignancies. Adverse cardiovascular effects have been observed in a significant proportion of IFN recipients. In two extensive reviews of IFN-α tolerability, 5% to 15% of more than 2,000 patients in clinical trials were reported to have adverse cardiovascular effects.[1,2] Most of these were benign, and consisted primarily of hypotension (sometimes hypertension), tachycardia, and distal cyanosis of mild to moderate severity. These effects were dose-dependent and age-related (more severe in aged patients), and they occurred transiently during the acute flulike syndrome that almost invariably accompanies initial exposure to IFN.[3–5]

More serious cardiotoxicity, including arrhythmia, ischemic heart disease, and cardiomyopathy, has been reported to occur in 1% to 4% of patients receiving IFN.[6] These complications do not appear to be dose- or age-related. In a prospective study of 138 IFN-α recipients, cardiac complications were observed in 6 (4.3%), including septal hypokinesia compatible with myocardial infarction, angina pectoris, asymptomatic deterioration of cardiac function on echocardiography, complete atrioventricular block, and recurrent atrial fibrillation. The symptoms resolved after withdrawal of treatment, but only half the patients recovered fully.[7]

Arrhythmia

In a recent review, cardiac arrhythmias were found to be the most common manifestation of IFN-induced cardiotoxicity, occurring in 25 of 44 patients from 15 different studies who were reported to have cardiovascular complications following IFN therapy.[8] In one of these studies, the frequency of occurrence of arrhythmias was reported to be as high as 20%.[9] Most of these patients had underlying cardiac disease. Both supraventricular and ventricular arrhythmias have been described.[7,8] Atrial arrhythmias, including benign supraventricular tachycardia, atrial flutter, and atrial fibrillation, were not life-threatening. They were reversed with antiarrhythmic drugs, and IFN treatment could be safely continued or reintroduced. Ventricular tachycardia, which resolved after a reduction in the dose of IFN, has been described in one patient,[10] and fatal ventricular fibrillation occurred in another.[11] Neither patient had a history of heart disease. Atrioventricular block has also been reported.[7,12,13]

Ischemic Heart Disease

The first report of serious cardiotoxicity related to the use of IFN was of four French patients who died of myocardial infarction in 1982 after being treated with the agent.[14] Sonnenblick and colleagues[8] reported on five other patients who had symptomatic or asymptomatic myocardial ischemia or infarction, which proved fatal in two cases. All five patients had underlying coronary artery disease.

Cardiomyopathy

Cardiomyopathy with congestive heart failure has been observed following a few days or months of IFN-α therapy.[15-20] None of the patients in these case reports had prior evidence of cardiac disease, although some of them had been previously treated with doxorubicin (Adriamycin). In most cases, cardiac function improved after discontinuation of IFN therapy. However, irreversible cardiomyopathy has been reported to occur.[16] Deyton and coworkers[18] reported that three patients with AIDS and Kaposi's sarcoma developed severe cardiac dysfunction following treatment with IFN-α, and it was suggested that a synergistic interaction with HIV infection may have contributed to the cardiotoxicity.[18]

Risk Factors for Cardiotoxicity

Preexisting cardiac disease, such as arrhythmia or coronary artery disease, has been found to be a risk factor for IFN-induced arrhythmia or myocardial ischemia. Such patients should be carefully monitored during IFN-α therapy, or excluded if they have unstable angina.[8,9]

None of the patients who developed cardiomyopathy were known to have previous heart disease,[8,21] and although most of them had undergone prolonged therapy with high doses of IFN-α, one patient had received only 1 week of treatment.[15]

Some reports have suggested that previous treatment with doxorubicin (Adriamycin) may be a predisposing factor for cardiotoxicity.[7,9] However, Deyton and colleagues[18] reported that three patients with AIDS and Kaposi's sarcoma developed cardiac dysfunction after receiving INF-α alone, and Sartori and colleagues[21] found that a reduction in previously normal left ventricular ejection fraction occurred in 11 patients with chronic viral hepatitis C treated with INF-α who had never been previously treated with cardiotoxic drugs. This risk factor has yet to be critically assessed.

Mechanism of Cardiotoxicity

The exact mechanism of adverse cardiac effects is unknown, and the many and varied manifestations of cardiotoxicity may indicate that more than one mechanism is responsible. It has been suggested that IFN may exert its cardiotoxic effect through peripheral vascular events. Increased oxygen demand caused by fever, chills, and tachycardia, which are part of the flulike syndrome that usually accompanies initial exposure to IFN, may precipitate infarction or arrhythmia in patients with underlying cardiac disease. IFN-induced coronary artery spasm is another possible mechanism in these patients. Other investigators have postulated that IFN has a more direct effect on the myocardium. In a rodent model, arrhythmias were produced by infusions of human recombinant IFN-α, but no myocardial structural changes were seen on light and electron microscopy.[22] It has been suggested that impairment of myocyte metabolism rather than histologic damage may account for the reversibility of cardiac dysfunction in some patients with IFN-induced cardiomyopathy.[19] Several in vitro studies have investigated the effect of IFN on cardiac cells. In one, it was thought that adenosine triphosphate (ATP) levels were altered in IFN-treated cultured rat myocytes.[23] However, another study failed to demonstrate a reduction in ATP/protein ratios.[24] An autoimmune or inflammatory mechanism has been proposed[19] but lacks histologic confirmation.[18]

Interactions with Other Drugs Used to Treat HIV

Combination of IFN-α with interleukin-2 (IL-2) may increase the risk of cardiovascular complications due to synergism between the cytokines causing myocardial damage.[25] But most studies of the combination of IL-2 and IFN-α have not shown an increased frequency and severity of adverse cardiac events compared with that expected from administration of IL-2 alone.[26] This suggests that severe cardiac toxicity is related to the use of high-dose IL-2.

Interleukin-2

IL-2 has been repeatedly documented to cause adverse cardiovascular effects in cancer patients treated with the cytokine, either alone or in combination with other therapeutic agents such as lymphokine-activated killer cells, IFN-α, and cyclophosphamide.[26-31] The capillary leak syndrome, accompanied by hemodynamic disturbances similar

to those seen in septic shock, has been reported in 40% to 70% of patients and is the most frequent complication of IL-2 treatment.[32] Other documented cardiotoxic effects include arrhythmias,[27,29-31,33] myocardial ischemia and infarction,[27,29,30,34] myocarditis,[35-38] and cardiomyopathy.[25,39-41] In one large study of cancer patients treated with high-dose IL-2, 7.5 % of 1,039 treatment courses were complicated by arrhythmias, 2.1% by angina, and 0.6% by myocardial infarction.[42]

IL-2 cardiotoxicity is usually dose-related and is readily reversible once the agent is discontinued.[29,31,42] Cancer patients on low-dose IL-2 regimens experience little or no cardiac toxicity.[40,43] Similar findings have been reported in patients with AIDS and in asymptomatic HIV-infected persons treated with low-dose IL-2.[44] No cardiotoxicity was observed in AIDS patients receiving low-dose natural IL-2 in two studies.[45,46] Likewise, studies of two small series of HIV-infected patients failed to find serious cardiac side effects relating to the use of IL-2.[47,48] Hypotension occurred in 3% of HIV-infected patients receiving IL-2 and antiretroviral therapy in a recent study,[49] and has previously been reported in patients with AIDS.[50,51] Fluid retention has also been reported.[52]

Capillary Leak Syndrome With Hemodynamic Disturbances

The capillary or vascular leak syndrome is the most common major toxicity associated with IL-2 administration. It is caused by damage to the endothelial cells that results in an increase in vascular permeability, with extravasation of plasma proteins and intravascular fluid into the extravascular space. Its clinical manifestation is a third-space syndrome characterized by generalized edema, significant weight gain of >10% body weight, hypotension, oliguria, elevated serum creatinine levels, and respiratory distress arising from pulmonary interstitial edema and pleural effusions. A direct dose-response relationship between IL-2 and the extent of vascular leakage has been demonstrated in murine models.[53]

Several mechanisms have been proposed to explain the capillary leak syndrome. Lymphokines produced by lymphoid cells activated directly by

IL-2 may mediate the vascular leakage. Cytokines such as tumor necrosis factor-α (TNF-α), IFN-α, and IL-1 have been shown to induce vascular leak in mice when given in combination with IL-2.[54] Alternatively a mechanism involving lymphokine-activated killer (LAK) cells may be involved. LAK cells may be directly cytotoxic to endothelial cells, or they may produce some factor that, in turn, damages endothelium.[55]

Hemodynamic disturbances that occur following high-dose IL-2 administration include an increase in heart rate and cardiac output, a decrease in mean systolic arterial blood pressure, often below 100 mmHg, and a fall in systemic vascular resistance.[29,30,34,56] These findings are very similar to the hemodynamic pattern seen in the early stages of septic shock and usually occur within 24 hours of IL-2 administration, peak at days 3 to 5, and persist throughout IL-2 therapy.[56] A decrease in myocardial contractility has also been documented, with an average 30% to 40% reduction in the mean left ventricular stroke work index.[29,31,34,56,57] Hypotension is common and is often severe enough to require vasopressor therapy. Besana,[33] Rosenberg,[42] and others have reported that as many as 50% of patients receiving IL-2 had hypotension that required pressor support. Hypotension is multifactorial and can result from decreased intravascular volume secondary to the capillary leak syndrome, decreased peripheral resistance, or depressed cardiac contractility.

Arrhythmias

Cardiac arrhythmias have been reported in 9% to 21% of patients undergoing IL-2 therapy,[30,31,33] and in 6% to 13.9% of treatment courses.[27,29,31] The majority of arrhythmias are atrial in origin, including supraventricular tachycardia and atrial fibrillation. These tachyarrhythmias respond to conventional drug therapy (e.g., verapamil, digoxin) and, like the hemodynamic disturbances, resolve after discontinuation of IL-2. Some patients have had ventricular ectopy or ventricular tachycardia,[29,30] particularly in the setting of myocarditis or acute myocardial infarction.[31,34]

Unspecified bradycardia has been observed in two patients, both of whom responded to single doses of atropine.[27] Three cases of high-grade atrio-ventricular block have been reported.[31,33,58] One of these patients, who had a history of supraventricular tachycardia, required insertion of a permanent pacemaker.[58]

Several possible mechanisms may give rise to the arrhythmias. The proarrhythmic effect of IL-2 may be related to its action on human cardiac sodium channels. A recent study showed that recombinant IL-2 acts like a class I antiarrhythmic drug by inhibiting sodium currents in human myocytes.[59] Pressor agents used to treat the hypotension that accompanies the capillary leak syndrome may account for some of the arrhythmias.[54]

Myocarditis/Cardiomyopathy

Myocarditis has been reported in patients receiving IL-2. Endomyocardial biopsies or postmortem studies have demonstrated both lymphocytic and eosinophilic myocarditis, which supports a drug-related etiology.[26,36–38] In other studies, the diagnosis of myocarditis was based on echocardiographic evidence of myocardial dysfunction[25,40,41] or on cardiac enzyme elevation in the absence of angiographic evidence of coronary artery disease.[29,31,35]

The mechanism by which IL-2 causes myocyte inflammation is unclear. It has been suggested that IL-2 causes a de novo antimyocyte immune response that is part of a systemic immunologic activation,[36] or that IL-2 exacerbates clinically unsuspected myocarditis. Direct myocardial toxicity is less likely, as IL-2 receptors have not been isolated on human myocytes. However, IL-2 may stimulate cytokines or some other substance that acts as a myocardial depressant.[54,60]

Ischemic Heart Disease

Myocardial infarction was first reported in 4 of 157 patients receiving IL-2 for cancer, and it proved fatal in two patients.[27] Most large studies report an incidence of between 1% and 4%,[29,30] although 30% (3 of 10) of patients in one study had this complication.[34] It has been postulated that the profound hypotension associated with IL-2 precipitates myocardial ischemia and infarction in patients at risk. However, myocardial infarction has occurred even in the absence of preexisting atherosclerotic heart disease or coronary artery disease risk factors.[61]

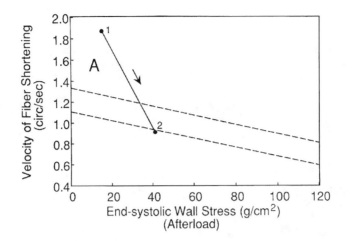

Figure 23-1.   Autonomic imbalance with high-grade ventricular ectopy in an 18-year-old hemophiliac with AIDS. Point 1 on part A illustrates enhanced contractility and reduced afterload with hyperdynamic LV function. Eight months after noting enhanced LV contractility with reduced afterload (point 1), the patient's ventricular function had dramatically fallen (point 2).

Sudden Death

There have been several reports of sudden death in patients on IL-2 therapy, which may have been related to the use of flecainide in one patient, who had a past history of supraventricular tachycardia,[26] and to myocarditis in the others.[62–64]

IL-2 in Pediatric Patients

Few studies have been published on the safety of IL-2 in children.[65,66] Most of the reported cardiac adverse effects were similar to those seen in adults, that is, hypotension and the capillary leak syndrome.[66–69] Only one death from cardiotoxicity has been reported.[70]

Antibiotics

Pentamidine

Pentamidine isethionate is commonly used to treat *Pneumocystis carinii* pneumonia in AIDS patients who fail to respond or develop adverse reactions to trimethoprim–sulfamethoxazole. It is also used as *P. carinii* pneumonia prophylaxis in HIV-positive patients with CD4+ lymphocyte counts <200 cells/mm^3 (0.2×10^9 cells per liter). Pentamidine may be administered intravenously, intramuscularly, or in an aerosolized form. Cardiac side

effects that have been reported with parenteral administration of pentamidine include hypotension, electrocardiographic (EKG) abnormalities, arrhythmias, and cardiac arrest. There have been no reports of cardiac toxicity in patients receiving aerosolized pentamidine.

Pentamidine has been associated with hypotension, tachycardia, cutaneous flushing, nausea, and vomiting.[71,72] It is unclear whether this is secondary to autonomic vasodilation or drug-induced histamine release.[73] We have reported a patient with intravenous pentamidine associated QTc prolongation who developed torsades de pointes. On further testing of that patient's cardiac autonomic system we determined that that patient had significant autonomic imbalance which may have contributed to the response to pentamidine (Figures 23-1 and 23-2).

Many case reports have documented prolongation of the QT interval in adult patients receiving pentamidine, which occasionally results in ventricular tachycardia[74,75] and torsades de pointes.[76–78] Although hypomagnesemia and hypokalemia may have predisposed some of these patients to the development of torsades de pointes,[79,80] the arrhythmia has also occurred when these electrolytes were normal.[73,75] Three studies have reported on the incidence of QT prolongation and ventricular arrhythmias in patients receiving intravenous pentamidine

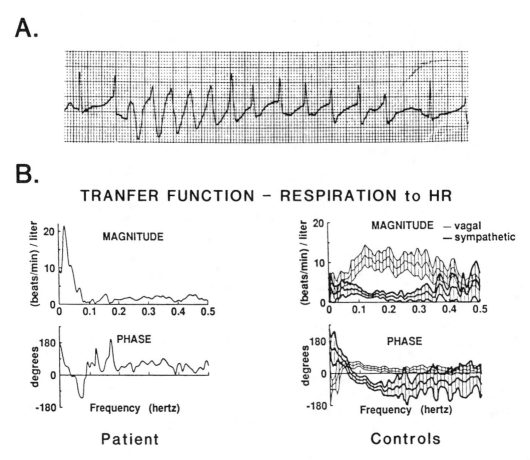

Figure 23-2. High-grade ventricular ectopy and autonomic imbalance in the same 18-year-old hemophiliac with AIDS described in Figure 23-1. **A**: A markedly prolonged QTc interval and torsades-de-pointes were noted while pentamidine isethionate was administered for *Pneumocystis carinii* at point 1, Figure 23-1. **B**: (*Patient*): Transfer function analysis of autonomic regulation at point 1, Figure 23-1 demonstrated virtually absent cardiac vagal activity and increased cardiac sympathetic activity in this patient. (*Controls*): This pattern was remarkably similar to the pure sympathetic activity in the group of normals treated with high doses of atropine. These results are consistent with inappropriate sympathetic activation and an appropriate vagal response, or abnormal central baroreflex sensitivity, and support the idea that the hyperdynamic LV function and QTc prolongation are related to increased cardiac sympathetic efferent activity. (Dr. J. Philip Saul and Dr. Edward Walsh were also involved in this work.)

for *P. carinii* pneumonia. In one study, 5 of 12 patients developed prolongation of the rate-corrected QT (QTc) interval.[81] In another study, 10 of 32 patients developed QTc prolongation (defined as QTc > 480 ms) despite intensive monitoring and correction of electrolyte abnormalities.[82] Two of these patients were found to have asymptomatic ventricular ectopy on screening ECGs. All cases of QTc prolongation developed within the first two weeks of therapy, and a significantly higher proportion of these patients had hypokalemia than those who did not have ECG abnormalities. A more recent study found that 5 of 14 patients receiving intravenous pentamidine developed QTc prolongation within 4 days of starting treatment.[83] Three of these patients (60%) developed torsades de pointes, which proved fatal in one case. None of these patients had significantly lowered serum potassium or magnesium levels.

Several reports have also documented cardiac arrest following pentamidine therapy for *P. carinii* pneumonia, both in adults[84] and in children.[85–87]

Wharton et al.[79] have suggested that the proarrhythmic effect of pentamidine may be related to its structural similarity to class Ia antiarrhythmic agents such as procainamide and phenylamine, both of which can induce torsades de pointes. Other proposed mechanisms include pentamidine-induced electrolyte abnormalities and HIV-mediated myocarditis.[83,85]

All patients receiving intravenous pentamidine should be monitored with serial ECGs, and the drug should be withheld if the QTc increases to above 480 ms or by more than 8 ms above baseline.[83] Potassium and magnesium levels should be closely followed and corrected where indicated. If a patient develops a ventricular arrhythmia during pentamidine treatment, the class Ia antiarrhythmics should be avoided.[88] Lidocaine has been used with success,[76] and bolus magnesium sulfate injections,[89] rapid overdrive pacing, or isoproterenol infusion may also be used.

Erythromycin

Erythromycin has been documented to cause arrhythmias and hypotension. Two recent reviews of the literature revealed 15 cases of erythromycin-induced torsades de pointes,[90,91] one of which resulted in the death of an 8-day-old neonate.[92] There has also been one report of ventricular tachycardia without QT prolongation.[93] The majority of cases were related to intravenous administration of erythromycin.[94–99] However, in one case, ventricular tachycardia occurred following oral administration of the drug.[100]

The proarrhythmic effect of erythromycin is thought to be a result of alteration of ion fluxes in the myocardium. Nattel and associates[101] showed that erythromycin prolonged the duration of the action potential in a canine model in a fashion similar to the fast sodium-channel blocking properties of the class IA antiarrhythmic drugs. In a more recent study, erythromycin induced phase 2 and 3 early-after depolarizations, suggesting a blockade of delayed rectifier potassium channels.[102] Further evidence of this has been provided in recently published work which showed that erythromycin blocks HERG (human ether-a-go-go related gene) and/or Kv1.5 potassium channels.[103]

Erythromycin-associated hypotension has been described in isolated case reports[104] and is thought to be related to histamine release.[105] In one instance, recurrent nodal bradycardia was also documented.[106]

Patients with idiopathic or acquired long QT syndromes are at higher risk of developing ventricular arrhythmias when given erythromycin. If possible, another antibiotic should be substituted, and if erythromycin has to be used, these patients should be carefully monitored during the infusion. Drug interactions with other arrhythmogenic drugs such as disopyramide and terfenadine may precipitate fatal arrhythmias, and their concomitant use should be avoided.[107,108]

Trimethoprim–Sulfamethoxazole

Trimethoprim–sulfamethoxazole is frequently used to treat or prevent bacterial and opportunistic infections in HIV-infected patients; the incidence of adverse reactions to trimethoprim–sulfamethoxazole appears to be higher in this group of patients than in those without HIV infection.[109,110] Drug hypersensitivity reactions resulting in cutaneous, hepatic, and hematologic abnormalities are common, but hemodynamic disturbances have also been noted.[109] Rare, severe, life-threatening reactions requiring cardiopulmonary resuscitation after administration of trimethoprim–sulfamethoxazole have been reported in both adults[111] and children.[112,113] Chanock and colleagues[113] described two HIV-infected children with life-threatening reactions after rechallenge with trimethoprim–sulfamethoxazole. Both children had evidence of cardiac abnormalities, suggesting a hyperadrenergic state before receiving the medication, and also had had a cutaneous reaction to this medication in the recent past.

Other Drugs

Amphotericin B has been documented to cause cardiac arrhythmias, hypertension, and cardiac arrest if infused too rapidly (<1 hour).[114]

Antiviral agents, such as foscarnet and ganciclovir, which are used to treat cytomegalovirus infection in HIV-infected patients, have cardiovascular side effects. There has been one case report of reversible cardiac failure associated with foscarnet therapy for cytomegalovirus esophagitis in a patient with AIDS.[115] Ganciclovir has been associated with ventricular tachycardia in adults with HIV infection and hypotension.[116,117]

Systemic corticosteroids have been shown to cause ventricular hypertrophy and abnormalities in left ventricular filling.[118,119] Doxorubicin, used for the treatment of AIDS-related Kaposi's sarcoma and malignant lymphomas, is well-known for causing cardiomyopathy and irreversible cardiac failure.[120–122]

Table 23-1 gives an overview of the important

Table 23-1. Cardiovascular Complications of Nonantiretroviral Pharmacotherapeutic Agents in Pediatric HIV Infection

Type of Drug (Ref.)	Primary Indication	Cardiac Side Effects
Antibiotics		
Erythromycin (90–108)	Bacterial and opportunistic infections	Hypotension
		Ventricular tachycardia/ torsades, bradycardia
Pentamidine (71–89)	*Pneumocystis carinii* pneumonia prophylaxis or treatment	Hypotension
		Prolonged QTc/torsades
		Cardiac arrest
Trimethoprim–sulfamethoxazole (109–113)	*P. carinii* pneumonia prophylaxis or treatment	Cardiac arrest/anaphylaxis
Antifungals		
Amphotericin B (114)	Disseminated fungal infections	Hypertension
		Arrhythmia/cardiac arrest
Antivirals		
Acyclovir	Inhibits herpes simplex virus/zoster	Unknown
Foscarnet (115)	Cytomegalovirus retinitis/other cytomegalovirus infections	Reversible cardiac failure
		Electrolyte abnormalities
Ganciclovir (116,117)	Cytomegalovirus infections	Ventricular tachycardia
		Hypotension
Ribavarin	Respiratory syncytial virus pneumonia (inhibits viral replication)	Unknown
Immunotherapy/biological response modifiers		
Immunoglobulin (123)	Infection prophylaxis	Anaphylactic reactions
	Myocarditis treatment	
Interferon-alfa (1–26)	Kaposi's sarcoma	Arrhythmia
		Myocardial infarction
		Cardiomyopathy
Interleukin-2 (27–70)	Activates T lymphocytes with zidovudine	Capillary leak/hypotension
		Arrhythmia/sudden death
		Myocardial infarction
		Myocarditis/cardiomyopathy
Other therapeutic agents		
Systemic corticosteroids (118,119)	Immunosuppression of viral damage	Ventricular hypertrophy/dysfunction
Doxorubicin (120–122)	Kaposi's sarcoma	Cardiac failure
	AIDS-related lymphoma	
Growth hormone (124,125)	Failure to thrive/wasting syndrome	Ventricular hypertrophy/dysfunction hypertension
		Activation of renin–angiotensin system
		Decreased low-density lipoproteins
Gene therapy (theoretical)	Inhibit viral replication	Unknown
	Enhance zidovudine efficacy	
	Block HIV receptor proteins	
HIV vaccines (theoretical)	Treatment and prevention of HIV infection	Anaphylaxis to vaccine components
Pentoxifylline (126,127)	Blocks tumor necrosis factor production	Decreases triglycerides

cardiovascular toxicities associated with therapeutic agents used in AIDS.

References

1. Jones GJ, Itri MI. Safety and tolerance of recombinant interferon alfa-2a (Roferon-A) in cancer patients. *Cancer* 1986;57:1709–1715.

2. Gauci L. Management of cancer patients receiving interferon alfa-2a. *Int J Cancer* 1987;(Supp)1: 21–30.

3. Quesada JR, Talpaz M, Rios A, et al. Clinical toxicity of interferons in cancer patients: a review. *J Clin Oncol* 1986;4:234–243.

4. Spiegel RJ. The alpha interferons: clinical overview. *Semin Oncol* 1987;14:1–12.

5. Mattson K, Niiranen A, Pyrhonen S, et al. Recombinant interferon gamma treatment in non-small cell lung cancer: antitumor effect and cardiotoxicity. *Acta Oncol* 1991;30:607–610.

6. Vial T, Descotes J. Clinical toxicity of the interferons. *Drug Safety* 1994;10:115–150.

7. Mansat-Kryzanowska E, Dreno B, Chiffoleau A, Litoux P. Manifestations cardiovasculaires associées à l'interfron α-2a. *Ann Med Int* 1991;142: 576–581.

8. Sonnenblick M, Rosin A. Cardiotoxicity of interferon: a review of 44 cases. *Chest* 1991;99: 557–561.

9. Martino S, Ratanatharathorn V, Karanes C, et al. Reversible arrhythmias observed in patients treated with recombinant alpha-2 interferon. *J Cancer Res Clin Oncol* 1987;113:376–378.

10. Grunberg SM, Kempf RA, Itri LM, et al. Phase II study of recombinant alpha interferon in the treatment of advanced non-small cell lung carcinoma. *Cancer Treat Rep* 1985;69:1031–1032.

11. Budd GT, Bukowski RM, Miketo L, et al. Phase I trial of ultrapure human leukocyte interferon in human malignancy. *Cancer Chemother Pharmacol* 1984;12:39–42.

12. Vadhan-Raj S, Al-Katib A, Bhalla R, et al. Phase I trial of recombinant interferon gamma in cancer patients. *J Clin Oncol* 1986;4:137–146.

13. Lee KH, Gutterman JU, Alil MK, Talpaz M. Cardiac arrhythmia in a CML patient treated with interferons. *Tex Med* 1989;4:36–38.

14. Dickson D. Death halts interferon trials in France. *Science* 1982;218:772.

15. Cohen MC, Huberman MS, Nesto RW. Recombinant alpha-2 interferon related cardiomyopathy. *Am J Med* 1988;85:549–550.

16. Zimmerman S, Adkins D, Graham M, et al. Irreversible severe congestive cardiomyopathy occurring in association with interferon alpha therapy. *Cancer Biother* 1994;9:291–299.

17. Simone G, Iaffaioli VR, La Mura G, et al. Reversible heart failure in a non-Hodgkin lymphoma patient being treated with alpha-interferon. *Curr Ther Res* 1988;44:78–85.

18. Deyton LR, Walker RE, Kovacs JA, et al. Reversible cardiac dysfunction associated with interferon alfa therapy in AIDS patients with Kaposi's sarcoma. *N Engl J Med* 1989;321:1246–1249.

19. Sonnenblick M, Rosenmann D, Rosin A. Reversible cardiomyopathy induced by interferon. *BMJ* 1990;300:1174–1175.

20. Guillot P, Barbuat C, Richard B, Jourdan J. Myocardiopathie reversible induite par l'interferon. *Therapie* 1993;48:65–66.

21. Sartori M, Andorno S, La Terra G, et al. Assessment of interferon cardiotoxicity with quantitative radionuclide angiocardiography. *Eur J Clin Invest* 1995;25:68–70.

22. Zbinden G. Effects of recombinant human alpha-interferon on a rodent cardiotoxicity model. *Toxicol Lett* 1990;50:25–35.

23. Lampidis TJ, Brouty-Boye D. Interferon inhibits cardiac function in vitro (41043). *Proc Soc Exp Biol Med* 1981;166:181–185.

24. Dorr RT, Shipp NG. Effect of interferon, interleukin-2 and tumour necrosis factor on myocardial cell viability and doxorubicin cardiotoxicity in vitro. *Immunopharmacology* 1989;18:31–38.

25. Azar JJ, Theriault RL. Acute cardiomyopathy as a consequence of treatment with interleukin-2 and interferon-α in a patient with metastatic carcinoma of the breast. *Am J Clin Oncol* 1991;14:530–533.

26. Kruit WH, Punt KJ, Goey SH, et al. Cardiotoxicity as a dose-limiting factor in a schedule of high dose bolus therapy with interleukin-2 and alpha-interferon: an unexpectedly frequent complication. *Cancer* 1994;74:2850–2856.

27. Rosenberg SA, Lotze MT, Muul LM, et al. A progress report on the treatment of 157 patients with advanced cancer using lymphokine-activated

killer cells and interleukin-2 or high-dose interleukin-2 alone. *N Engl J Med* 1987;316:889–897.

28. Isner JM, Dietz WA. Cardiovascular consequences of recombinant DNA technology: interleukin-2. *Ann Intern Med* 1988;109:933–935.

29. Lee RE, Lotze MT, Skibber JM, et al. Cardiorespiratory effects of immunotherapy with interleukin-2. *J Clin Oncol* 1989;7:7–20.

30. Margolin KA, Rayner AA, Hawkins MJ, et al. Interleukin-2 and lymphokine-activated killer cell therapy of solid tumors: analysis of toxicity and management guidelines. *J Clin Oncol* 1989;7: 486–498.

31. White RL, Schwartzentruber DJ, Guleria A, et al. Cardiopulmonary toxicity of treatment with high dose interleukin-2 in 199 consecutive patients with metastatic melanoma or renal cell carcinoma. *Cancer* 1994;74:3212–22.

32. Vial T, Descotes J. Clinical toxicity of interleukin-2. *Drug Safety* 1992;7:417–433.

33. Besana C, Borri A, Bucci E, et al. Treatment of advanced renal cell cancer with sequential intravenous recombinant interleukin-2 and subcutaneous α-interferon. *Eur J Cancer* 1994;30A:1292–1298.

34. Nora R, Abrams JS, Tait NS, et al. Myocardial toxic effects during recombinant interleukin-2 therapy. *J Natl Cancer Inst* 1989;81:59–63.

35. Osanto S, Cluitmans FHM, Franks CR, et al. Myocardial injury after interleukin-2 therapy. *Lancet* 1988;2:48–49.

36. Samlowski WE, Ward JH, Craven CM, Freedman RA. Severe myocarditis following high dose interleukin-2 administration. *Arch Pathol* 1989;113: 838–841.

37. Schuchter LM, Hendricks CB, Holland KH, et al. Eosinophilic myocarditis associated with high dose interleukin-2 therapy. *Am J Med* 1990; 88:439–440.

38. Kragel AH, Travis WD, Steis RG, et al. Myocarditis or acute myocardial infarction associated with interleukin-2 therapy for cancer. *Cancer* 1990;66: 1513–1516.

39. Beck AC, Ward JH, Hammond EH, et al. Cardiomyopathy associated with high-dose interleukin-2 therapy. *West J Med* 1991;155:293–296.

40. Goel M, Flaherty L, Lavine S, Redman BG. Reversible cardiomyopathy after high-dose interleukin-2 therapy. *J Immunother* 1992;11:225–229.

41. Du Bois JS, Udelson JE, Atkins MB. Severe reversible global and regional ventricular dysfunc-tion associated with high-dose interleukin-2 immunotherapy. *J Immunother* 1995;18:119–123.

42. Rosenberg SA, Lotze MT, Yang JC, et al. Experience with the use of high-dose interleukin-2 in the treatment of 652 cancer patients. *Ann Surg* 1989;210:474–484.

43. Eberlein TJ, Schoof DD, Jung SE, et al. A new regimen of interleukin-2 and lymphokine-activated killer cells: efficacy without significant toxicity. *Arch Intern Med* 1988;148:2571–2576.

44. Smith KA. Lowest dose interleukin-2 immunotherapy. *Blood* 1993;81:1414–1423.

45. Mertelsmann R, Welte K, Sternberg C, et al. Treatment of immunodeficiency with interleukin-2: initial exploration. *J Biol Res Modifiers* 1984;4:483.

46. Lane HC, Siegel JP, Rook AH, et al. Use of interleukin-2 in patients with acquired immunodeficiency syndrome. *J Biol Res Modifiers* 1984; 3:512.

47. Schwartz DH, Skowron G, Merigan TC. Safety and effects of interleukin-2 plus zidovudine in asymptomatic individuals infected with human immunodeficiency virus. *J Acquir Immune Defic Syndr* 1991;4:11–23.

48. Teppler H, Kaplan G, Smith K, et al. Efficacy of low-doses of the polyethylene glycol derivative of interleukin-2 in modulating the immune response of patients with human immunodeficiency virus type 1 infection. *J Infect Dis* 1993;167: 291–298.

49. Kovacs, JA, Vogel S, Albert JM, et al. Controlled trial of interleukin-2 infusions in patients infected with the human immunodeficiency virus. *N Engl J Med* 1996;335:1350–1356.

50. Volberding P, Moody DJ, Beardslee D, et al. Therapy of acquired immune deficiency syndrome with recombinant interleukin-2. *AIDS Res Hum Retrov* 1987;3:115–124.

51. Wood R, Montoya JG, Kundu SK, et al. Safety and efficacy of polyethylene glycol-modified interleukin-2 and zidovudine in human immunodeficiency virus type 1 infection: a phase I/II study. *J Infect Dis* 1993;167:519–525.

52. Mazza P, Bocchia M, Tumietto F, et al. Recombinant interleukin-2 (rIL-2) in acquired immune deficiency syndrome (AIDS): preliminary report in patients with lymphoma associated with HIV infection. *Eur J Hematol* 1992;49:1–6.

53. Ettinghausen SE, Puri RK, Rosenberg SA. Increased vascular permeability in organs mediated

by the systemic administration of lynphokine-activated killer cells and recombinant interleukin-2 in mice. *J Natl Cancer Inst* 1988;80:177–187.

54. Siegel JP, Puri RK. Interleukin-2 toxicity. *J Clin Oncol* 1991;9:694–704.

55. Damle NK, Doyle LV. IL-2 activated human killer lymphocytes but not their secreted products mediate an increase in albumin flux across cultured endothelial monolayers : implications for vascular leak syndrome. *J Immunol* 1989;142:2660–2669.

56. Gaynor ER, Vitek L, Sticklin L, et al. The hemodynamic effects of treatment with interleukin-2 and lymphokine-activated killer cells. *Ann Intern Med* 1988;109:953–958.

57. Ognibene FP, Rosenberg SA, Lotze MT, et al. Interleukin-2 administration causes reversible hemodynamic changes and left ventricular dysfunction similar to those seen in septic shock. *Chest* 1988;94:750–754.

58. Vaitkus PT, Grossman D, Fox KR, et al. Complete heart block due to interleukin-2 therapy. *Am Heart J* 1990;119:978–980.

59. Proebstle T, Mitrovics M, Schneider M, Hombach V, Rudel R. Recombinant interleukin-2 acts like a class I antiarrhythmic drug on human cardiac sodium channels. *Pfluegers Arch* 1995;429:462–469.

60. Zhang J, Yu ZX, Hilbert SL, et al. Cardiotoxicity of human recombinant interleukin-2 in rats: a morphological study. *Circulation* 1993;87:1340–1353.

61. Kragel AH, Travis WD, Feinberg L, et al. Pathologic findings asssociated with interleukin-2-based immunotherapy for cancer: a postmortem study of 19 patients. *Hum Pathol* 1990;21:493–502.

62. Weiss GR, Margolin KA, Aronson FR, et al. A randomized phase II trial of continuous infusion interleukin-2 or bolus injection interleukin-2 plus lymphokine-activated killer cells for advanced renal cell carcinoma. *J Clin Oncol* 1992;10:275–281.

63. Sleijfer DT, Janssen RA, Buter J, et al. Phase II study of subcutaneous interleukin-2 in unselected patients with advanced renal cell cancer on an outpatient basis. *J Clin Oncol* 1992;10:1119–1123.

64. Shulman KL, Stadler WM, Vogelzang NJ. High-dose continuous intravenous infusion of interleukin-2 therapy for metatstatic renal cell carcinoma. *Urology* 1996;47:194–197.

65. Chien CH, Hsieh KH. Interleukin-2 immunotherapy in children. *Pediatrics* 1990;86:937–943.

66. Cochat P, Floret D, Bouffet E, et al. Renal effects of continuous infusion of recombinant interleukin-2 in children. *Pediatr Nephrol* 1991;5:33–37.

67. Pais RC, Abdel-Mageed A, Ghim TT, et al. Phase I study of recombinant interleukin-2 for pediatric malignacies: feasibility of outpatient therapy: a Pediatric Oncology Group Study. *J Immunother* 1992;12:138–146.

68. Roper M, Smith MA, Sondel PM, et al. A phase I study of interleukin-2 in children with cancer. *Am J Pediatr Hematol Oncol* 1992;14:305–311.

69. Ribeiro RC, Rill D, Roberson PK, et al. Continuous infusion of interleukin-2 in children with refractory malignancy. *Cancer* 1993;72:623–628.

70. Negrier S, Michon J, Floret D, et al. Interleukin-2 and lymphokine-activated killer cells in 15 children with advanced metastatic neuroblastoma. *J Clin Oncol* 1991;9:1363–1370.

71. Helmick CG, Green JK. Pentamidine associated hypotension and route of administration. *Ann Intern Med* 1985;103:480.

72. Cheung TW, Matta R, Neibart E, et al. Intramuscular pentamidine for the prevention of *Pneumocystis carinii* pneumonia in patients infected with human immunodeficiency virus. *Clin Infect Dis* 1993;16:22–25.

73. Bibler MR, Chou TC, Toltzis RJ, Wade PA. Recurrent ventricular tachycardia due to pentamidine-induced cardiotoxicity. *Chest* 1988;94:1303–1306.

74. Loescher T, Loeschke K, Niebel J. Severe ventricular arrhythmia during pentamidine treatment of AIDS-associated *Pneumocystis carinii* pneumonia. *Infection* 1987;15:455.

75. Pujol M, Carratala J, Mauri J, Viladrich PF. Ventricular tachycardia due to pentamidine isethionate. *Am J Med* 1988;84:980.

76. Stein KM, Haronian H, Mensah GA, et al. Ventricular tachycardia and torsades de pointes complicating pentamidine therapy of *Pneumocystis carinii* pneumonia in the acquired immunodeficiency syndrome. *Am J Cardiol* 1990;66:888–889.

77. Farquhar ZLA, Oliphant CM. Pentamidine-induced torsades de pointes. *Ann Pharmacother* 1994;28:282–283.

78. Cortese LM, Gasser RA Jr, Bjornson DC, et al. Prolonged recurrence of pentamidine-induced

torsades de pointes. *Ann Pharmacother* 1992;26: 1365–1369.

79. Wharton JM, Demopulos PA, Goldschlager N. Torsade de pointes during administration of pentamidine isethionate. *Am J Med* 1987;83:571–576.

80. Mitchell P, Dodek P, Lawson L, et al. Torsades de pointes during intravenous pentamidine isethionate therapy. *Can Med Assoc J* 1989;140: 173–174.

81. Thalhammer E, Arasteh K, Hess F, et al. Systemic pentamidine therapy induces QT-prolongation. [Abstract]. *Proc STD World Congress* 1992;3: B140.

82. Stein KM, Fenton C, Lehany AM, et al. Incidence of QT interval prolongation during pentamidine therapy of *Pneumocystis carinii* pneumonia. *Am J Cardiol* 1991;68:1091–1094.

83. Eisenhauer MD, Eliasson AH, Taylor AJ, et al. Incidence of cardiac arrhythmias during intravenous pentamidine therapy in HIV-infected patients. *Chest* 1994;105:389–394.

84. Balslev U, Berild D, Nielsen TL. Cardiac arrest following pentamidine isethionate treatment of *Pneumocystis carinii* pneumonia. *Scand J Infect Dis* 1992;24:111–112.

85. Lipshultz SE, Chanock S, Sanders SP, et al. Cardiovascular manifestations of human immunodeficiency virus infection in infants and children. *Am J Cardiol* 1989;63:1489–1497.

86. Harrel H, Scott WA, Szeinberg A, Barzilay Z. Pentamidine-induced torsades de pointes. *Pediatr Infect Dis J* 1993;12:692–694.

87. Miller HC. Cardiac arrest after intravenous pentamidine in an infant. *Pediatr Infect Dis J* 1993;12: 694–696.

88. Leenhardt A, Coumel P, Slama R. Torsades de pointes. *J Cardiovasc Electrophysiol* 1992;3: 281–292.

89. Tzivoni D, Banai S, Schuger C, et al. Treatment of torsade-de-pointes with magnesium sulfate. *Circulation* 1988;77:392–397.

90. Brandriss MW, Richardson WS, Barold SS. Erythromycin-induced QT prolongation and polymorphic ventricular tachycardia (torsades de pointes): case report and review. *Clin Infect Dis* 1994;18: 995–998.

91. Rezkalla MA, Pochop C. Erythromycin induced torsades de pointes: case report and review of the literature. *S D J Med* 1994;47:161–164.

92. Benoit A, Bodiou C, Villain E, et al. QT prolongation and circulatory arrest after an injection of erythromycin in a newborn infant. *Arch Fr Pediatr* 1991;48:39–41.

93. Chennareddy SB, Siddique M, Karim MY, Kudesia V. Erythromycin-induced polymorphous ventricular tachycardia with normal QT interval. *Am Heart J* 1996;132:691–694.

94. Guelon D, Bedock B, Chartier C, Habere J-P. QT prolongation and recurrent "torsades de pointes" during erythromycin lactobionate infusion. *Am J Cardiol* 1984;54:666.

95. McComb JM, Campbell NPS, Cleland J. Recurrent ventricular tachycardia associated with QT prolongation after mitral valve replacement and its association with intravenous administration of erythromycin. *Am J Cardiol* 1984;54:922–923.

96. Lindsay J, Smith MA, Light JA. Torsades de pointes associated with antimicrobial therapy for pneumonia. *Chest* 1990;98:222–223.

97. Schoenenberger RA, Haefeli WE, Weiss P, Ritz RF. Association of intravenous erythromycin and potentially fatal ventricular tachycardia with QT prolongation. *BMJ* 1990;300:1375–1376.

98. Haefeli WE, Schoenenberger RA, Weiss P, Ritz R. Possible risk of cardiac arrhythmia related to intravenous erythromycin. *Intens Care Med* 1992; 18:469–473.

99. Gitler B, Berger LS, Buffa SD. Torsades de pointes induced by erythromycin. *Chest* 1994;105: 368–372.

100. Freedman RA, Anderson KP, Green LS, Mason JW. Effect of erythromycin on ventricular arrhythmias and ventricular repolarization in idiopathic long QT syndrome. *Am J Cardiol* 1987;59: 168–169.

101. Nattel S, Ranger S, Talajic M, et al. Erythromycin induced long QT syndrome: concordance with quinidine and underlying cellular electrophysiologic mechanism. *Am J Med* 1990;89:235–238.

102. Rubart M, Pressler ML, Pride HP, Zipes DP. Electrophysiological mechanisms in a canine model of erythromycin-associated long QT syndrome. *Circulation* 1993;88:1832–1844.

103. Roy ML, Kiehn J, Dumaine R, Brown AM. Ketoconazole, erythromycin, and terfenadine block HERG currents, suggesting multiple mechanisms for cardiotoxicity. *Circulation* 1996;94(Suppl 1): 3753.

104. Dan M, Feigl D. Erythromycin-associated hypotension. *Pediatr Infect Dis J* 1993;12:692.

105. Keller RS, Parker JL, Adams HR. Cardiovascular toxicity of antibacterial antibiotics. In: Acosta D Jr (ed). *Cardiovascular Toxicology.* New York: Lippincott-Raven, 1992:165–195.

106. Fichtenbaum CJ, Babb JD, Baker DA. Erythromycin-induced cardiovascular toxicity. *Conn Med* 1988;52:135–136.

107. Honig PK, Woosley RL, Zamani K, et al. Changes in the pharmacokinetics and electrocardiographic pharmacodynamics of terfenadine with concomitant administration of erythromycin. *Clin Pharmacol Ther* 1992;52:231–238.

108. Ragosta M, Weihl AC, Rosenfeld LE. Potentially fatal interaction between erythromycin and disopyramide. *Am J Med* 1989;86:464–466.

109. Bayard PJ, Berger TG, Jacobson MA. Drug hypersensitivity reactions and human immunodeficiency virus disease. *J Acquir Immune Defic Syndr* 1992;5:1237–1257.

110. Gordin FM, Simon GL, Wofsy CB, Mills J. Adverse reactions to trimethoprim–sulfamethoxazole in patients with the acquired immunodeficiency syndrome. *Ann Intern Med* 1984;100:495–499.

111. Kelly JW, Dooley DP, Lattuada CP, Smith CE. A severe, unusual reaction to trimethoprim–sulfamethoxazole in patients infected with human immunodeficiency virus. *Clin Infect Dis* 1992;14:1034–1039.

112. McSherry G, Wright M, Oleske J, et al. Frequency of serious adverse reactions to trimethoprim–sulfamethoxazole and pentamidine among children with human immunodeficiency virus 1 infection. [Abstract]. *Proc Int Conf Antimicrob Agents Chemother*, 1988;••:1357.

113. Chanock SJ, Luginbuhl LM, McIntosh K, Lipshultz SE. Life-threatening reaction to trimethoprim-sulfamethoxazole in pediatric human immunodeficiency virus infection. *Pediatrics* 1994;93:519–520.

114. Kinney EL, Monsuez JJ, Kitzis M, Vittecoq DE. Treatment of AIDS-assoiciated heart disease. *J Vasc Dis* 1989;40:970–976.

115. Brown DL, Sather S, Cheitlin MD. Reversible cardiac dysfunction associated with foscarnet therapy for cytomegalovirus esophagitis in an AIDS patient. *Am Heart J* 1993;125:1439–1441.

116. Cohen AJ, Weiser B, Afzal Q, Fuhrer J. Ventricular tachycardia in two patients with AIDS receiving ganciclovir (DHPG). *AIDS* 1990;4:807–809.

117. Faulds D, Heel RC. Ganciclovir: a review of its antiviral activity, pharmacokinetic properties and therapeutic efficacy in cytomegalovirus infections. *Drugs* 1990;39:597–638.

118. Werner JC, Sicard RE, Hansen TWR, et al. Hypertrophic cardiomyopathy associated with dexamethasone therapy for bronchopulmonary dysplasia. *J Pediatr* 1992;120:286–291.

119. Bensky AS, Kothadia JM, Covitz W. Cardiac effect of dexamethasone in very low birth weight infants. *Pediatrics* 1996;97:818–821.

120. Lipshultz SE, Colan SD, Gelber RD, et al. Late cardiac effects of doxorubicin therapy for acute lymphoblastic leukemia in childhood. *N Engl J Med* 1991;324:808–815.

121. Lipshultz SE, Lipsitz SR, Mone SM, et al. Female sex and drug dose as risk factors for late cardiotoxic effects of doxorubicin therapy for childhood cancer. *N Engl J Med* 1995;332:1738–1743.

122. Lipshultz SE. Dexrazoxane for protection against cardiotoxic effects of anthracyclines in children. *J Clin Oncol* 1996;14:328–331.

123. Lipshultz SE, Orav EJ, Sanders SP, Colan SD. Immunoglobulins and left ventricular structure and function in pediatric HIV infection. *Circulation* 1995;92:2220–2225.

124. Barton JS, Gardineri HM, Cullen SM, et al. The growth and cardiovascular effects of high dose growth hormone therapy in idiopathic short stature. *Clin Endocrinol* 1995;42:619–626.

125. Daubeney PE, McCaughey ES, Chase C, et al. Cardiac effects of growth hormone in short normal children: results after 4 years of treatment. *Arch Dis Child* 1995;72:337–339.

126. Ambrus JL, Lillie MA. Pentoxifylline in treatment of acquired immunodeficiency syndrome. *Blood* 1992;79:535–536.

127. Dezube BJ, Sherman ML, Fridovich-Keil JL, et al. Down-regulation of tumor necrosis factor expression by pentoxifylline in cancer patients: a pilot study. *Cancer Immunol Immunother* 1993;36:57–60.

24

Cardiovascular Monitoring of HIV-Infected Patients

L. Nandini Moorthy, M.B.B.S., and Steven E. Lipshultz, M.D.

This chapter establishes recommendations for the cardiovascular monitoring of patients with human immunodeficiency virus (HIV) infection. With longer survival[1-4] cardiovascular abnormalities become more advanced.[4-10] In order to develop a monitoring strategy, we first review types and frequencies of HIV-associated abnormalities in HIV-infected adults and children. We then discuss the risk factors and their correlation with noncardiac status and establish signs and symptoms associated with cardiovascular disease and factors that may be important for the detection of clinically inapparent symptomatic heart disease. Based on the types of heart disease, we offer suggestions on how to efficiently detect and treat the heart disease. Finally, we review data relating to treatment of cardiovascular disease in HIV-infected patients, since it appears that early detection and appropriate interventions can significantly improve the cardiovascular status of HIV-infected patients, thereby justifying cardiovascular monitoring.

Prevalence of HIV-Associated Cardiovascular Disease in Adults

Cardiovascular involvement in HIV-infected adults is uniformly found in studies throughout the world.[3,11,12-29] It is progressive and is frequently associated with significant morbidity and mortality. In one study, the annual incidence of symptomatic cardiovascular involvement in HIV-infected adults was found to be 6%.[30]

The cardiac abnormalities include pericardial effusions, biventricular dysfunction, segmental wall motion abnormalities, endocarditis, mitral valve prolapse, and cardiac masses. The most frequently observed cardiac abnormalities in patients with HIV infection are dilated cardiomyopathy, pericarditis, myocarditis, and endocarditis.[21,22,24,26,31]

Specific Cardiovascular Abnormalities in HIV-Infected Adults

Heart Muscle Disease

Heart muscle disease is one of the most common abnormalities in patients with HIV infection.[3,6,32,33] It is often progressive and may lead to dilated cardiomyopathy, which is associated with adverse outcomes (Table 24-1). It may be caused by many factors, such as myocarditis and chronic lung disease. In this section, we will discuss ventricular dysfunction and myocarditis.

Table 24-1. Longitudinal Prospective Studies of Cardiovascular Involvement of HIV-Infected Adults

Study (Ref.)	Patients	Cardiac Abnormalities Before Follow-up	Subsequent Echocardiogram	Follow-up Period	Cardiac Abnormalities After Follow-up	Major Finding
Hsia et al., Washington DC, 1993 (30)	343 HIV+	Echocardiographic abnormalities 19% (66/343) Cardiomyopathy 9.3% (32/343) Pericardial effusion 4.4% (15/343) Diastolic dysfunction 0.8% (3/343) Left ventricular dilatation 4.4% (15/343) Right ventricular dilatation 0.3% (1/343)	235	560 patient-yr	Echocardiographic abnormalities 24% (57/235) Congestive heart failure symptoms 6% (14/235) Pericardial effusion requiring drainage 3.4% (8/235) Obstructive intracardiac mass 0.4% (1/235) Ventricular tachycardia symptoms 0.4% (1/235) Aborted sudden death 1.3% (3/235)	Clinically significant heart disease developed in 11% of HIV+ patients over 21 months; incidence of clinically important heart disease is 6% per year
Herskowitz et al., Baltimore, 1993 (34)	69 HIV+ (no clinically suspected heart disease)	Echocardiographic abnormalities 14.5% (10/69) Left ventricular hypokinesis 14.5% (10/69) Normal echocardiograms 86% (59/69)	69	18 mo	Congestive heart failure symptoms 5.8% (4/69) New global left ventricular dysfunction 18% (11/59)	Prevalence of global left ventricular hypokinesia = 14.5% Incidence of global left ventricular hypokinesia = 18%/year
Herskowitz et al., Baltimore, 1993 (34)	N = 39 (of 1,819 HIV+ patients referred to cardiomyopathy service)	Echocardiographic abnormalities 100% (39/39) All had left ventricular dysfunction and symptomatic congestive heart failure				Crude rate of global ventricular dysfunction = 2.1%

Reference	Subjects	Findings	Duration	Clinical manifestations	Results
Currie et al., Scotland, 1994 (6)	296 (10 HIV+, 100 AIDS, 134 HIV+ with symptoms) (A contempory classification was not available for 52 subjects)	Echocardiographic abnormalities 15% (44/296) Dilated cardiomyopathy 4.4% (13/296) Isolated right ventricular dysfunction 4% (12/296) Borderline left ventricular dysfunction 19% (19/296)	4 yr	*Clinical manifestations of heart failure were found in:* 69% (9/13) patients with dilated cardiomyopathy 37% (7/19) patients with borderline left ventricular dysfunction 50% (6/12) patients with isolated right ventricular dysfunction *Mortality in:* 92% (12/13) patients with dilated cardiomyopathy 42% (5/12) patients with isolated right ventricular dysfunction 42% (8/19) patients with borderline left ventricular dysfunction	Prevalence of heart muscle disease = 15% Decrease in the survival of patients with dilated cardiomyopathy Survival significantly decreased with cardiac findings ($P < .001$)
Himelman et al., California, 1989 (49)	6 AIDS		7 yr	6 of 1200 patients (longitudinally followed) developed pulmonary hypertension	Incidence of pulmonary hypertension = 0.5%
Heidenreich et al., California, 1995 (57)	231 (59 asymptomatic HIV+, 62 ARC, 74 AIDS, 21 HIV-negative healthy homosexual men, 15 non-HIV end-stage medical illness)	Effusions present on the subjects' first echocardiograms as AIDS subjects 7% (5/74)	Recruited over a 5 yr period	Total echocardiograms performed = 601 Developed an effusion after an initial negative echocardiogram as AIDS subjects = 8	Prevalence of pericardial effusion = 5% Incidence of pericardial effusion in surviving AIDS subjects = 11%/ year over a 2-year period

Left Ventricular
and Biventricular Dysfunction

Left ventricular dysfunction is widely prevalent[3,11,12,15,21,25,31,34-42] and consistently progressive (Tables 24-1 and 24-2). Its associated risk factors and pathophysiology are discussed in other chapters of the book.

Cardiac dysfunction occurs in homosexual men,[3,11] intravenous drug users,[12,39,40] women,[43] and children,[37,38,42] the major risk groups for HIV infection. In HIV-positive patients, the prevalence of left ventricular dysfunction is estimated to vary from 2% to over 40%,[6,8,12,15,18,25,34,44] with clinically significant heart failure in 6% of patients,[34] most of whom have end-stage acquired immunodeficiency syndrome (AIDS).[3,13,15,34]

Dilated cardiomyopathy is now recognized as an important HIV-related cardiac complication in the Western world.[6,15,18,34,45,46] Severe left ventricular global hypokinesis along with congestive heart failure is the most frequent presentation of symptomatic HIV-associated heart disease.[1] Clinically evident signs and symptoms of decreased cardiac output are often attributed to AIDS.[1] Coughing and breathlessness with diffuse pulmonary rales are assumed to be due to *Pneumocystis carinii* pneumonia or some other opportunistic pulmonary infection.[3]

Decreased left ventricular fractional shortening percentage, owing to decreased contractility is the most common sign of cardiac dysfunction. The progressive deterioration of left ventricular function is characterized by left ventricular wall thinning and dilatation until finally the left ventricle assumes a globular shape. It is often accompanied by pericardial effusion.[47]

Myocarditis

Myocarditis is seen in 5.5% to 53% of HIV-infected patients[15,18,21,22,24,26,31,36,48] who have had autopsies and is frequently associated with ventricular dysfunction and arrhythmias (Table 24-3).[21,26,48] The most common cause is infection, but there are numerous other causes. Myocarditis may occur as a self-limited brief episode[40] or may be chronic.

Right Ventricular Dysfunction

Right ventricular dysfunction is one of the most frequently found cardiac complications[11,25,39,40,49] in HIV-infected patients (Tables 24-1 and 24-2). It may occur as an isolated process or as a part of biventricular dysfunction and four-chamber dilatation.[35,36,38]

Isolated right ventricular dysfunction may result from changes in the pulmonary circulation or primary myocardial pathology,[11,49-51] as discussed in the chapter devoted exclusively to this topic and is not consistently associated with clinically severe primary myocardial disease.[11] If present, it may lead to recurrent pulmonary emboli that may be fatal.[11,31]

A longitudinal study (Table 24-1) estimated the incidence of pulmonary hypertension and cor pulmonale to be 0.5% in HIV-infected patients.[49] Pulmonary hypertension was echocardiographically detected in 13% of hospitalized HIV-infected African-Americans.[52] Some studies[11,40] have suggested that right ventricular dilatation is reversible after a follow-up period.

Pericardial Effusion

Pericardial effusion occurs in 4.3% to 53% of HIV-infected adults (Tables 24-1 to 24-4).[6,28] AIDS is an important cause of large, clinically significant pericardial effusions.[53] Mycobacterial pericarditis, which often occurs during the early stages of HIV infection, may be considered an index condition of AIDS in Africa.[54,55]

Pericardial effusion is seen more often in patients with AIDS than in patients with AIDS-related complex or in asymptomatic HIV-positive patients (Table 24-4).[28,56] Pericardial effusion occurs more often in patients with end-stage AIDS. Most effusions are small and asymptomatic; they usually do not get larger but are adversely associated with survival.[57] A 5% prevalence of pericardial effusion was found among 99 HIV-positive patients on their first echocardiogram and a 7% prevalence in patients with end-stage AIDS.[57] The incidence of pericardial effusion in surviving AIDS patients was 11% per year over a 2-year period (Table 24-1). No effusions were found in healthy HIV-negative patients.[57] Development of an effusion serves as a marker for undiagnosed opportunistic infections and are sometimes indicative of a patient's function of the immune status. Significantly reduced CD4+ lymphocyte counts[11,13,57] and albumin levels,[58] both

Table 24-2. Prospective Studies of Cardiovascular Involvement in HIV-Infected Adults

Study (Ref.)	N	Patients	Abnormal Echocardiogram	Congestive Heart Failure	Pericardial Effusion	Cardiac Abnormalities
Corallo et al., Italy, 1988 (12)	102	100% AIDS 29 ± 7 yr 78% male 70% IVDA	54% (55/102)	17% (17/102)	38% (39/102) (9 large effusions)	Persistent tachycardia 54% (55/102) Sinus tachycardia 54% (55/102) S3 gallop 47% (48/102) Reduced left ventricular fractional shortening 54% (55/102) Increased left ventricular end-diastolic dimension, decreased left ventricular wall thickness, and left ventricular % fractional shortening 54% (55/102) Globular left ventricle with diffuse reduction of wall motion 41% (42/102) Valvular vegetations 3.9% (4/102): all IVDA Intracardiac mass 2.9% (3/102) Globular and poorly contracting left ventricle 18% (18/102)
Corallo et al., Italy, 1987 (47)	70	100% AIDS 29 yr 78% male	70% (49/70)		40% (28/70)	Globular and poorly contracting left ventricle 36% (25/70) On autopsy, globular heart, 4-chamber dilatation, and left ventricular thinning 67% (12/18) Cardiac abnormalities (left ventricular wall thickness, systolic thickening, and left ventricular fractional shortening reduction) 70% (49/70) Intracardiac mass 1% (1/70)
Fink et al., Pennsylvania 1984 (31)	15	100% AIDS 26–49 yr 93% male 20% IVDA	67% (10/15)		43% (6/14) On one patient, echocardiography was not performed, hence the denominator is 14.	Cardiac abnormalities 73% (by echocardiography or autopsy) Left ventricular hypokinesis 23% (3/13) Mitral valve prolapse with mitral regurgitation 17.7% (1/13) Dilated right ventricle 15% (2/13) Sudden death (cardiac tamponade) 13% (2/15)

Continued

Table 24-2. *Continued*

Study (Ref.)	N	Patients	Abnormal Echocardiogram	Congestive Heart Failure	Pericardial Effusion	Cardiac Abnormalities
Himelman et al., California, 1989 (3)	70	73% AIDS 37 yr 97% male 4% IVDA	22.8% (16/70)		10% [impending tamponade 1% (1/70)]	Dilated cardiomyopathy 11% (8/70) Abnormal echocardiogram in 25 hospitalized patients 64% (16/25) Mediastinal mass 1% (1/70) Abnormal echocardiogram in 45 ambulatory patients 7% (3/45) (only abnormality: mitral valve prolapse) (P < .001) Trend: more cardiac abnormalities in hospitalized patients (P < .0001)
Levy et al., Washington DC, 1988 (15)	60	58% AIDS 98% male Age information not available	35% (21/60)		15% (9/60)	Left ventricular dilatation 15% (9/60) Decreased left ventricular fractional shortening 15% (9/60)
DeCastro et al., Italy, 1992 (18)	114	63% AIDS 34.6 ± 5.4 yr 74% IVDA	65% (47/72) in AIDS patients		18% (13/72) in AIDS patients	Cardiac involvement in AIDS patients 65% (47/72) Dilated cardiomyopathy in AIDS patients 17% (12/72) Mitral valve prolapse in AIDS patients 4% (3/72) Myocarditis in AIDS patients 6% (4/72) Valvular bacterial endocarditis in AIDS patients 7% (5/72) Alterations of left ventricular regional contractility in AIDS patients 14% (10/72) Mortality during a mean-follow up of 44 months in AIDS patients 40% (includes 4 deaths due to cardiac events) Cardiac involvement in HIV-infected patients 46%

Reference	n	Characteristics				Findings
Jacob et al., Scotland, 1992 (40)	173	100% HIV+ 69% IVDA	54% (7/13 patients with dilated cardiomyopathy)	15% (26/173)		Abnormalities of ventricular size or function or both 15% (26/173) Dilated cardiomyopathy 8% (13/173) Left ventricular dilatation without loss of function 3% (6/173) Isolated right ventricular dilatation 4% (7/173) Borderline left ventricular dysfunction 2% (3/173)
Blanchard et al., California, 1991 (11)	70	63% AIDS 38.1 ± 9.3 yr 99% male		48% (33/70)	21% (15/70)	Any abnormality 49% (34/70) Mitral valve prolapse 10% (7/70) Excluding mitral valve prolapse 44% (31/70) Left ventricular dysfunction (ejection fraction <45%, fractional shortening <28%) 11% (8/70) Right-sided cardiac enlargement 24% (17/70)
Monseuz et al., USA and France, 1988 (29)	85	49% AIDS 91% Male 34% IVDA		5% (4/85)	Pericardial tamponade = 13% (11/85)	Arrhythmia = 3.5% (3/85) New murmur = 1.2% (1/85: due to Kaposi's sarcoma) Cryptococcal myocarditis = 2.3% (2/85) Toxoplasma myocarditis = 1.2% (1/85) Salmonella endocarditis = 1.2% (1/85) Cardiogenic deaths = 36%
Cardoso et al., Portugal, 1994 (28)	137	42% AIDS (118 HIV-1, 114 HIV-2, 1 both) 33 ± 10 yr 76% male 45% IVDA	7% (10/137)	76% (104/137), 25% (34/137) severe	43% (59/137)	Dilated cardiomyopathy 5% (7/137) Left ventricular hypokinesis 7% (9/137) Left ventricular segmental wall motion abnormalities 12% (17/137) Right ventricular dilatation 17% (23/137) Trend: HIV-1 worse than HIV-2

Continued

351

Table 24-2. *Continued*

Study (Ref.)	N	Patients	Abnormal Echocardiogram	Congestive Heart Failure	Pericardial Effusion	Cardiac Abnormalities
Steffen et al., Germany, 1990 (61)	92	36 yr 90% male 12% IVDA	13% (12/92)		13% (12/92)	Left ventricular dilatation 1% (1/92) Tumor compression 1% (1/92)
Sztajzel et al., Switzerland, 1993 (186)	23	31.7 ± 7.4 yr Asymptomatic HIV+ 8.7% IVDA 887% Male				Left ventricular dysfunction or enlargement 26% Disorder of right ventricular size or function 60%
Mota-Miranda, Portugal, 1992 (187)	30	14 AIDS 63% male 37 ± 88 yr		10% (3/30)		Left ventricular hypokinesis 13% (4/30)
Fong et al., Canada, 1993 (19)	101	71 AIDS, 30 pre-AIDS 24 healthy controls	HIV+ 29% (29/101) controls 12.5% (3/24). P < .003	Abnormal cardiac findings on physical exam 6% (6/101) vs. 0% (0/24) in controls	9% (9/102)	Any abnormality in HIV+ patients 41% (41/101) vs. controls 12.5% (3/24) P < .003 Left ventricular dysfunction 5% (5/102) Fractional shortening decrease 10% (10/102) Wall thickness increase 8% (8/102) Electrocardiologic abnormalities 11% (11/102) Clinical abnormalities 6% (6/102)
Raffanti et al., New York, 1988 (39)	12	100% AIDS				Echocardiographic, electrocardiographic, or ventriculographic abnormalities 75% (9/12) Significant ventricular dysfunction 42% (5/12)

Reitano et al., New York, 1984 (23)	25	84% AIDS 100% male 27–67 yr	48% (10/21) AIDS patients	33% (7/21) AIDS patients Required drainage 10% AIDS patients (2/21)	Prodrome patients ($n = 4$) had normal studies

In AIDS patients ($n = 21$):

Echocardiographic abnormalities
Total abnormal 48% (10/21)
Left ventricular end-diastolic dimension >65 mm 14% (3/21)
Fractional shortening <28%, 10% (2/21)
Right ventricular end-diastolic dimension > 25 mm 29% (6/21)

Electrocardiographic abnormalities
Total abnormal 19% (4/21)

Abnormal resting radionuclide angiogram
Total abnormal 67% (6/9)
Decreased right ventricular ejection fraction 44% (4/9)
Dilated right ventricle 22% (2/9)
Dilated left ventricle 11% (1/9)
Of 21 AIDS patients
Isolated right ventricular abnormality 33% (7/21)
Biventricular dysfunction 14% (3/21)

ARC, AIDS-related complex; IVDA, intravenous drug abuser.

Table 24-3. Retrospective Studies of Cardiovascular Involvement in HIV-Infected Adults

Study (Ref.)	Type	Patients	Findings
Lewis, California 1989 (25)	Autopsy study	$N = 115$ (111 AIDS 4 ARC) 38.3 ± 9.3 yr	*Cardiac findings = 51% (59/115)* Pericardial effusion 63% (37/59) Right ventricular hypertrophy 31% (18/59) Kaposi's sarcoma 12% (7/59) Nonbacterial thrombotic endocarditis 10% (6/59) Infiltrates 10% (6/59) Opportunistic infection 7% (4/59) Cardiomyopathy 3% (2/59) Abscess 2% (1/59)
Reynolds et al., New York 1991 (53)	Review of records of 50 patients undergoing pericardiocentesis	$N = 50$ undergoing pericardiocentesis AIDS in 28% (14/50)	Diagnostic pericardiocentesis in 21% (3/14) of AIDS patients In 57% (8/14), some evidence of tuberculosis
Reilly et al., Baltimore 1988 (48)	Review of autopsies	$N = 58$ AIDS	*Histological myocarditis = 45%* ≥1 clinical abnormality 58% (15/26) Ventricular tachycardia 15% (4/26) Electrocardiological abnormalities 38% (10/26) Pericardial abnormalities 15% (4/26) *No myocarditis = 55% (32/58)* Pericardial or electrocardiologic abnormalities or both = 19% (6/32) (No congestive cardiac failure or ventricular tachycardia or left ventricular dysfunction)
Petiperez et al., France, 1993 (225)		$N = 20$ HIV+ patients with pulmonary hypertension	Death in 80% (8/10) of HIV+ patients within 1 year of diagnosis of pulmonary hypertension

ARC, AIDS-related complex.

adverse predictors of survival, were found in patients with effusion (Table 24-5). When survival was controlled for these two factors, it was found that the development of pericardial effusion adversely affected survival.[57]

Most of the pericardial effusions found in HIV-infected adults are clinically occult and are detected incidentally by echocardiography.[1] The prevalence would be overestimated in hospitalized patients, as they more frequently get an echocardiographic examination for cardiac or pulmonary abnormalities.[2] Continued monitoring should be provided not only for hospitalized patients but also for ambulatory patients and outpatients.

No risk factors have been determined for the development of tamponade.[59] Tamponade due to symptomatic pericardial effusion is frequent in AIDS-infected patients.[1] The occurrence of pericardial effusion in association with global left ventricular dysfunction indicates the involvement of different layers of the heart.[1]

Endocarditis

Endocarditis is more common in adults than in children and in HIV-infected than in noninfected persons.[1] Further, the occurrence of infective endocarditis is correlated with intravenous drug abuse (Table 24-5).[1,18] Autopsy studies have suggested a 10% occurrence of endocarditis in HIV-positive patients.[2,8,21,22,24,25] The prevalence of valvular vegetations ranges from 4% to 19.3% (Tables 24-2 and 24-4).[12,18,31,60,61] It has been recognized as a potentially fatal complication in HIV-positive adults, adversely affecting survival.[1]

Rhythm Disturbances and Sudden Death

It has been estimated that more than one-fifth of cardiac disease-related deaths in HIV-positive patients are sudden deaths, caused by ventricular arrhythmia.[3]

Cardiac arrhythmias may be consequent to other cardiac pathology, autonomic dysfunction, or treat-

Table 24-4. Cardiovascular Abnormalities in HIV-Infected Adults: Correlation With Stage of HIV Infection

| Study (Ref.) | Factors Assessed | Stage of HIV Infection | | | P | |
		AS (%)	ARC (%)	AIDS (%)	AIDS vs AS	AIDS vs ARC
Cardoso et al., Portugal 1994 (28)	Cardiac symptoms	0	5.6	13.8	<.05	NS
	Abnormal echocardiogram	65	72.2	96	<.0005	<.005
	Severely abnormal echocardiogram	50	22.2	41.3	<.00005	<.05
	Left ventricular dilatation	10		31	<.05	
	Interventricular septum thickness (mm)	9 ± 1.2		9.9 ± 1.4	<.01	
	Left ventricular mass index (g/m^2)	117 ± 24		138 ± 32	<.01	
	Left ventricular fractional shortening	34 ± 5		31 ± 6	<.05	
	Ejection fraction	70 ± 8		62 ± 12	<.01	
	Right ventricular dilatation	5		25.8	<.05	
	Pericardial effusion	27.5		65.5	<.0005	
Blanchard et al., California, 1991 (11)	Any abnormality	40		52	*	
	Mitral valve prolapse	10		10	*	
	Excluding mitral valve prolapse as the sole abnormality	35		48	*	
	Left ventricular dysfunction (ejection fraction < 45%, fractional shortening < 28%)	5		14	*	
	Right heart enlargement	35		20	*	
	Pericardial effusion	220		22	*	
Monseuz et al., France, 1988 (29)	Any abnormality		4	12	*	
La Font et al., France, 1988 (60)	Normal echocardiogram	66	69	28	<.01	
	Cardiomyopathy (decreased shortening fraction with or without left ventricular dilatation)	8	4	30	*	
	Pericardial effusion	7	4	34	*	
	Endocarditis	25	23	10	*	
Kinney et al., Florida, 1989 (16)	Abnormal echocardiogram		>21	>47	*	
Levy et al., Washington, DC, 1988 (15)	Any abnormality	36		66	*	
	Abnormal echocardiogram	28		40	*	
	Increased left ventricular diastolic dimension/body surface area	12		17	<.05 compared to patients with pre-AIDS	
	Decreased left ventricular shortening fraction	8		20	*	
	Pericardial effusion	8		20	*	
	Abnormal electrocardiogram	28		53	*	
	Abnormal ambulatory electrocardiographic monitor	0		14	*	

Continued

Cardiology in AIDS

Table 24-4. *Continued*

Study (Ref.)	Factors Assessed	AS (%)	ARC (%)	AIDS (%)	AIDS vs AS	AIDS vs ARC
			Stage of HIV Infection		*P*	
Akhras et al., England, 1994 (226)	Normal echocardiogram	61		31	*	
	Pericardial effusion	9		44	*	
	Dilated cardiomyopathy (ejection fraction < 35%)	0		16	*	
	Left ventricular dysfunction (normal size, ejection fraction <35%)	0		4	*	
	Isolated right ventricular dilatation	4		4	*	
	Intracardiac echogenic masses	4		7	*	

AS, asymptomatic; ARC, AIDS-related complex; NS, not significant.
*No *P* values given.

ment modality. The association of untreatable ventricular tachycardia and sudden death in patients with myocarditis or congestive heart failure has been demonstrated by many studies.[15,31,62] Atrial and ventricular ectopics,[37] ventricular tachycardia,[15] and sudden death[48,62] have all been reported in patients with HIV-associated myocarditis or heart muscle disease (Tables 24-1 to 24-4).

Prolongation of the QT interval with hypomagnesemia, and torsades de pointes due to pentamidine isothionate for treatment of *P. carinii* pneumonia, are the most frequent drug-induced ventricular arrhythmias in HIV-positive patients.[3,9,63–67] Ganciclovir, a nucleoside employed in the treatment of cytomegalovirus infection, has been reported to cause rhythm abnormalities.[68]

It has been suggested that autonomic dysfunc-tion, a frequent condition in HIV-positive patients,[69] increases the risk of syncopal events and death.[70,71]

Vascular Disease

HIV-infected patients of all ages show evidence of vascular disease that manifests clinically as reduced microcirculatory perfusion.[72,73] Arteries in almost any part of the body may be affected by vasculitis. Stroke, coronary artery disease, vascular aneurysms, eosinophilic vasculitis, Kawasaki disease, and polyarteritis nodosa have been seen in young HIV-infected adults.[74–81]

Cardiac Tumors

Kaposi's sarcoma, B-lymphocyte lymphoma, and other tumors of the lymphoid system are associ-

Table 24-5. Risk Factors for Cardiovascular Disease in Adults With HIV Infection

Risk Factor	Clinical Correlate (Ref.)
Advanced state of HIV infection	
Low CD4+ lymphocyte counts	Dilated cardiomyopathy (3,11,15,28,29,60)
Low albumin	Pericardial effusion (adversely affects survival) (13,57)
Opportunistic infections	Pericardial effusion (adversely affects survival) (58)
Oral candidiasis	Increase in the progression from asymptomatic HIV-1 infection to AIDS (6)
Hairy leukoplakia	
Herpes zoster	
Intravenous drug abuse	Infectious endocarditis (1,18)
Infection with HIV-1 versus HIV-2	Greater left ventricular dilatation and hypertrophy (28)
Malnutrition and wasting	
Selenium deficiency	Heart muscle disease, immune dysfunction, Keshan disease (33,123)
Carnitine deficiency	Left ventricular dysfunction

ated with immunodeficiency states, most frequently with AIDS (Tables 24-2 and 24-4).[5,13,22,24,26,48,82–86] Kaposi's sarcoma is the most common AIDS-associated neoplastic condition and is found in 25% to 35% of patients,[87,88] male homosexuals being at the greatest risk. Tachyarrhythmias, heart block, right ventricular hypokinesis, pericardial effusion, fatal tamponade,[59,84] and congestive heart failure in the absence of ventricular dilatation[89,90] can be clinical indicators of underlying Kaposi's sarcoma[59,84] or lymphoma.[5,91,92] The prognosis is poor.

Lymphoma may occur more frequently in patients with mononuclear infiltrative lung disease.[90–95] In HIV-infected patients with a sudden onset and a rapid progression of cardiac symptoms, the possibility of a malignant cardiac lymphoma should be entertained.[96] This tumor, though rare, is occurring with increasing frequency.[96]

Risk Factors in HIV-Infected Adults

Stage of Disease and Low CD4+ Lymphocyte Counts

Cardiac abnormalities increase in frequency and severity as HIV infection progresses.[3,11,15,28,29,60] Female sex, opportunistic infection, and advanced HIV disease are all factors that increase the likelihood of developing symptomatic cardiac disease.[13,18,97] Dilated cardiomyopathy and pericardial effusion are more common in patients with AIDS than in those with asymptomatic HIV infection or AIDS-related complex[60] and are associated with low CD4+ lymphocyte counts[40] (Tables 24-4 and 24-5). The isolated dilatation of either ventricle, is generally transient and occurs in the earlier stages.[40] The prevalence of cardiac abnormalities is higher in adults who have advanced HIV disease, who are inpatients rather than outpatients, who have *P. carinii* pneumonia, or who have a CD4+ lymphocyte count less than 100/mm[3].[3,6,13,15,17,28,34,40] Opportunistic infection with *Mycobacterium avium-intracellulare* frequently occurs in HIV-positive patients with CD4+ lymphocyte counts $<50 \times 10^6$ cells per liter.[53]

Dilated cardiomyopathy independently predicts a poor outcome[3,6,25,34,36] and is strongly correlated with very low CD4+ lymphocyte counts[6] (Table 24-5). Some studies have stated that 50% of HIV-infected adults with dilated cardiomyopathy will die within 6 months.[3,98] Some of these patients develop clinically evident congestive heart failure.[33,34] Persistent left ventricular dysfunction, characterized by a low ejection fraction (<45%), observed on two consecutive echocardiograms is associated with a grim prognosis of 100% mortality in 1 year.[11]

Opportunistic Infections

Opportunistic infection is responsible for cardiac complications in 45.6% of HIV-positive patients in the later stages.[18] Hairy leukoplakia, oral candidiasis, and herpes zoster have been shown to play an essential role in the rapid progression of asymptomatic HIV infection to later stages of AIDS[6] (Table 24-5).

Fungal infections in HIV-infected patients[19,33,40,56,83,97,99–102] may result in endocarditis, myocarditis, pericarditis, abscesses, congestive heart failure, and dilated cardiomyopathy.

A correlation between ventricular dysfunction and *P. carinii* pneumonia has been documented.[3] *P. carinii* pneumonia causes pulmonary pathology and is a sign of advanced HIV infection, where cardiac lesions and abnormalities of pulmonary hypertension are common.[49]

Toxoplasma gondii infection tends to be associated with left ventricular dysfunction and is said to be the most common cause of myocarditis in HIV-infected adults.[26,44,103–105] However, in a recent study of HIV-infected subjects, no evidence of *T. gondii* was documented.[40]

Several bacteria are known to infect the heart.[106,107] Longevity of HIV-infected patients increases the risk of *M. avium-intracellulare* infection.[102,106] Patients with later stages of HIV infection should be evaluated for the presence of *M. avium-intracellulare* co-infection, which may be difficult to diagnose.[102]

Cytomegalovirus inclusions have been demonstrated in cardiac myocytes of HIV-infected adults with congestive heart failure, pericarditis, and rhythm disturbances.[44,48,99,108,109] The absence of inclusions did not exclude cytomegalovirus infection.[109] However, a recent study failed to demonstrate any serologic evidence of cytomegalovirus infection in patients with myocardial dysfunction.[40]

HIV-1 Versus HIV-2

With HIV-1 infection, patients had significantly greater left ventricular dilatation and hypertrophy than with HIV-2 infection patients.[28]

Therapy

Studies of the cardiotoxic effects of zidovudine have produced conflicting results. Improvement, preservation, or worsening of ventricular function with this drug has been reported.[110–112] Zidovudine may also lead to a dose-dependent abnormality in mitochondrial replication, causing reversible skeletal myopathy.[113] Evidence points to zidovudine as a causative agent for heart muscle disease, as cardiac function is seen to improve on withdrawal of the drug in some cases.[111] Conversely, HIV-associated heart muscle disease has been documented in patients who have never taken the drug.[40] Agents other than nonretroviral agents may cause cardiovascular or hemodynamic compromise.

Malnutrition and Wasting

Nutritional deficiencies frequently affect HIV-positive patients. They may be due to malabsorption or decreased food intake. Deficiencies of selenium, carnitine, B group vitamins, and zinc are reported to lead to a deterioration of cardiac function. Zinc may be associated with high levels of circulating tumor necrosis factor, which may lead to immune dysfunction or cardiac compromise.[114–117] The consequences of selenium and carnitine deficiency have been investigated (see below).

Loss of lean body mass is seen frequently in HIV-positive patients.[118] Wasting is a predictor of mortality in HIV-infected adults in the intensive care unit.[119] Severe anemia may also lead to further deterioration of cardiac health in this population.[120,121]

Selenium Deficiency

Selenium, the trace element indispensable for the activity of glutathione, is thought to be important in the development of heart muscle disease. Lack of this antioxidant has been implicated in Keshan disease, a type of dilated cardiomyopathy first observed in China.[33] The low levels of selenium

in the serum and myocardium of AIDS patients further confirm the correlation between the lack of this trace element and heart muscle disease (Table 24-5).[122,123]

This deficiency may be correlated with heart muscle disease and immune dysfunction (Table 24-5), including oral candidiasis, abnormal phagocyte function, and low CD4+ lymphocyte counts. Low levels of selenium have been documented in the red blood cells and plasma of AIDS patients.[123] Subjects with advanced HIV disease are more likely to have greater deficits. The relation between the selenium level and the serum albumin and lymphocyte count has been documented. Malabsorbtion or decreased intake in the diet might cause this deficiency and lead to cardiac and immunologic abnormalities in HIV-positive patients.[123]

Carnitine Deficiency

Deficiency of L-carnitine was observed in 72% of HIV-infected adults with malnutrition, some of whom had symptoms of heart disease (Table 24-5).[124] Carnitine administration may reverse clinically significant left ventricular dysfunction in some patients.

Specific Clinical Cardiovascular Syndromes in HIV-Infected Children

HIV-seropositive children often develop a broad spectrum of cardiac lesions, ranging from congenital heart disease to other potentially serious complications that occur with the advancement of HIV disease.[125]

Congenital Cardiovascular Effects of Maternal HIV Infection

A higher rate of occurrence of congenital cardiac defects in children born to HIV-infected mothers has been suggested.[126–128]

Left Ventricular Dysfunction

Left ventricular dysfunction is evolving as the most prominent cardiac manifestation of pediatric HIV disease.[23,129–133] Left ventricular dysfunction is found in 29% to 74% of HIV-infected pediatric patients and is significantly more frequent in patients with clinically manifest disease (Tables 24-6 to 24-8).[37,56,128,134–147] A significant deterioration of left ventricular function has been observed in children with progression of HIV infection.[4,125,144,148,149] In a setting of dilated cardiomyopathy it frequently leads to symptomatic heart disease, such as congestive heart failure.[144] Often, marked deterioration of left ventricular performance and contractility occurs in a period of few months.[143]

Left ventricular abnormalities are more often clinically symptomatic and persistent than right ventricular abnormalities or pericardial effusions.[149]

Congestive Heart Failure

Formerly most children with congestive heart failure were diagnosed later in the course of HIV infection in the setting of acute severe intercurrent illness, and suffered fatal consequences within a couple of months after diagnosis. Longer survival

Table 24-6. Prospective Studies of Cardiovascular Involvement in Pediatric HIV Infection

Study	N	Patients	Follow-up	Major Findings
Lipshultz (P^2C^2), USA, 1996 (227)	197	Vertical transmission Median age 2.1 yr	39 mo (median)	Depressed LVFS predicts mortality independent of CD4+ lymphocyte count and encephalopathy
Starc (P^2C^2), USA, 1996 (141)	86 HIV+ 419 HIV-newborns born to HIV+ mothers	Vertical transmission Followed since birth	1.1 yr (mean)	LVFS < 19% = 1.7% (9/505) LVFS < 25% = 8.6% (42/505) LVEDD (z score > 1.5) = 5.8% Cardiomegaly (x-ray) = 13.7%
Lipshultz (P^2C^2), USA, 1995 (142)	34	Vertical transmission Followed since birth	4.1 mo (mean)	LVFS initially depressed and remained so LV contractility depressed LVEDD increased (all $P < .003$ compared to 285 controls)
Lipshultz (P^2C^2), USA, 1993 (143)	130	Vertical transmission Mean age 2.0 yr	4.1 mo (mean)	Initially depressed contractility 42% (55/130) Initially increased LV afterload 20% (26/130) Initially decreased FS 25% (32/130) On follow-up: progressive deterioration of LV performance with reduced contractility and increased afterload (all $P < .02$)
Ruga, Italy, 1993 (144)	41	Vertical transmission 1 mo–8 yr	14.1 mo	Dilated cardiomyopathy 10% (4/41) LV hypertrophy by ECG 29% (12/41) Decreased LVFS 5% (2/41)
Dolfus, Paris, 1993 (145)	31	3 mo–10 yr All HIV+ with symptoms All on zidovudine	3–23 mo	Dilated cardiomyopathy 32% (10/31) Severe heart failure 6% (2/31)
De Simone, Italy, 1992 (146)	20	Vertical transmission Followed since birth	3.7 yr	LV dilatation 10% (2/20) Gallop rhythm 5% (1/20)
Lipshultz, Boston, 1989 (147)	31	3 mo–22.5 yr 11 HIV+, 20 HIV+ with symptoms	Variable	New/progressive changes in 84% (16/19) of patients followed with ECG L/RV hypertrophy = 48% (15/31) Decreased contactility = 26% (8/31) Increased contractility = 32% (10/31) Pericardial effusion = 26% (8/31)

LV, left ventricular; RV, right ventricular; EDD, end-diastolic dimension; FS, fractional shortening.

Table 24-7. Cross-Sectional Studies of Cardiovascular Involvement in Pediatric HIV Infection

Study (Ref.)	N	Patients	Testing Modality	Major Findings
Kavanaugh-McHugh (ACTG043), Baltimore, 1991 (228)	88	Echocardiogram on enrollment and at 6-mo intervals (a prospective study reported as a cross-sectional study)	ECHO	Ventricular dilatation 34% (30/88) Pericardial effusion 16% (14/88) Decreased ventricular function 20% (18/88) Atrial dilatation 11% (10/88)
Kavanaugh-McHugh, Baltimore, 1990 (140)	34	1 mo–18 yr	ECHO	Total abnormalities 62% (21/34) LV dilatation 26% (9/34) LV dysfunction 9% (3/34) RV dilatation 6% (2/34) Pericardial effusion 44% (15/34)
Issenberg, New York, 1985 (139)	22	6 mo–6 yr 12 AIDS, 10 ARC	ECHO	LV dilatation/dysfunction 45% (10/22) RV dilatation 9% (2/22) Pericardial effusion 18% (4/22)
Sherron, Miami, 1985 (138)	23	4–48 mo All with ARC or AIDS	ECHO	LV dysfunction 74% (17/23) Decreased fractional shortening 65% (15/23) Pericardial effusion 18% (4/22) Pulmonary artery hypertension 17% (4/23)
Lindvig, Denmark, 1990 (20)	24	All with AIDS	ECHO	Total abnormalities 54% (13/24) RV diameter > 26 mm 37.5% (9/24) Dilated LA or LV 12.5% (2/24) Pericardial effusion 21% (5/24)

(more than 1 year after diagnosis) and a better quality of life have been achieved after the institution of early appropriate therapy for congestive heart failure diagnosed in the setting of a less severe illness.[38]

A high percentage of HIV-positive children have been reported to develop heart failure. Prospective studies on children with HIV infection have observed congestive heart failure in 10% to 13% of patients.[4] At Children's Hospital in Boston, 10% displayed evidence of transient congestive heart failure accompanying systemic illness that responded in less than 30 days to treatment.[71,134,150] Chronic cardiac failure was observed in 10% (Table 24-8).[134,150] This high cumulative incidence, when extrapolated to the global situation, suggests that the incidence of congestive heart failure in the world pediatric population may surpass that in the entire adult population of the United States by the year 2000.[129,151]

Electrocardiographic Abnormalities

High-grade arrhythmias are more frequently found in HIV-infected patients than in healthy patients and are associated with symptomatic heart disease or poor outcomes. From 30% to 65% of HIV-infected children have been reported to have abnormal electrocardiographic findings (Tables 24-9 and 24-10).[5,37,71,125,128,134,139,140,152]

The most frequently observed abnormalities are tachycardia, seen in 49% to 70% of HIV-infected children,[37,153,154] and ventricular hypertrophy, seen in 20% to 30% of these patients.[125,148,153,155] ST-T wave changes are seen in 7% to 33% of HIV-infected children.[152,155] Rhythm disturbances,[134,153] including sinus arrhythmias, atrial ectopy, and ventricular arrhythmias, have been documented.

Dysrhythmias and conduction abnormalities have been reported in patients with abnormal electrocardiographic findings, possibly related to small-vessel vasculitis, neural tissue fibrosis, autonomic dysfunction,[5,37] or myocarditis.[73,156]

Cardiac Arrests

At Children's Hospital, 7 of 81 HIV-infected children developed 8 unexpected cardiorespiratory arrests, one of which was fatal (Table 24-8).[37,134,157] Causes of the arrests included flushing of a central line, medication, respiratory infection, or sepsis.

Table 24-8. Retrospective Studies of Cardiovascular Abnormalities in Pediatric HIV Infection

Study (Ref.)	N	Patients	Testing Modality	Major Findings
Domanski, Washington, DC, 1995 (137)	137	All ages and risk factors Reviewed 1 month–5 yr	ECHO	Cardiomyopathy 14% (19/137) 6% avg decrease in FS units/yr
Al-Attar, Boston, 1995 (136)	68	All ages and risk factors All with AIDS Reviewed since AIDS diagnosis	Survival study	Serious cardiac event (CHF, tamponade, CVA, arrest) 28% (19/68) (CMV+/prior CV abnormality predictive) 35% (15/43) of deaths in setting of significant cardiac disease (encephalopathy, male sex, wasting predictive of cardiac death)
Grenier, Washington, DC, 1994 (135)	95	4 mo–12 yr 15 HIV+, 80 HIV+ with symptoms Reviewed for average 10 mo	ECHO	ECHO abnormalities 25% (24/95) Increased LV contractility 75% (18/24) Cardiomyopathy 87.5% (21/24) 92% of deaths had abnormal heart Cardiac cause for 25% (3/12) of deaths
Tripp, Durham, NC 1993 (128)	129	All ages	ECHO	Cardiomyopathy 9% (11/129) Pericadial effusion 2% (2/129)
Luginbuhl, Boston, 1993 (134)	81	Mean age 4.1 yr Mean f/u = 1.8 yr 8 HIV+, 73 HIV+ with symptoms	ECHO	Chronic CHF 10% (8/81) Transient CHF 10% (8/81) Cardiopulmonary arrest 9% (7/81) 33% (10/30) of deaths with cardiac dysfunction
Mast, New York, 1992 (56)	45	0–8 yr All with autopsy or ECHO	ECHO/CXR 21 autopsied	Pericardial effusion 58% (26/45) Tamponade 8% (2/26) Normal CXR 50% (13/26) Ventricular dilatation or hypertrophy 43% (9/21)

FS, fractional shortening; CHF, congestive heart failure; CVA, cerebrovascular accident; CV, cardiovascular; ECHO, echocardiogram; CMV, cytomegalovirus; CXR, chest x-ray.

Sudden death was reported in five children who had a history of myopericardial pathology.[158] Examination of myocytes from some of these children revealed evidence of HIV infection.

A remarkable 15-fold increase in the relative risk of postneonatal mortality (4% compared to 0.3% in the general population) was found in the Swiss Neonatal HIV Prospective Study of 286 children of HIV-infected mothers; the mortality was due equally to AIDS and sudden death.[159] The postneonatal mortality of infants born to HIV-infected mothers was 0.7% and 0.5% in two studies.[160,161]

Since these fatalities occurred between 6 and 10 weeks of age in children weighing at least 2,800 g, authors have suggested a role of fetal hypoxia in utero. It has also been demonstrated that HIV-positive patients are less likely to survive a cardiorespiratory arrest.[162]

Cardiac Death

Cardiac abnormalities are significantly associated with a high mortality rate in pediatric HIV infection (Table 24-8).[134,136] Death was related to

Table 24-9. Longitudinal Studies of Electrocardiographic Abnormalities in Pediatric HIV Infection

Study	N	Patients	Follow-up	Major Findings
Grenier, Washington, DC, 1994 (125)	95	4 mo–12 yr	10 mo (mean) Range 1–24 mo (retrospective)	30% (24/80) with AIDS had ECG changes Ventricular hypertrophy 21% (20/95) RBBB: atrial flutter; prolonged QTc; frequent VPBs 1% (1/95) Nonspecific ST/T changes 6% (6/95)
Luginbuhl, Boston, 1993 (134)	81	Mean age at entry = 1.5 yr 8 HIV+, 38 ARC, 35 AIDS	2.1 yr (mean) (retrospective)	Tachycardia 64% (52/81) Bradycardia 11% (9/81) Atrial ectopy 25% (20/81) Premature junctional beats 4% (3/81) VPBs 15% (12/81) Marked sinus arrhythmia 17% (14/81) Ventricular tachycardia 2% (2/81) Ventricular fibrillation 1% (1/81)
Tripp, Durham, NC 1993 (128)	129	All ages		Myocardial dysfunction or ECG changes 14% (18/129) 19% (17/90) surviving to 3 years had these findings
De Simone, Italy, 1992 (152)	20	All vertically infected	3.7 yr (mean) (prospective)	ST/T changes 20% (4/20)
Lipshultz, Boston, 1991 (71)	105	All with AIDS		Tachycardia 47% (49/105) Bradycardia 7% (7/105) Marked sinus arrhythmia 15% (16/105) including 30% of patients with unexpected arrest High-grade ventricular ectopy 5% (5/105) including 30% of patients with unexpected arrest
Kavanaugh-McHugh/ ACTG043/ Baltimore, 1991 (228)	88	All symptomatic with HIV	Prospective	Rhythm disturbances 24% (21/88) Conduction abnormalities 48% (42/88) Ventricular hypertrophy 17% (15/88) ST/T changes 33% (29/88) Atrial enlargement 5% (4/88)

RBBB, right bundle branch block; VPBs, ventricular premature beats.

cardiac dysfunction in 25% of HIV-infected children at Children's Hospital[5] and of HIV-infected children at Children's National Medical Center.[135]

Autonomic Dysfunction

A wide spectrum of central and peripheral nervous system disorders, including autonomic dysfunction, may occur in HIV-positive patients of all ages at any stage of infection, and may have a significant effect on cardiovascular reflexes.[5,37,69,70,134,163–165] The most frequent echocardiographic finding in HIV-infected children is increased left ventricular performance, suggesting a hyperadrenergic state.[37,151,166–168] High-grade ectopy, sudden unexplained death, myocarditis, pericarditis, and inflammation of the cardiac conduction tissue are more likely to occur in these patients. Since neural tissue is affected early in HIV infection, these cardiovascular manifestations may be due to an underlying autonomic neuropathy.[5]

The magnitude of clinical problems associated with autonomic dysfunction in children with symptomatic (CDC Class P-2) HIV infection is significant. Hemodynamic abnormalities, dysrhythmias, unexplained arrests, and sudden death are frequently noted in HIV-infected children, especially when acute deterioration, interventions, or neuro-

Table 24-10. Cross-Sectional Studies of Electrocardiographic Abnormalities in Pediatric HIV Infection

Study	N	Patients	Major-Findings
Kavanaugh-McHugh, Baltimore, 1990 (140)	34	1 mo–18 yr	ECG abnormalities 65% (15/23) LV hypertrophy 26% (9/34) Sinus tachycardia 26% (9/34) Nonspecific ST/T changes 21% (7/34) Right axis deviation 9% (3/34) RV hypertrophy 6% (2/34) Right atrial enlargement 3% (1/34) Rhythm disturbances 9% (3/34)
Lipshultz, Boston, 1989 (37)	30	3 mo–22.5 yr 11 HIV+, 20 HIV+ with symptoms	Sinus tachycardia 77% (23/30) LV hypertrophy 37% (11/30) RV hypertrophy 13% (4/30) ST/T changes 50% (15/30) Atrial ectopy 40% (12/30) Ventricular ectopy 30% (9/30) Normal 7% (2/30)
Issenberg, New York, 1985 (139)	22	6 mo–6 yr	ECG abnormalities 55% (12/22) Ventricular hypertrophy 36% (8/22) RBBB 5% (1/22)

LV, left ventricular; RV, right ventricular; RBBB, right bundle branch block.

logic involvement is observed.[71,134,150] Abnormal cardiac autonomic regulation probably contributes to these problems and should be assessed.[5]

Myocarditis

Infectious organisms have been less commonly identified in the myocytes, and their relation to HIV-associated heart disease has been indirect.[169] Histopathologic evidence of myocarditis, characterized by a preponderance of mononuclear and lymphocytic infiltrates and myocyte necrosis, has been documented in some HIV-infected patients. It may be infectious in origin and is often associated with ventricular dysfunction.[169]

Other factors implicated in this condition are therapeutic or illicit drug use, postviral cardiac autoimmunity, and selenium deficiency.[1] However, no definite correlation with any of these factors has been established.

Vascular Disease

Vascular disease is often present in HIV-infected children[73] and may present as myocardial infarction,[170] coronary dilatation associated with ventricular dysfunction,[170] vascular aneurysms,[171] stroke,[172] or cardiomyopathy.[172] An association between HIV-

1-infected children with parvovirus B19 coinfection and recurrent Kawasaki disease has been found.[173]

Pulmonary Hypertension

Symptomatic HIV-infected children often present with pulmonary hypertension.[138,139] It may result from thromboembolic phenomena, left ventricular dysfunction, or recurrent respiratory infections.[5]

Pericardial Disease

HIV infection is less often associated with pericardial effusion in children than in adults, but complications of tamponade and sudden death have been reported in several children with HIV disease. A prevalence of 16% to 26% of pericardial effusion in HIV-infected children has been documented (Tables 24-6 to 24-8) but the 1-year cumulative incidence is 0.6%.[37,56,128,138–140,147] Despite a high prevalence, most of the effusions are transient, as shown by echocardiography.[149]

Endocarditis

Endocarditis is less common in HIV-infected children than in adults, probably because most children are not in the high-risk category.[169] Endocarditis of the aortic valve was documented in an HIV-infected child with congestive heart failure at 4 months of age,[38] and nonbacterial thrombotic endocarditis of the mitral valve was found in another HIV-positive child.[139]

Risk Factors in HIV-Infected Children

Stage of HIV Disease and Low CD4+ Lymphocyte Counts

Cardiac abnormalities occur more often during the later stages of HIV infection.[4,71,134,150] Patients with AIDS-related complex have the highest risk of sinus arrhythmias with significant heart rate variability and have higher odds of developing tachycardia, bradycardia, and cardiac arrest. CDC class P-2C (symptomatic HIV infection with lymphoid interstitial pneumonitis) is associated with cardiac arrest, sinus arrhythmias and tachycardia. Nonneurologic, nonlymphocytic interstitial pneumonia AIDS, CDC classes P-2D1 and P-2D2, is associated with many adverse cardiac outcomes (death with cardiac dysfunction, abnormalities of blood pressure and heart rate).[4]

Ventricular dysfunction, tachycardia, higher left ventricular afterload, and decreased left ventricular contractility were found more frequently in HIV-infected children with CD4+ lymphocyte counts two standard deviations below normal.[143,174] The estimated median time to death was 3 months for a child with encephalopathy, wasting, and a CD4+ lymphocyte count z score three standard deviations below normal, as compared with more than 64 months for a child with none of these risk factors[136] (Table 24-11).

A correlation between CD4+ lymphocyte counts of 100 cells/mm^3 or less and cardiomyopathy is observed in the pediatric age group[4,128,141,174] (Table 11).

Length of Time Infected

A decade ago, children with AIDS succumbed to fatal infections before the clinical manifestation of cardiac complications.[5] With newer medical interventions for treating infections, better nutrition, and closer surveillance, HIV-infected patients will probably survive longer, and cardiac complications will comprise a significant proportion of their clinical problems.[19] As a result, there may be an increase in the number of HIV-infected patients with heart disease. Cardiomyopathy was nonfatal and was more likely to be reversible in 12 HIV-infected children younger than 3 years, compared to children dying after the age of 3 years.[128]

Encephalopathy

As discussed in the previous section, encephalopathy is an important predictor of adverse cardiac outcomes.[134,136,175] It is associated with left ventricular dysfunction.[174] Encephalopathy along with wasting and male sex, has been shown to be an important marker of "cardiac death"[134,136] (Table 24-11).

The strongest correlate of cardiorespiratory arrest was found to be encephalopathy, perhaps reflecting autonomic nervous system dysfunction.[134,157] After adjusting for CDC classification, encephalopathy was still significantly correlated with marked sinus arrhythmia, bradycardia, tachycardia, hypotension, death due to a noncardiac cause, and death due to any cause. Encephalopathy significantly increases the risk of chronic heart failure in pediatric HIV infection (Table 24-11). Other AIDS-defining illnesses did not have such a significant association.[134]

Coinfections

Viral infections

Viruses in pediatric HIV infection exhibit tropism to the heart and are also markers of cardiac disease. Infection with Epstein-Barr virus and cytomegalovirus is briefly described here. Other viruses, such as adenovirus, coxsackievirus, herpesvirus, and parvovirus, have been associated with frequent high-grade ventricular arrhythmia, dilated cardiomyopathy, pericardial involvement, and fatal myocarditis.[176–178]

Epstein-Barr virus infection. HIV-infected children with evidence of Epstein-Barr virus infection are at a greater risk of developing cardiac abnormalities, especially congestive cardiac failure, chronic heart failure, bradycardia and other abnormalities

Table 24-11. Predictors of Cardiovascular Morbidity and Mortality: Pediatric HIV Infection

Cardiovascular Morbidity and Mortality (Ref.)	Predictors
Overall mortality (228)	Decreased left ventricular fractional shortening
	Increased age
	Reduced height
	Encephalopathy
	Low CD4+ lymphocyte count
Cardiac mortality (226)	Encephalopathy
	Wasting
	Low CD4+ lymphocyte count
	Nonneurologic, non-LIP AIDS*
Cardiac death (134,136)	Male sex
	Encephalopathy
	Wasting
	Low CD4+ lymphocyte count
	Nonneurologic, non-LIP AIDS*
Serious cardiac events (136)	Wasting
(Heart failure, significant dysrrhythmias, tamponade,	Positive cytomegalovirus status
stroke with hemodynamic instability and arrest)	History of cardiovascular abnormalities before the diagnosis of AIDS
Cardiorespiratory arrest (134)	Encephalopathy, LIP
Chronic congestive heart failure (134)	Epstein-Barr virus coinfection
Rhythm Disturbances (134)	
Sinus arrhythmia	Encephalopathy, LIP
Bradycardia	Encephalopathy*, Epstein-Barr virus infection
Tachycardia	Nonneurologic, non-LIP AIDS*
	Encephalopathy, LIP
	Nonneurologic, non-LIP AIDS*
Hemodynamic abnormalities (134,136)	Recurrent bacterial infections
	1 yr of age at AIDS diagnosis
	Hispanic ethnicity, positive cytomegalovirus status
Hypertension	Nonneurologic, non-LIP AIDS*
Hypotension	Encephalopathy*
	Nonneurologic, non-LIP AIDS*

LIP, lymphocytic interstital pneumonitis.

*Nonneurologic, non-LIP AIDS as defined by opportunistic and severe bacterial infections (CDC Class P2D1 and P2D2, respectively)

of heart rate, and blood pressure. They also have higher overall cardiac and noncardiac mortality.[37,134,153] Epstein-Barr virus infection is the strongest correlate of congestive heart failure and may be used as a marker for identifying patients with deteriorating cardiac health[134] (Table 24-11).

Epstein-Barr virus infection is associated with leiomyomas and leiomyosarcomas in children who have AIDS or are otherwise immunosuppressed.[179]

Cytomegalovirus infection. A longitudinal study of HIV-positive children demonstrated that positive cytomegalovirus status, wasting, and a prior history of cardiovascular abnormalities were significant

predictors of serious cardiac events[136] (Table 24-11).

Other Infections

Cardiac involvement with bacterial, fungal, and protozoal agents has been documented.[19,37,56,99,100] In 78% of HIV-positive children, *M. avium-intracellulare* coinfection was associated with cardiomyopathy.[180] The increased lifespan of HIV-positive children is placing them at a greater risk of developing *M. avium-intracellulare* coinfection, and most of them succumb to progressive ventricular dysfunction and cardiac failure.[5] It is recommended that children in the later stages of HIV infection who have unexplained symptomatic ventricular dysfunction be assessed for the presence of *M. avium-intracellulare* coinfection.[5]

P. carinii pneumonia may occur in the early months of life and often has a fulminant course in children with perinatally acquired HIV-1 infection.[181]

T. gondii appears to affect children less frequently than adults, probably because children are less likely to be exposed to the infection.[169] However, congenital cardiac toxoplasmosis was found at death in a child with AIDS who also had unexplained hypertrophic cardiomyopathy.[182]

Antiretroviral Therapy

There are conflicting reports about the clinical cardiac effects of zidovudine. Echocardiographic evaluation of 24 HIV-positive children revealed progressive ventricular dilatation and inadequate ventricular hypertrophy (although normal contractility was maintained) that were not significantly changed during treatment with zidovudine.[183] Moreover, congestive heart failure was not reported in any of the zidovudine-treated patients with advanced HIV disease. This was a surprising finding, since 20% of HIV-infected children at our hospital had congestive heart failure.[134] Another study in our institution demonstrated a decrease in cardiac morbidity and mortality in children in whom zidovudine therapy was initiated.[184] In contrast, according to a recent retrospective study of 137 HIV-infected children, a decrease in fractional shortening and an increase in the odds of developing cardiomyopathy were associated with zidovudine treatment.[137] This result may not be conclusive, because of several confounding factors: the study was not randomized and was mostly cross-sectional, the subjects were patients with advanced disease, and no consistent pattern of association with other variables was seen.

No evidence of cardiotoxicity associated with dideoxyinosine (ddI) has been found.[137]

Wasting and History of Prior Cardiac Abnormalities

In HIV-infected children, wasting is an important predictor of adverse cardiac outcomes. The median time to the occurrence of a serious cardiac event was estimated to be 8 months in the setting of a history of prior cardiac abnormalities and wasting, in contrast to more than 64 months in their absence[136] (Table 24-11).

Diagnosis and Monitoring of Cardiovascular Complications in HIV-Infected Patients

The incidence of cardiac symptoms ranges from less than 10% to 25% in HIV-infected patients.[12,13,34,146] Although rare, they nevertheless, indicate worsening cardiac health. The most common signs and symptoms are associated with congestive cardiac failure, which may serve as an important marker of left ventricular dysfunction.[5,37,38,62,185] Early detection and appropriate therapy results in a significant improvement in these patients.

Subclinical Cardiac Involvement

Cardiac involvement is frequently present in asymptomatic patients and can cause diverse complications affecting the different layers of the heart.[2,3,11,14,28,34,186,187] Echocardiographic lesions were reported in 48% of clinically asymptomatic patients.[14] Since cardiac complications occur at all stages of HIV disease and may lead to a fatal outcome, it may be worthwhile to start cardiovascular monitoring in the early stages of the disease.[18]

"Masking" of Cardiac Signs and Symptoms

Often cardiac symptoms in HIV-infected children and adults are undetected, especially in patients with an intercurrent systemic illness.[3,38,125,134,185,188] Hospitalized patients with AIDS are often afflicted with cardiovascular signs and symptoms that are attributed to the disease of another organ system.[1,3] Often, symptomatic HIV-infected patients have echocardiographic and electrocardiographic evidence of cardiac abnormalities that may lead to fatal complications.[38,125] An early cardiac evaluation is recommended in all symptomatic patients, as it is helpful in diagnosing cardiac dysfunction, valvular abnormality, and potentially fatal tamponade.[31] Evaluation with echocardiography is recommended in patients presenting with fatigue, severe dyspnea out of proportion to diagnosed pulmonary disease, gallop rhythm, pulmonary rales, pallor, hepatosplenomegaly, respiratory failure, or sepsis.[3,38,125,188] These physical findings may mask the underlying cardiac pathology and be attributed to extracardiac lesions.[38] An S_3 gallop may be an indicator of cardiac dysfunction in this patient population.[38]

Changes in feeding patterns, diaphoresis, growth failure, respiratory difficulties, perfusion, edema, diastolic filling sounds, and hepatomegaly are all signs and symptoms associated with cardiac failure in the pediatric age group.[4] Exercise dysfunction with a limitation of oxygen delivery to exercising muscles has been detected in HIV-infected adults and may represent an important and more accurate way to evaluate functional cardiovascular involvement in older children, because HIV-infected patients with cardiac symptoms may have exercise limitations.[189] Clinical signs and symptoms of significant pericardial disease may be difficult to detect in children because of the age of the child, the chronicity of the process, low-pressure tamponade, or concurrent signs and symptoms of other ongoing processes in the child.[5]

Detection of Cardiac Abnormalities

Noninvasive Techniques

Echocardiography

Cardiac pathology is detectable in 45% of HIV-infected patients.[18] Echocardiography has been shown to be the most suitable diagnostic tool for HIV-associated cardiac disease.[1,3,12,15,18,19,28,31,33,40,60,187] It was observed that after anticongestive therapy, all patients demonstrated marked improvement in fractional shortening as well as clinical symptoms, suggesting that, for at least half of these patients, multisystem noncardiac factors had a significant adverse effect on ventricular preload, heart rate, and afterload. Because half the children with HIV infection who have depressed shortening fractions have normal or enhanced contractility, we prefer the use of load-independent measurements of con-

tractility for greater sensitivity and specificity.[37,151,153,166–168,190] Echocardiography is the tool of choice for diagnosis and monitoring, as it provides a quantitative assessment of cardiac structure and function.[1,5]

Ventricular function. Echocardiography detects the extent of left ventricular dysfunction in HIV-seropositive patients. Quantification of contractility is done in the form of fractional shortening. Although electrocardiographic changes may reflect right ventricular hypertrophy, right ventricular function may be assessed by echocardiography. Right ventricular systolic pressure may be determined by Doppler studies.[49]

Ventricular dimension. Echocardiography assesses ventricular dilatation and hypertrophy.

Cardiac anatomy. Echocardiography detects structural abnormalities, vegetations, thrombi, and intracardiac masses.

Pericardial disease. Echocardiography is the most sensitive and specific method of detection of pericardial disease.[1] Right ventricular compression or collapse can be detected by echocardiography and indicates invasive intervention. Testing for infectious agents (for example, skin testing for tuberculosis) should be initiated if pericardial disease is detected.[5] Echocardiography is important and is recommended early, as effusion may often be due to malignancy (missed during pericardial fluid sampling) or infection.[2]

Coronary arteries. Echocardiography has proved to be useful in assessing coronary dilatation and aneurysms in HIV-infected children.[5]

The value of echocardiography in detecting clinically occult cardiac disease has been recognized by several previous studies.[12,18,28] Echocardiography demonstrated cardiac lesions in 72% of patients with AIDS, and therefore serial echocardiographic examination is recommended.[60]

Echocardiography, an important noninvasive tool, provides a better diagnostic yield than chest radiography or electrocardiography. A prospective echocardiographic study demonstrated evidence of cardiac disease in 44 patients (13 with dilated cardiomyopathy, 12 with right ventricular dilatation,

19 with borderline left ventricular dysfunction). Chest x-ray showed cardiomegaly in 6 of 13 patients with cardiomyopathy (46%). Electrocardiography showed nonspecific T wave changes in only one patient with isolated left ventricular dysfunction out of 44 patients with cardiac dysfunction.[6] That the chest x-ray is not a uniformly dependable tool for detecting pericardial effusion is reflected by a study in which half of the 26 HIV-infected children with effusion had normal roentgenograms.[56]

Echocardiography is very useful in detecting pericardial or myocardial involvement, intracardiac masses, and associated pericardial effusions. For identifying more diffuse cardiac involvement, radionuclide[94] and molecular resonance imaging scans may occasionally be helpful.[191]

Electrocardiography

Electrocardiography assesses heart rate, arrhythmias, atrial enlargement and ventricular hypertrophy, ischemic heart disease, the conduction system, and various ST and T wave changes, including ischemia and strain.[4,5] It has been found more useful in children than adults. Electrocardiographic abnormalities due to chamber enlargement and T wave changes have frequently been found in HIV-infected children with congestive cardiac failure.[38]

A prospective study over a 22-month follow-up period of HIV-positive patients with normal echocardiograms and abnormal electrocardiograms, showed that 14% developed new echocardiographic abnormalities. Therefore, if electrocardiographic abnormalities developed before echocardiographic abnormalities, screening with electrocardiography would be useful.[2] Although significant dysfunction occurrs in only a small number of patients, evaluation of patients with abnormal electrocardiographic findings has been recommended.[39] Electrocardiographic monitoring may contribute significantly in the detection of clinically occult cardiac abnormalities.[192]

Holter Monitoring

Holter monitoring is the next step if arrhythmias are found on physical examination or ectopy is found on the echocardiogram. Holter monitoring

determines the heart rate and rhythm, and the presence and types of different arrhythmias, conduction disorders, or ST and T-wave changes (ischemia, strain).[5] To estimate the occurrence of clinically silent arrhythmia, HIV-infected patients were subjected to 24-hour Holter monitoring. Though ventricular tachycardia was detected in many subjects, all of them had electrocardiographically and echocardiographically evident cardiac abnormalities.[2]

Cardiac Event Recorders

A transtelephonic postevent recorder is a hand-held device that is used to study intermittent palpitations. It is handed over to the patient, who applies it to the chest when the symptoms occur. The patient presses a button to record 30 seconds of the cardiac rhythm, which is stored in the memory of the device. The recording is later transmitted over the telephone for printing and interpretation.[193] In a recent study, event recorders detected 19% of patients with significant arrhythmias, in contrast to Holter monitors, which failed to detect any clinically important rhythm disturbances ($P < .005$). These event monitors were twice as likely to provide a diagnostic rhythm strip electrocardiogram during symptoms as 48-hour Holter monitoring and were also more cost-effective.[193]

Invasive Techniques

Pericardiocentesis

Of the patients who had pericardial effusion, 40% demonstrated evidence of clinical pericarditis, and 32% of the patients had tamponade.[194] Exudative fluid was found in 10 patients in whom pericardiocentesis was performed.[194] The yield of pericardiocentesis varies from 0% to 100%,[90,91] and large pericardial effusion may be the cause of circulatory compromise.[41,195-197] One study reported the yield of pericardiocentesis to be 36%.[198] Potentially treatable opportunistic infections or malignancies can be diagnosed by culture of pericardial biopsy or fluid from clinically manifest effusions.[93] It is a long-term (more than five years) effective palliative measure in patients with tamponade.[199] Therefore, pericardiocentesis serves diagnostic and therapeutic purposes.[1,16]

Endomyocardial Biopsy

Myocarditis has been detected in more than 52% of HIV-infected adults.[21] Endomyocardial biopsy has helped in detecting the treatable infections, such as *T. gondii.*[103] This procedure may be indicated in patients with severe intractable left ventricular dysfunction (congestive heart failure unresponsive to anticongestive therapy) demonstrated by serial echocardiography or in patients with refractory ventricular tachycardia.[1,5] In such cases it might be helpful in detecting the cause and provoking the initiation of appropriate therapy.[2] Molecular biological assay techniques, such as in situ hybridization for pathogens and the polymerase chain reaction, have been shown to increase the sensitivity of endomyocardial biopsy. Currently, endomyocardial biopsy may aid in diagnosing: inflammatory heart disease, reversible mitochondrial myopathy caused by zidovudine, and infectious heart disease.[5]

Assessment of Micronutrient Deficiencies

Selenium and carnitine deficiencies are reported to cause reversible ventricular dysfunction. Their assessment should be considered in the event of ventricular dysfunction. In selenium deficiency, the levels of selenium in the heart, plasma, and red blood cells are low and the activity of glutathione is decreased.[5]

Monitoring Recommendations

A number of studies have recognized the significant morbidity and mortality associated with cardiac disease and recommended systematic cardiac evaluation and HIV monitoring. The occurrence of subclinical cardiac abnormalities is common in this population. Both adult and pediatric studies have established that this could lead to fatal consequences. Therefore, early and periodic echocardiographic assessment may be beneficial.[18,23,28,60,187]

Several clinical investigators consider echocardiography to be the ideal modality for screening and monitoring of HIV-associated cardiac disease. In one study, all symptomatic patients had abnormal echocardiograms. Echocardiographic abnormalities occurred at early stages, before clinically obvious symptoms appeared.[28] Abnormalities at the asymptomatic stage can be diagnosed by echocardiography, thus providing a sensitive monitoring method.[18]

Relevance of Detection to Treatment Modality

Apart from directing the choice of treatment, echocardiography is useful in determining cardiac function in the event of administration of medications that might lead to the deterioration of cardiac functional status. Detection of clinically evident or asymptomatic cardiomyopathy in HIV-infected subjects is helpful when considering treatment options for opportunistic infections or secondary malignancies.[1,3] Some medicines, such as intravenous trimethoprim–sulfamethoxazole, should be administered with a large fluid load.[3] Antitumor agents could cause further cardiac compromise due to their own cardiotoxic properties.[1]

Monitoring Guidelines

Periodic and systematic monitoring of cardiac status is essential for the care of HIV-infected adults and children to rule out cardiac dysfunction and to detect cardiac disease early.[5,37] A comprehensive history and thorough cardiac examination may help in the differentiation of cardiac from noncardiac symptoms.[4]

Cardiac involvement is frequently present in asymptomatic patients and can cause diverse complications affecting the different layers of the heart. All patients who are *seropositive for HIV infection* (irrespective of stage or manifestation of disease progression) should be evaluated with baseline echocardiography, electrocardiography, and Holter monitoring.

Asymptomatic patients should have echocardiography once a year, and electrocardiography and Holter examination every 2 years. For patients with *noncardiac symptoms* (apparently due to systemic intercurrent illness such as lymaphadenopathy, wasting, neurologic diseases, serious infections, and malignancies),[5] a formal cardiac assessment (echocardiography, electrocardiography, and Holter monitoring) may reveal the presence of an abnormality. If no abnormality is found, follow-up echocardiography at 8-month intervals and annual electrocardiography and Holter monitoring are recommended.

If an HIV-infected patient has any one of the 10 criteria listed in Table 24-12, echocardiography every 6 months and electrocardiography and Holter monitoring every 9 months are advised. If two or more of the above criteria are present, then echocardiography every 4 months and electrocardiography and Holter monitoring every 6 months are recommended.

If any of the following is noted in an HIV-infected subject, a formal cardiac assessment is recommended:

1. Dyspnea out of proportion to the diagnosed pulmonary disease, unexpected or unresponsive respiratory symptoms lasting for more than 7 days, cough, oxygen desaturation, and diffuse pulmonary rales.[1,6,38,125,188]

2. Signs and symptoms of congestive heart failure: tachycardia, respiratory distress, diaphoresis, hypoxia, poor peripheral perfusion, edema, and (especially in case of children) poor sucking, growth failure, hepatosplenomegaly, changes in feeding pattern, weak cry, mottled extremities, decreased peripheral pulses, decreased urine output (<1 ml /kg /h), decreased blood pressure, activity intolerance, or prolonged QTc interval.[1,4,6,34,38,125,138,188,192] (See the subsections Cardiac Tumors, Congestive Heart Failure, Subclinical Cardiac Involvement in this chapter.)

3. History or presence of left ventricular dysfunction or dilatation or structural abnormalities.[47,136]

4. History or presence of frequent arrhythmias or inappropriate tachycardia.[134] (See the subsections Rhythm Disturbances and Sudden Death AND Cardiac Tumors in this chapter.)

5. History or presence of cyanotic episodes, seizures, syncope, or autonomic dysfunction.[69–71] (See the subsection Autonomic Dysfunction in this chapter.)

6. Severe intercurrent illness or hospitalization.[3,15,28,38,125,134,188] (See the subsections Opportunistic Infections AND Coinfections in this chapter.)

7. Evidence of clinical coinfections. (See the subsections Pericardial Effusion, Opportunistic Infections AND Coinfections in this chapter.)

8. Evidence of AIDS encephalopathy.[134,136,157,200]

9. CDC-defined AIDS stage. (See the subsection Stage of Disease and Low CD4+ Lymphocyte Counts in this chapter.)

Table 24-12. Recommendations for Monitoring of HIV-Infected Patients Without Symptomatic Cardiovascular Disease

HIV Disease Status	Frequency of Echocardiographic Monitoring	Frequency of Electrocardiographic and Holter Monitoring
Asymptomatic	Annually	Every 2 yr
Symptomatic HIV infection	Every 8 mo	Annually
Symptomatic HIV infection with the following:	Any 1 factor: every 6 mo	Any 1 factor, every 9 mo
Wasting	≥2 factors: every 4 mo	≥2 factors: every 6 mo
Encephalopathy (especially children)		
Coinfections (e.g., cytomegalovirus, Epstein-Barr virus)		
CD4+ lymphocyte counts >2 standard deviations below normal		
Significant illness warranting hospitalization		
Intravenous illicit drug abuse or symptoms of infectious endocarditis (especially adults)		
Left ventricular dysfunction (fractional shortening ≤ 25%, ejection fraction ≤ 50%)		
Pericardial effusion (more than trivial)		
History of cardiac dysrhythmias		
Cardiac malignancy		

10. Treatment with intravenous pentamidine, foscarnet, or ganciclovir.[3,9,63–67] (See the subsections Electrocardiographic Abnormalities AND Rhythm Disturbances and Sudden Death in this chapter.)

11. Treatment with antiretroviral drugs (zidovudine for more than 1 year or interferon therapy).[3,9,63–67] (See the subsections Antiretroviral Therapy AND Immunomodulatory Therapy in this chapter.)

12. Wasting and malnutrition: L-carnitine or selenium deficiency, hypoalbuminemia, anemia, etc.[136] (See the subsection Malnutrition and Wasting in this chapter.)

13. Decreased CD4+ lymphocyte count.[3,6,11,25,36,128,141,174,200] (See the subsection Stage of Disease and Low CD4+ Lymphocyte Counts in this chapter.)

14. Treatment with a chemotherapeutic agent or a drug that requires a large volume load[1,3] or is known to be cardiotoxic (e.g., anthracyclines).

15. History of intravenous drug abuse.[12,39,40,49,201] (See the subsection Endocarditis in this chapter.)

16. Symptoms of right ventricular dysfunction, pulmonary hypertension, or frequent bronchopulmonary infections: blue spells, dyspnea, syncope, chest pain, dry cough, vomiting, narrow second heart sound with a loud P2 component, right ventricular failure.[4,49]

17. Vague chest pain, constitutional signs and symptoms such as malaise, fatigue, lethargy, weakness, and tiredness.[11,38,125,188]

18. Signs and symptoms of pericardial effusion: inappropriate tachycardia, high cardiothoracic ratio by radiograph, dyspnea out of proportion to the diagnosed pulmonary disease, precordial or left shoulder pain, signs of right-sided heart failure, friction rub, distant heart sounds, hypotension, decreased cardiac output, or pulsus paradoxus.[1,4,198] (See the subsections Cardiac Tumors AND Pericardial Effusion in this chapter.)

If an HIV-infected patient presents with conditions 1, 2, 3, 6, 7, 8, 9, 11, 12, 14, 15, 16, 17, or 18, an echocardiogram is most useful in detecting the lesion and monitoring the effectiveness of treatment. These conditions are found in patients with pericardial effusion, left ventricular dysfunction, and structural heart diseases that can be diagnosed and appropriately treated (Figure 24-1). Conditions 1, 2, 4–10, and 16–18 are usually

found in HIV-infected patients with conduction abnormalities, and electrocardiography, Holter monitoring, or cardiac event recording may prove helpful (Figure 24-1).

Although we have suggested evaluations for symptomatic ventricular dysfunction, pericardial effusion, structural heart disease, and electrocardiographic abnormalities, HIV-infected patients are also at risk for symptomatic vascular disease. An algorithm for that is not included, since symptoms of vascular insufficiency can occur in any part of the body, and specific vascular events should be considered when any unexpected problem occurs.

Patients with *P. carinii* Pneumonia on Pentamidine Therapy

P. carinii pneumonia affects more than 60% of patients with AIDS.[202] The drug of choice, trimethoprim–sulfamethoxazole, is associated with many adverse effects and many patients are given pentamidine isethionate in the intravenous, intramuscular, or aerosolized form.[169] However, a prolonged QTc interval, sometimes leading to torsades de pointes has been described in several case reports of adults on pentamidine.[9,66,67,203,204] Several case reports have documented a probable cause-effect relationship between pentamidine and torsades de pointes.[9,63–65,67,205] Torsades de pointes or cardiac arrest[37,204,206,207] due to pentamidine has also been reported in children. Reversible pentamidine-induced cardiac adverse effects are seen electrocardiographically as QT prolongation, T-wave inversion, and electrical alternans of the U wave.[9] The patient had recurrent ventricular tachycardia that led to torsades de pointes. According to case reports and studies, the incidence of prolonged QTc in patients treated with intravenous pentamidine is 27%, and the risk of developing potentially fatal arrhythmias is greater. A study reported a 60%–75% incidence.[205] The criteria followed were QTc interval > 0.48 seconds or increase in QTc interval > 0.08 seconds. In that study, 36% of patients had a prolonged QTc interval within 4 days of treatment, and torsades de pointes developed in 60% of those patients. One of the patients with torsades de pointes died.[205]

In the setting of *P. carinii* pneumonia with pentamidine treatment, it would be worthwhile to mon-

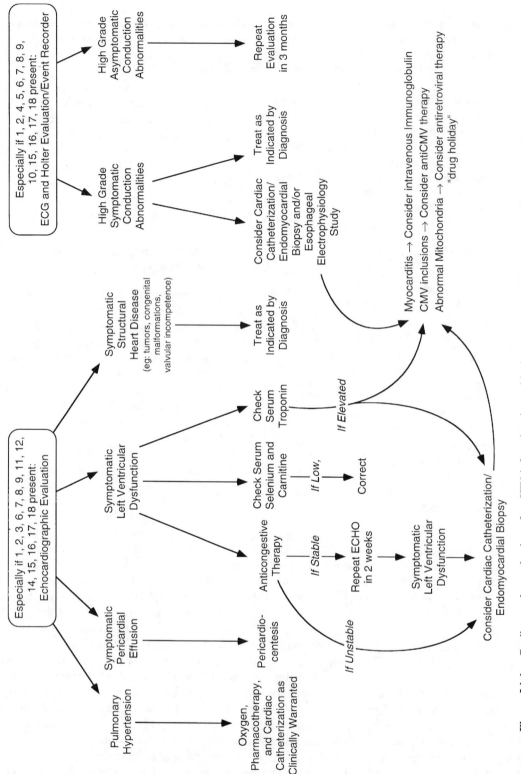

Figure 24-1. Cardiovascular evaluation of an HIV-infected patient with signs or symptoms consistent with cardiovascular involvement.

itor the patient closely electrocardiographically for the development of QTc interval prolongation.[9] An initial baseline electrocardiogram followed by daily electrocardiographic monitoring of patients on intravenous pentamidine for at least the first week of therapy is recommended.[205] Monitoring of potassium, calcium, and magnesium is important because reduced concentrations can be associated with prolongation of the QTc interval, and low glucose can affect it indirectly as well.[205] A QTc interval of more than 0.48 seconds or more than 0.08 seconds over baseline should be considered a significant indicator of arrhythmia. In the event of a prolonged QTc interval, continuous electrocardiographic monitoring or discontinuation of pentamidine is advocated[205] (Figure 24-2).

It is proposed that the structure of pentamidine, which is similar to that of the class I antiarrhythmics, is responsible for its cardiotoxic effects. Therefore the concurrent administration of drugs

causing a prolonged QT interval (procainamide, quinidine, disopyramide, and aprindine) is contraindicated, as they would increase the risk of development of torsades de pointes.[9] Lidocaine, bretylium, or isoproterenol is useful for the treatment of pentamidine-induced malignant ventricular tachyarrythmias.[9] Aerosolized pentamidine has not been reported to be associated with cardiac toxicity.[208]

Treatment Conditions

General Supportive Treatment

Early detection would initiate the correction of factors that might cause cardiac compromise, such as selenium deficiency,[209] dehydration, malnutrition, and electrolyte imbalance.[5]

Specific Therapy

Antiinfective Treatment

At least in the short term, it appears that some infectious causes of HIV-associated heart disease are amenable to antiinfective treatment.[5] HIV-associated opportunistic infections such as *Salmonella* endocarditis, cryptococcal myopericarditis, *Toxoplasma* myocarditis,[210] and tuberculous or *M. avium-intracellulare*[19] pericarditis have responded to appropriate antiinfective treatment with considerable success.[211]

We have noted significant improvement in ventricular function and clinical heart failure in HIV-infected children with cytomegalovirus coinfection after treatment of cytomegalovirus with a combination of ganciclovir and cytomegalovirus hyperimmunoglobulin.[5]

Some reports have suggested that zidovudine improves cardiac function.[1,112]

Anticongestive Treatment

In HIV-infected adults, cardiac function has been seen to improve significantly with medical therapy.[11,37,38,40,41] Digoxin may improve the quality of life for a patient with congestive heart failure even if it does not prolong life.[5] Afterload reduction therapy with angiotensin-converting enzyme inhibitors has been shown to reduce progression to death

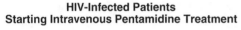

HIV-Infected Patients
Starting Intravenous Pentamidine Treatment

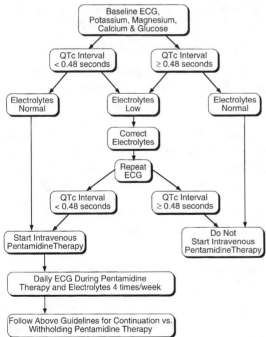

Figure 24-2. Recommendations for HIV-infected patients starting intravenous pentamidine treatment. (Modified from Ref. 205.)

in adults with congestive heart failure.[5] Occasionally, patients with refractory severe symptomatic ventricular dysfunction despite maximal conventional anticongestive therapy will achieve improved ventricular performance and a better quality of life, sometimes lasting for several weeks, after several days of palliative inpatient therapy with intravenous dobutamine.[5]

Treatment of Pulmonary Hypertension

Treatment of pulmonary hypertension with continuous intravenous infusion of epoprostenol plus conventional therapy (anticoagulants, oral vasodilators, diuretic agents, cardiac glycosides, and supplemental oxygen) has resulted in better hemodynamics, exercise endurance, quality of life, and survival than conventional therapy alone. In severe cases, cardiac catherization is recommended.[212]

Immunoglobulins

Several reports have documented immunoglobulin therapy to be effective in HIV-infected patients.[213] We found that HIV-infected children receiving monthly intravenous immunoglobulin therapy had fewer cardiac abnormalities than those not receiving intravenous immunoglobulin therapy; this was also true for those children with higher endogenous serum IgG and IgA levels.[200] Intravenous immunoglobulin therapy has resulted in improvement of left ventricular function[200] and improved survival[214] in patients with inflammatory heart disease, the acute phase of pediatric Kawasaki syndrome,[215] congestive cardiac failure refractory to anticongestive therapy,[200] and acute congestive cardiomyopathy.[214] Immunoglobulin therapy has also resulted in improvement in HIV-associated polymyositis.[216] Children with HIV infection and CD4+ lymphocyte counts $\geq 0.2 \times 10^9$ cells per liter who were not consistently receiving zidovudine or trimethoprim-sulfamethoxazole had beneficial effects from intravenous immunoglobulin therapy that included reductions in serious bacterial and minor viral and bacterial infections.[217,218]

Antihypertensive Therapy

Antihypertensive therapy and a search for treatable causes of hypertension are indicated in HIV-infected patients because their cardiovascular substrate may be compromised and they are less able to utilize cardiovascular reserves necessary to maintain cardiac function in the setting of severe hypertension.[5]

Immunomodulatory Therapy

Discontinuation of interferon alfa has been shown to correlate with significant improvement in myocardial function.[195]

Immunosuppressive Therapy

One HIV-infected adult with endomyocardial biopsy-proven myocarditis and ventricular dysfunction showed resolution of myocarditis and was not on medication for this problem after treatment with prednisone and azathioprine.[62] However, it is unclear whether immunosuppressive therapy alters the course of myocarditis in this population.[5]

Antiarrhythmic Therapy

Antiarrhythmic therapy in children with symptomatic arrhythmias is appropriate. Patients receiving intravenous or intramuscular pentamidine should have regular electrocardiographic measurement of QTc intervals (Figure 24-2).[5]

Micronutrient Replacement Therapy

Selenium-deficient HIV-infected patients with symptomatic ventricular dysfunction poorly responsive to conventional anticongestive therapy have improved cardiac function after selenium replacement.[219] Carnitine deficiency is another potentially reversible cause of symptomatic ventricular dysfunction in other populations.[220] For HIV-infected children with worsening or symptomatic ventricular dysfunction, it appears prudent to determine micronutrient status, and if the status is reduced, to initiate micronutrient replacement therapy.[5]

Treatment of Pericardial Effusion

Pericardial disease is frequently amenable to treatment when managed early.[13,31,36,49,53,56,201,221] In one study, 18% of patients were affected by pericardial effusion that was amenable to treatment with nonsteroidal antiinflammatory drugs.[18] An invasive approach was warranted in only one patient. In some cases a 50% resolution of pericardial effusion was observed over the follow-up period.[11] The use of steroids or anticoagulants may be contraindicated for HIV-infected patients with pericardial involvement,[19] and pericardiocentesis may be a more suitable alternative.

Surgery for Congenital and Acquired Heart Disease

HIV-positive patients seem to be at a higher risk than noninfected patients for hemodynamically significant reactions to medical or surgical therapeutic interventions.[37,67,68,70,71,134] A case series of 40 HIV-infected adults who underwent cardiopulmonary bypass (38 for valve replacement, 33 for endocarditis) found the actual survival to be the same as for other patients with AIDS, suggesting that surgery does not hasten the progression of AIDS.[82] A similar conclusion was reached by a study of six HIV-infected patients undergoing cardiopulmonary bypass surgery for infectious endocarditis (due to *Staphylococcus aureus* in all six cases).[222] Positive outcomes after surgery have been reported in several studies. Valve replacement for endocarditis in 10 HIV-positive patients[223] and surgical intervention in an HIV-infected adult with an atrial lymphoma[224] have been documented as being successful.

Evidence of Beneficial Effects of Cardiovascular Monitoring in HIV-Infected Patients

A retrospective review of medical records at Children's Hospital, Boston over a 10-year period revealed a later onset of AIDS in recent years in patients with vertically transmitted HIV infection.[184] As we had previously encountered problems of decreased survival of HIV-positive patients, we started monitoring patients more closely. Lower age-adjusted CD4+ lymphocyte counts, more anemia, and more wasting at the time of diagnosis of AIDS were seen in the more recently diagnosed patients with AIDS. In spite of these poor prognostic factors, these recent patients had a longer survival period, and the in odds of cardiac death and adverse cardiac outcomes were lower.[184]

This study found that AIDS patients diagnosed recently were older, were more likely to have had prior medical management, and have led longer lives, with significantly lower cardiac morbidity and mortality. These results imply that survival has improved in the recent years because patients have been more closely followed and cared for. It may be inferred that early detection, prompt institution of therapy, and close monitoring would all have a favorable impact on the survival of children with AIDS.[184] This supports the use of cardiac monitoring in patients with HIV infection.

Conclusion

About 5,000 patients per year in the United States may have cardiac complication resulting from HIV infection.[132] Better treatment and surveillance of opportunistic infection and the use of antiretroviral agents have contributed to the prolonged survival of patients with AIDS.[28] As the life span of HIV-infected patients is over 10 years, there exist substantial grounds to justify cardiovascular monitoring and care of HIV-infected subjects and improve their quality of life.[2] With the availability of effective treatment modalities, it is therefore imperative to consider periodic monitoring of HIV-infected patients at an early stage for the detection of subclinical cardiovascular complications.

References

1. Herskowitz A, Baughman KL. Effect of HIV infection on the heart. *Heart Dis* 1994;24:495–504.

2. Hsia J. Cardiovascular consequences of AIDS. In: Rapaport E (ed). *Cardiology and Coexisting Disease.* New York: Churchill Livingstone, 1994: 349–370.

3. Himelman RB, Chung WS, Chernoff DN, et al. Cardiac manifestations of human immunodeficiency virus infection: a two-dimensional echocardiographic study. *J Am Coll Cardiol* 1989;13: 1030–1036.

4. Lane-McAuliffe, E Lipshultz SE. Cardiovascular complications in pediatric HIV infection. *Nurs Clin North Am* 1995;30:291–316.

5. Lipshultz SE. Cardiovascular manifestations of pediatric HIV infection. In: Pizzo PA Wilfert CM (eds). *The Challenge of HIV Infection in Infants, Children and Adolescents.* Baltimore: Williams & Wilkins, 1994:483–511.

6. Currie PF, Jacob AH, Foreman AR, et al. HIV-related heart muscle disease: prognostic implications. *BMJ* 1994;309:1605–1607.

7. Tovo PA, de Martino M, Gabiano C, et al. Prognostic factors and survival in children with perinatal HIV-1 infection. *Lancet* 1992;339:1249–1253.

8. Anderson DW, Virmani R. Emerging patterns of heart disease in human immunodeficiency virus infection. *Hum Pathol* 1990;21:253–259.

9. Bibler MR, Chou TC, Toltzis RJ, Wade PA. Recurrent ventricular tachycardia due to pentamidine-induced cardiotoxicity. *Chest* 1988;94:1303–1306.

10. Italian Register for HIV Infection in Children . Features of children perinatally infected with HIV-1 surviving longer than 5 years. *Lancet* 1994; 343:191–195.

11. Blanchard DG, Hagenhoff C, Chow LC, et al. Reversibility of cardiac abnormalities in human immunodeficiency virus (HIV)-infected individuals: a serial echocardiographic study. *J Am Coll Cardiol* 1991;17:1270–1276.

12. Corallo S, Mutinelli MR, Lazzarin A, et al. Echocardiography detects myocardial damage in AIDS: prospective study in 102 patients. *Eur Heart J* 1988;9:887–892.

13. Monsuez JJ, Kinney EL, Vittecoq D, et al. Comparison among acquired immune deficiency syndrome patients with and without clinical evidence of cardiac disease. *Am J Cardiol* 1988;62:1311–1314.

14. Hecht SR, Berger M, Van Tosh A, Croxson S. Unsuspected cardiac abnormalities in the acquired immune deficiency syndrome: an echocardiographic study. *Chest* 1989;96:805–808.

15. Levy WS, Simon GL, Rios JC, Ross AM. Prevalence of cardiac abnormalities in human immunodeficiency virus infection. *Am J Cardiol* 1989; 63:86–89.

16. Kinney EL, Brafman D, Wright RJ. Echocardiographic findings in patients with acquired immunodeficiency syndrome (AIDS) and AIDS related complex (ARC). *Cathet Cardiovasc Diagn* 1989; 16:182–185.

17. Lassaigne D, Greder A, Hedoire F, et al. Myocardial involvement during AIDS: echographic eval-uation of 85 HIV infected patients. *Ann Med Interne* 1991;142:205–208.

18. DeCastro S, Migliau G, Silvestri A, et al. Heart involvement in AIDS: a prospective study during various stages of the disease. *Eur Heart J* 1992; 13:1452–1459.

19. Fong IW, Howard R, Elzawi A, et al. Cardiac involvement in human immunodeficiency virus-infected patients. *J Acquir Immune Defic Syndr* 1993;6:380–385.

20. Lindvig K, Nielsen TL, Videbaek R, Pedersen C. Echocardiographic screening in 24 consecutive AIDS patients. *Dan Med Bull* 1990;37:449–451.

21. Anderson DW, Virmani R, Reilly JM, et al. Prevalent myocarditis at necropsy in the acquired immunodeficiency syndrome. *J Am Coll Cardiol* 1988; 11:792–799.

22. Cammarosano C, Lewis W. Cardiac lesions in acquired immune deficiency syndrome (AIDS). *J Am Coll Cardiol* 1985;5:703–706.

23. Reitano J, King M, Cohen H, et al. Cardiac function in patients with acquired immune deficiency syndrome (AIDS) or AIDS prodrome. [Abstract]. *J Am Coll Cardiol* 1984;3:525.

24. Roldan EO, Moskowitz L, Hensley GT. Pathology of the heart in acquired immunodeficiency syndrome. *Arch Pathol* 1987;111:943–946.

25. Lewis W. AIDS: cardiac findings from 115 autopsies. *Prog Cardiovasc Dis* 1989;32:207–215.

26. Baroldi G, Corallo S, Moroni M, et al. Focal lymphocytic myocarditis in acquired immunodeficiency syndrome (AIDS): a correlative morphologic and clinical study in 26 consecutive fatal cases. *J Am Coll Cardiol* 1988;12:463–469.

27. Hofman P, Michiels JF, Saint-Paul MC, et al. An autopsy study of the cardiac lesions in 25 patients with AIDS. *Ann Pathol* 1990;10:247–257.

28. Cardoso JS, Miranda AM, Moura B, et al. Cardiac morbidity in the human immunodeficiency virus infection. *Rev Port Cardiol* 1994;13:901–911.

29. Monsuez JJ, Kinney EL, Vittecoq D, et al. AIDS heart disease: results in 85 patients. [Abstract]. *J Am Coll Cardiol* 1988;11:195A.

30. Hsia J, Adams S, Mohanty N, Ross A. Human immunodeficiency virus-related heart disease during 560 patient-years of follow-up. *Circulation* 1992;86:I-795–I-790.

31. Fink L, Reichek N, St John Sutton MG. Cardiac abnormalities in acquired immune deficiency syndrome. *Am J Cardiol* 1984;54:1161–1163.

32. Willoughby SB, Vlahov D, Herskowitz A. Frequency of left ventricular dysfunction and other echocardiographic abnormalities in human immunodeficiency virus seronegative intravenous drug users. *Am J Cardiol* 1993;71:446–447.

33. Currie PF, Boon NA. Cardiac involvement in human immunodeficiency virus infection. *Q J Med* 1993;86:751–753.

34. Herskowitz A, Vlahov D, Willoughby S, et al. Prevalence and incidence of left ventricular dysfunction in patients with human immunodeficiency virus infection. *Am J Cardiol* 1993;71:955–958.

35. Corboy JR, Fink L, Miller T. Congestive cardiomyopathy in association with AIDS. *Radiology* 1987;16:139–141.

36. Cohen IS, Anderson DW, Virmani R, et al. Congestive cardiomyopathy in association with the acquired immunodeficiency syndrome. *N Engl J Med* 1986;315:628–630.

37. Lipshultz SE, Chanock S, Sanders SP, et al. Cardiovascular manifestations of human immunodeficiency virus infection in infants and children. *Am J Cardiol* 1989;63:1489–1497.

38. Stewart JM, Kaul A, Gromisch DS, et al. Symptomatic cardiac dysfunction in children with human immunodeficiency virus infection. *Am Heart J* 1989;117:140–144.

39. Raffanti SP, Chiaramida AJ, Sen P, et al. Assessment of cardiac function in patients with the acquired immunodeficiency syndrome. *Chest* 1988;93:592–594.

40. Jacob AJ, Sutherland GR, Bird AG, et al. Myocardial dysfunction in patients infected with HIV: prevalence and risk factors. *Br Heart J* 1992;68:549–553.

41. Steinherz LJ, Brochstein JA, Robins J. Cardiac involvement in congenital acquired immunodeficiency syndrome. *Am J Dis Child* 1986;140:1241–1244.

42. Joshi VV, Gadol C, Connor E, et al. Dilated cardiomyopathy in children with acquired immunodeficiency syndrome: a pathologic study of five cases. *Hum Pathol* 1988;19:69–73.

43. Cusi MV, Lewis W. Cardiac changes in women with AIDS. *Mod Pathol* 1994;7:27A.

44. Klatt EC, Meyer PR. Pathology of the heart in acquired immunodeficiency syndrome (AIDS). *Arch Pathol* 1988;112:114–110.

45. DeCastro S, D'Amati G, Gallo P, et al. Frequency of development of acute global left ventricular dysfunction in human immunodeficiency virus infection. *J Am Coll Cardiol* 1994;24:1018–1024.

46. Herskowitz A, Willoughby SB, Vlahov D, et al. Dilated heart muscle disease associated with HIV infection. *Eur Heart J* 1995;16:50–55.

47. Corallo S, Mutinell M, Moroni M, et al. Echocardiography detects cardiac involvement in acquired immunodeficiency syndrome: study in 70 patients. [Abstract]. *Proc Int Conf AIDS* 1987;3:191.

48. Reilly JM, Cunnion RE, Anderson DW, et al. Frequency of myocarditis, left ventricular dysfunction and ventricular tachycardia in the acquired immune deficiency syndrome. *Am J Cardiol* 1988;62:789–793.

49. Himelman RB, Dohrmann M, Goodman P, et al. Severe pulmonary hypertension and cor pulmonale in the acquired immunodeficiency syndrome. *Am J Cardiol* 1989;64:1396–1400.

50. Coplan NL, Shimony RY, Ioachim HL, et al. Primary pulmonary hypertension associated with human immunodeficiency viral infection. *Am J Med* 1990;89:96–99.

51. Mohanty N, Adams S, Hsia J. Cardiac problems in persons with AIDS. *Choices Cardiol* 1993;6:1.

52. Webber JD, Lewis JF, Mody V. Cardiovascular abnormalities by echocardiography in patients with human immunodeficiency virus infection: influence of race and gender. [Abstract]. *J Am Coll Cardiol* 1993;21:395A.

53. Reynolds MM, Hecht SR, Berger M, et al. Large pericardial effusions in the acquired immunodeficiency syndrome. *Chest* 1992;102:1746–1747.

54. Cegielski JP, Ramaiya K, Lallinger GJ, et al. Pericardial disease and human immunodeficiency virus in Dar es Salaam, Tanzania. *Lancet* 1990;335:209–212.

55. Taelman H, Kagame A, Batungwanayo J, et al. Pericardial effusion and HIV infection. [Letter; Comment]. *AIDS* 1990;4:807–809.

56. Mast HL, Haller JO, Schiller MS, Anderson VM. Pericardial effusion and its relationship to cardiac disease in children with acquired immunodeficiency syndrome. *Pediatr Radiol* 1992;22:548–551.

57. Heidenreich PA, Eisenberg MJ, Kee LL, et al. Pericardial effusion in AIDS: incidence and survival. *Circulation* 1995;92:3229–3234.

58. Guenter P, Muurahainene N, Simons G, et al. Relationships among nutritional status, disease

progression, and survival in HIV infection. *J Acquir Immune Defic Syndr* 1993;6:1130–1138.

59. Stotka JL, Good CB, Downer WR, Kapoor WN. Pericardial effusion and tamponade due to Kaposi's sarcoma in acquired immunodeficiency syndrome. *Chest* 1989;951:1359–1361.

60. Lafont A, Darwiche H, Sayegh F, et al. At which stage of human immunodeficiency virus infection is echocardiography useful in diagnosing cardiac injury? [Abstract]. *Circulation* 1988;78:II458.

61. Steffen HM, Muller R, Schrappe-Bacher M, et al. The heart in HIV-infection: preliminary results of a prospective echocardiographic investigation. *Acta Cardiol* 1990;45:529–535.

62. Levy WS, Barghese PJ, Anderson DW, et al. Myocarditis diagnosed by endomyocardial biopsy in human immunodeficiency virus infection wtih cardiac dysfunction. *Am J Cardiol* 1988;62:658–659.

63. Mitchell P, Dodek P, Lawson L, et al. Torsades de pointes during intravenous pentamidine isethionate therapy. *Can Med Assoc J* 1989;140:173–174.

64. Pujol M, Carratala J, Mauri J, Viladrich P. Ventricular tachycardia due to pentamidine isethionate. *Am J Med* 1988;84:980.

65. Stein KM, Haronian H, Mensah GA, et al. Ventricular tachycardia and torsades de pointes complicating pentamidine therapy of *Pneumocystis carinii* pneumonia in the acquired immunodeficiency syndrome. *Am J Cardiol* 1990;66:888–890.

66. Stein KM, Fenton C, Lehany AM, et al. Incidence of QT interval prolongation during pentamidine therapy of *Pneumocystis carinii* pneumonia. *Am J Cardiol* 1991;68:1091–1094.

67. Wharton JM, Demopulos PA, Goldschlager N. Torsades de pointes during administration of pentamidine isethionate. *Am J Med* 1987;83:571–576.

68. Cohen AJ, Weiser B, Afzal Q, Fuhrer J. Ventricular tachycardia in two patients with AIDS receiving ganciclovir (DHPG). *AIDS* 1990;4:807–809.

69. Freeman R, Roberts MS, Friedman LS, Broadbridge C. Autonomic function and human immunodeficiency virus infection. *Neurology* 1990;40:575–580.

70. Craddock C, Bull R, Pasvol G, et al. Cardiorespiratory arrest and autonomic neuropathy in AIDS. *Lancet* 1987;2:16–18.

71. Lipshultz SE, Luginbuhl LM, Saul P, McIntosh K. Dysrhythmias, unexpected arrest and sudden death in pediatric HIV infection. [Abstract]. *Circulation* 1991;84:II-660.

72. Xiu RJ, Jun C, Berglund O. Microcirculatory disturbances in AIDS patients: a first report. *Microvasc Res* 1991;42:151–159.

73. Bharati S, Joshi VV, Connor EM, et al. Conduction system in children with acquired immunodeficiency syndrome. *Chest* 1989;96:406–413.

74. Tabib A, Greenland T, Mercier I, et al. Coronary lesions in young HIV-positive subjects at necropsy. *Lancet* 1992;340:730.

75. Berger JR, Harris JO, Gregorios J, Norenberg M. Cardiovascular disease in AIDS: a case-control study. *AIDS* 1990;4:239–244.

76. Boggian K, Leu HJ, Schneider J, et al. True aneurysm of the ascending aorta in HIV infection. *Schweiz Med Wochenschr* 1994;124:2083–2087.

77. Carrel T. True aneurysm of the ascending aorta in HIV infections. [Letter]. *Schweiz Med Wochenschr* 1995;125:706–707.

78. Schwartz ND, So YT, Hollander H, et al. Eosinophilic vasculitis leading to amaurosis fugax in a patient with acquired immunodeficiency syndrome. *Arch Intern Med* 1986;146:2059–2060.

79. Yoganathan K, Goodman F, Pozniak A. Kawasaki-like syndrome in an HIV positive adult. *J Infection* 1995;30:165–166.

80. Porneuf M, Sotto A. Kawasaki syndrome in an adult AIDS patient. *Int J Dermatol* 1996;35:292–294.

81. Aladhami SMS, Arrowsmith WA, Ingis J, Madlom MM. A young child with Kawasaki syndrome and AIDS. *Lancet* 1996;347:912–913.

82. Aris A, Pomar ML, Saur E. Cardiopulmonary bypass in HIV-positive patients. *Ann Thorac Surg* 1993;55:1104–1108.

83. Lewis W, Lipsick J, Cammarosano C. Cryptococcal myocarditis in acquired immune deficiency syndrome. *Am J Cardiol* 1985;55:1238–1239.

84. Steigman CK, Anderson DW, Macher AM, et al. Fatal cardiac tamponade in acquired immunodeficiency syndrome with epicardial Kaposi's sarcoma. *Am Heart J* 1988;116:1105–1106.

85. Silver MA, Macher AM, Reichert CM, et al. Cardiac involvement by Kaposi's sarcoma in acquired immune deficiency syndrome (AIDS). *Am J Cardiol* 1984;53:983–985.

86. Autran BR, Gorin I, Leibowitz M, et al. AIDS in a Haitian woman with cardiac Kaposi's sarcoma and Whipple's disease. *Lancet* 1983;1:767–768.

87. Moskowitz L, Hensley GT, Chan JC, Adams K. Immediate causes of death in acquired immunodeficiency syndrome. *Arch Pathol* 1985;109: 735–738.

88. Ambros RA, Lee E-Y, Sharer LR, et al. The acquired immunodeficiency syndrome in intravenous drug abusers and patients with a sexual risk. *Hum Pathol* 1987;18:1109–1114.

89. Welch K, Finkbeiner W, Alpers CE, et al. Autopsy findings in the acquired immune deficiency syndrome. *JAMA* 1984;252:1152–1159.

90. Guarner J, Brynes RK, Chan WC, et al. Primary non-Hodgkin's lymphoma of the heart in two patients with the acquired immunodeficiency syndrome. *Arch Pathol* 1987;111:254–256.

91. Balasubramanyam A, Waxman M, Kazal HL, Lee MH. Malignant lymphoma of the heart in acquired immune deficiency syndrome. *Chest* 1986;90: 243–246.

92. Kelsey RC, Saker A, Morgan M. Cardiac lymphoma in a patient with AIDS. *Ann Intern Med* 1991;115:370–371.

93. Andress JD, Polish LB, Clark DM, Hossack KF. Transvenous biopsy diagnosis of cardiac lymphoma in an AIDS patient. *Am Heart J* 1989;118: 421–423.

94. Constantino A, West TE, Gupta M, Loghmanee F. Primary cardiac lymphoma in a patient with acquired immune deficiency syndrome. *Cancer* 1987;60:2801–2805.

95. Ioachim HL, Cooper MC, Hellman GC. Lymphomas in men at high risk for acquired immune deficiency syndrome (AIDS): a study of 21 cases. *Cancer* 1985;56:2831–2842.

96. Holladay AO, Siegel RJ, Schwartz DA. Cardiac malignant lymphoma in acquired immune deficiency syndrome. *Cancer* 1992;70:2203–2207.

97. Schuster M, Valentine F, Holzman R. Cryptococcal pericarditis in an intravenous drug user. *J Infect Dis* 1985;153:842.

98. Factor SM. Acquired immune deficiency syndrome: the heart of the matter. *J Am Coll Cardiol* 1989;13:1037–1038.

99. Niedt GW, Schinella RA. Acquired immunodeficiency syndrome: clinicopathologic study of 56 autopsies. *Arch Pathol* 1985;109:727–734.

100. Henochowicz S, Mustafa M, Lawinson WE, et al. Cardiac aspergillosis in acquired immune deficiency syndrome. *Am J Cardiol* 1985;55:1239–1240.

101. Lafont A, Wolff M, Marche C, et al. Overwhelming myocarditis due to *Cryptococcus neoformans* in an AIDS patient. *Lancet* 1981;1145:1146–1140.

102. Brivet F, Livertowski J, Herve P, et al. Pericardial cryptococcal disease in acquired immune deficiency syndrome. [Letter]. *Am J Med* 1987;821: 1273–1270.

103. Grange F, Kinney EL, Monsuez JJ, et al. Successful therapy for *Toxoplasma gondii* myocarditis in acquired immunodeficiency syndrome. *Am Heart J* 1990;120:443–444.

104. Guarda LA, Luna MA, Smith LJ, et al. Acquired immune deficiency syndrome: postmortem findings. *Am J Clin Pathol* 1984;81:549–557.

105. Adair OV, Randive N, Krashow N. Isolated toxoplasma myocarditis in acquired immune deficiency syndrome. *Am Heart J* 1989;118:856–857.

106. Klatt EC, Nichols L, Noguchi TT. Evolving trends revealed by autopsies of patients with the acquired immunodeficiency syndrome. *Arch Pathol* 1994; 118:884–890.

107. Hofman P, Michiels JF, Rosenthal E, et al. Myocardite aigue à *Staphylococcus aureus* au cours du SIDA. *Arch Mal Coeur* 1993;86:1765–1768.

108. Wu TC, Pizzorno MC, Hayward GS, et al. In situ detection of human cytomegalovirus immediate-early gene transcripts within cardiac myocytes of patients with HIV-associated cardiomyopathy. *AIDS* 1992;6:777–785.

109. Nathan PE, Arsula EL, Zappi M. Pericarditis with tamponade due to cytomegalovirus in the acquired immunodeficiency syndrome. *Chest* 1991;99: 765–766.

110. Hsia J, Adams S, Ross AM. Natural history of human immunodeficiency virus (HIV) associated heart disease. *Circulation* 1991;84:2–3.

111. Herskowitz A, Willoughby SB, Baughman KL, et al. Cardiomyopathy associated with antiretroviral therapy in patients with HIV infection: a report of six cases. *Ann Intern Med* 1992;116:311–313.

112. Wilkins CE, Sexton DJ, McAllister HA. HIV-associated myocarditis treated with zidovudine (AZT). *Tex Heart Inst J* 1989;16:44–46.

113. Simpson MV, Chin CD, Keilbaugh SA, et al. Studies on the inhibition of mitochondrial DNA replication by 3′-azido–3′-deoxythymidine and other dideoxynucleoside analogs which inhibit HIV-1 replication. *Biochem Pharmacol* 1989;38:1033–1036.

114. Dworkin BM, Antonecchia PP, Smith F, et al. Reduced cardiac selenium content in the acquired immunodeficiency syndrome. *J Parenter Enter Nutr* 1989;13:644–647.

115. Baum MK, Mantero-Atienza E, Shor-Posner G, et al. Association of vitamin B_6 status with parameters of immune function in early HIV-1 infection. *J Acquir Immune Defic Syndr* 1991;4:1122–1132.

116. Lahdevirta J, Maury CPJ, Teppo A-M, Repo H. Elevated levels of circulating cachectin/tumor necrosis factor in patients with acquired immunodeficiency syndrome. *Am J Med* 1988;85:289–291.

117. Beutler B. The presence of cachectin/tumor necrosis factor in human disease states. *Am J Med* 1988;85:287–288.

118. Miller TL, Winter HS, Orav EJ, et al. Preservation of cardiac function and mass in pediatric HIV infection accompanied by skeletal muscle wasting and malnutrition. [Abstract]. *Pediatr Res* 1990; 27:177A.

119. De Palo VA, Millstein BH, Mayo PH, et al. Outcome of intensive care in patients with HIV infection. *Chest* 1995;107:506–510.

120. Graettinger JS, Parsons RL, Campbell JA. A correlation of clinical and hemodynamic studies in patients with mild and severe anemia with and without congestive failure. *Ann Intern Med* 1963;58: 617–626.

121. Duke M, Abelmann WH. The hemodynamic response to chronic anemia. *Circulation* 1969;39: 503–515.

122. Cegielski JP, Lwakatare J, Dukes CS, et al. Tuberculous pericarditis in Tanzanian patients with and without HIV infection. *Tuber Lung Dis* 1994; 75:429–434.

123. Dworkin BM. Selenium deficiency in HIV infection and the acquired immunodeficiency syndrome (AIDS). *Chem-Biol Interact* 1994;181:186–180.

124. De Simone C, Tzantzoglou S, Santini G, et al. Clinical and immunologic effects of combination therapy with intravenous immunoglobulins and AZT in HIV-infected patients. *Immunopharmacol Immunotoxicol* 1991;13:447–458.

125. Grenier MA, Karr SS, Rakusan TA, Martin GR. Cardiac disease in children with HIV: relationshiip of cardiac disease to HIV symptomatology. *Pediatr AIDS HIV Infect* 1994;5:174–179.

126. Vogel RL. Cardiac manifestations of pediatric acquired immunodeficiency syndrome. In: Yogev R, Connor E (eds). *Management of HIV Infection in Infants and Children*. St. Louis, MO: Mosby-Year Book, 1992:357–370.

127. Vogel RL, Alboliras ET, McSherry GD, et al. Congenital heart defects in children of human immunodeficiency virus positive mothers. [Abstract]. *Circulation* 1988;78:II–17.

128. Tripp ME, McKinney RE, Katz SL. Cardiac complications of human immunodeficiency virus (HIV) infection in children. *Pediatr Res* 1993; 33:185A.

129. Bestetti RB. Cardiac involvement in the acquired immune deficiency syndrome. *Int J Cardiol* 1989; 22:143–146.

130. Johnson JE, Slife DM, Anders GT, et al. Cardiac dysfunction in patients seropositive for the human immunodeficiency virus. *West J Med* 1991;155: 373–379.

131. Kaminski HJ, Katzman M, Wiest PM, et al. Cardiomyopathy associated with the acquired immune deficiency syndrome. *J Acquir Immune Defic Syndr* 1988;1:105–110.

132. Kaul S, Fishbein MC, Siegel RJ. Cardiac manifestations of acquired immune deficiency syndrome: a 1991 update. *Am Heart J* 1991;122:535–544.

133. Kinney EL. Cardiac findings in AIDS. *Chest* 1988; 94:1113–1114.

134. Luginbuhl LM, Orav EJ, McIntosh K, Lipshultz SE. Cardiac morbidity and related mortality in children with HIV infection. *JAMA* 1993;269: 2869–2875.

135. Grenier MA, Karr SS, Rakusan TA, Martin GR. Cardiac disease in children with human immunodeficiency virus: relationship of cardiac disease to virus symptoms. [Abstract]. *Pediatr Res* 1993; 33:21A.

136. Al-Attar I, Orav EJ, Exil V, Lipshultz SE. Predictors of cardiac morbidity and related mortality in children with the acquired immunodeficiency syndrome. [Abstract]. *Pediatr Res* 1995;37:169A.

137. Domanski MJ, Sloas MM, Follmann DA, et al. Effect of zidovudine and didanosine treatment on heart function in children infected with human immunodeficiency virus. *J Pediatr* 1995;127: 137–146.

138. Sherron P, Pickoff AS, Ferrer PL, et al. Echocardiographic evaluation of myocardial function in pediatric AIDS patients. [Abstract]. *Am Heart J* 1985;110:710.

139. Issenberg HJ, Charytan M, Rubinstein A. Cardiac involvement in children with acquired immune deficiency. *Am Heart J* 1985;710.

140. Kavanaugh-McHugh AL, Rowe SA, Hutton N, et al. Prevalence of cardiac involvement in human immunodeficiency virus (HIV) infection. [Abstract]. *Pediatr Res* 1991;29:176A.

141. Starc TJ, Lipshultz S, Easley K, et al. Cardiac complications in HIV infected children: the NHLBI P2C2 study. [Abstract]. *Pediatr Res* 1995; 37:189A.

142. Lipshultz SE, Easley K, Kaplan S, et al. Abnormal left ventricular structure and function shortly after birth in infants of HIV-infected mothers: the prospective NHLBI P2C2 study. *Circulation* 1995; 92:I–581.

143. Lipshultz SE, Pediatric Pulmonary and Cardiovascular Complications of Vertically Transmitted HIV Infection Study G. Progressive cardiac dysfunction in HIV-infected children: the prospective NHLBI P2C2 HIV study. [Abstract]. *Proc Int Conf AIDS* 1993;9:48.

144. Ruga E, Cozzani S, Secchieri S, et al. Cardiac abnormalities and HIV infection: follow-up of forty-one pediatric patients. [Abstract]. *Proc Int Conf AIDS* 1993;9:463.

145. Dollfus C, Bancillon A, Tillous-Borde I, Lasfargues G. Cardiac abnormalities and immunologic status in children with HIV infection treated with zidovudine. [Abstract]. *Proc Int Conf AIDS* 1993;9:463.

146. De Simone C, Tzantzoglou S, Jirillo E, et al. L-Carnitine deficiency in AIDS patients. *AIDS* 1992;6:203–205.

147. Lipshultz SE, Sanders SP, Colan SD, McIntosh K. Enhanced cardiac function in pediatric HIV infection. [Abstract]. *Proc Int Conf AIDS* 1989; 5:311.

148. Issenberg HJ, Cho S, Rubinstein A. Cardiac pathology in children with acquired immune deficiency syndrome. [Abstract]. *Pediatr Res* 1986; 20:295A.

149. Kavanaugh-McHugh AL, Hutton N, Holt E, et al. Echocardiographic abnormalities in pediatric HIV infection: prevalence and serial changes. [Abstract]. *Pediatr Res* 1992;31:166A.

150. Lipshultz SE, Luginbuhl LM, McIntosh K, Orav EJ. Cardiac morbidity and mortality in children with symptomatic HIV infection. [Abstract]. *Circulation* 1992;86:I–362.

151. Lipshultz S, Fox CH, Perez-Atayde AR, et al. Identification of human immunodeficiency virus-1 RNA and DNA in the heart of a child with cardiovascular abnormalities and congenital acquired immune deficiency syndrome. *Am J Cardiol* 1990;66:246–250.

152. De Simone L, Galli L, Manetti A, et al. Long-term cardiac follow-up in children with perinatal HIV 1 infection. [Abstract]. *Proc STD World Congr* 1992;3:B205.

153. Lipshultz SE, Orav EJ, Sanders SP, et al. Cardiac structure and function in children with human immunodeficiency virus infection treated with zidovudine. *N Engl J Med* 1992;327:1260–1265.

154. Lipshultz SE, Miller TL, Orav EJ, McIntosh K. Exaggerated myocardial hypertrophic responses in pediatric HIV infection. [Abstract]. *Circulation* 1990;82:III-11.

155. Kavanaugh-McHugh AL, Ruff AJ, Rowe SA, et al. Cardiac abnormalities in a multicenter interventional study of children with symptomatic HIV infection. *Pediatr Res* 1991;28:1040.

156. Bharati S, Lev M. Pathology of the heart in AIDS. *Prog Cardiol* 1989;2:261–272.

157. Chanock S, Luginbuhl LM, McIntosh K, Lipshultz SE. Life-threatening reactions to trimethoprim–sulfamethoxazole in children with HIV infection. *Pediatrics* 1994;93:519–521.

158. Kovacs A, Hinton D, Wong W, et al. HIV infection of myocytes and sudden death in pediatric AIDS. *Pediatr Res* 1992;31:167A.

159. Kind C, Brandle B, Wyler CA, et al. Epidemiology of vertically transmitted HIV-1 infection in Switzerland: results of a nationwide prospective study. *Eur J Pediatr* 1992;151:442–448.

160. Bulterys M, Lepage P, Hitimana DG, et al. Sudden infant death among children born to women with human immunodeficiency virus type 1 infection. *Pediatr Infect Dis J* 1993;12:172–170.

161. European Collaborative Study. Children born to women with HIV-1 infection: natural history and risk of transmission. *Lancet* 1991;337:253–250.

162. Raviglione MC, Battan R, Taranta A. Cardiopulmonary resuscitation in patients with the acquired immunodeficiency syndrome. *Arch Intern Med* 1988;148:2602–2605.

163. Cohen J, Laudenslager M. Autonomic nervous system dysfunction in human immunodeficiency virus. *Neurology* 1989;8:111–112.

164. Ruttimann S, Hilti P, Spinas GA, Dubach UC. High frequency of human immunodeficiency virus-associated autonomic neuropathy and more severe involvement in advanced stages of human

immunodeficiency virus disease. *Arch Intern Med* 1991;151:2441–2443.

165. Ioachim HL, Adsay V, Giancotti FR, et al. Kaposi's sarcoma of internal organs: a multiparameter study of 86 cases. *Cancer* 1995;75:1376–1385.

166. Lipshultz SE, Sanders SP, Colan SD, McIntosh K. Enhanced left ventricular function in pediatric human immunodeficiency virus infection. [Abstract]. *Pediatr Res* 1989;25:153A.

167. Lipshultz SE, Chanock S, Sanders SP, et al. Cardiac manifestations of pediatric human immunodeficiency virus (HIV) infection. [Abstract]. *Circulation* 1987;76:IV-515.

168. Lipshultz SE, Sanders SP, Colan SD, et al. The use of left ventricular fractional shortening as an index of contractility in HIV-infected children. [Abstract]. *Am J Cardiol* 1990;66:521.

169. Lipshultz SE, Bancroft EA, Boller A-M. Cardiovascular manifestations of HIV infection in children. In: Bricker JT (ed). *The Science and Practice of Pediatric Cardiology.* Baltimore: Williams & Wilkins, 1996.

170. Paton P, Tabib A, Loire R, Tete R. Coronary artery lesions and human immunodeficiency virus infection. *Res Virol* 1993;144:225–231.

171. Husson RN, Saini R, Lewis LL, et al. Cerebral artery aneurysms in children infected with human immunodeficiency virus. *J Pediatr* 1992;121:927–930.

172. Park YD, Belman AL, Kim TS, et al. Stroke in pediatric acquired immunodeficiency syndrome. *Ann Neurol* 1990;28:303–311.

173. Nigro G, Pisano P, Krzysztofiak A. A recurrent Kawasaki disease associated with coinfection with parvovirus B19 and HIV-1. *AIDS* 1993;7:288–290.

174. Lipshultz SE, Easley K, Kaplan S, et al. The relation between progressive immune dysfunction and ventricular dysfunction: the prospective NHLBI P_2C_2 study. *Proc Natl Conf Retrov* 1995;2:90.

175. Lobato MN, Caldwell B, Ng P, Oxtoby MJ. Encephalopathy in children with perinatally acquired human immunodeficiency virus infection. *J Pediatr* 1995;126:710–715.

176. Towbin JA, Ni J, Demmler G, et al. Evidence for adenovirus as a common cause of myocarditis in children using polymerase chain reaction (PCR). [Abstract]. *Pediatr Res* 1993;33:27A.

177. Dittrich H, Chow L, Denaro F, Spector S. Human immunodeficiency virus, coxsackievirus, and cardiomyopathy. *Ann Intern Med* 1988;108:308–309.

178. Freedberg RS, Gindea AJ, Dieterich DT, Greene JB. Herpes simplex pericarditis in AIDS. *NY State J Med* 1987;87:304–306.

179. McClain KL, Leach CT, Jenson HB, et al. Association of Epstein-Barr virus with leiomyosarcomas in young people with AIDS. *N Engl J Med* 1995;332:12–18.

180. Gesner M, Pollack H, Lawrence R, et al. Clinical and laboratory correlates of *Mycobacterium avium* infection (MAI) in HIV-infected children. [Abstract]. *Pediatr Res* 1992;31:163A.

181. Scott GB, Hutto C, Makuch RW, et al. Survival in children with perinatally acquired human immunodeficiency virus type 1 infection. *N Engl J Med* 1989;321:1791–1796.

182. Medlock MD, Tilleli JT, Pearl GS. Congenital cardiac toxoplasmosis in a newborn with acquired immunodeficiency syndrome. *Pediatr Infect Dis J* 1990;9:129–132.

183. Levi G, Patrizio M, Bernardo A, et al. Human immunodeficiency virus coat protein gp120 inhibits the adrenergic regulation of astroglial and microglial functions. *Proc Natl Acad Sci USA* 1993;90:1541–1545.

184. Al-Attar I, Orav EJ, Exil V, et al. Survival patterns of pediatric patients with the acquired immunodeficiency syndrome. *Pediatr Res* 1995;37:169A.

185. Bierman FS. Guidelines for diagnosis and management of cardiac disease in children with HIV infection. *J Pediatr* 1991;119:S53-S56.

186. Sztajzel J, Doat M, Ricou F, et al. Heart involvement in asymptomatic HIV patients. [Abstract]. *Int Conf AIDS* 1993;9:66.

187. Mota-Miranda A, Cardoso S, Gomes HM, et al. Heart involvement in HIV disease. *Proc STD World Congr* 1992;3:B124.

188. Croft NM, Jacob AJ, Godman MJ, et al. Cardiac dysfunction in paediatric HIV infection. *J Infect* 1993;26:191–194.

189. Johnson JE, Anders GT, Blanton HM, et al. Exercise dysfunction in patients seropositive for the human immunodeficiency virus. *Am Rev Respir Dis* 1990;141:618–622.

190. Lipshultz SE, Sanders SP, Colan SD. Cardiac structure and function in HIV-infected children (response). *N Engl J Med* 1993;328:513–514.

191. Goldfarb A, King CL, Rosenzweig BP, et al. Cardiac lymphoma in the acquired immunodeficiency syndrome. *Am Heart J* 1989;118:1340–1344.

192. Walsh CA, Better D, Adam HM, et al. Holter monitor and ECG abnormalities in children with HIV. [Abstract]. *Am J Dis Child* 1990;144:434.

193. Kinlay S, Leitch JW, Neil A, et al. Cardiac event recorders yield more diagnoses and are more cost-effective than 48-hour Holter monitoring in patients with palpitations. *Ann Intern Med* 1996; 124:16–20.

194. Galli FC, Cheitlin MD. Pericardial disease in AIDS: frequency of tamponade and therapeutic and diagnostic use of pericardiocentesis. [Abstract]. *J Am Coll Cardiol* 1992;19:266A.

195. Deyton LR, Walker RE, Kovacs JA, et al. Reversible cardiac dysfunction associated with interferon alfa therapy in AIDS patients with Kaposi's sarcoma. *N Engl J Med* 1989;321:1246–1249.

196. Venable RS, Yanda RL. Cardiopulmonary manifestations in HIV-infected patients. *Top Emerg Med* 1994;16:17–23.

197. Dalli E, Quesada A, Gustavo J, et al. Tuberculous pericarditis as the first manifestation of acquired immunodeficiency syndrome. *Am Heart J* 1987; 114:905–906.

198. Hsia J, Ross AM. Pericardial effusion and pericardiocentesis in human immunodeficiency virus infection. *Am J Cardiol* 1994;74:94–96.

199. DeMaria A. President's page: ethical activism. *J Am Coll Cardiol* 1988;12:1146–1147.

200. Lipshultz SE, Orav EJ, Sanders SP, Colan SD. Immunoglobulins and left ventricular structure and function in pediatric HIV-infection. *Circulation* 1995;92:2220–2225.

201. Acierno LJ. Cardiac complications in acquired immunodeficiency syndrome. *J Am Coll Cardiol* 1989;13:1144–1154.

202. Conte JE Jr, Hollander H, Golden JA. Inhaled or reduced-dose intravenous pentamidine for *Pneumocystis carinii* pneumonia. *Ann Intern Med* 1987; 107:495–498.

203. Loescher T, Loeschke K, Niebel J. Severe ventricular arrhythmia during pentamidine treatment of AIDS-associated *Pneumocystis carinii* pneumonia. *Infection* 1987;15:455–450.

204. Balslev U, Berild D, Nielsen TL. Cardiac arrest during treatment of *Pneumocystis carinii* pneumonia with intravenous pentamidine isethionate. *Scand J Infect Dis* 1992;24:111–112.

205. Eisenhauer MD, Eliasson AH, Taylor AJ, et al. Incidence of cardiac arrhythmias during intravenous pentamidine therapy in HIV-infected patients. *Chest* 1994;105:389–394.

206. Harel H, Scott WA, Szeinberg A, Barzilay Z. Pentamidine-induced torsades de pointes. *Pediatr Infect Dis J* 1993;12:692–694.

207. Miller HC. Cardiac arrest after intravenous pentamidine in an infant. *Pediatr Infect Dis J* 1993; 12:694–696.

208. Thalhammer E, Arasteh K, Hess F, et al. Systemic pentamidine therapy induces QT-prolongation. [Abstract]. *Proc STD World Congr* 1992;3:B140.

209. Dworkin BM, Rosenthal WS, Wormser GP, Weiss L. Selenium deficiency in the acquired immunodeficiency syndrome. *J Parenter Enter Nutr* 1986; 10:405–407.

210. Albrecht H, Stellbrink HJ, Fenske S, et al. Successful treatment of *Toxoplasma gondii* myocarditis in an AIDS patient. *Eur J Clin Microbiol Infect Dis* 1994;13:500–504.

211. Kinney EL, Monsuez JJ, Kitzis M, Vittecoq DE. Treatment of AIDS-associated heart disease. *J Vasc Dis* 1989;40:970–976.

212. Barst RJ, Rubin LJ, Long WA, et al. Comparison of continuous intravenous epoprostenol (prostacyclin) with conventional therapy for primary pulmonary hypertension. *N Engl J Med* 1996;334: 296–301.

213. Mofenson LM, Moye JJr, Bethel J, et al. Prophylactic intravenous immunoglobulin in HIV-infected children with CD4+ counts of 0.20×10^6/ L or more: effect on viral, opportunistic, and bacterial infection. *JAMA* 1992;268:483–488.

214. Drucker NA, Colan SD, Wessel DL, et al. Use of intravenous gamma globulin in acute congestive cardiomyopathy. [Abstract]. *Circulation* 1992; 86:I–363.

215. Newburger JW, Sanders SP, Burns JC, et al. Left ventricular contractility and function in Kawasaki syndrome: effect of intravenous γ-globulin. *Circulation* 1989;79:1237–1246.

216. Viard J-P, Vittecoq D. Response of HIV-1-associated polymyositis to intravenous immunoglobulin. *Am J Med* 1992;92:580–581.

217. National Institute of Child Health and Human Development Intravenous Immunoglobulin Study Group. Intravenous immune globulin for the prevention of bacterial infections in children. *N Engl J Med* 1991;325:73–80.

218. Mofenson LM, Moye J, Bethel J, et al. Prophylactic intravenous immunoglobulin in HIV-infected children with CD4+ counts of $0.20 \times 10^9/l$ or more. *JAMA* 1992;268:483–488.

219. Kavanaugh-McHugh AL, Ruff A, Perlman E, et al. Selenium deficiency and cardiomyopathy in acquired immunodeficiency syndrome. *J Parenter Enter Nutr* 1991;15:347–349.

220. Waber LJ, Valle D, Neill C, et al. Carnitine deficiency presenting as familial cardiomyopathy: a treatable defect in carnitine transport. *J Pediatr* 1982;101:700–705.

221. Herskowitz A, Willoughby SB, Ansari AA, et al. High risk profile for the development of congestive heart failure in HIV-related cardiomyopathy. [Abstract]. *Circulation* 1991;84:II-I3.

222. Lemma M, Vanelli P, Botta BM, et al. Cardiac surgery in HIV-positive intravenous drug addicts: influence of cardiopulmonary bypass on the progression to AIDS. *Thorac Cardiovasc Surg* 1992; 40:279–282.

223. Uva MS, Jebara VA, Fabiani JN, et al. Cardiac surgery in patients with human immunodeficiency virus infection: indications and results. *J Cardiac Surg* 1992;7:240–244.

224. Horowitz MD, Cox MM, Neibart RM, et al. Resection of right atrial lymphoma in a patient with AIDS. *Int J Cardiol* 1992;34:139–142.

225. Petitpretz P, Brenot F, Azarian R, et al. Pulmonary hypertension in patients with human immunodeficiency virus infection: comparison with primary pulmonary hypertension. *Circulation* 1994; 89:2722–2727.

226. Akhras F, Dubrey S, Gazzard B, Noble MIM. Emerging patterns of heart disease in HIV infected homosexual subjects with and without opportunistic infections; a prospective colour flow Doppler echocardiographic study. *Eur Heart J* 1994;15: 68–75.

227. Lipshultz SE for the P_2C_2 Study Group. Cardiac dysfunction predicts mortality in HIV-infected children. The Prospective NHLBI P_2C_2 Study. [Abstract]. *Proc Conf Retrovir Opportun Infect* 1996;65:415.

228. Kavanaugh-McHugh AL, Ruff AJ, Rowe SA, et al. Cardiac abnormalities in a multicenter interventional study of children with symptomatic HIV infection. [Abstract]. *Pediatr Res* 1991; 29:176A.

Part 4
Diagnosis and Management

25

Cardiac Therapeutics in HIV-Infected Patients

Amy L. Giantris and Steven E. Lipshultz, M.D.

Symptomatic heart disease is common in children and adults infected with human immunodeficiency virus (HIV), as illustrated elsewhere in this book. Cardiac involvement can occur at any stage of HIV infection and may be difficult to diagnose clinically. Further, cardiac involvement may be life-threatening, even though it is generally not clinically significant. Progressive left ventricular dysfunction and congestive heart failure are the most prominent and threatening cardiac complications in HIV-infected patients. Arrhythmias are also of significant concern for these patients. Although therapeutic intervention for cardiac complications may not prolong life in HIV-infected patients, prompt initiation of treatment usually helps to alleviate symptoms and improve the patient's quality of life.

Therapy for many of the cardiac complications encountered by HIV-infected patients is similar to that for noninfected patients, and as with noninfected patients, it is essential to reassess the accuracy of diagnosis and the efficacy of therapy frequently. This chapter discusses therapeutic options for cardiac problems that may occur during the course of HIV infection, including adverse effects of treatment, drug dosages, toxicities, and relevant drug interactions, with an emphasis on outpatient care. We review some of the nonpharmaceutical therapeutic measures involving lifestyle modifica-

tions and supportive care. Finally, this chapter addresses the pharmacologic management of asymptomatic left ventricular function and congestive heart failure, and makes recommendations for immunoglobulin, immunosuppressive, antiarrhythmic, antiinfective, antihypertensive, and micronutrient replacement therapies.

Treatment of Asymptomatic Left Ventricular Dysfunction

Left ventricular dysfunction is emerging as the most important cardiac manifestation of HIV infection for both adult and pediatric populations[1-9] and can be an early indicator of congestive heart failure.[9-13] Autopsy studies indicate that up to 25% of HIV-infected adults have dilated cardiomyopathy[14] and up to 52% have myocarditis[9,15] at death. There are fewer data on cardiac disease in HIV-infected children than in HIV-infected adults.[8] However, the preliminary results of the Prospective Pediatric Pulmonary and Cardiovascular Complications of Vertically Transmitted HIV Infection Study (P²C²) noted that depressed left ventricular function was common and progressive in children without clinically apparent congestive heart failure.[16] The left ventricular dysfunction was due both to intrinsic cardiomyopathy (depressed contractility) and to factors that were either intrinsic or extrinsic to the heart (e.g., elevated afterload). In another study evaluating zidovudine, serial echocardiographic studies of 88 children with advanced symptomatic HIV infection showed that 21% had decreased left ventricular dysfunction and 34% had ventricular dilitation; 14% of these children required medical therapy for cardiac abnormalities.[17]

In addition, left ventricular dysfunction related to therapy for HIV infection has been noted in the literature. Foscarnet therapy for cytomegalovirus infection in an adult with acquired immunodeficiency syndrome (AIDS) was associated with reversible episodes of congestive heart failure.[18] Interferon alpha therapy was correlated with the development of reversible congestive cardiomyopathy in three adults with AIDS and Kaposi's sarcoma.[19] Life-threatening reactions requiring cardiopulmonary resuscitation after the administration of trimethoprim–sulfamethoxazole occurred in HIV-infected children.[20,21] These children had evidence of cardiac abnormalities before receiving the medication, suggesting a hyperadrenergic state. These children also had had a recent cutaneous reaction to this drug. It has also been suggested that systemic corticosteroids, used to treat some infected children, may result in ventricular hypertrophy and ventricular dysfunction.[22] Conflicting reports of various studies suggest that the potential cardiotoxic effects of zidovudine are not clearly defined. One study suggests there is a relationship between the administration of zidovudine and improvement of ventricular function,[23] while others suggest the drug is associated with deterioration of function.[24,25] Still others maintain that zidovudine use can be associated with the preservation of ventricular function[26,27] and have shown patients to have normal left ventricular contractility during and following zidovudine therapy.[7,8]

Treatment Objectives

The primary goal of the treatment of left ventricular dysfunction is the prevention of further deterioration of left ventricular performance. Serial monitoring of left ventricular function in HIV-infected patients is critical both for the early diagnosis of cardiac dysfunction and for ruling it out. With a comprehensive cardiovascular history and a baseline cardiac physical examination, one can begin to differentiate between cardiac and noncardiac symptoms.[22] Echocardiography appears to be the most effective and routinely used noninvasive test for the evaluation of cardiac status. It provides information on ventricular function, chamber dimension, and the motion and composition of heart valves and other cardiac structures (such as the pericardium and the coronary arteries) that allows the clinician to diagnose abnormalities early. Studies have demonstrated the utility of echocardiograms in the management of HIV-infected patients.[28–30]

Assessment

The frequency of screening for the assessment of cardiac status varies among institutions. For asymptomatic HIV-infected infants and children at Children's Hospital in Boston, an echocardiogram is generally performed annually, and electrocardiographic (EKG) and Holter monitor examinations every 2 years. Symptomatic HIV-infected patients (e.g., presenting with lymphadenopathy, wasting, neurologic disease, serious infections, or malignancies) with no cardiac abnormalities generally receive an echocardiogram at 8-month intervals and an EKG and Holter monitor study annually. Symptomatic HIV-infected patients with cardiac abnormalities receive a baseline echocardiogram, EKG, and Holter monitor study, and subsequent examinations as clinically indicated. It is also recommended at this institution that baseline studies be performed at diagnosis of HIV infection. A more detailed discussion of cardiac monitoring can be found in Chapter 24 of this book.

Treatment

Early treatment of left ventricular dysfunction with angiotensin-converting enzyme (ACE) inhibitors has been shown to have beneficial effects on the clinical course.[31–33] The ACE catalyzes two important reactions: the conversion of angiotensin I to angiotensin II, a strong vasoconstricting hormone, and the breakdown of bradykinin, a vasodilator agent. In addition to vasoconstriction, angiotensin II stimulates the release of aldosterone from the adrenal cortex, thereby inducing salt and water retention. The potential combined effect of these reactions is increased systemic vascular resistance and edema, which increase the physiologic demands on the heart. ACE inhibitors reduce the production of angiotensin II by inhibiting its conversion from angiotensin I. The overall effect of the drug is a reduction in systemic vascular resistance and arterial pressure through vasodilation, and the inhibition of salt and water retention by the kidneys, resulting in lower ventricular filling pressure, increased venous capacitance and increased cardiac output. It has been suggested that there may be effects on cellular growth in addition to alterations in vascular resistance levels[34] and neurohormonal alterations.[35] The findings of a Veterans Administration Cooperative Vasodilator Heart Failure Trial showed that the most beneficial response to ACE inhibition occurred in patients with neurohormonal activation, emphasizing the importance of the relationship between neurohormonal activity and mortality, and the relevance of neurohormonal blockade to improved survival.[36] Enalapril, captopril, and lisinopril are three of the most commonly administered drugs of the ACE inhibitor class.

Enalapril therapy can help reduce the likelihood of the otherwise intractable progression of severe left ventricular dysfunction to overt heart failure, according to results of the prevention arm of the National Heart, Lung and Blood Institute (NHLBI) Studies of Left Ventricular Dysfunction (SOLVD), a multicenter randomized trial of enalapril versus placebo in adults with ventricular dysfunction.[31] This study included 4,228 patients with left ventricular ejection fraction less than 35% and without manifest heart failure. A significant 37% reduction in the risk of developing heart failure with enalapril was noted, with the curves diverging early and continuing to diverge over the 48-month study (Figure 25-1). For every 1,000 patients treated, 90 were prevented from developing heart failure and 65 were prevented from being hospitalized during the study period.[31]

In this trial, adult patients were started on 2.5 mg twice daily and titrated as tolerated to a targeted daily dose of 20 mg, in divided doses. Other sources have published slightly different dosage regi-

mens.[37,38] No pediatric dosages have been specified by the manufacturer for the use of enalapril in the treatment of asymptomatic left ventricular function. Dosages for infants and children are generally based on weight. An oral dosage of 0.1 to 0.4 mg kg^{-1} day^{-1} has been suggested by one source,[38] although another has noted effective pediatric enalapril dosages.[39]

Similar results were obtained in another study of the efficacy of captopril in the prevention of further ventricular remodeling after myocardial enlargement in a group of patients with some systolic dysfunction but without severe left ventricular dilatation.[32] This Survival and Ventricular Enlargement (SAVE) trial demonstrated a significant reduction in overall mortality of 19% with captopril compared with placebo. The development of severe heart failure and hospitalization due to heart failure were also reduced by captopril.[32] These findings suggest that initiating treatment with an ACE inhibitor before any left ventricular dilatation occurs might be expected to prevent myocardial remodeling, resulting in improved survival. In this trial, the initial dosage of captopril was 6.25 mg three times daily. The dosage was increased to 25 mg and later to 50 mg three times daily.[32]

A randomized, double-blind, placebo-controlled trial with 6-week treatment periods examined the effects of another ACE inhibitor, lisinopril, in adults with untreated, symptom-free left ventricular systolic dysfunction.[33] Lisinopril significantly improved cardiac function as measured by an improvement in the cardiopulmonary response to exercise (e.g., increased peak oxygen consumption during exercise) compared with controls. However, lisinopril did not improve indices of cardiac function at rest.[33] In this study, asymptomatic adult patients received 10 mg lisinopril or matching placebo once daily by mouth.

It is recommended that the patient be observed under medical supervision for at least two hours after the initial ACE inhibitor dose and until blood pressure has stabilized for at least an hour. Also, the clinician may want to be aware of low carnitine, selenium, or thyroid levels during ACE inhibitor therapy. In such cases, replacement therapy is often administered. A cardiac examination (e.g., echocardiogram, EKG, and Holter monitor) before the

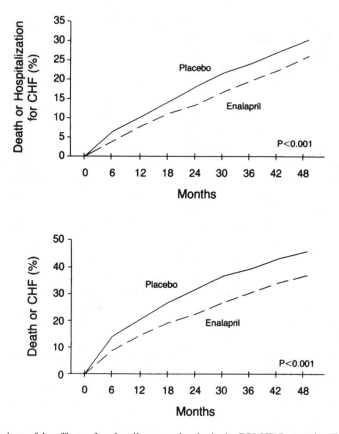

Figure 25-1. Comparison of the effects of enalapril versus placebo in the SOLVD Prevention Trial. **Top**: The number of patient deaths or hospitalizations for congestive heart failure. **Bottom**: The number of deaths or development of heart failure. Enalapril was associated with significant reductions in the incidence of heart failure and in deaths and hospitalizations due to heart failure. (From Ref. 31, with permission.)

initiation of ACE inhibitor therapy is recommended to assess baseline status. In addition, it is often useful for the patient's caregiver to be supplied with information regarding the signs and symptoms of congestive heart failure outlined later in this chapter so that patients can be regularly monitored for subtle changes from their baseline cardiac function.

Diuretics are not normally prescribed for the treatment of asymptomatic left ventricular dysfunction, because studies have shown them to be of greatest use for symptomatic relief. It is generally accepted that if mild symptoms develop (e.g., fatigue or exertional dyspnea without other overt signs of heart failure), the clinician may want to consider the addition of diuretics and/or digoxin therapy, as described below.

Anticongestive Treatment

Management of Symptomatic Left Ventricular Dysfunction and Congestive Heart Failure

General Aspects

In this chapter *congestive heart failure* refers to the inadequate perfusion of the body's tissues as a result of an abnormality of cardiac function. The heart fails to pump blood at the rate needed to meet the metabolic requirements of the body, including, in a child, the requirements of the growth process. For infants and children, respiratory distress and increased work of breathing resulting from heart failure produces a further increase in the metabolic requirements, which may worsen the metabolic deficit that he body must overcome before growth and weight gain can be established.[40]

Many reports have considered the frequency of cardiovascular involvement in HIV-infected adults.[1,4,15,27,41–43] The most frequently observed abnormalities include dilated cardiomyopathy and myocarditis.[4,6,15,27] One source concluded that dilated cardiomyopathy was a feature of advanced HIV disease and affected members of all major risk groups for HIV infection.[27] These cardiac abnormalities can progress to heart failure and can be associated with significant morbidity and mortality. Studies have demonstrated that cardiac function in HIV-infected adult patients can improve significantly with medical therapy.[11,31,44–46] In addition, HIV infection is likely to be the leading global cause of acquired cardiovascular disease in childhood at this time.[22] One source described two types of congestive heart failure in HIV-infected children.[12] The majority of the patients followed were children diagnosed with heart failure during severe, acute systemic illness. In general, these patients were later in the course of HIV infection, had a more fulminant course at the time of diagnosis with congestive heart failure, and died 2 months after the diagnosis of multisystem organ failure. A more indolent course, with survival for more than one year after diagnosis, resulted from prompt treatment of congestive heart failure during less severe illness. The quality of life was also significantly improved for these patients.

The management of heart failure presented in this chapter is a summarization of the recommendations made by both the consensus committee of the Canadian Cardiovascular Society's Consensus Conference and the expert panel for the Agency for Health Care Policy and Research Heart Failure Guidelines. These recommendations are based on a review of current studies of heart failure therapeutics. Figure 25-2 from the Canadian Cardiovascular Society's Consensus Conference shows an example of the treatment algorithm that can be used to determine the appropriate choice of therapeutic agents based on the clinical findings and the results of noninvasive tests. We recommend that this type of algorithm be used in conjunction with the nonpharmaceutical treatments summarized in this chapter.

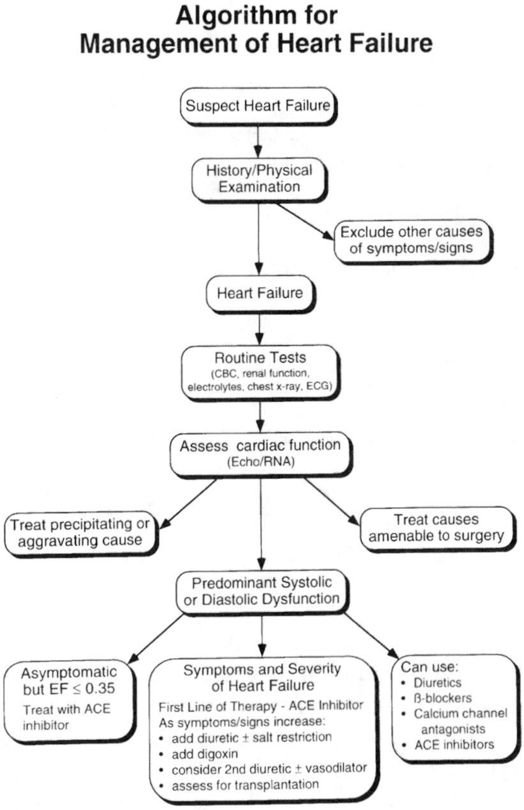

Although an extensive review of the pathophysiology and clinical manifestations of heart failure is beyond the scope of the chapter, a brief overview is warranted for the consideration of therapeutic options.

Algorithm for Management of Heart Failure

Figure 25-2. Algorithm for the management of heart failure as recommended by the Canadian Cardiovascular Society Consensus Conference on the Diagnosis and Management of Heart Failure. (Adapted from Ref. 47.)

Signs and Symptoms

The degree of symptoms of adult heart failure has been classified in the widely used New York Heart Association (NYHA) classification system found in Table 25-1. The Canadian Cardiovascular Society's Consensus Conference summarized these criteria as follows:[47]

Class I:	No symptoms
Class II:	Symptoms with ordinary activity
Class III:	Symptoms with less than ordinary activity
Class IV:	Symptoms at rest

Table 25-1. New York Heart Association Classification For Adults

Functional Capacity

Class I: Patients with cardiac disease but without resulting limitation of physical activity. Ordinary physical activity does not cause undue fatigue, palpitation, dyspnea, or anginal pain.

Class II: Patients with cardiac disease resulting in slight limitation of ordinary physical activity. They are comfortable at rest. Ordinary physical activity results in fatigue, palpitation, dyspnea, or anginal pain.

Class III: Patients with cardiac disease resulting in marked limitation of physical activity. They are comfortable at rest. Less than ordinary activity causes fatigue, palpitation, dyspnea, or anginal pain.

Class IV: Patients with cardiac disease resulting in inability to carry on any physical activity without discomfort. Symptoms of heart failure or of the anginal syndrome may be present even at rest. If any physical activity is undertaken, discomfort is increased.

Objective Assessment

A: No objective assessment of cardiovascular disease.
B: Objective evidence of minimal cardiovascular disease.
C: Objective evidence of moderately severe cardiovascular disease.
D: Objective evidence of severe cardiovascular disease.

From Ref. 158, with permission.

Symptoms in adults generally include peripheral edema, fatigue, dyspnea, orthopnea, nocturia, paroxysmal nocturnal dyspnea, cough, weight gain, abdominal discomfort, and pulmonary and systemic venous congestion.[47–49] These and other signs and symptoms are listed in Table 25-2, and may provide important information on the heart failure status of the patient. The signs and symptoms of pediatric heart failure differ in a few important ways,[47] namely, that rales, neck vein distention, and peripheral edema are rarely heard or seen in newborns and infants. In addition, the NYHA classification of heart failure is not generally considered practical to determine the severity of heart failure for younger pediatric patients. The Canadian Cardiovascular Society's Consensus Conference[47] outlined a classification system[50] to address this problem. This system is an adaptation of the adult NYHA classification for infants. However, this system is not standard for pediatric heart failure assessment:

Class I: No symptoms
Class II: Mild tachypnea and/or diaphoresis with feeds in infants; dyspnea on exercise in older children. No growth delay
Class III: Marked tachypnea and/or diaphoresis with feeds or exertion and increased feeding time, and poor weight gain
Class IV: Tachypnea, retractions, grunting, and diaphoresis at rest, plus poor weight gain

In addition, determination of positional blood pressure, temperature, blood pressure response to Valsalva's maneuver, proportional pulse pressure, pulse rate, rhythm and quality may be useful in the examination of the status of a patient with heart failure. Abnormal findings should be followed up without hesitation for these patients.

Nonpharmaceutical Therapeutic Measures: Lifestyle Modifications

The improvement of the patient's quality of life is one of the principal therapeutic goals with HIV-infected patients. Although the physiologic dimensions of treatment are crucial for patient survival, not all lives can be prolonged by therapy. For these patients especially, which include a large portion of the individuals infected with HIV, quality of life is an extremely important consideration.

Physical activity.   The amount of tolerable exercise and physical activity for HIV-infected patients may be dependent on many physiological and emotional factors, such as stage of HIV infection, severity of cardiac dysfunction, and psychologic depression. The role of symptoms such as lethargy and fatigue in the process of wasting, often associated with HIV infection, is becoming increasingly noted in the literature.[51–53] One source noted that even short periods of bed rest result in reduced exercise tolerance and aerobic capacity, as well as muscular

Table 25-2. Signs and Symptoms Associated
With Heart Failure

Pulmonary and Respiratory Signs

Wheezing	Costal retractions (infants
Dyspnea	and children)
Paroxysmal nocturnal	Tachypnea
dyspnea	Ronchi
Orthopnea	Pleural effusion
Cough	Friction rub
Cheyne-Stokes respiration	Dullness to percussion
Rales	Diaphragmatic impairment
Grunting (infants and	Pulmonary venous con-
children)	gestion

Cardiovascular Signs

Neck-vein distention	Heart murmurs
Abdominal-jugular neck	Diminished S_1 or S_2
vein reflex	Prominent P_2
Cardiomegaly on palpita-	Friction rub
tion/percussion	
Chest wall pulsatile activity	
Gallop rhythm (S_3, S_4)	

Abdominal Signs

Abdominal discomfort	Hepatosplenomegaly
Decreased bowel sounds	Ileus
Ascites	

Neurologic Signs

Mental status abnormalities	Irritability
Anxiety	Fatigue

Systemic Signs

Growth failure (infants and	Edema
children)	Rash
Changes in feeding pattern	Systemic venous congestion
(infants and children)	Petechiae/ecchymosis
(e.g., increased feeding	Arthritis
time, tiredness while feed-	Diaphoresis
ing, shortness of breath,	Cool extremities
decreased volume intake)	Poor peripheral perfusion
Adult weight gain	
Nocturia	
Cachexia	

Metabolic Signs

Metabolic/gas exchange abnormalities (e.g., azotemia, hyponatremia, acidosis/alkalosis, hypoxia/oxygen desaturation, decreased myocardial oxygen consumption)

atrophy and weakness.[54] Decreased muscle mass
can lead to physical debilitation, in that inadequate
strength increases the frequency of fatigue, making
activities such as food preparation and eating even
more difficult.[51,53]

The level of recommended physical activity for

HIV-infected patients with cardiac dysfunction can
be difficult to determine, since patients with severe
left ventricular dysfunction and congestive heart
failure often have a limited tolerance for physical
exertion. Some sources have recommended bed rest
for patients suffering from heart failure, particularly
when they are ill, to avoid an excessive load on
the already compromised myocardium.[34] Especially
with young children, such limitations may cause
restlessness.[34] Distractions such as television and
reading may be helpful for both children and adults
who are confined to bed. However, in the HIV-
infected population, where malnutrition may be of
serious concern, it is unclear if bed rest is the most
appropriate approach. If the patient responds favor-
ably to pharmacologic therapy, the clinician might
allow increased physical activity.

Alternatively, several studies have demonstrated
the safety of exercise rehabilitation programs to
improve the exercise capacity of patients with severe left ventricular dysfunction.[55–62] An increase
in exercise capacity may be beneficial to the HIV-
infected patient who is at risk for the wasting syndrome. Depending on the degree of cardiac dysfunction the patient is struggling with, walking may
be advantageous for both physical and mental
health.

Diet. A patient's diet can have a considerable
effect on quality of life. Although it is common to
restrict sodium intake for a patient suffering from
heart failure, low-sodium foods may be unpalatable.
This is of particular importance for patients who
suffer from other maladies that may be associated
with diminished food consumption and wasting,
such as HIV infection or AIDS. It has been suggested that digitalis and diuretic therapy can be
carried out without significant alteration of dietary
composition,[34] although a reduced-sodium diet is
common in managing heart failure. No studies have
evaluated specific dietary recommendations, making it unclear whether mild or moderate salt restriction (e.g., 2 or 3 g per day) is more appropriate.[54]

Dietary requirements differ for each patient. The
following are some suggestions from a collection
of sources that may serve as a guide for establishing
an appropriate diet for a particular patient. For infants, it has been recommended that fortified breast

milk or simulated breast milk preparations be concentrated to provide 24 to 27 calories per ounce.[34] In addition, low-sodium formulas that are available may provide too little sodium to satisfy growth requirements and may be associated with electrolyte disturbances. They may also be unpalatable.

A low- or no-sodium diet is often prescribed for children with signs or symptoms of venous congestion and peripheral edema, but such extreme sodium restriction may not be healthy for the child on both a mental and a physical level. The child may feel deprived of the right to enjoy food and refuse to eat.[34] It is recommended that the clinician modify the dietary program in accordance with the child's response to salt restriction.

A diet containing 2 g sodium per day has been described as unpalatable for most adult patients.[54] Such a diet may also be too costly for disadvantaged patients. Instead, a 3-g diet is generally thought to be reasonable and viable for patients with mild to moderate heart failure. There are a number of ways to modify the amount of salt a patient consumes. One way is not to add salt to food during preparation and after cooking. In addition, the patient may avoid salty foods, as well as milk, milk products, and canned and prepared foods. It has been suggested that if salt intake is excessive, larger diuretic doses may be necessary and potassium wasting may be exacerbated. Patients who require larger doses of diuretics (e.g., greater than 80 mg furosemide per day) may require a reduction in sodium intake to 2 g per day or less.

Excessive fluid intake should be generally avoided in patients with symptomatic severe cardiac dysfunction, although some clinicians feel fluid restriction is not advisable unless hyponatremia is present.[54] For some patients, vitamin supplementation may be beneficial because of the loss of water-soluble vitamins that may result from diuresis and problems with gastrointestinal absorption of fat-soluble vitamins.[54]

For HIV-infected patients with congestive heart failure, quality of life is at least as important as the control of excess salt and water. The clinician should avoid decreasing the quality of life of the patient by excessive dietary restrictions when pharmacologic treatment methods are available. One source noted that although the elimination of dietary salt may be necessary in patients with severe heart failure, this can result in severe anorexia and a marked reduction in caloric intake, contributing to malnutrition and cardiac cachexia,[37] a situation obviously to be avoided. The clinician may work individually with the patient and the family to help them understand the guidelines of the nutritional regimen.

Drug use. For adolescent and adult patients with cardiac dysfunction, the effects of alcohol use are undetermined. Acute alcohol ingestion depresses myocardial contractility in patients with known cardiac disease,[54] although the clinical significance of this is not known. It is generally believed that alcohol consumption should be discouraged. One source specifies that the patient consume no more than one drink per day (30 ml of liquor or its equivalent in beer or wine).[54]

Cocaine is a commonly used drug among HIV-infected individuals. Cocaine can cause coronary artery spasms, and it has been described as causing myocarditis and reversible cardiomyopathy.[63] Other cocaine-related medical complications, including ischemic stroke, coronary ischemia, ischemia-based renal failure, myocardial infarction, and ventricular fibrillation have been reviewed.[23,64] Patients should be warned of the hazards of cocaine and encouraged to limit or discontinue its use. Although the management of substance abuse is beyond the scope of this chapter, other authors have addressed this issue and related social implications of living with HIV infection.[65]

Oxygen support. Oxygen support may be necessary to relieve pulmonary and cardiac stressors that affect patients with cardiac dysfunction. It is generally agreed that adequate humidification can be effective in loosening pulmonary secretions. For an infant, this may be achieved by using a conventional oxygen tent. Oxygen may be bubbled through a nebulizer and supplied through a face mask or nasal prongs, depending on what is most comfortable for the patient. The temperature in the tent can be adjusted so that the infant's body temperature is maintained within a normal range. For the older child and adult, supplemental oxygen may be given by a nasal cannula or, if necessary, a face mask.

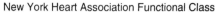

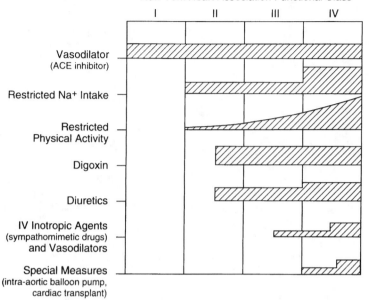

Figure 25-3. Overview of the treatment of heart failure caused by systolic dysfunction. (From Ref. 181, with permission.)

Position. The position of a patient with severe left ventricular dysfunction is important for respiratory ease and for the improvement of pulmonary function. It is generally recommended that infants be positioned in a modified cardiac chair that puts the patient in a semi-Fowler position, achieved by elevating the head and shoulders to a 45° angle with a pillow behind the back or an infant seat. For older children and adults, it is recommended that the head of the bed be elevated. This position will ease respiration and allow for peripheral rather than pulmonary pooling.

Pharmacologic Treatment

The primary goals in the pharmacologic treatment of HIV-infected patients with chronic heart failure include symptomatic relief, improvement of the quality of life, and prevention of the progression of left ventricular dysfunction. Furthermore, treatment can increase the patient's physical activity and sense of well-being and help the patient avoid hospitalization, even though it may not prolong life. The improvement of myocardial performance and, ideally, the reversal of the underlying disease process with the early use of interventional procedures

or surgical approaches,[34] are also primary objectives for patients with congestive heart failure. Different strategies for the management of heart failure have been described in the literature.[34,37,47,48,66–71] Figure 25-3 summarizes the common treatment of heart failure for different NYHA functional classes. A thorough medical history, physical examination, echocardiogram, EKG and chest radiograph are most often employed for diagnosis and management of heart failure.

ACE inhibition. The mildest manifestations of heart failure are often treated with ACE inhibitors alone, and as symptoms increase diuretic and digoxin therapy are added.[37,47] ACE inhibitors have been shown to reduce mortality in adults with mild to moderate and severe congestive heart failure. Studies have shown that enalapril and captopril enhance functional status in adults, where 40% to 80% of patients showed an improvement in NYHA functional classes.[72–81] Figures 25-4 and 25-5 demonstrated the mortality results of the SOLVD[72] and CONSENSUS[46] trials, which evaluated enalapril in the treatment of patients with congestive heart failure. Figure 25-6 demonstrates the efficacy of

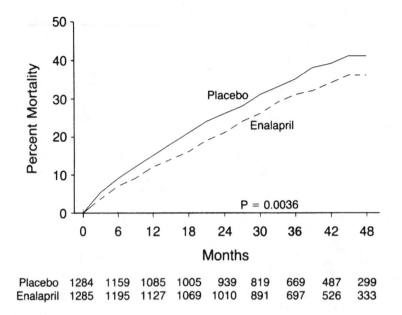

Placebo	1284	1159	1085	1005	939	819	669	487	299
Enalapril	1285	1195	1127	1069	1010	891	697	526	333

Figure 25-4. Comparison of the effects of enalapril versus placebo on percent mortality in the SOLVD Treatment Trial. Enalapril was associated with a significant decrease in mortality compared with placebo. (From Ref. 72, with permission.)

captopril in improving cardiac functional performance in the first placebo-controlled exercise study patients with heart failure, performed by the Captopril Multicenter Research Group. The results of some of these studies have also supported the use of ACE inhibitors for marked left ventricular dysfunction even if no signs and symptoms of congestive heart failure are apparent. The benefits of ACE inhibitor therapy in children have not been as extensively documented as for adults.[31,46,72] Although only a limited number of studies have examined the effects of this therapy with pediatric heart failure, ACE inhibitor therapy is becoming more widely accepted in the pediatric heart failure population.[82-84]

Before ACE inhibitor therapy is initiated, the clinician may want to assess the patient for volume depletion (e.g., orthostatic hypotension, prerenal azotemia, or metabolic alkalosis).[68] Sensitivity to potential first-dose hypotension for both pediatric and adult patients is important when therapy is initiated. Patients with congestive heart failure or excessively high afterload can be carefully monitored for blood pressure fluctuations generally for

the first 2 weeks of treatment and whenever the dosage of ACE inhibitors or diuretics is increased. Transient hypotension can occur after administration of the drug and is usually well tolerated, producing either no symptoms or a brief, mild lightheadedness.

Currently, enalapril maleate, captopril, lisinopril, and quinapril hydrochloride are the ACE inhibitors approved by the Food and Drug Administration (FDA) for the treatment of heart failure. Enalapril is the most frequently administered agent of this class for adults with heart failure. Although enalapril is not FDA-approved for patients under 12 years of age for any cause, it is often prescribed to infants and children for the treatment of congestive heart failure. Both lisinopril and quinapril hydrochloride are indicated as adjunctive therapy with diuretics and digitalis.

The following dosage schedules for enalapril are recommended by the manufacturer, although other regimens for adult patients have been noted in the literature.[48,68-70] The recommended initial dose of enalapril for adult patients is 2.5 mg. As a precaution, it is advisable for patients to be observed under

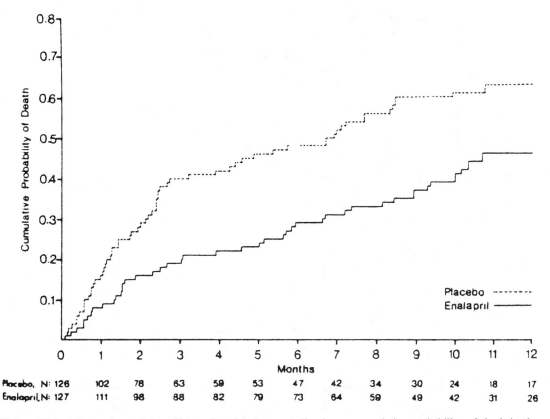

Figure 25-5. Comparison of the effects of enalapril versus placebo on cumulative probability of death in the CONSENSUS Trial. Enalapril was associated with a significant reduction in mortality due to the progression of heart failure in the enalapril-treated group. (From Ref. 46, with permission.)

medical supervision for at least 2 hours and until blood pressure has stabilized for at least an hour. Doses can then be titrated upward as needed and tolerated over a period of a few days or weeks, with a recommended dosing range of 2.5–20 mg given twice a day. If the patient is already taking a diuretic, the likelihood of hypotension may be minimized if the diuretic dose can be reduced; ACE inhibition will inhibit salt and water retention and thus decrease systemic blood volume.

Even though captopril and enalapril are frequently used for the treatment of infants and children, recommended dosages for both of these agents are not specified by the manufacturer because safety and effectiveness for pediatric use have not been established. Pediatric dosages may be determined on a body weight basis and are generally

reported to be comparable to or less than those used in adults.

Many studies have demonstrated the efficacy of enalapril in the treatment of heart failure in infants and children.[82–84] In one study, eight children with congestive heart failure received enalapril instead of captopril because of the advantage of once-a-day administration.[82] Enalapril resulted in diminished afterload, reflected in lower blood pressure and decreased heart volume, suggesting that enalapril is an effective option in the treatment of children with heart failure. In another study, eight infants between the ages of 4 days and 12 weeks with severe heart failure refractory to diuretic therapy were treated with enalapril, and within 2 weeks of the initiation of treatment the clinical features of heart failure had improved in all the infants.[83] In both of these

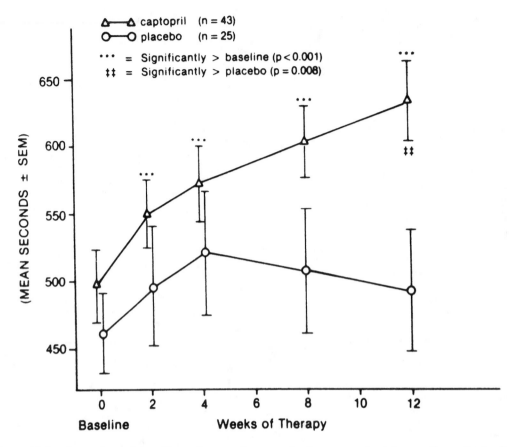

Figure 25-6. Comparison of the effects of captopril versus placebo on exercise tolerance times. Captopril was associated with a significant increase in exercise tolerance times from baseline, and patients receiving captopril had significantly greater exercise tolerance than patients receiving placebo. (From Ref. 112, with permission.)

studies, patients were started on 0.1 mg kg^{-1} day^{-1} of enalapril and titrated upward as tolerated to a maximum of 0.5 mg kg^{-1} day^{-1}. Other sources have recommended weight-determined dosages for this population.[38]

Hydralazine is another effective vasodilator for pediatric congestive heart failure,[34,85] acting directly on the arteriolar smooth muscle. The peripheral vasodilating effects of hydralazine result in decreased arterial blood pressure (primarily diastolic), decreased peripheral vascular resistance, and increased heart rate, stroke volume, and cardiac output. The pediatric starting dosage recommended by the manufacturer is 0.75 mg/kg body weight daily in four divided doses. The dosage may be increased gradually over the next 3 to 4 weeks to a maximum of 7.5 mg/kg or 200 mg daily. Side effects of hydra-

lazine include headache, nausea and vomiting, diarrhea, anorexia, palpitations, tachycardia, and angina pectoris.

Renal function, serum potassium, serum creatinine, blood pressure, and symptoms of hypotension are generally assessed after one week of ACE inhibitor therapy. In addition, reassessment of volume status may be beneficial for patients who develop renal insufficiency or hypotension. In patients who cannot tolerate an ACE inhibitor, a combination of hydralazine and isosorbide dinitrate may be considered as an alternative therapy for mild heart failure.

Hypersensitivity to ACE inhibitors, a history of angioedema related to previous treatment with an ACE inhibitor, and detected pregnancy are absolute contraindications for ACE inhibitors. Other contraindications have been noted in the literature.[68] It is recommended that ACE inhibitors be used with caution if the patient has increased levels of serum creatinine or decreased levels of serum potassium. ACE inhibitors attenuate potassium loss. Unless hypokalemia is observed, potassium supplements are also generally withheld.

Patients with asymptomatic hypotension should continue with therapy but require close follow-up, since, as described above, ACE inhibitors may induce further hypotension. Patients should be cautioned that excessive perspiration, dehydration, diarrhea, or vomiting may lead to an excessive fall in blood pressure because of decreased blood volume and should consult a physician if any of these occur. One source has noted that orthostatic hypotension is an indication for dose reduction and consideration of discontinuation of treatment.[68] In addition, the manufacturer advises that infants, especially newborns, may be more susceptible to the adverse hemodynamic effects of captopril and that excessive, prolonged, and unpredictable decreases in blood pressure and associated complications, including oliguria and seizures, have been reported.

Specific drug interactions with ACE inhibitors have been noted.[47,68,86] Patients taking diuretics, especially those who have recently begun diuretic therapy, may occasionally experience excessive reduction of blood pressure after initiating ACE inhibitor therapy. The possibility of hypotensive effects may be minimized by decreasing or discontinuing diuretic treatment or by increasing salt intake before initiating ACE inhibitor treatment. It is generally recommended that potassium-sparing agents not be routinely used in patients taking ACE inhibitors because of the known attenuation of potassium loss by ACE inhibitors. Concomitant use of ACE inhibitors and potassium-sparing agents (e.g., spironolactone, amiloride hydrochloride, triamterene, and other diuretics; potassium supplements; or salt-containing substitutes) may lead to significant increases in serum potassium.[47,68,86,87] These potassium-sparing agents are often discontinued upon initiation of ACE inhibitor therapy to avoid hyperkalemia. Lithium toxicity has been reported in patients receiving lithium concomitantly with ACE inhibitors.[86] Serum lithium levels are generally monitored routinely during the administration of this concurrent therapy. The antihypertensive efficacy of ACE inhibitors, particularly captopril, has been reportedly reduced by nonsteroidal antiinflammatory drugs.[88] No drug interactions have been noted with β-adrenergic antagonists, methyldopa, nitrates, calcium-blocking agents, hydralazine, prazosin, and digoxin.

Some of the major adverse reactions encountered during ACE inhibitor therapy are cough, hypotension, hyperkalemia, renal insufficiency, skin rash, angioedema, neutropenia, and dizziness.[68,86,89] A recent study investigated a possible underlying mechanism of the cough reported by patients receiving ACE inhibitors. The inflammatory peptide bradykinin, which is normally degraded by ACE, caused a sensitization of airway sensory nerves and an enhancement of the cough reflex in unanesthetized guinea pigs.[90] This mechanism could account for the enhanced cough seen with ACE inhibitor therapy, and the persistent spontaneous cough may reflect an increased irritability of the sensitized sensory nerves.[90] Although it is generally thought that most patients will tolerate a mild cough in exchange for the benefits of these agents, which include, in some cases, prolongation of life, the investigators in this study suggested that bradykinin receptor antagonists may be of benefit in treating the chronic cough seen with this condition.[90] Dizziness is usually mild and may often be managed by reducing the dose of ACE inhibitor.

The caregiver may want to strongly consider the importance of the quality of life of the HIV-infected patient who experiences side effects from ACE inhibition therapy. The goal of anticongestive treatment for this patient may not include prolongation of life, but may necessarily focus solely on the improvement of symptoms and quality of life.

Diuretics. Salt and water retention, commonly associated with congestive heart failure, is an effect of the activation of the renin–angiotensin–aldosterone system and decreased renal perfusion. This causes an increase in intravascular volume, leading to increased left and right heart filling pressures. The resulting pulmonary and systemic venous congestion is responsible for many of the symptoms of congestive heart failure. Diuretic therapy reduces filling pressures in the pulmonary and systemic venous beds, which ultimately will provide considerable and expeditious symptomatic relief to the patient. Generally, continued diuretic use leads to decreased symptoms of heart failure, vasodilation, and improved cardiac performance. Patients generally take diuretics until edema and other signs of volume overload are no longer evident.

It has been suggested that some beneficial effects of diuretics may be a result of increased concentrations of prostaglandins.[91] For example, renal prostaglandins help to maintain renal blood flow in the presence of countervailing influences.[91] Another reported important benefit of diuresis is its association with a decrease in catecholamines, since it is believed that catecholamines are responsible for cardiac deterioration.[91,92]

Thiazide and thiazide-related diuretics.   Patients with mild heart failure, requiring more gradual or less diuresis, are often treated with thiazide or thiazide-related diuretics.[37,48,68,93,94] These agents prevent reabsorption of sodium at the distal tubule of the nephron.[95] Thiazide use is limited, however, since renal clearance decreases with congestive heart failure.[96,97] Thiazides become ineffective when the glomerular filtration rate is less than approximately 30 ml/min.[48,91]

Hydrochlorothiazide is the most frequently used agent of this class. The manufacturer recommends an initial dosage of 25–100 mg daily for adults administered as a single or a divided dose. An intermittent schedule (e.g., administration on alternate days or on 3 to 5 days each week) may minimize excessive response to the drug or undesirable electrolyte imbalances. Whenever possible, the dosage should be tailored to the individual diuretic needs of the patient, with the goal of maximizing diuretic effects with the minimum required dose. The usual pediatric dosage is based on 1.0 mg hydrochlorothiazide per pound of body weight per day in two doses. For infants less than 6 months of age, up to 1.5 mg/lb body weight per day in two doses may be required.

Metolazone, a thiazide-related diuretic, is also effective in the management of fluid retention in both pediatric and adult patients with heart failure. It has been described as particularly useful in combination with a loop diuretic.[98,99] As with all diuretic agents, the dosage should be modified according to the individual patient requirements. The usual recommended dosage for edema of cardiac failure in adults is 5–20 mg once daily, but the safety and efficacy guidelines in children have not yet been established.

The diuresis produced by these agents may result in fluid or electrolyte imbalances, including hyponatremia, hypochloremic alkalosis, hyperglycemia, hypercalcemia, hypomagnesemia, and hypokalemia. The caregiver should be aware of the warning signs or symptoms of these adverse effects, which include dryness of the mouth, thirst, weakness, lethargy, drowsiness, restlessness, confusion, seizures, muscle pains or cramps, muscular fatigue, hypotension, oliguria, tachycardia, and gastrointestinal disturbances such as nausea and vomiting. It is recommended that appropriate therapy be initiated if any of these signs or symptoms develop during diuresis, including supplementation of depleted electrolytes and treatment of disturbances such as metabolic alkalosis.

Loop diuretics.   Loop diuretics are generally prescribed for patients with severe volume overload, persistent edema, or renal insufficiency who do not sufficiently respond to thiazide diuretics, or who require a more potent diuretic during the initiation of treatment. Loop diuretics are the most commonly used diuretics in the treatment of congestive heart failure because of their potency and efficacy. Loop diuretics act on the ascending limb of the loop of Henle to inhibit the transport of salt and water, resulting in the alteration of diluting and concentrating capabilities of the kidneys.[95] The net result is an increase in free water excretion, thereby reducing the edema and volume overload that frequently accompany congestive heart failure. Clinicians should be aware that congestive heart failure may have an effect on diuretic therapy.[91,96,97] Specifically, congestive heart failure may suppress renal function, thus reducing the response to the diuretic.[87] Therefore, the clinician should be aware of the pharmocokinetics of these agents, tailor therapy according to individual patient requirements, and monitor each patient closely for both sufficient and excessive diuresis. More detailed accounts of the pharmocokinetics of these agents are given elsewhere.[87,91,96,97,100]

The most commonly administered loop diuretic for both adult and pediatric patients is furosemide. As recommended by the manufacturer, therapy with this agent should be individualized according to patient response to obtain a maximum therapeutic response. A single initial dose of 20–80 mg is usually given. Diuresis generally follows promptly. However, if needed, the same dose or one increased by 20–40 mg may be administered at 6- to 8-hour intervals until the desired diuretic effect is obtained. Because of the hemodynamic effects of diuresis, careful laboratory monitoring and clinical observation during diuresis are normally employed, especially when the cumulative daily dose exceeds 80 mg. The usual dose for oral furosemide in infants and children is 1 mg/kg body weight per dose. The doses are generally administered one to four times per day, and the amount per dose may be increased up to 2 mg/kg. It is recommended that the dose maintenance level be adjusted to achieve the minimum effective level. If the initial furosemide dose does not provide sufficient diuresis, it is generally agreed that the dosage should be increased no sooner than 6 to 8 hours after the previous dose.

The principal signs and symptoms of overdosage with furosemide are dehydration, blood volume reduction, hypotension, electrolyte imbalance, hypokalemia, and hypochloremic alkalosis. Other toxicities are listed in Table 25-3. It is recommended that caregivers be sensitive to the potential for diuretic overdosage and respond promptly if any signs or symptoms become apparent. Treatment of overdosage generally consists of replacement of excessive electrolyte losses. Furosemide should not be taken concomitantly with certain other drugs, including use with aminoglycoside antibiotics, ethacrynic acid, turbocurarine, and lithium. Furosemide may

enhance the therapeutic effects of antihypertensive agents.

Bumetamide is another loop diuretic used to treat adults heart failure. Bumetamide and furosemide have only minimal clinically significant differences, with bumetamide having a slightly shorter duration of action.[101] The usual total daily adult dose of bumetamide is 0.5–2.0 mg, given to most patients as a single dose. Patients who require additional diuresis are often prescribed second or third doses given at 4- to 5-hour intervals up to a maximum daily dose of 10 mg. The safest and most effective method for the continued control of edema is an intermittent dosing schedule. This would entail the administration of bumetamide on alternate days, or for 3 to 4 days with rest periods of 1 to 2 days in between. The safety and efficacy of bumetamide in children below the age of 18 have not yet been established, and no recommended dosages are offered by the manufacturer.

Potassium-sparing diuretics. Potassium-sparing diuretics are used in the management of congestive heart failure when serum potassium levels are low and potassium supplementation is required.[34,68] By inhibiting the secretion of potassium, these agents avoid the hypokalemia that might be caused by other diuretics. This agent is a specific aldosterone antagonist, competitively binding receptors at the aldosterone-dependent sodium-potassium exchange site in the distal convoluted renal tubule.[34] It acts to reduce the reabsorption of sodium, thus affecting plasma volume, body weight, and blood pressure. This agent has no effect on free water production or absorption because it acts beyond the site where free water formation takes place.[34] Spironolactone, triamterene, and amiloride hydrochloride are three examples of these agents, spironolactone being the most commonly used for this purpose. They are most often used in conjunction with loop diuretics. The manufacturer recommends an initial daily dose of 100 mg spironolactone administered either as a single or a divided dose for adult patients. However, the dosage may range from 25 to 200 mg daily, depending on the amount of diuresis desired. Spironolactone is also the principal potassium-sparing diuretic agent used for infants and children with heart failure. The usual pediatric

Table 25-3. Common Toxicities Associated with Furosemide

Principal Signs and Symptoms of Overdosage	*Other Toxicities*
Dehydration, blood volume reduction	Various skin rashes
	Interstitial nephritis
Hypotension	Deafness
Electrolyte imbalance	Hyperuricemia, gout
Hypokalemia	Carbohydrate intolerance
Hypochloremic alkalosis	

daily dose of spironolactone is 0.75–1.5 mg/lb body weight (1.65–3.3 mg/kg). As with the loop diuretics, it is recommended that patients receiving spironolactone be carefully evaluated for disturbances in fluid and electrolyte balance.

The principal complication encountered during the administration of potassium-sparing diuretics is hyperkalemia.[102] Concomitant use of ACE inhibitors and potassium-sparing agents may lead to a significant increase in serum potassium and is generally avoided during the management of heart failure.

General diuresis considerations. If the initial oral dose of a diuretic agent is inadequate, there are two ways to increase diuresis. Some prefer to increase diuresis by increasing the individual dose,[68] whereas others prefer to increase the frequency of administration (e.g., to twice a day). If patients are resistant to both of these methods, the clinician may want to consider using a combination of diuretics. As previously mentioned, loop diuretics plus metolazone has proven to be a potent combination.[98,99] These synergistic agents may provide effective diuresis for those patients for whom single agents have been insufficient.

Some have suggested that the addition of dobutamine to a diuretic regimen may be beneficial, increasing diuresis in patients whose renal function is limited by severe heart failure.[91] Dobutamine alone improves left ventricular filling pressure and cardiac output. Low-dose dopamine added to dobutamine can increase glomerular filtration rate, urine flow rate, and fractional excretion of sodium by direct vasodilatory actions on the renal vasculature.[91]

Patients on diuretics can be monitored for significant weight change relative to their baseline weight. Significant weight change may reflect fluid status, which would allow excessive diuresis to be controlled. For patients whose baseline is unknown, caregivers should attempt to identify other indicators of excessive fluid loss, such as dehydration.

Diuretic-induced electrolyte abnormalities, particularly hypokalemia, are commonly seen during chronic diuretic therapy. Because depleted serum potassium may raise the potential for cardiac arrhythmias, it is generally recommended that potassium levels be checked regularly. One source defines a potassium level of less than 4.0 mmol/l as an indication to give potassium supplements or a potassium-sparing agent,[68] administered with caution for patients on ACE inhibitor therapy.

Digitalis. For some clinicians, the cornerstone of symptomatic heart failure treatment remains the combination of diuretics and digitalis glycosides. However, others have noted that digitalis has not been shown to affect the natural history of heart failure, and it is generally reserved for patients who remain symptomatic after treatment with ACE inhibitors and diuretics.[47,68,103] In the Randomized Assessment of the Effect of Digoxin on Inhibitors of the Angiotensin-Converting Enzyme (RADIANCE) trial, adult patients with chronic heart failure were given diuretics and ACE inhibitors plus digoxin.[104] Patients who were withdrawn from digoxin experienced a worsening of symptoms and underwent more hospitalizations (Figure 25-7), suggesting that patients with severe chronic congestive heart failure that is unresponsive to the combination of ACE inhibitors and diuretics would benefit from treatment with a combination of three drugs: an ACE inhibitor, a diuretic, and digoxin. Placebo-controlled trials of the effects of digoxin in patients with congestive heart failure appear to indicate that the patients most likely to benefit from digoxin are those with mild or severe heart failure who remain symptomatic despite optimal treatment with ACE inhibitors and diuretics.[74,105,106]

Digoxin, the most commonly prescribed digitalis agent, has a positive inotropic and electrophysiologic effect on the heart. The positive inotropic effect on the ventricle is the reduction of left ventricular volume in addition to the increase in stroke volume. Digoxin may also benefit patients through its effects on the autonomic nervous system, which may modulate neurohormonal factors in patients with heart failure.[103] Ultimately, cardiac output is increased, filling pressures decrease, and the characteristic disturbances of heart failure (such as venous congestion, edema, dyspnea, orthopnea, and cardiac asthma) are ameliorated,[86] especially when digoxin is used in conjunction with ACE inhibitors and diuretics. The role of digoxin has been de-

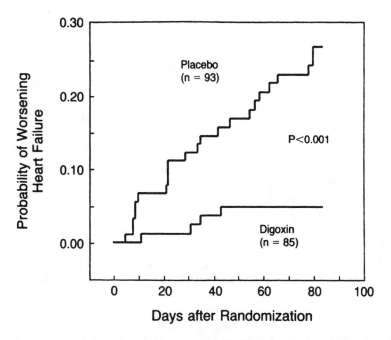

Figure 25-7. Kaplan-Meier analysis of the cumulative probability of worsening heart failure in patients continuing to receive digoxin and patients switched to placebo in the RADIANCE Trial. Patients continuing to receive digoxin remained stable during combined treatment with ACE inhibitors and diuretics, but there was a high risk of worsening heart failure in patients receiving ACE inhibitors, diuretics, and placebo. (From Ref. 104, with permission.)

scribed as support, taking the form of a relatively mild inotropic agent, for the damaged myocardium to counteract the compensatory increases in intravascular volume by ACE inhibitors and stimulation of the renin–angiotensin system by diuretics.[107] In addition, tachycardia and swelling, which are adaptive responses to decreased cardiac output and heart failure, decrease with digitalis therapy. Renal and hepatic function are restored as a result of improved organ perfusion, and systemic vascular resistance decreases. It is recommended that electrolytes be assessed regularly while the patient is on combination treatment.

The influence of digitalis glycosides on the heart is dose-related and involves both a direct action on the cardiac muscle and the specialized conduction system, and indirect actions on the cardiovascular system mediated by the autonomic nervous system.[86] The pharmacologic consequences of these direct and indirect effects are an increase in the force and velocity of myocardial systolic contraction, or positive inotropic action, a slowing of heart

rate, and decreased conduction velocity through the atrioventricular node.[86] The following is a brief review of the dosing schedule requirements for digoxin. Daily maintenance dose calculations, as specified by the manufacturer, are based on lean body weight and renal function. An important factor requiring modification of the recommended doses is diminished renal function, which decreases elimination of the agent from the body. Decreased elimination creates the potential for digitalis toxicity.

Peak body digoxin stores of 0.008–0.012 mg/kg should provide a therapeutic effect with minimum risk of toxicity in most adult patients with heart failure and normal sinus rhythm. The loading dose is normally administered in several portions, with approximately half of the total given as the first dose. Additional fractions of the total planned dose may be given at 6- to 8-hour intervals. If the patient's initial clinical response requires a change from the original calculated dose of digoxin, then the calculation of the maintenance dose should be based upon the amount actually given. The maintenance dose is generally calculated according to the following equation:

$$\text{Maintenance dose} = \text{peak body stores} \times \frac{\% \text{ daily loss}}{100}$$

where peak body stores = loading dose, and % daily loss = 14 + creatinine clearance/5. Table 25-4 provides the usual daily maintenance dose requirements for adults for estimated peak body stores of 0.010 mg/kg body weight as recommended by the manufacturer. A slight modification of these recommendations, provided by the Digitalis Investigation Group, is currently in press.[108]

Digoxin is also widely used in the treatment of heart failure in infants and children, and it is available in oral and parenteral forms. The pediatric dosages presented in this chapter are average values recommended by the manufacturer and may require significant modification because of individual patient sensitivity or associated conditions.

The manufacturer recommends that children over the age of 10 years receive adult dosages in proportion to their body weight, while infants and children under 10 years generally receive divided daily dosing. Table 25-5 lists the recommended usual digitalizing and maintenance dosages in children with normal renal function based on lean body weight.

The elimination of digoxin has been noted to decrease with renal failure and with excessive use of diuretics, indomethacin, cyclosporine, spironolactone, verapamil, quinidine, and propafenone.[34] Care should be taken when digoxin is used in combination with these agents, since decreased elimination increases the risk of digitalis toxicity. Diarrhea with dehydration can also result in toxicity by increasing the serum concentration of digoxin. By contrast, diarrhea without dehydration can reduce intestinal absorption, and vasodilators increase elimination.

The distinction between optimally therapeutic and toxic doses of digitalis can be difficult to make and is patient-specific. One source defines a toxicity range of 4–5 ng/ml for infants and 3 ng/ml for children.[34] However, this range may vary considerably, depending on the patient's age, electrolyte composition, concomitant drug use, and individual susceptibility. The toxicity level may also deviate from this range with the presence of inflammatory myocardial disease.[34] Although the toxicity of digitalis is fairly low, the effects can be life-threatening. Anorexia, nausea, vomiting, and arrhythmias, as well as visual disturbances and behavioral alterations, may be indications of digitalis toxicity. A clinical evaluation of the cause of any of these symptoms might be valuable before proceeding

Table 25-4. Usual Digoxin Tablet Daily Maintenance Dose Requirements (mg) for Estimated Peak Body Stores of 0.01 mg/kg in Adults

Corrected creatinine clearance (ml/min per 70 kg)	Lean Body Weight (kg/lb)						Number of days before steady-state achieved
	50/110	60/132	70/154	80/176	90/198	100/220	
0	.063*	.125	.125	.125	.188†	.188	22
10	.125	.125	.125	.188	.188	.188	19
20	.125	.125	.188	.188	.188	.250	16
30	.125	.188	.188	.188	.250	.250	14
40	.125	.188	.188	.250	.250	.250	13
50	.188	.188	.250	.250	.250	.250	12
60	.188	.188	.250	.250	.250	.375	11
70	.188	.250	.250	.250	.250	.375	10
80	.188	.250	.250	.250	.375	.375	9
90	.188	.250	.250	.250	.375	.500	8
100	.250	.250	.250	.375	.375	.500	7

*0.5 of .125 mg tablet or .125 mg every other day.

†1.5 of .125 mg tablet.

Table 25-5. Usual Digitalizing and Maintenance Dosages for Lanoxin Elixir Pediatric in Children with Normal Renal Function Based on Lean Body Weight

Age	Digitalizing* Dose (mg/kg)	Daily† Maintenance Dose (% of oral loading dose‡)
Premature	0.02–0.03	20–30
Full term	0.025–0.035	25–35
1–24 mo	0.035–0.06	25–35
2–5 yr	0.03–0.04	25–35
5–10 yr	0.02–0.035	25–35
Over 10 yr	0.01–0.015	25–35

*Intravenous digitalizing doses are 80% of oral digitalizing doses.

†Divided daily dosing is recommended for children under 10 years of age.

‡Projected or actual digitalizing dose providing clinical response.

Table 25-6. Drug Interactions With Digoxin

Decrease Digoxin Blood Levels	Increase Digoxin Blood Levels
Antacids	Quinidine
Kaolin	Amiodarone
Pectin	Erythromycin
Cholestyramine	Propafenone
Colestipol	Flecainide
Bran	Verapamil
Psyllium	Nicardipine
Phenytoin	Tiapamil
Propafenone	Spironolactone
Sulfasalazine	Triamterene
Bepridil	Indomethacin
Neomycin	Cyclosporine
Cathartics	
Tetracyclines	

with digoxin administration. Newborns show considerable variability in their tolerance to digoxin, and premature and immature infants are especially sensitive. It is recommended that dosages be reduced for these patients and individualized according to their degree of maturity.[86]

Digoxin therapy may result in hypokalemia, which may be accompanied by prolonged vomiting and diarrhea, and long-standing heart failure. Hypokalemia may also be associated with the malnutrition often seen in AIDS patients. Potassium depletion sensitizes the myocardium to digoxin, creating the potential for conduction alterations, which are generally manifested clinically as arrhythmias. Bradyarrhythmias are more common in children and supraventricular tachycardias, ectopic activity, and ventricular tachyarrhythmias are more common in adults.[34] Ventricular fibrillation and death are equally frequent in adults and children.[34]

Hypokalemia, hypercalcemia, hypomagnesemia, and hyponatremia have been shown to increase sensitivity to digoxin and can lead to digitalis toxicity. Acid and base changes secondary to changes in potassium and calcium levels, hypothyroidism, advanced pulmonary disease, and renal failure also increase sensitivity to digoxin. Clinicians should be cautious of these factors throughout digoxin administration. Specific drug interactions with digoxin have been noted in the literature[40,109,110] and are listed in Table 25-6.

Two approaches are generally considered when serum digoxin or creatinine levels are elevated, or

when significant conduction abnormalities or increased arrhythmias are identified: temporarily discontinuing digitalis therapy or decreasing the dose to avoid adverse effects. As mentioned above, caregivers should be aware of possible signs and symptoms associated with digoxin toxicity, which include ventricular tachycardia and other arrhythmias, anorexia, nausea, vomiting, confusion, dizziness, and visual disturbances (Table 25-7). These

Table 25-7. Signs and Symptoms of Digoxin Toxicity

Cardiac arrhythmias, most commonly:
  Unifocal or multiform ventricular premature contractions
  Ventricular tachycardia
  Atrioventricular dissociation
  Accelerated junctional rhythm
  Atrial tachycardia with block
  (The manufacturer recommends that any arrhythmia in children initially be assumed to be a consequence of digoxin intoxication)
Excessive slowing of pulse
Anorexia*
Nausea*
Vomiting*
Diarrhea*
Visual disturbances*
Headache*
Weakness*
Dizziness*
Apathy*
Psychosis*

*Rare as initial symptoms of toxicity in infants.

can be identified by regular clinical examination, EKG, and blood serum analysis.

Vesnarinone. A new synthetic oral inotropic agent, vesnarinone, may be an alternative in the treatment of stable heart failure. Vesnarinone is a quinolinone derivative currently under investigation for its ability to augment myocardial contractility in model systems with minimal effect on heart rate or myocardial oxygen consumption. In one study, 477 adults with congestive heart failure were randomized to receive either 60 mg of vesnarinone or a placebo for 6 months.[111] Patients receiving vesnarinone had fewer deaths or worsening heart failure during the study period than patients receiving the placebo (Figure 25-8).[111] The reduction in risk was 50%. Patients treated with vesnarinone also had a 62% reduction in the risk of dying from any cause.[111] In addition, the improvement in quality of life over a 12-week period was greater in the group treated with vesnarinone than in the placebo group.[111]

In a recent study, 21 NYHA class III and class IV patients with dilated cardiomyopathy were randomized to receive either 30 mg per day or 60 mg per day of vesnarinone. Chronic vesnarinone treatment yielded mild, positive inotropic changes without altering heart rate and lowered afterload in a dose-dependent manner.[112]

Vesnarinone treatment of murine myocarditis resulted in improved survival and reduced myocardial damage as a result of the drug's immunomodulatory effects, which suppressed tumor necrosis factor-α (TNF-α) production and natural killer cell activity.[113] It has also been suggested that vesnarinone may be therapeutically useful in patients infected with HIV-1, especially to reduce the frequency and magnitude of HIV-associated cardiovascular disease.

The mechanism of the effects of vesnarinone in the treatment of heart failure is unclear, but it may involve a decrease in the delayed outward and inward rectifying potassium currents, an increase in intracellular sodium caused by prolonged opening of sodium channels, and an increase in the inward calcium current attributable to the mild inhibition of phosphodiesterase.[111]

β-Adrenergic antagonists. β-Adrenergic antagonist therapy has recently been shown to be a potentially effective approach to patients with severe heart failure, perhaps by decreasing endocrine excitation, myocardial ischemia, and ventricular arrhythmias.[47] Carvedilol and metoprolol are β-adrenergic antagonists that have been shown to be beneficial in reducing mortality and clinical deterioration and improving symptoms and cardiac function.[114]

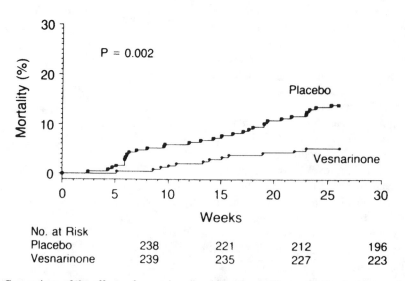

Figure 25-8. Comparison of the effects of vesnarinone and placebo on the cumulative incidence of mortality from any cause. Vesnarinone was associated with a significant reduction in the risk of death from any cause. (From Ref. 111, with permission.)

A recent double-blind, placebo-controlled trial examined the effects of the β-adrenergic antagonist carvedilol in 1,094 adult patients with chronic heart failure.[115] Patients with mild, moderate, or severe heart failure were randomly assigned to receive either a placebo or carvedilol in addition to background therapy with digoxin, diuretics, and an ACE inhibitor. The risk of both death and hospitalization for cardiovascular causes in patients with severe chronic heart failure was reduced with the addition of carvedilol to conventional therapy (Figure 25-9). The initial carvedilol dose for all patients was 12.5 mg twice daily which was increased, if tolerated, to 25–50 mg twice daily in addition to their usual medication. No dosage information for pediatric patients is available at this time.

In a multicenter study examining the effects of metoprolol in adult patients with idiopathic cardiomyopathy, 383 patients were randomized to receive placebo or drug in addition to conventional medications.[114] All patients were started at a test dose of 5 mg twice daily for 2 to 7 days and the 96% who tolerated the drug were randomized to receive placebo or drug. The dose of metoprolol was increased slowly from 10 mg to 100–150 mg daily.

Metoprolol prevented clinical deterioration, improved symptoms and cardiac function, and was well tolerated. The usual initial dosage of metoprolol is 100 mg daily in single or divided doses, with a usual effective dose range of 100–450 mg/day.

Removal of underlying cause. Chronic heart failure may often be controlled by medical treatment of the underlying cause, such as hypertension, infective endocarditis, arrhythmias, or common HIV-related infections such as cytomegalovirus (see below).

Worsening heart failure. Some conditions commonly associated with worsening heart failure have been cited in the literature, including failure to take adequate doses of prescribed drugs, dietary noncompliance, cardiac arrhythmias, emotional and environmental issues, inadequately conceived drug therapy, pulmonary infections and thyrotoxicosis.[116]

Refractory heart failure. If combination therapy does not control the symptoms of heart failure, it may be helpful to check that all medications are being taken properly and the conditions commonly associated with worsening heart failure have been

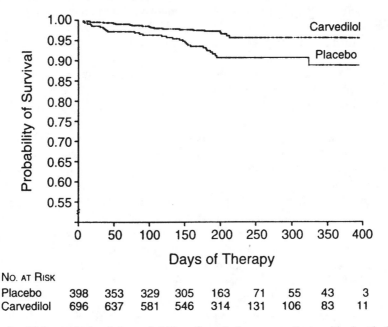

No. at Risk									
Placebo	398	353	329	305	163	71	55	43	3
Carvedilol	696	637	581	546	314	131	106	83	11

Figure 25-9. Kaplan-Meier analysis of the probability of survival among patients with chronic heart failure in carvedilol and placebo groups. Patients receiving carvedilol had a significantly lower risk (65%) of death than patients receiving the placebo. (From Ref. 115, with permission.)

considered. Factors that can exacerbate heart failure, such as electrolyte imbalance, should also be controlled if possible. If therapy is still ineffective, a number of alternatives have been suggested.[37,47,68,107] Vasodilators have been used for the treatment of refractory heart failure seen with cardiomyopathies. By relaxing the vascular smooth muscle, these drugs alter the loading conditions on the heart which subsequently modifies cardiac performance.[34,71,117] The decrease in systemic vascular resistance ameliorates the decrease in cardiac output that would result from the increased resistance. Vasodilators that relax arterial smooth muscle increase cardiac output. Conversely, venodilitation increases capacitance of the systemic vascular bed and lowers filling volumes. The result is diminished pulmonary and systemic venous congestion.

Some have recommended adding a direct-acting vasodilator like flosequinan, a quinolone derivative, since ACE inhibitors are only weak vasodilators.[68,107] There is evidence that this drug improves exercise performance and symptomatic status when added to the ACE inhibitor-diuretic-digoxin therapy.[118–123] However, flosequinan for the treatment of patients with heart failure was withdrawn[108] as a result of a study that demonstrated excess mortality in patients randomized to receive the drug in addition to the combination ACE inhibitor-diuretic-digoxin therapy.[124] An alternative may be the combination of hydralazine and isosorbide dinitrate.[107] Both flosequinan and hydralazine-isorbide dinitrate are frequently prescribed for patients who cannot tolerate ACE inhibitors. Hydralazine-isorbide dinitrate provides a combination of venous and arterial dilators, though there tend to be more side effects associated with this combination.[107] For patients with refractory volume overload, salt restriction can be reemphasized and furosemide dose increased.[68]

If maximum doses of ACE inhibitors or other direct vasodilators do not sufficiently reduce blood pressure, the clinician may want to consider initiating an α-adrenergic antagonist (e.g., prozasin) or a centrally acting α-antagonist (e.g., clonidine, α-methyldopa).[68] For further positive inotropic and vasodilatory treatment of heart failure, amrinone injection is available to increase the patient's cardiac output at rest and with exercise and to improve renal perfusion. It is the only nonglycosidal, noncat-

echolamine agent available at this time for the treatment of heart failure in all age groups.[34,40,125] The clinical experience of this agent is primarily for the management of adult patients with dilated cardiomyopathy but has also been recommended for pediatric patients to improve ventricular systolic function.[40] It has some serious side effects, such as fever, thrombocytopenia, and hepatotoxicity. Also, the combination of nitroprusside or nitroglycerin with dobutamine or dopamine for patients with severe heart failure insufficiently responsive to other treatment regimens may prove beneficial.[37] Many of these pharmacologic options are available only for intravenous administration.

A number of supportive measures have been suggested for patients with refractory severe symptomatic ventricular dysfunction despite maximal anticongestive therapy.[34,37,47,48,69,107] An example is intravenous dobutamine administered in the hospital, either alone or in combination with amrinone.[37] Dobutamine may improve ventricular performance up to several weeks. The primary function of this therapy is to improve quality of life. Dobutamine in low doses is often used for its beneficial effects on renal vasculature, improving renal blood flow and, subsequently, glomular filtration rate.[40] The result is improved urine output. Home dobutamine infusions have been used as well, often to stabilize patients with cardiomyopathy and worsening heart failure. Because dobutamine does not appear to cause systemic vasoconstriction, it may be better suited than dopamine for the treatment of myocardial dysfunction in absence of any systemic hypertension.[40]

For patients at risk for cardiac cachexia, or for newborns and young infants, there are generally three options to minimize energy expenditure: continuous nasogastric feeding (continuous or bolus infusion),[37,47] surgical insertion of a feeding tube, or parenteral hyperalimentation. Enteral feeding has reduced morbidity in children with symptomatic HIV infection. One study demonstrated the efficacy of gastrostomy tube supplementation for HIV-infected children in improving weight and fat mass when oral methods failed.[126] Supplemental oxygen therapy at night has been shown to offer benefit by reducing Cheyne-Stokes respiration, correcting hypoxia, and consolidating sleep by reducing arousals caused by the hyperpneic phase of the Cheyne-

Stokes cycle.[37] Both of these supportive measures can generally only be carried out in the hospital because of the need to carefully monitor filling pressures, cardiac output, and arterial pressure. If this support is successful, the patient can be weaned from intravenous treatment.

A transfusion may be a therapeutic option for anemic patients, increasing blood oxygen levels to potentially decrease the heart failure symptoms. HIV-infected patients may be at increased risk for premature coronary artery disease, and non-HIV-infected patients with significant coronary artery obstruction would normally be considered for surgical revascularization when medical treatment remains unsuccessful in the management of severe heart failure. As described later in this chapter, studies have shown that an HIV-positive status should not preclude cardiac surgery.[127–131] However, the utility of surgical treatment is necessarily dependent on the stage of HIV infection in the patient and must be considered on an individual basis. Critical care and inpatient therapy are beyond the scope of this chapter. A more extensive discussion may be found elsewhere.

Emergency Management of Severe Heart Failure

Severe heart failure can be paroxysmal and transient, in that there may be a rapid onset of inadequate tissue perfusion, which results in an inability to meet the oxygen requirements of the tissues. The course of heart failure has been described as rarely smoothly progressive; rather, it is usually punctuated by a series of abrupt downward steps due to acute decompensation.[37] Often with immediate initiation of treatment, this type of episode of severe heart failure can be short in duration and is referred to as acute failure. Sometimes acute heart failure represents only a reduction in cardiac output, while the oxygen demand of the tissues remains normal.[132] For some patients, circulatory failure can occur without overt contractile dysfunction of the myocytes. Sudden pressure or volume overload, as sometimes is seen with a sudden onset of malignant hypertension, pulmonary embolism, or valvular regurgitation, may present with acute cardiac failure regardless of normal myocardial contractility. In addition, some types of chronic pressure overload, such as septal defects, aortic stenosis, or arteriovenous fistulae, can cause heart failure in the presence of normal myocyte function. Arrhythmias and mechanical obstructions such as pulmonary emboli can also cause circulatory failure even though contractile function of the myocyte is normal. Other common conditions associated with acute heart failure include ventricular rupture, mitral or aortic valvular disruption, myocarditis and cardiomyopathy, uncontrolled severe systemic hypertension, pulmonary hypertension, and pericardial tamponade. The pathogenesis of sudden-onset failure may therefore have important therapeutic implications, and the clinician is encouraged to evaluate for readily reversible causes of acute failure, such as cardiac arrhythmias and pericardial tamponade, so that the appropriate intervention is initiated.

The signs and symptoms associated with acute heart failure include tachycardia, respiratory distress (e.g., dyspnea, tachypnea), diaphoresis, hypoxia, poor peripheral perfusion, edema, and hepatosplenomegaly. In addition, as seen with chronic congestive heart failure, infants and children may also present with growth failure and changes in feeding patterns (e.g., tiring easily during feeding and becoming short of breath).

HIV-infected patients are often at risk of acute cardiac decompensation, which results in episodes of severe heart failure. These patients, who may not have any signs or symptoms of heart failure, could suffer from this rapid onset of symptoms in the setting of infection or other stressors. Although inpatient care is generally beyond the scope of this chapter, a brief overview of the treatment options for emergency management of severe heart failure is warranted. A more thorough discussion of this type of management can be found elsewhere.[37,47,68,100,132]

The two primary objectives in the treatment of acute heart failure are the restoration of adequate perfusion of the tissues and the reduction of symptoms. Oxygen administration is generally the first step, and may be effective in improving symptoms, especially for hypoxic patients. β-Adrenergic and dopaminergic agonists (e.g., dobutamine, dopamine, and epinephrine) are used in adult and pediatric patients.[40,68,132] They interact with the β-adrenergic or dopaminergic receptors of the myocardium to increase atrial and ventricular contractility, increase heart rate, and enhance atrioventricular conduction. Intravenous dobutamine is most frequently administered in adult patients. It causes less tachycardia and fewer systemic vascular effects than other agents of its class, while still exerting a strong inotropic effect on the myocardium. The immediate cardiac output response with the use of dobutamine can sometimes be related to a significant increase in arterial pressure, although changes in arterial pressure are generally modest.[133] Dopamine is frequently used for pediatric patients with reduced cardiac output, although dobutamine is also considered for patients with contractility-based cardiac dysfunction.[40,100]

Some sources recommend that diuretics be used cautiously in hemodynamically unstable patients such as those with acute heart failure,[132] since they lead to the failure of other organs by limiting cardiac output. Intravenous vasodilators with short half-lives are often used for the treatment of heart failure that is related to increased afterload for both adults and children. Commonly administered agents of this class are nitroglycerin (or dinitrate isosorbide) and sodium nitroprusside in both adult and pediatric populations. Prozasin, captopril, phentolamine, and hydralazine are also frequently used for pediatric patients.[134]

It has been noted that patients acutely ill with anemia should be transfused.[132] However, caution is advised for patients with severe heart failure who may poorly tolerate the increased intravascular volume. Increasing the length of transfusion, decreasing the volume of transfusion, administering diuretics with transfusion, or performing an exchange transfusion should be considered for these patients. One study has shown beneficial effects of digitalis glycosides for patients with severe heart failure.[133] Caregivers are encouraged to consult other sources for a more detailed examination of the treatment of acute heart failure.

Intravenous Immunoglobulin Treatment

Intravenous immunoglobulins are immunomodulatory agents appropriate for a variety of conditions, and have been shown to be effective in patients with HIV infection.[135] Outlined below are a few of the most common applications of these agents.

Intravenous immunoglobulins have been used in the management of acute congestive cardiomyopathy and nonspecific myocarditis in HIV-negative children.[136] Studies have also shown that they are useful in the treatment of idiopathic or viral myocarditis and dilated cardiomyopathy in children.[137] Monthly infusions of immunoglobulin to HIV-infected children appear to be associated with more normal left ventricular structure and function compared with untreated infected children, suggesting that immunoglobulins may influence mechanisms of left ventricular function and hypertrophy.[138] The analysis showed an increase in wall thickness and a reduction in peak cardiac wall stress with immunoglobulin treatment.

In addition, these agents may be useful for patients with congestive heart failure who are unresponsive to anticongestive therapy and for patients with inflammatory heart disease according to endomyocardial biopsy.[138] Immunoglobulins have also been prescribed for the improvement of HIV-associated polymyositis, an inflammatory skeletal muscle disorder.[13,139] Immunoglobulins had beneficial effects in HIV-infected children with CD4+ lymphocyte counts of greater than 0.2×10^9 cells per liter who were not consistently receiving zidovudine or trimethoprim–sulfamethoxazole, including reductions in serious bacterial infections and minor viral and bacterial infections.[135,140]

Immunoglobulin therapy has also been shown to be beneficial in the treatment of the myocarditis of Kawasaki disease. Patients who were treated during the acute phase had demonstrated accelerated recovery of early abnormalities of left ventricular contractility and function.[14]

The mechanism of action of immunoglobulin agents is unknown. It has been suggested that these agents alter the secretion or effects of excessively produced cytokines and cellular growth factors,[141,142] which are known to affect the cardiovascular system adversely.[138,143,144] Another view holds that these agents may work by the presence of anti-idiotypic antibodies in the infusion, specific antibodies to a toxin or infectious agent, or antigens that behave as superantigens.[141] Other postulates have been noted in the literature.[138] Whether immunoglobulin therapy improves cardiomyopathy and myocarditis in patients with HIV disease is still unknown.

Immunosuppression Treatment

Resolution of myocarditis was observed in one HIV-infected adult with endomyocardialbiopsy-proven myocarditis and ventricular dysfunction after having been treated with prednisone plus azathioprine.[145] This patient was reported to be alive and off medication after 15 months of follow-up. A patient with a similar diagnosis treated with prednisone alone showed resolution of the myocardial infiltrate after 1 month of therapy.[6] In addition, a small, uncontrolled trial of immunosuppressive therapy for the management of acute myocarditis in children noted an improvement of clinical course and cardiac function with prednisone use.[146] A larger controlled trial in adult patients failed to demonstrate benefits from this therapy.[147] Therefore, it is not clear whether immunosuppressive therapy affects the course of myocarditis in HIV-infected patients.

Antiarrhythmic Treatment

Electrocardiographic abnormalities are not uncommon in HIV-infected patients. Rhythm disturbances have been reported in 44% of adults[41] and 55% to 93% of children with HIV infection.[45] In addition to the reported 47% to 77% prevalence of ECG abnormalities in HIV-infected pediatric patients,[8,10,20,148] arrhythmias have been noted in 24% to 35% of infected children.[22] Ventricular tachycardia has also been reported in this population and has been associated with autonomic dysfunction.[10,13] Further, in a nonrandomized prospective study of HIV-infected adults receiving intravenous pentamidine, there was a 60% to 75% incidence of potentially life-threatening arrhythmias, depending on the QTc criteria used.[149] Intravenous pentamidine is often used to treat *Pneumocystis carinii*, a common infection in HIV positive patients.

Although the management of chronic arrhythmia

is beyond the scope of this chapter, consideration of acute management is warranted. Torsades de pointes have been associated with pentamidine therapy.[149,150] This therapy has been associated with life-threatening hyperkalemia[151] and may prolong the QT interval, increasing the potential for torsades de pointes. It is recommended that patients who receive prophylactic or therapeutic pentamidine, or patients with a prolonged QTc interval, undergo serial electrocardiography in an attempt to prevent pentamidine-induced arrhythmias. If a prolonged QTc interval or torsades de pointes develops, it is generally recommended that pentamidine treatment be discontinued and normal electrolyte levels be restored. In addition, the use of type I antiarrhythmic agents such as quinidine and procainamide to treat torsades de pointes has been reported to exacerbate the arrhythmia[9,152] and therefore should be avoided.

Other transient forms of antiarrhythmic therapy include QRS-synchronized cardioversion for patients suffering from intolerable supraventricular tachycardia.[107] Alternative therapy for this problem is the administration of verapamil, a calcium entry blocker, which will temporarily slow the patient's heart rate. The manufacturer recommends intravenous verapamil be administered as a slow bolus injection over at least a two-minute period under continuous ECG and blood pressure monitoring. The recommended adult dose is 5–10 mg initially, followed by a 10-mg dose 30 minutes later if the initial dose is inadequate. Pediatric dosing is weight-based. Infants aged 0 to 1 would receive 0.1–0.2 mg/kg body weight initially, and the same dose if the initial dose proves to be inadequate. Pediatric patients between 1 and 15 years of age would require 0.1 to 0.3 mg/kg body weight for both the initial and the repeat doses. If an alternative treatment is required, amiodarone is often used because of its safety and effectiveness without the strong myocardial depressant qualities of verapamil.

Antiinfective Treatment

The infectious causes of HIV-associated heart disease have been successfully treated in both adult and pediatric patients. Conventional antiinfective therapy resulted in the significant improvement of cardiac status for HIV-infected adults with cardiac symptoms who had tuberculosis pericarditis, cryptococcal myopericarditis, or salmonella endocarditis.[153] Other preliminary results involved adults with active myocarditis or dilated cardiomyopathy, and cytomegalovirus identified by endomyocardial biopsy.[154] After treatment with cytomegalovirus hyperimmunoglobulin, these patients demonstrated significant elimination of cytomegalovirus from the myocardium.[154] Improvement in ventricular function and clinical heart failure in HIV-infected children with cytomegalovirus coinfection was also noted following treatment with ganciclovir and/or cytomegalovirus hyperimmunoglobulin.[9]

Zidovudine therapy improved cardiac function for some HIV-infected patients.[23,24] One source noted two patients with severe left ventricular dysfunction related to HIV infection who responded to zidovudine.[24] A case study of one HIV-positive patient with retractable diffuse lymphocytic myocarditis who did not respond to conventional treatment reported definite clinical improvement three months following the initiation of zidovudine therapy.[23]

Surgical Treatment

The effect of the virus on the outcome of cardiac surgery has been a concern in the treatment of HIV-infected patients. Studies have shown that an HIV-positive status should not preclude cardiac surgery in adults.[127–131] Aris and colleagues[128] examined the effect of cardiopulmonary bypass on the development of AIDS in 40 HIV-infected adults. The actuarial progression to AIDS was the same as that in infected patients who did not undergo cardiac surgery, suggesting that surgery is unrelated to AIDS progression and does not accelerate the development of the disease. In another study, six HIV-infected adults underwent surgery for infective endocarditis.[130] No correlation was found between the temporary lymphopenia, an immune dysregulation, induced by cardiopulmonary bypass and progression to AIDS. Another study reported good results in 10 HIV-infected adults who received valve replacements for endocarditis,[127] and a fourth demonstrated successful surgery in an HIV patient with

atrial lymphoma.[129] Further, open cardiac surgery was performed for endocarditis 11 times in HIV-positive adults who appeared to have a normal response to the surgery in the absence of uncontrolled infection.[131]

Although we are unaware of any trial that has specifically examined pediatric surgery as related to progression to AIDS, the studies of adult patients suggest that HIV-positive children should have the same operations for the same indications as noninfected patients.

Antihypertensive Treatment

Systemic Hypertension

The primary goal in the treatment of hypertension in HIV-infected patients is to identify the cause so that the appropriate therapy may be initiated. The cardiovascular substrate of these patients may be compromised and less able to utilize the cardiovascular reserves necessary to maintain cardiac function in the setting of severe hypertension.[13] Hypertension can be refractory to treatment in this patient population, leading to clinically significant hypertensive sequelae, including end-organ damage and death. Pharmacologic and nonpharmacologic treatment options for systemic hypertension have been noted in the literature[38,155,156] and are summarized in Table 25-8.

Pulmonary Hypertension

It is not uncommon for both adult and pediatric patients with symptomatic HIV infection to present with pulmonary hypertension.[157–162] Pulmonary hypertension is often a consequence of left ventricular dysfunction, repeated respiratory infections, or thromboembolic disease; occasionally it is a primary process without any identifiable cause.[9] Epoprostenol, formerly known as prostacyclin or prostaglandin-2 (PG2), has been shown to improve exercise capacity and survival in patients with severe primary pulmonary hypertension refractory to conventional therapy.[163] In this randomized controlled trial, improvement in hemodynamic function, exercise capacity and survival were consistently greater for patients receiving epoprostenol

Table 25-8. Treatment Options for Systemic Hypertension in HIV-Infected Patients

Nonpharmacologic	Pharmacologic
Dietary modification	Vasodilators (e.g., hydralazine, minoxidil)
Cessation of smoking, excessive alcohol consumption, and drug use (e.g., cocaine)	β-Adrenergic antagonists† (e.g., propranolol, atenolol)
Regular exercise (e.g., walking, swimming, bicycling)	Calcium channel blockers† (e.g., nifedipine, verapamil, diltiazem)
Micronutrient supplementation (e.g., calcium, potassium, magnesium)	ACE inhibitors (e.g., enalapril, captopril)
Stress management	α-Adrenergic blocking agents (e.g., prozasin)
	Central sympatholytics* (e.g., clonidine, α-methyldopa)
	Diuretics (e.g., thiazides, loop diuretics, potassium-sparing diuretics)

*Normally initiated only when high blood pressure is refractory to other treatment.

†Concomitant administration of β-adrenergic antagonists and calcium channel blockers may have an additive negative inotropic and chronotropic effect. It is recommended that this combination be used cautiously.

‡Caution is advised when potassium-sparing diuretics are prescribed in conjunction with ACE inhibitors.

than for patients receiving conventional therapy alone. Conventional therapy consisted of anticoagulants, oral vasodilators, diuretic agents, cardiac glycosides, and supplemental oxygen. Treatment with epoprostenol also resulted in better quality of life, a primary concern in the management of HIV-infected patients. A more detailed discussion of pulmonary hypertension can be found in Chapter 12 of this book.

Micronutrient Replacement

Deficiencies of selenium[164–166] and L-carnitine[43] have been noted in malnourished HIV-infected patients. In addition, a common and progressive problem associated with pediatric HIV infection is abnormality in growth and body composition.[167] It has been suggested that selenium deficiency[164–166] and malnutrition[168,169] may be causes of cardiac disease, but the role of selenium deficiency remains unclear. Poor dietary intake and malabsorption can lead to decreased serum albumin levels and total lymphocyte counts, which correlate with the selenium deficit in the blood.[170] It has been suggested that this deficiency may result in progression of HIV disease by increasing the oxidative stress of the patient.[42] It has also been associated with reversible ventricular dysfunction in uninfected patients.[171]

However, another study reported that there was no correlation between left ventricular function and reduced selenium content in several HIV-infected adults.[166] Further, a prospective assessment of selenium levels, nutritional status, severity of infection, and cardiac function in HIV-infected children showed no significant positive associations between selenium and ventricular function and contractility.[172] Nevertheless, selenium repletion has been shown in selenium-deficient pediatric and adult patients with symptomatic ventricular dysfunction poorly responsive to conventional anticongestive therapy to improve cardiac function.[164,173]

Carnitine deficiency was noted in 72% of malnourished HIV-infected adults in one study, and some of these patients did have cardiac symptoms.[43] This deficiency has been described as another potentially reversible cause of symptomatic ventricular dysfunction.[174] Case reports also suggest that reversible cardiomyopathy can result from carnitine deficiency.[175] In patients with low plasma carnitine levels, carnitine administration may partially or completely reverse myocardial dysfunction.

Regular assessment of micronutrient status may be advantageous for both adult and pediatric HIV-infected patients who demonstrate worsening or symptomatic ventricular dysfunction. Although replacement efforts have not been proved effective for HIV-infected patients, replacement therapy may be considered if decreased micronutrient levels are found, since other populations have demonstrated the reversal of cardiac dysfunction with this treatment.

Pericardiocentesis and Treatment of Pericardial Effusion

Pericardiocentesis has been used in the diagnosis of pericardial effusion in HIV-infected patients[176] and has been recommended as a therapeutic option for pericardial disease and tamponade.[22,177] Supportive nonspecific treatment for patients may be instituted if no tamponade is present. In addition, pharmaceutic agents such as aspirin or indomethacin may be useful in the management of chest pain.

It is not uncommon for HIV-infected patients to have effusions with or without symptoms (e.g., dyspnea, peripheral edema). Pericardial effusion, most often detected incidentally by echocardiogram, can generally be controlled when treatment is initiated early.[178,179] However, the presence of a pericardial effusion may be associated with an adverse prognosis.[176]

Steroids and oral anticoagulants may be contraindicated for HIV-infected patients with pericardial involvement.[177] One source suggested that steroid therapy be avoided in patients with AIDS because of the possibility of concurrent infection (such as tuberculosis) that could be exacerbated by steroids.[177] It was also noted that because of the risk of intrapericardial hemorrhage, central nervous system bleeding, and mycotic aneurysm, oral anticoagulants may not be appropriate for AIDS-related pericardial disease.

Early detection of pericardial involvement in AIDS and prompt initiation of treatment are beneficial for both adult and pediatric patients. Because of the potential for hemodynamic disturbances in patients with pericardial disease, close monitoring of progression and therapeutic efficacy may be helpful in the management of these patients.

Conclusion

The treatment of cardiac problems in HIV-infected adults and children is difficult because the patient usually has multiple health problems. We are beginning to understand the role cardiac problems play in the natural history and prognosis of AIDS. If, as one source suggested, the number of deaths of HIV-infected patients by opportunistic infection is declining, and both the morbidity of the disease and the survival time are increasing,[180] the need to address cardiac-related morbidity is critical. This chapter has described some ways in which caregivers may not only address specific cardiac complications such as congestive heart failure, but also slow the progression of cardiac dysfunction (Figure 25-10). In addition, because the improvement of quality of life is often the only reachable goal, we have introduced some nonpharmacologic treatments. By incorporating these treatment options into practice and remaining informed of ongoing randomized trials of cardiac therapy for children and adults with HIV infection and AIDS, caregivers will be more adequately prepared to support these patients.

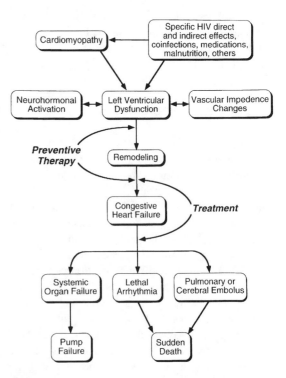

Figure 25-10. Progression of cardiac dysfunction in HIV-infected patients.

References

1. Johnson JE, Slife DM, Anders GT, et al. Cardiac dysfunction in patients seropositive for the human immunodeficiency virus. *West J Med* 1991;155: 373–379.

2. Kinney EL. Cardiac findings in AIDS. *Chest* 1988;94:1113–1114.

3. Reitano J, King M, Cohen H, et al. Cardiac function in patients with acquired immune deficiency syndrome (AIDS) or AIDS prodrome. [Abstract]. *J Am Coll Cardiol* 1984;3:525–520.

4. Kaminski HJ, Katzman M, Wiest PM, et al. Cardiomyopathy associated with the acquired immune deficiency syndrome. *J Acquir Immune Defic Syndr* 1988;1:105–110.

5. Bestetti RB. Cardiac involvement in the acquired immune deficiency syndrome. *Int J Cardiol* 1989; 22:143–146.

6. Kaul S, Fishbein MC, Siegel RJ. Cardiac manifestations of acquired immune deficiency syndrome: a 1991 update. *Am Heart J* 1991;122:535–544.

7. Lipshultz SE, Sanders SP, Colan SD. Cardiac structure and function in HIV-infected children. [Response]. *N Engl J Med* 1993;328:513–514.

8. Lipshultz SE, Orav EJ, Sanders SP, et al. Abnormalities of cardiac structure and function in HIV-infected children treated with zidovudine. *N Engl J Med* 1992;327:1260–1265.

9. Lipshultz SE, Bancroft EA, Boller A-M. Cardiovascular manifestations of HIV infection in children (in press). In: Bricker JT (ed). *The Science and Practice of Pediatric Cardiology*. Baltimore: Williams & Wilkins, 1996.

10. Lipshultz SE, Chanock S, Sanders SP, et al. Cardiovascular manifestations of human immunodeficiency virus infection in infants and children. *Am J Cardiol* 1989;63:1489–1497.

11. Bierman FS. Guidelines for diagnosis and management of cardiac disease in children with HIV infection. *J Pediatr* 1991;119:S53-S56.

12. Stewart JM, Kaul A, Gromisch DS, et al. Symptomatic cardiac dysfunction in children with human immunodeficiency virus infection. *Am Heart J* 1989;117:140–144.

13. Lipshultz SE. Cardiovascular problems. In: Pizzo PA, Wilfert CM (eds). *Pediatric AIDS: The Challenge of HIV Infection in Infants, Children, and Adolescents*. Baltimore: Williams & Wilkins, 1994:483–511.

14. Newburger JW, Sanders SP, Burns JC, et al. Left ventricular contractility and function in Kawasaki syndrome: effect of intravenous γ-globulin. *Circulation* 1989;79:1237–1246.

15. Anderson DW, Virmani R, Reilly JM, et al. Prevalent myocarditis at necropsy in the acquired immunodeficiency syndrome. *J Am Coll Cardiol* 1988; 11:792–799.

16. Lipshultz SE for the Pediatric Pulmonary and Cardiovascular Complications of the Vertically Transmitted HIV Infection Study. Progressive left ventricular dysfunction in HIV-infected children: the prospective NHLBI P2C2 HIV study. [Abstract]. *Circulation* 1993;88:I.

17. Kavanaugh-McHugh AL, Ruff AJ, Rowe SA, et al. Cardiac abnormalities in a multicenter interventional study of children with symptomatic HIV infection. *Pediatr Res* 1991;28:1040.

18. Brown DL, Sather S, Cheitlin MD. Reversible cardiac dysfunction associated with foscarnet therapy for cytomegalovirus esophagitis in an AIDS patient. *Am Heart J* 1993;125:1439–1440.

19. Deyton LR, Walker RE, Kovacs JA, et al. Reversible cardiac dysfunction associated with interferon alfa therapy in AIDS patients with Kaposi's sarcoma. *N Engl J Med* 1989;321:1246–1249.

20. Luginbuhl LM, Orav EJ, McIntosh K, Lipshultz SE. Cardiac morbidity and related mortality in children with HIV infection. *JAMA* 1993;269: 2869–2875.

21. Chanock S, Luginbuhl LM, McIntosh K, Lipshultz SE. Life-threatening reactions to trimethoprim–sulfamethoxazole in children with HIV infection. *Pediatrics* 1994;93:519–521.

22. Lane-McAuliffe E, Lipshultz SE. Cardiovascular complications in pediatric HIV infection. *Nurs Clin North Am* 1995;30:291–316.

23. Wilkins JN. Brain, lung, and cardiovascular interactions with cocaine and cocain-induced catecholamine effects. [Review]. *J Addict Dis* 1992; 11:9–19.

24. Herskowitz A, Willoughby SB, Baughman KL, et al. Cardiomyopathy associated with antiretroviral therapy in patients with HIV infection: a report of six cases. *Ann Intern Med* 1992;116:311–313.

25. D'Amati G, Kwan W, Lewis W. Dilated cardiomyopathy in a zidovudine-treated AIDS patient. *Cardiovasc Pathol* 1992;1:317–320.

26. Hsia J, Adams S, Ross AM. Natural history of human immunodeficiency virus (HIV) associated heart disease. *Circulation* 1991;84:2–3.

27. Jacob AJ, Sutherland GR, Bird AG, et al. Myocardial dysfunction in patients infected with HIV: prevalence and risk factors. *Br Heart J* 1992; 68:549–553.

28. Corallo S, Mutinelli MR, Lazzarin A, et al. Echocardiography detects myocardial damage in AIDS: prospective study in 102 patients. *Eur Heart J* 1988;9:887–892.

29. DeCastro S, Migliau G, Silvestri A, et al. Heart involvement in AIDS: a prospective study during various stages of the disease. *Eur Heart J* 1992; 13:1452–1459.

30. Coudray N, De Zuttere D, Force G, et al. Left ventricular diastolic function in asymptomatic and symptomatic human immunodeficiency virus carriers: an echocardiographic study. *Eur Heart J* 1995;16:61–76.

31. The SOLVD Investigators . Effect of enalapril on mortality and the development of heart failure in asymptomatic patients with reduced left ventricular ejection fractions. *N Engl J Med* 1992;327: 685–691.

32. Pfeffer MA, Braunwald E, Moye LA, et al. Effect of captopril on mortality and morbidity in patients with left ventricular dysfunction after myocardial infarction. *N Engl J Med* 1992;327:669–677.

33. Cleland JGF, Shah D, Krikler S, et al. Effects of lisinopril on cardiorespiratory, neuroendocrine, and renal function in patients with reduced left ventricular dysfunction. *Br Heart J* 1993;69: 512–515.

34. Talner HS. Heart failure. In: Emmanouilides GC, Riemenschneider TA, Allen HD, Gutgusell HP (eds). *Moss and Adams' Heart Disease in Infants, Children, and Adolescents Including the Fetus and Young Adult,* 5th Ed. Baltimore: Williams and Wilkins, 1995:1746–1773.

35. Sharpe N. Beta blockers in heart failure. *Eur Heart J* 1996;17(Suppl B):39–42.

36. Cohn JN, Simon A, Johnson G, the VHeFT Study Group. Relationship of plasma norepinephrine and plasma renin activity to mortality in heart failure: V-HeFT II. [Abstract]. *Circulation* 1991;84 (Suppl II):II310.

37. Smith TW, Braunwald E, Kelly RA. The management of heart failure. In: *Heart Disease: A Textbook of Cardiovascular Medicine.* Philadelphia: WB Saunders, 1992:464–519.

38. Artman M. Appendix: drugs and dosages. In: Emmanouilides GC, Riemenschneider TA, Allen HD

Gutgusell HP (eds). *Moss and Adams' Heart Disease in Infants, Children, and Adolescents Including the Fetus and Young Adults.* Baltimore: Williams and Wilkins, 1995:1813–1824.

39. Schneeweiss A. Cardiovascular drugs in children: II. Angiotensin-converting enzyme inhibitors in pediatric patients. *Pediatr Cardiol* 1990;11: 199–207.

40. Parikh SR, Girod DA. Treatment of heart failure in the pediatric and young adult patient. *Contemp Treat Cardiovasc Dis* 1996;1:3–32.

41. Levy WS, Simon GL, Rios JC, Ross AM. Prevalence of cardiac abnormalities in human immunodeficiency virus infection. *Am J Cardiol* 1989; 63:86–89.

42. Baruchel S, Wainberg MA. The role of oxidative stress in disease progression in individuals infected by the human immunodeficiency virus. *J Leukocyte Biol* 1992;52:111–114.

43. DeSimone C, Tzantzoglou S, Jirillo E. L-Carnitine deficiency in AIDS patients. *AIDS* 1992;6: 203–205.

44. Vogel RL. Cardiac manifestations of pediatric acquired immunodeficiency syndrome. In: Yogev R, Connor E (eds). *Management of HIV Infection in Infants and Children.* St. Louis, MO: Mosby-Year Book, 1992:357–370.

45. Kavanaugh-McHugh A, Ruff AJ, Rowe SA, et al. Cardiovascular manifestations. In: Pizzo PA Wilfert CM (eds). *Pediatric AIDS: The Challenge of HIV Infection in Infants, Children, and Adolescents.* Baltimore: Williams & Wilkins, 1991: 355–372.

46. CONSENSUS Trial Study Group . Effects of enalapril on mortality in severe congestive heart failure. *N Engl J Med* 1987;316:1429–1435.

47. Johnstone DE, Abdulla A, Arnold JMO, et al. Diagnosis and management of heart failure. *Can J Cardiol* 1994;10:613–631.

48. Smith TW. Heart failure. In: Bennett JC, Plum F (eds). *Cicil's Textbook of Medicine.* Philadelphia: WB Saunders, 1996:211–231.

49. Young JB. Assessment in heart failure. In: Braunwald E (ed). *Atlas of Heart Diseases,* Vol IV: *Heart Failure: Cardiac Function and Dysfunction.* St. Louis, MO: Mosby-Year Book, 1995:7.1–7.20.

50. Ross RD, Bollinger RO, Pinsky WW. Grading the severity of congestive heart failure in infants. *Pediatr Cardiol* 1992;13:72–75.

51. Grunfeld C, Schambelan M. The wasting syndrome: pathophysiology and treatment. In: Broder S, Merigan TC, Bolognesi D (eds). *Textbook of AIDS Medicine*. Baltimore: Williams & Wilkins, 1994:637–649.

52. Grunfeld C, Kotlet DP. Wasting in the acquired immunodeficiency syndrome. *Semin Liver Dis* 1992;12:175–187.

53. Grunfeld C, Feingold KR. Metabolic disturbances and wasting in the acquired immunodeficiency syndrome. *N Engl J Med* 1992;327:329–337.

54. Dracup K, Baker DW, Dunbar SB. Management of heart failure: II. counseling education, and lifestyle modifications. *JAMA* 1994;18:1442–1446.

55. Conn EH, Williams RS,Wallace AG. Exercise responses before and after physical conditioning in patients with severely depressed left ventricular function. *Am J Cardiol* 1982;49:296–300.

56. Lee AP, Ice R, Blessey R, Sanmarco ME. Long-term effects of physical training on coronary patients with impaired ventricular function. *Circulation* 1979;60:1519–1526.

57. Kellerman JJ, Ben-Ari E, Fisman E, et al. Physical training in patients with ventricular impairment. *Adv Cardiol* 1986;34:131–147.

58. Kellerman JJ, Shemesh J, Fisman EZ, et al. Arm exercise training in the rehabilitation of patients with impaired ventricular function and heart failure. *Cardiology* 1990;77:130–138.

59. Coats AJS, Adamopolous S, Mayer TE, et al. Effects of physical training in congestive heart failure. *Lancet* 1990;335:63–66.

60. Kochj M, Douard H, Broustet JP. The benefit of graded physical exercise in congestive heart failure. *Chest* 1992;101:231S–235S.

61. Meyer TE, Casadei B, Coats AJS, et al. Angiotensin-converting enzyme and physical training in chronic heart failure. *J Intern Med* 1991;230:407–413.

62. Scalvini S, Marangoni S, Volterrani M, et al. Physical rehabilitation in coronary patients who have suffered from episodes of cardiac failure. *Cardiology* 1993;80:417–423.

63. Chokshi SK, Moore R, Pandian NG, Isner JN. Reversible cardiomyopathy associated with cocaine intoxication. *Ann Intern Med* 1989;111:1039–1040.

64. Billman GE. Cocaine: a review of its toxic actions and cardiac function. *Crit Rev Toxicol* 1995;25:113–132.

65. Boland MG, Harris DM. Living with HIV infection. In: Yogev R, Connor E (eds). *Management of HIV-Infected Infants and Children*. St. Louis, MO: Mosby-Year Book, 1992:533–550.

66. Carson P. Pharmacologic treatment of heart failure. *Clin Cardiol* 1996;19:271–277.

67. Taylor SH. Towards a comprehensive treatment. *Eur Heart J* 1996;17(Suppl B):43–56.

68. Baker DW, Konstam MA, Bottoroff M, Pitt B. Management of heart failure (I): pharmacologic treatment. *JAMA* 1994;17:1361–1366.

69. Noonan JA. Congestive heart failure. In: Burg FD, Wald ER, Ingelfinger JR, Polin RA (eds). *Gellis and Kagan's Current Pediatric Therapy*. Philadelphia: WB Saunders, 1996:173–175.

70. Abrams J. Congestive heart failure. In: Rakel RE (ed). *Conn's Current Therapy*. Philadelphia: WB Saunders, 1996:281–284.

71. Smith TW, Kelly RA. Therapeutic strategies for CHF in the 1990's. *Hosp Pract* 1991;Nov:69–86.

72. The SOLVD Investigators. Effect of enalapril on survival in patients with reduced left-ventricular ejection fractions and congestive heart failure. *N Engl J Med* 1991;325:293–302.

73. Cohn JN, Johnson G, Zieschem S. A comparison of enalapril with hydralazine-isosorbide dinitrate in the treatment of chronic congestive heart failure. *N Engl J Med* 1991;325:303–310.

74. The Captopril-Digoxin Multicenter Research Group. A placebo-controlled trial of captopril in refractory chronic congestive heart failure. *J Am Coll Cardiol* 1983;2:755–763.

75. Franciosa JA, Wilen MM, Jordan RA. Effects of enalapril, a new angiotensin-converting enzyme inhibitor, in a controlled trial in heart failure. *J Am Coll Cardiol* 1985;5:101–107.

76. Jennings G, Kiat H, Nelson L, et al. Enalapril for severe congestive heart failure: a double-blind study. *Med J Aust* 1984;141:723–726.

77. Kleber FX, Niemoller L, Fischer M, Doering W. Influence of severity of heart failure on the efficacy of angiotensin-converting enzyme inhibition. *Am J Cardiol* 1991;68:121–126.

78. Magnani B, Magelli C. Captopril in mild heart failure; preliminary observations of a long-term double-blind, placebo-controlled study. *Postgrad Med J* 1986;62:153–158.

79. McGrath BP, Arnolda L, Matthews PG, et al. Controlled trial of enalapril in congestive heart failure. *Br Heart J* 1985;54:405–414.

80. Remes J, Nikander P, Rehnberg S, et al. Enalapril in chronic heart failure: a double-blind placebo-controlled study. *Ann Clin Res* 1986;18:124–128.

81. Sharpe D, Murphy J, Coxon R, Hannan SF. Enalapril in patients with chronic heart failure: a placebo-controlled, randomized, double-blind study. *Circulation* 1984;70:271–278.

82. Eronen J, Personen E, Wallgren EI, et al. Enalapril in children with congestive heart failure. *Acta Paediatr Scand* 1991;80:555–558.

83. Frenneaux M, Stewart RAH, Newman CMH, Hallidie-Smith KA. Enalapril for severe heart failure in infancy. *Arch Dis Child* 1989;64:219–223.

84. Lloyd TR, Mahoney LT, Kneodel PAC, et al. Orally administered enalapril for infants with congestive heart failure: a dose-finding study. *J Pediatr* 1989;114:650–654.

85. Artman M, Parrish MD, Appleton S, et al. Hemodynamic effects of hydralazine in infants with idiopathic dilated cardiomyopathy and congestive heart failure. *Am Heart J* 1987;113:144–150.

86. Physician's Desk Reference, 49th Ed. Montevale, NJ: Medical Economics, 1995. Ed. 49

87. Nies AS. Clinical pharmacokinetics in congestive heart failure. In: Hosenpud JD, Greenberg BH (eds). *Congestive Heart Failure: Pathophysiology, Diagnosis, and Comprehensive Approach to Management.* New York: Springer-Verlag, 1994:323–340.

88. Breckenridge AM. Drug interactions with ACE inhibitors. *J Hum Hypertens* 1989;3:133–138.

89. Massie BM, Amidon T. Angiotensin-converting enzyme inhibitor therapy for congestive heart failure: rationale, results, and current recommendations. In: Hosenpud JD, Greenberg BH (eds). *Congestive Heart Failure: Pathophysiology, Diagnosis and Comprehensive Approach to Management.* New York: Springer-Verlag, 1994:380–399.

90. Fox AJ, Lalloo UG, Belvisi MG, et al. Bradykinin-evoked sensitization of airway sensory nerves: a mechanism for ACE-inhibitor cough. *Nature Med* 1996;2:814–817.

91. Gottlieb SS. Diuretics. In: Hosenpud JD, Greenberg BH (eds). *Congestive Heart Failure: Pathophysiology, Diagnosis, and Comprehensive Management.* New York: Springer-Verlag, 1994:341–353.

92. Packer M, Lee WH, Kessler PD, et al. Role of neurohormonal mechanisms in determining survival in patients with severe chronic heart failure. *Circulation* 1987;75:IV-80–IV-92.

93. Kupper AJ, Fintelman H, Huige MC, et al. Crossover comparison of the fixed combination of hydrochlorothiazide and triampterene and the free combination of furosemide and triampterene in the maintenance treatment of congestive heart failure. *Eur J Clin Pharmacol* 1986;30:342–343.

94. Whight C, Morgan T, Carney S, Wilson M. Diuretics, cardiac failure, and potassium depletion: a rational approach. *Med J Aust* 1974;2:831–833.

95. Kokko JP. Diuretics. In: Schlant RA, Alexander W (eds). *The Heart.* New York: McGraw-Hill, 1994:595–609.

96. Shammas FVG, Dickstein K. Clinical pharmacokinetics in heart failure: an updated review. *Clin Pharmakokinet* 1988;15:94–113.

97. Beermann B, Groschinsky-Grind M. Pharmacokinetics of hydrochlorothiazide in patients with congestive heart failure. *Br J Clin Pharmacol* 1979;7:579–583.

98. Ghose RR, Gupta SK. Synergistic actions of metolazone with "loop" diuretics. *BMJ* 1981;812:1432–1433.

99. Kiyingi A, Field MJ, Pawsel CC, et al. Metolazone in treatment of severe refractory congestive heart failure. *Lancet* 1990;335:29–31

100. Artman M. Pharmacologic therapy. In: Emmanouilides GC, Riemenschneider TA, Allen HD, Gutgusell HP (eds). *Moss and Adams' Heart Disease in Infants, Children and Adolescents Including the Fetus and Young Adult.* Baltimore: Williams & Wilkins, 1995:375–398.

101. Brater DC, Day B, Burdette A, Anderson S. Butanemide and furosemide in heart failure. *Kidney Int* 1984;26:183–189.

102. Greenblatt DJ, Koch-Weiser J. Adverse reactions to spironolactone: a report from the Boston collaborative drug surveillance program. *JAMA* 1973;225:40–43.

103. Ott P, Marcus FI. The role of digoxin in the treatment of chronic congestive heart failure. *J Cardiovasc Pharmacol Ther* 1996;1:259–264.

104. Packer M, Gheorghiade M, Young JB, et al. Withdrawal of digoxin from patients with chronic heart failure treated with angiotensin converting enzyme inhibitors. *N Engl J Med* 1993;329:1–7.

105. Jaeschke R, Oxman AD, Guyatt GH. To what extent do congestive heart failure patients in sinus rhythm benefit from digoxin therapy?: a system-

atic overview and meta-analysis. *Am J Med* 1990; 88:279–286.

106. Di Bianco R, Shabetai R, Kostuk W, et al. A comparison of oral milrinone, digoxin, and their combination in the treatment of patients with chronic heart failure. *N Engl J Med* 1989;321:476.

107. Greenberg BH. The medical management of chronic congestive heart failure. In: Hosenpud JD, Greenberg BH (eds). *Congestive Heart Failure: Pathophysiology, Diagnosis and Comprehensive Approach to Management.* New York: Springer-Verlag, 1994:628–644.

108. Cohn JN. The management of chronic heart failure. *N Engl J Med* 1996;335:490–498.

109. Kelly RA, Smith TW. Digitalis glycosides. In: Hosenpud JD, Greenberg BH (eds). *Congestive Heart Failure: Pathophysiology, Diagnosis and Comprehensive Approach to Management.* New York: Springer-Verlag, 1994:354–379.

110. Rahimtoola SH, Tak T. Digitalis in heart failure. In: McCall D, Rahimtoola SH (eds). *Heart Failure.* New York: Chapman and Hall, 1995:229–269.

111. Feldman AM, Bristow MR, Parmley WW, et al. Effects of vesnarinone on morbidity and mortality in patients with heart failure. *N Engl J Med* 1993;329:149–155.

112. Captopril Multicenter Research Group. A placebo-controlled trial of captopril in refractory heart failure. *J Am Coll Cardiol* 1983;2:755–763.

113. Matsui S, Matsumori A, Matoba Y, et al. Treatment of virus-induced myocardial injury with a novel immunomodulatory agent, vesnarinone: suppression of natural killer cell activity and tumor necrosis factor-alpha production. *J Clin Invest* 1994;94:1212–1217.

114. The MDC Trial Study Group. Metoprolol in dilated cardiomyopathy. *Lancet* 1993;342:1141–1146.

115. Packer M, Bristow MR, Cohn NJ, et al. The effect of carvedilol on morbidity and mortality in patients with chronic heart failure. *N Engl J Med* 1996;334:1349–1355.

116. Ghali JK, Kadakia S, Cooper R, Ferlinz J. Precipitating factors leading to decompensation of heart failure: traits among urban blacks. [Review]. *Arch Intern Med* 1988;148:2013–2016.

117. Artman M, Graham TP Jr. Guidelines for vasodilator therapy of congestive heart failure in infants and children. *Am Heart J* 1987;113:994–1005.

118. Cowley AJ, Wynne RD, Hampton JR. The effects of BTS 4946S on blood pressure and peripheral arteriolar and venous tone in normal volunteers. *J Hypertens* 1984;2:547–549.

119. Elborne J, Sanford C, Nocholls D. Effect of flosequinan on exercise capacity and symptoms in severe heart failure. *Br Heart J* 1989;61:331–335.

120. Packer M, Narahar KA, Eklayam U, et al. Double-blind, placebo-controlled study of the efficacy of flosequinan in patients with chronic heart failure. *J Am Coll Cardiol* 1993;22:65–72.

121. Pitt B, on behalf of the Reflect II Study Group. A randomized, multicenter, double-blind placebo controlled study of the efficacy of flosequinan in patients with chronic heart failure. [Abstract]. *Circulation* 1991;84:II-311.

122. Silke B, Tennet H, Fisher-Hansen, et al. A double-blind parallel-group comparison of flosequinan and enalapril in the treatment of chronic heart failure. *Eur Heart J* 1992;13:1092–1100.

123. Massie BM, Berke MR, Brozena SC, et al. Can further benefit be achieved by adding a vasodilator to a diuretic, digoxin and angiotensin converting enzyme inhibitor therapy in patients with congestive heart failure: results of the flosequinan plus ACE inhibitor trial (FACET). *Circulation* 1993; 88:492–501.

124. Packer M, Rouleau J, Swedberg K, et al. Effects of flosequinan on survival in chronic heart failure: preliminary results of the PROFILE study. [Abstract]. *Circulation* 1993;88:(Suppl I):I-301.

125. Lejemtel TH, Keung E, Sonnenblock EH, et al. Amrinone: a new non-glycosidal nonadrenergic cardiotonic agent effective in the treatment of intractable myocardial failure in man. *Circulation* 1979;59:1098–1104.

126. Miller TL, Awnetwant EL, Evans S, et al. Gastronomy tube supplementation for HIV-infected children. *Pediatrics* 1995;96:696–702.

127. Uva MS, Jebara VA, Fabiani JN, et al. Cardiac surgery in patients with human immunodeficiency virus infection: indications and results. *J Cardiac Surg* 1992;7:240–244.

128. Aris A, Pomar ML, Saur E. Cardiopulmonary bypass in HIV-positive patients. *Ann Thorac Surg* 1993;55:1104–1108.

129. Horowitz MD, Cox MM, Neibart RM, et al. Resection of right atrial lymphoma in a patient with AIDS. *Int J Cardiol* 1992;34:139–142.

130. Lemma M, Vanelli P, Botta BM, et al. Cardiac surgery in HIV-positive intravenous drug addicts:

influence of cardiopulmonary bypass on the progression to AIDS. *Thorac Cardiovasc Surg* 1992; 40:279–282.

131. Frater RWM, Sisto D, Condit D. Cardiac surgery in human immunodeficiency virus (HIV) carriers. *Eur J Cardio thorac Surg* 1989;3:146–151.

132. Vincent JL. Hemodynamic monitoring, pharmacological therapy, and arrhythmia management in acute congestive heart failure. In: Hosenpud JD, Greenberg BH (eds). *Congestive Heart Failure: Pathophysiology, Diagnosis, and Comprehensive Approach to Management.* New York: Springer-Verlag, 1994:509–521.

133. Rackow EC, Packman MI,Weil MH. Hemodynamic effects of digoxin during acute cardiac failure: a comparison in patients with and without acute myocardial infarction. *Crit Care Med* 1996; 15:1001–1005.

134. Moore JW. Afterload manipulation. In: Garson A, Bricker JT, McNamara DG (eds). *The Science and Practice of Pediatric Cardiology,* Vol 3. Philadelphia: Lea & Febiger, 1990:2086–2098.

135. Mofenson LM, Moye J Jr, Bethel J, et al. Prophylactic intravenous immunoglobulin in HIV-infected children with CD4+ counts of 0.20×10/L or more: effect on viral, opportunistic, and bacterial infections. *JAMA* 1992;268:483–488.

136. Kaplan S, Lipshultz SE. Cardiovascular complications of HIV infection in children. *Cardiol Rev* 1995;3:99–105.

137. Drucker NA, Colan SD, Lewis A, et al. Gamma-globulin treatment of acute myocarditis in the pediatric population. *Circulation* 1994;89:252–257.

138. Lipshultz SE, Orav EJ, Sanders SP, Colan SD. Immunoglobulins and cardiac structure and function in HIV-infected children. *Circulation* 1995; 92:2220–2225.

139. Viard JP, Vittecoq D, Lacroix C, Bach JF. Response of HIV-1-associated polymyositis to intravenous immunoglobulin. *Am J Med* 1992;92: 580–581.

140. National Institute of Child Health and Human Development Intravenous Immunoglobulin Study Group . Intravenous immune globulin for the prevention of bacterial infections in children. *N Engl J Med* 1991;325:73–80.

141. Dwyer JM. Manipulating the immune system with immune globulin. *N Engl J Med* 1992;326: 107–116.

142. Matsuyama T, Kobayashi N, Yamamoto N. Cytokines and HIV infection: is AIDS a tumor necrosis factor disease? *AIDS* 1991;5:1405–1417.

143. Odeh M. The role of tumour necrosis factor-alpha in acquired immunodeficiency syndrome. *J Intern Med* 1990;228:549–556.

144. Parker TG, Schneider MD. Growth factors, proto-oncogenes, and plasticity of the cardiac phenotype. *Annu Rev Physiol* 1991;53:179–200.

145. Levy WS, Barghese PJ, Anderson DW, et al. Myocarditis diagnosed by endomyocardial biopsy in human immunodeficiency virus infection with cardiac dysfunction. *Am J Cardiol* 1988;62:658–659.

146. Chan KY, Iwahara M, Benson LN, et al. Immunosuppressive therapy in the management of acute myocarditis in children: a clinical trial. *J Am Coll Cardiol* 1991;17:458–460.

147. Mason JW, O'Connell JB, Herskowitz A, et al. The myocarditis treatment trial investigators: a clinical trial of immunosuppressive therapy for myocarditis. *N Engl J Med* 1995;333:269–275.

148. Lipshultz SE, Luginbuhl LM, Saul JP, McIntosh K. Dysrhythmias, unexpected arrest and sudden death in pediatric HIV infection. [Abstract]. *Circulation* 1991;84:II-660.

149. Eisenhauer MD, Eliasson AH, Taylor AJ, et al. Incidence of cardiac arrhythmias during intravenous pentamidine therapy in HIV-infected patients. *Chest* 1994;105:389–394.

150. Wharton JM, Demopulos PA, Goldschlager N. Torsades de pointes during administration of pentamidine isethionate. *Am J Med* 1987;83:571–576.

151. Kleyman TR, Roberts C, Ling BN. A mechanism for pentamidine-induced hyperkalemia: inhibition of distal nephron sodium transport. *Ann Intern Med* 1995;122:103–106.

152. Smith WM, Gallagher JJ. "Les torsades de pointes": an unusual ventricular arrhythmia. *Ann Intern Med* 1980;93:578–584.

153. Kinney EL, Monsuez JJ, Kitzis M, Vittecoq DE. Treatment of AIDS-associated heart disease. *J Vasc Dis* 1989;40:970–976.

154. Maisch B, Schonian U. Elimination of cytomegalovirus DNA by hyperimmunoglobulin therapy in active myocarditis and dilated heart muscle disease. [Abstract]. *J Am Coll Cardiol* 1993;21: 21A-210.

155. Atiyeh B, Dabbagh S, Fleischymann LE, Gruskin AB. Systemic hypertension. In: Burg FD, Wald ER, Ingelfinger JR, Polin RA (eds). *Gellis and*

Kagan's Current Pediatric Therapy. Philadelphia: WB Saunders, 1996:200–205.

156. Oparil S. Arterial hypertension. In: Bennett JC, Plum F (eds). *Cicil's Textbook of Medicine.* Philadelphia: WB Saunders, 1996:256–271.

157. Issenberg HJ, Charytan M, Rubinstein A. Cardiac involvement in children with acquired immune deficiency. [Abstract]. *Am Heart J* 1985;110:710.

158. Sherron P, Pickoff AS, Ferrer PL, et al. Echocardiographic evaluation of myocardial function in pediatric AIDS patients. [Abstract]. *Am Heart J* 1985;110:710.

159. Himelman RB, Dohrmann M, Goodman P, et al. Severe pulmonary hypertension and cor pulmonale in the acquired immunodeficiency syndrome. *Am J Cardiol* 1989;64:1396–1400.

160. Arunabh S, Edasery B. Human immunodeficiency virus and primary pulmonary hypertension. *West J Med* 1993;159:708–709.

161. Petitpretz P, Brenot F, Azarian R, et al. Pulmonary hypertension in patients with human immunodeficiency virus infection: comparison with primary pulmonary hypertension. *Circulation* 1994;89: 2722–2727.

162. Aarons EJ, Nye FJ. Primary pulmonary hypertension and HIV infection. *AIDS* 1991;5:1276–1277.

163. Barst RJ, Rubin LJ, Long WA, et al. Comparison of continuous intravenous epoprostenol (prostacyclin) with conventional therapy for primary pulmonary hypertension. *N Engl J Med* 1996;334: 296–301.

164. Kavanaugh-McHugh AL, Ruff A, Perlman E, et al. Selenium deficiency and cardiomyopathy in acquired immunodeficiency syndrome. *J Parenter Enter Nutr* 1991;15:347–349.

165. Dworkin BM, Rosenthal WS, Wormser GP, Weiss L. Selenium deficiency in the acquired immunodeficiency syndrome. *J Parenter Enter Nutr* 1986; 10:405–407.

166. Dworkin BM, Antonecchia PP, Smith F, et al. Reduced cardiac selenium content in the acquired immunodeficiency syndrome. *J Parenter Enter Nutr* 1989;13:644–647.

167. Miller TL, Evans SJ, Orav EJ, et al. Growth and body composition in children infected with the human immunodeficiency virus-1. *Am J Clin Nutr* 1993;57:588–592.

168. Webb JG, Kiess MC, Chan-Yan CC. Malnutrition and the heart. *Can Med Assoc J* 1986;135:753–750.

169. Alden PB, Madoff RD, Stahl TJ, et al. Cardiac function in malnutrition. *Nutr Heart Dis* 1987; 2:71–81.

170. Dworkin BM. Selenium deficiency in HIV infection and the acquired immunodeficiency syndrome (AIDS). *Chem Biol Interact* 1994;91:181–186.

171. Oster O, Prellwitz W. Selenium and cardiovascular disease. *Biol Trace Element Res* 1990;24: 91–103.

172. Miller TL, Orav EJ, McIntosh K, Lipshultz SE. Is selenium deficiency clinically significant in pediatric HIV infection? [Abstract]. *Gastroenterology* 1993;104:A746–A740.

173. Lafonte A, Zazzo JF, Chappuis P, et al. Are cardiomyopathies in acquired immunodeficiency syndrome dependent on selenium deficiency? [Abstract]. *Circulation* 1988;78:II-375.

174. Waber LJ, Valle D, Neill C, et al. Carnitine deficiency presenting as familial cardiomyopathy: a treatable defect in carnitine transport. *J Pediatr* 1982;101:700–705.

175. Zales VR, Benson DW. Reversible cardiomyopathy due to carnitine deficiency from renal tubular wasting. *Pediatr Cardiol* 1995;16:76–78.

176. Hsia J, Ross AM. Pericardial effusion and pericardiocentesis in human immunodeficiency virus infection. *Am J Cardiol* 1994;74:94–96.

177. Francis CK. Cardiac involvement in AIDS. In: O'Rourke RA, McCall D, Beller GA, et al. (eds). *Current Problems in Cardiology.* St. Louis, MO: Mosby-Year Book, 1990:571–639.

178. Mast HL, Haller JO, Schiller MS, Anderson VM. Pericardial effusion and its relationship to cardiac disease in children with acquired immunodeficiency syndrome. *Pediatr Radiol* 1992;22:548–551.

179. Reynolds MM, Hecht SR, Berger M, et al. Large pericardial effusions in the acquired immunodeficiency syndrome. *Chest* 1992;102:1746–1747.

180. Peters BS, Beck EJ, Coleman DG, et al. Changing disease patterns in patients with AIDS in a referral centre in the United Kingdom: the changing face of AIDS. *BMJ* 1991;302:203–207.

181. Kelly RA, Smith TW. Treatment of stable heart failure: digitalis and diuretics. In: Braunwald E (ed). *Atlas of Heart Diseases,* Vol. 4: *Heart Failure: Cardiac Function and Dysfunction.* St. Louis, MO: Mosby-Year Book, 1995:10.1–10.16.

26

Diagnosis and Course of Other Viral Heart Disease in Patients with HIV Infection

Jeffrey A. Towbin, M.D.

Human immunodeficiency virus (HIV) infection has been associated with significant cardiovascular disease, including myocarditis and dilated cardiomyopathy. It is unclear, however, how this retroviral infection leads to myocardial dysfunction. The purpose of this chapter is to review the reported data concerning cardiac dysfunction in HIV, as well as to outline the current knowledge regarding viral disorders of the heart and the diagnostic approaches available.

Viral Myocarditis

The defining features of active myocarditis in non-HIV-infected patients include an interstitial mononuclear cell infiltrate and myocyte necrosis as seen by histopathology[1,2] (Figure 26-1). One or both ventricles (predominantly the left ventricle) and/or the pericardium, may be affected by this multifocal, patchy disease. Two stages of myocarditis are usually described: (1) an acute stage characterized by virus-induced myocyte necrosis and (2) a chronic stage with autoimmunity-mediated myocyte destruction. Although most patients recover clinically from acute myocarditis, a significant number develop chronic myocarditis and dilated cardio-

myopathy. It has been reported that as many as 63% of patients with dilated cardiomyopathy have active myocarditis detectable by endomyocardial biopsy.[3] However, a significant number of patients die, either suddenly or from chronic heart failure. The underlying causes of myocarditis are many (Table 26-1), but viruses appear to be the most common.[4]

Etiology of Myocarditis

Most cases of myocarditis in immunocompetent patients in the United States and Western Europe result from viral infections (Table 26-2), most commonly thought to be enteroviruses (coxsackievirus, echovirus, poliovirus).[4,5] These nonenveloped viruses contain a single strand of RNA in their genome. All enteroviruses are cardiotropic but produce myocarditis only in a susceptible, genetically predisposed host. Usually no virus is isolated, but when it is, coxsackievirus, particularly coxsackie B virus, is the most common. More recently, adenoviruses, double-stranded DNA viruses that commonly infect children (70–80% of children at 5 years of age have neutralizing antibody to adenovirus types 1 and 2 and 50% to type 5),[6] have been shown to be frequently associated with myocarditis

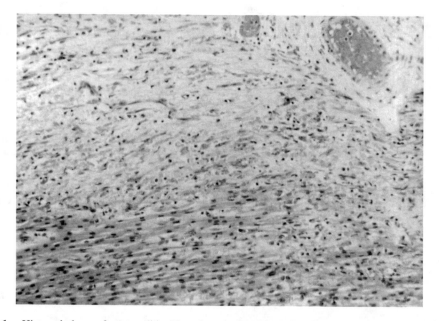

Figure 26-1. Histopathology of myocarditis. Note the mononuclear cell infiltrate, edema, and myocyte necrosis, consistent with active myocarditis (Hematoxylin and eosin; ×56.)

in children.[7,8] HIV has also been identified in a significant number of patients with myocarditis.[9–14] Other viruses have less commonly been reported to be responsible for myocarditis.[4]

Initial evidence indicating that there is a connection between viruses and inflammatory heart disease was circumstantial and based on identification of a viral infection in patients with a clinical diagnosis of myocarditis.[15,16] The diagnosis of a viral infection relied on identification of a virus by peripheral cultures (blood, stool, nasopharyngeal fluid, urine, or cerebrospinal fluid) or serial serology. Repeated attempts to isolate virus from the myocardium were

typically unsuccessful. Except for the rare reports of myocardial cultures of enterovirus, direct evidence of an association between enteroviruses and myocarditis was not found until the recent development of molecular methods.[17–20] The earliest evidence suggesting direct HIV infection of the myocardium was provided by Calabrese and colleagues[21] when they were able to culture the virus from an endomyocardial biopsy specimen obtained from an HIV-infected patient with cardiomyopathy. Myocyte degeneration was seen on electron microscopy, but no inflammatory infiltrate or viral particles were identified.

Table 26-1. Causes of Myocarditis

Infectious etiologies	Noninfectious etiologies
Viral	Collagen-vascular
Rickettsial	Granulomatous disease
Bacterial	Pharmacologic agents
Mycobacterial	Physical agents (e.g., radiation)
Spirochetal	Chemicals
Fungal	Metabolic disorders
Parasitic	

Table 26-2. Viral Causes of Myocarditis

Enterovirus	Epstein-Barr virus
Coxsackie A	Varicella
Coxsackie B	Mumps
Echovirus	Rabies
Poliovirus	Hepatitis
Adenovirus	Rubella
Cytomegalovirus	Rubeola
Herpesvirus	Parvovirus
Influenza	HIV

Pathogenesis of Myocarditis

The pathogenetic mechanism of myocarditis has been best studied in mouse models of disease using various cardiotropic viruses.[22-25] In these models, two stages of myocarditis are seen. The acute stage, which occurs in the initial 5 to 7 days of infection, is followed by a chronic stage 9 to 45 days later. The major feature of the acute stage is multiple foci of myocyte necrosis. Simultaneous active viral replication within the myocytes is also present, but inflammatory cells are not. Myocyte necrosis occurs when the mature virus lyses the myocyte.

After activation of the mouse immune system, viral replication is terminated by natural killer cells, macrophages, and virus-specific cytotoxic T-lymphocytes, and the virus is removed by neutralizing antibody[15]; recovery follows in most mice. Those mice that do not recover develop a chronic stage, even though virus is no longer identified by culture. Active myocyte necrosis continues, and an interstitial cellular infiltrate composed of autoimmune cytotoxic T lymphocytes develops and results in lysis of uninfected myocytes. Heart-reactive autoantibodies, another feature of autoimmunity, are commonly found in the chronic stage. These autoantibodies are directed against different components of the myocyte, including cardiac myosin.

Myocarditis in humans is very similar to that seen in mice, with acute and chronic stages. The isolated myocyte necrosis that occurs during the acute stage is usually not observed unless the patient dies or rapidly deteriorates. More often, the patient is not "ill enough" to warrant a biopsy. Some investigators, therefore, believe that active myocarditis detected by endomyocardial biopsy most likely represents the chronic stage of myocarditis. Support for this hypothesis comes from several lines of evidence. First, the interstitial mononuclear cell infiltrate adjacent to necrotic myofibers is virtually identical to that seen in murine models. These inflammatory cells have been identified as T-lymphocytes. Second, the inability to culture virus from the myocardium is also consistent with the hypothesis of chronic myocarditis. Third, heart-specific autoantibodies are frequently found in patients with active myocarditis and dilated cardiomyopathy.

Abnormally high levels of major histocompatibility complex (MHC) class I and class II antigens have been found on myocytes and microvascular endothelium from biopsy samples of patients with active myocarditis.[26] These findings all support the idea that chronic myocarditis in humans is caused by autoimmunity.

Many investigators also support the hypothesis that idiopathic dilated cardiomyopathy occurs as a late sequela of acute or chronic viral myocarditis,[3,27-30] due either to persistence of virus or to an autoimmune phenomenon occurring secondary to previous exposure to the inciting virus. Children with dilated cardiomyopathy may require long-term medical therapy for congestive heart failure and, in many cases, may require cardiac transplantation; sudden cardiac death, especially in athletes, may occur. Evidence supporting the hypothesis of myocarditis-induced dilated cardiomopathy includes: (1) the presence of scattered foci of inflammatory cells on myocardial histologic examination in patients with dilated cardiomyopathy; (2) the clinical and pathologic similarities between dilated cardiomyopathy and acute myocarditis; and (3) data obtained from animal models of myocarditis, particularly the murine viral myocarditis model.

Susceptibility to Myocarditis

Several factors, including the genetic composition of the host,[15,23] sex hormones,[15] exercise,[15,31] malnutrition,[15] and a variety of drugs, appear to influence susceptibility. The genetic composition of the host appears to be the most important factor determining susceptibility; it is strongly influenced by the MHC, which, in turn, controls the immune response. Men are at greater risk, since testosterone increases the number of viral receptor sites, making the myocyte more vulnerable to infection. Conversely, estrogen increases the number of suppressor T lymphocytes, reducing the risk of autoimmunity. Postpartum women or those in the last trimester of pregnancy are more susceptible because of increased levels of progesterone. Exercise greatly increases the severity of myocyte necrosis and mortality by changing the immune response, which is induced by increased levels of norepinephrine and cyclic guanosine 3,5′-monophosphate (cGMP). Although both corticosteroids and cyclosporine (i.e., immunosuppressant drugs) have been proposed as possible treatments for active myocarditis, both types of drug increase myocyte necrosis and mortality in mice.

Diagnosis of Myocarditis

Traditionally, the diagnosis of myocarditis has been made clinically when new cardiac abnormalities appear during an acute viral infection in a previously healthy,[1-3] often young, person. Several studies have shown that clinical predictions of the presence of myocarditis are often inaccurate. The diagnosis of myocarditis requires a high index of suspicion based upon symptoms and/or compatible physical findings (signs of heart failure, pericardial rub). Echocardiography is required to clinically define the ventricular dilatation and dysfunction associated with myocarditis. Echocardiography may demonstrate a pericardial effusion, left ventricular dysfunction, and/or left ventricular dilatation. Echocardiography, however, cannot differentiate between myocarditis and dilated cardiomyopathy due to other causes.[3] Chest x-ray and electrocardiography are also used for screening. Nonspecific electrocardiographic changes may occur, such as sinus tachycardia, conduction defects, and repolarization abnormalities, and there may be x-ray evidence of cardiac enlargement or pulmonary edema.

Demonstration of the presence of a virus by culture of all body fluids and by titration of antibodies for selected viruses (hepatitis virus, Epstein-Barr virus, cytomegalovirus) is supportive (albeit circumstantial) evidence of myocarditis. Measurement of neutralizing antibodies is not recommended unless the virus is isolated by culture; false positive and false negative results are common. Serologic studies, in general, are time-consuming, usually requiring serial analysis over several weeks.

The procedure of endomyocardial biopsy was developed to better diagnose myocarditis.[32-34] However, the specific criteria used to define myocarditis varied among different pathologists, creating problems with diagnostic disagreement. For this reason,

a simplified uniform histologic classification of myocarditis was developed at a meeting of cardiac pathologists in Dallas in 1984 (the "Dallas criteria") (Table 26-3).[35]

Limited sensitivity remains the major problem of endomyocardial biopsy, however, and this has been attributed to restricted availability of biopsy sites and the multifocal, patchy nature of myocarditis.[36-38] Sampling error in myocarditis has been documented, demonstrating a sensitivity of 63% for the right ventricle and 55% for the left ventricle when 10 samples are obtained; when the usual 4 or 5 samples are obtained (as suggested by the Dallas criteria), only 50% sensitivity is demonstrated. In HIV-induced myocarditis these criteria may be particularly inaccurate, since the HIV-infected patient may be unable to mount an appropriate immune response.

Although HIV is primarily an infection of the immune system, it is now apparent that many organs can be damaged directly or indirectly by the virus.[39-42] Diverse effects on a number of organs, including the central nervous system,[39] gastrointestinal tract,[40] and cardiovascular system,[41] have been described. Cardiac disease, in fact, has emerged as a significant cause of morbidity and mortality in HIV-infected patients. All portions of the heart can be affected, including the myocardium. The myocardial abnormality may be caused by viral myocarditis or may be considered a dilated cardiomyopathy. Although it is likely that HIV itself plays a major role in myocardial dysfunction, infection with other viruses may be important in the develop-

Table 26-3. Dallas Criteria: Working Histopathologic Diagnostic Criteria for Myocarditis

---

General definition: Myocardial cell injury with degeneration or necrosis with inflammatory infiltrate, not due to ischemia.

Active myocarditis: Both myocyte degeneration or necrosis and definite cellular infiltrate; ± fibrosis.

Borderline myocarditis: Definite cellular infiltrate without myocyte injury.

Persistent myocarditis: Continued active myocarditis on repeat right ventricular endomyocardial biopsy.

Resolving/resolved myocarditis: Diminished or absent infiltrate with evidence of connective tissue healing.

---

ment of myocarditis. The remainder of this chapter will outline the spectrum of associated viral causes of myocarditis in children with HIV and the current methods available to diagnose the etiologic agents involved in the underlying process.

Heart Disease in Patients with HIV Infection

The etiology of HIV heart muscle disease is unknown. The most likely causative factors are preceding myocarditis attributable to HIV itself or secondary to other infectious agents, nutritional deficiencies, excessive sympathetic drive, or the effects of drugs used in the treatment of HIV disease and its complications.

The hypothesis that HIV heart muscle disease is caused by a preceding myocarditis is supported by postmortem studies that have demonstrated myocarditis in hearts with structural disease,[9-12,43-46] and by considerable experimental evidence based on human, animal, and in vitro studies of the pathogenetic role of myocarditis in idiopathic dilated cardiomyopathy in patients without HIV infection.[29,47,48] The demonstration that some cases of HIV-related left ventricular dysfunction resolve spontaneously[49] is also consistent with the idea that myocarditis, which is potentially self-limiting, serves as the substrate for the subsequent development of HIV heart muscle disease. Some groups have demonstrated left ventricular dyskinesis,[11,13] or increase in four-chamber wall thickness. Lipshultz and colleagues[50] showed hyperdynamic left ventricular performance in some children with myocarditis and HIV infection.

The reported prevalence of myocarditis associated with HIV heart muscle disease varies widely, ranging from essentially nonexistent[51-53] to nearly 100% of patients.[9,43] As previously noted, it is possible that the Dallas criteria are not appropriate diagnostic criteria to use in HIV patients because they are based on inflammatory infiltrate and adjacent myocardial necrosis and HIV impairs the capacity to mount an immune response.

In 1986, Cohen and associates[43] described three HIV-infected patients who presented with the symptoms and signs of heart failure. Two of these patients

underwent postmortem examinations that showed global dilatation of the cardiac chambers without evidence of coronary artery disease or myocarditis. Since then, a number of in vivo studies[14,49-59] and retrospective postmortem analyses[9,45,60] have confirmed the existence of "HIV heart muscle disease" (also known as HIV cardiomyopathy) and myocarditis. In some cases HIV has been identified in the myocardium, suggesting a direct action by the virus itself. Another possibility is that a secondary infection is responsible for myocardial inflammation. HIV may be the principal cause of myocyte damage in cases of myocarditis detected at postmortem in which there is no evidence of secondary infection.[9-11]

The evidence that heart muscle disease is a specific phenomenon associated with HIV infection, as opposed to a nonspecific manifestation of chronic disease in a dying patient, is based on two observations:

1. Cardiac dysfunction has been documented in apparently healthy, well-nourished patients.[13]

2. Himelman and coworkers[59] studied 70 ambulatory and hospitalized HIV-infected patients and compared them with 20 inpatients with acute leukemia. The hospital patients with HIV had more advanced disease than their ambulatory counterparts and were of similar nutritional status to those with leukemia, as evidenced by percentage of predicted ideal body weight and serum albumin. Eight patients with heart muscle disease were identified by echocardiography, and, in these cases, four-chamber enlargement and diffuse left ventricular hypokinesia were seen. All eight were HIV-positive and were hospitalized. None of the leukemia patients had myocardial dysfunction. Within 6 months, four of the eight patients with heart muscle disease died.

The pathogenetic mechanisms responsible for myocarditis due solely to HIV have not been established, although a number of theories have been proposed. HIV may enter cardiac myocytes and cause damage either directly or indirectly. For example, by analogy with T-helper lymphocytes, HIV-induced destruction may take place by initiation of an intrinsic cellular process leading to apoptosis.[61] The evidence for such viral entry is based upon culture and in situ techniques.[21,42,62,63] However, these methods are potentially unreliable because of the possibility of contamination of cardiac muscle preparations by blood cells containing HIV. Furthermore, contradictory results have been obtained from workers who have failed to demonstrate HIV in myocardial biopsies[64] and from in vitro experiments using skeletal muscle cell lines[65] that have shown that HIV is unable to gain entry into myocytes.

In the majority of patients, however, no viral agent is found within the heart, consistent with an indirect viral etiology due to an autoimmune process. HIV-induced myocyte damage, therefore, could result from various autoimmune mechanisms. Herskowitz and associates[66,67] found high levels of cardiac autoantibodies in HIV-infected patients with myocarditis and heart muscle disease. These were accompanied by induction of class I MHC antigens within the myocardium, suggesting that the autoantibodies were involved in the inflammatory process. It is possible that HIV enters myocytes and either modifies existing surface antigens or exposes previously hidden epitopes, provoking the immune system to generate anti-heart antibodies. Another possible mechanism of autoimmune myocyte damage is by "innocent bystander" destruction, a hypothesis proposed by Ho and coworkers[68] to explain central nervous system destruction in HIV infection. Here, blood cells carrying HIV enter the tissue and release proteolytic enzymes and lymphokines, which first cause cell destruction and then promote the ingress of inflammatory cells, which augment the destructive process. Lymphokines such as tissue necrosis factor (TNF) are found in abnormally high concentrations in the blood of HIV-infected patients[69] and have been shown to cause skeletal myocyte death in vitro.[65]

Molecular Methods of Diagnosis of Myocarditis

The ability to diagnose viral infection in cardiac tissue appeared to improve significantly with the advent of in situ hybridization by Bowles and co-workers.[17] The method of in situ hybridization utilizes radioactively labeled nucleic acid probes,

which are hybridized directly to the endomyocardial specimen to identify any viral sequences within the myocardium. Support for the utility of this technique in diagnosing enteroviral infection of the heart was provided by confirmatory data from several laboratories.[70,71] Bowles and colleagues[17] found enteroviral genomic sequences in 52% of total nucleic acid extracts from myocardial biopsy specimens in non-HIV infected patients with myocarditis and dilated cardiomyopathy. However, 28.5% of recipients' hearts removed at transplant in patients with dilated cardiomyopathy, and approximately 5% of "controls," also showed the presence of enteroviral RNA, thus bringing into question the diagnostic accuracy of this moderately sensitive technique. The results of these studies, despite concerns about the method, led to the hypothesis that enteroviral persistence occurred in patients with dilated cardiomyopathy and supported the view that dilated cardiomyopathy is a late sequela of viral myocarditis. Grody and colleagues,[62] Lipshultz and colleagues,[63] and others[72] later used in situ hybridization with HIV probes to demonstrate the HIV genome in the myocardium of affected patients. However, this method came into question when others were not able to duplicate these results.[12,21]

More recently, the polymerase chain reaction (PCR) has been employed in the rapid detection of viral sequences in many tissues and body fluids, including enteroviral sequences in the myocardium of patients with suspected myocarditis or dilated cardiomyopathy.[18-20] These PCR studies use oligonucleotide primers approximately 20 to 25 nucleotides in length, which are synthesized on the basis of the known sequence of the virus to be amplified. For RNA viruses such as enterovirus, reverse transcriptase PCR (RT-PCR) is required. During RT-PCR, the viral RNA is converted into complementary DNA (cDNA) before amplification of a specific region of the viral sequence occurs. This amplification process is driven by a DNA polymerase and has become automated with the help of a thermostable DNA polymerase derived from the bacterium *Thermus aquaticus* and known as Taq polymerase. Using this method, Jin and coworkers[18] identified enteroviral RNA in 5 of 48 patients with myocarditis and/or dilated cardiomyopathy, including 3 of

20 patients with dilated cardiomyopathy. Chapman and colleagues[19] confirmed that PCR can amplify enteroviral genome from cardiac tissue by showing that 5 of 11 patients with dilated cardiomyopathy amplified enteroviral nucleic acid. However, Weiss and associates[20] initially were unable to identify enteroviral nucleic acid sequences in 11 patients with DCM using coxsackie B3 virus-specific primers and probes, but subsequently this group was able to amplify enteroviral genome in 9 of 24 control patients. Grasso and coworkers[73] also were unable to demonstrate PCR-positive product in 40 explants (21 with dilated cardiomyopathy, 19 with coronary artery disease). These conflicting studies led to questions about the usefulness of PCR in the diagnosis of viral infection of the heart, as well as the concept of viral persistence in dilated cardiomyopathy. More recently, however, Martin and colleagues[7] and Griffin and colleagues[8] were able to demonstrate adenovirus and enterovirus genome (as well as other viral genomes) consistently in the myocardium of children (frozen and formalin-fixed tissue) with myocarditis in nearly 50% of patients. Factor and colleagues[74] provided evidence for direct invasion of the myocardium in patients with HIV myocarditis when they demonstrated HIV-1 DNA sequences within the myocardium of three HIV-infected patients by PCR and Southern blot analysis. Rodriguez et al.[75] analyzed 215 HIV-infected patients, 15 of whom underwent endomyocardial biopsy. Using PCR, they found that 8 of 15 biopsy samples had HIV-1 proviral genomic sequences within myocytes. Several of these patients were also found to have HIV-1 sequences within dendritic cells. No correlation between symptomatic and asymptomatic heart disease was found, however. Interestingly, light microscopic results were normal in all cases, and immunohistochemical analysis failed to demonstrate inflammatory cells. MHC class II antigens were detected in interstitial cells of the myocardium around capillaries and larger vessels (venules and arterioles), however. Currently PCR is the molecular method of choice for the identification of viral genome from the myocardium, but it should be used in conjunction with standard diagnostic methods (histopathology, viral culture, serology).

Interactions Between HIV and Other Viruses

A variety of viral infections have been identified in patients with HIV. The most common agents are the viruses in the herpes family, including herpes simplex virus,[76] (Figure 26-2) cytomegalovirus,[72,77] (Figure 26-3) varicella-zoster virus, and Epstein-Barr virus (Figure 26-4).[78] More recently human herpes virus 6[79] has been reported in HIV-infected individuals. These secondary viral infections typically affect mucocutaneous sites, the lungs, or the central nervous system, or can be disseminated.

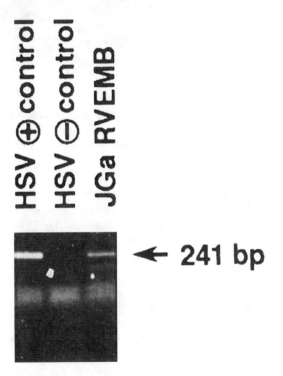

Figure 26-2.   Herpes simplex myocarditis. Polymerase chain reaction (PCR) analysis of a right ventricular endomyocardial biopsy specimen (RVEMB, lane 3) reveals a 241-bp band on agarose gel electrophoresis consistent with herpes simplex virus (HSV). This same size band is seen in the HSV-positive control lane but is absent in the HSV-negative control lane, excluding contamination. The negative control lane contains a PCR reaction utilizing the same substrate as in the positive control and patient lane, with the exception of the nucleic acid, which is excluded.

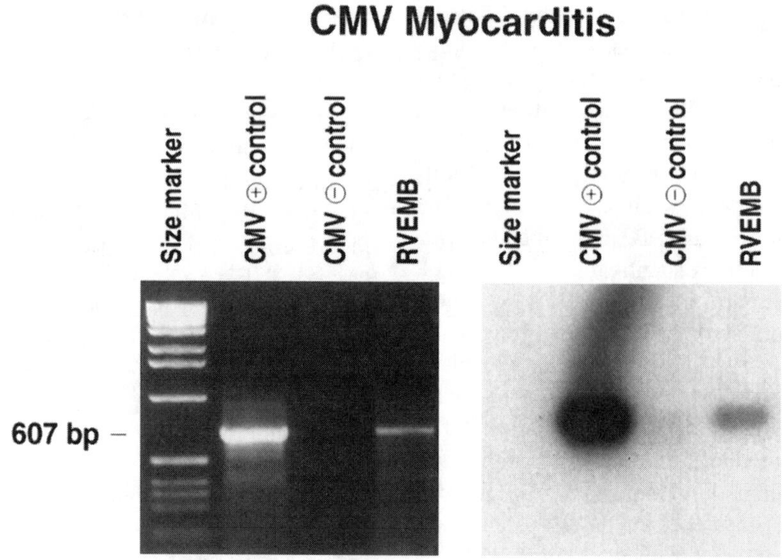

CMV Myocarditis

Figure 26-3. Polymerase chain reaction (PCR) analysis of a right ventricular endomyocardial biopsy (RVEMB) specimen for cytomegalovirus (CMV). **Left**: The CMV-positive control band is 607 bp in size as seen on this agarose gel after electrophoresis. The patient RVEMB specimen, from a 3-year-old child with AIDS, amplified the same 607-bp band; the cytomegalovirus negative control is devoid of this band. **Right**: Southern blot analysis and hybridization using a radioactively labeled cytomegalovirus probe identifies the CMV-positive control and patient RVEMB bands specifically, with no cross-hybridization to the negative control.

Other viruses, such as polyoma virus and poxvirus, have also been identified.[41] Like other immunocompromised hosts, HIV-infected patients should be excellent targets for a wide variety of viral and other infectious agents. These secondary infections are expected to cause a wide spectrum of end organ abnormalities, including myocarditis. Serologic techniques are of limited diagnostic value in patients with HIV disease because of widespread immunologic dysfunction[80] which may prevent development of the immune response to both primary and secondary opportunistic infections.

Other Organisms As Causes of Myocarditis in HIV-Infected Patients

Many opportunistic agents[81] have been implicated in the development of myocarditis in patients infected with HIV, including *Toxoplasma gondii*,[82–85] *Cryptococcus neoformans*,[44,86] *Histoplasma capsulatum*,[83] and *Aspergillus fumigatus*.[87,88] *Mycobacte-rium avium-intracellulare* complex, which is a relatively common cause of systemic infection in patients with AIDS, has been cultured from the myocardium of HIV-infected patients.[9,10,43] Another opportunistic agent, *Mycoplasma*, has been implicated in HIV damage to the kidney, liver, and spleen, but not the heart.[89] Other agents are also likely to emerge as causes of inflammatory heart disease. These diverse organisms might cause myocyte damage through the same mechanisms as HIV or by acting synergistically with the virus.[64,81]

Anderson and coworkers[9] reported a characteristically focal, mild, mononuclear myocarditis in 37 of 71 (52%) consecutive AIDS patients; 7 of these (10%) had biventricular dilatation. Opportunistic cardiac pathogens were identified as the cause of 7 of 37 cases of myocarditis; these included *H. capsulatum*, *M. avium-intracellulare*, and cytomegalovirus. Although the etiology was not determined in the remaining 30 cases, histologic findings were suggestive of viral infection.

T. gondii is one of the myocardial pathogens

Epstein-Barr Virus Pneumonitis/Myocarditis

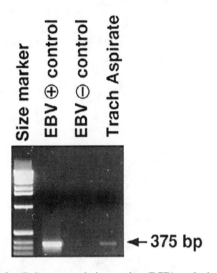

Figure 26-4. Polymerase chain reaction (PCR) analysis of a tracheal aspirate specimen from a child with pneumonitis and myocarditis using primers for Epstein-Barr virus (EBV) reveals the expected 375-bp band in the positive control and patient tracheal aspirate lanes. The negative control lane is devoid of contamination. Subsequent endomyocardial biopsy and PCR analysis confirmed EBV in the myocardium.

identified most frequently in patients with HIV infection.[81–85] AIDS patients are particularly susceptible to toxoplasma encephalitis, but pneumonitis, hepatitis, pericarditis, and myocarditis have also been reported. Roldan and associates[85] described six cases of toxoplasma myocarditis recognized at autopsy; five of these patients had previous toxoplasma encephalitis with or without pneumonitis, and the cardiac lesions were felt to be asymptomatic. The sixth patient, however, died of overwhelming toxoplasma myocarditis without evidence of concomitant central nervous system or pulmonary involvement.

Cytomegalovirus has been identified infrequently in the myocardium of AIDS patients.[9,46,90–93] Despite positive cytomegalovirus cultures or the identification of cytomegalovirus inclusion bodies in cardiac tissue of patients with AIDS, it has been somewhat controversial whether cytomegalovirus has been directly responsible for myocardial dysfunction. Anderson and coworkers[9] demonstrated distant cytomegalovirus infection serologically in 28 of 37 cases of myocarditis or biventricular enlargement, possibly consistent with a causal role of cytomegalovirus in the disease. The demonstration of myocardial necrosis and inflammation in experimentally infected animal models of cytomegalovirus and enteroviral (coxsackie B virus) myocarditis at late time points after infection, when the virus can no longer be cultured from cardiac tissue,[23,70,94] prompted Wu and collaborators[72] to postulate that nonpermissive or latent cytomegalovirus infection may play a role in the pathogenesis of HIV-associated myocarditis and cardiomyopathy. In 6 of 12 endomyocardial biopsy samples, myocyte nuclear and perinuclear hybridization for transcripts of cytomegalovirus immediate early (IE) gene was seen, whereas hybridization was not seen in control samples from HIV-infected patients without heart disease using in situ hybridization. All six patients presented with unexplained heart failure and had CD4+ lymphocyte $< 100 \times 10^6$ cells per liter, and five of them had active or borderline myocarditis on biopsy according to histopathologic findings. Immunohistochemical studies showed that all six patients had extensive myocardial MHC class I expression, a finding typically seen in non-HIV myocarditis.[26,95] As expected in nonpermissive infection, no patient had intranuclear cytomegalovirus inclusions; only two of six patients who specifically hybridized to cytomegalovirus IE probes (within the myocytes) had clinical evidence of solid organ infection with cytomegalovirus at the time of cardiovascular presentation. Lack of cytopathic changes in the myocyte and lack of specific hybridization suggests no active viral replication or so-called permissive infection.

Another virus implicated as a cause of myocarditis in children with HIV infection is Epstein-Barr virus. Luginbuhl and colleagues[96] reported that, after adjusting for disease classification, Epstein-Barr virus coinfection had the strongest correlation for development of chronic heart failure. In addition, cytomegalovirus was not independently correlated with any adverse cardiac outcomes. Importantly, Epstein-Barr virus was also correlated with total deaths.

Unfortunately, no PCR or in situ hybridization studies searching for known viral causes (or unsuspected causes) of myocarditis have been reported. On the basis of previous studies of children with myocarditis, and of immunocompromised patients with cancer, it is likely that the gamut of viruses (i.e. adenovirus, enterovirus, cytomegalovirus, herpes simplex virus, human herpes viruses 6 and 8) will be identified as responsible for cardiac dysfunction. Thus far, our laboratory has identified cytomegalovirus and herpes simplex virus in the formalin-fixed autopsy myocardial tissue of some patients with HIV infection and myocarditis.[8] We have begun a prospective pilot project using PCR analysis of myocardial specimens, and it appears that such agents as adenovirus and enterovirus, which are commonly seen in non-HIV-infected children with myocarditis, are also involved in cardiac disease in children with HIV. In addition, polyviral infection, particularly involving cytomegalovirus and adenovirus also appears to be an important cause of morbidity and mortality in HIV-infected patients with myocardial involvement.

Future Directions

It is likely that PCR will become an important diagnostic method in the identification of the cause of viral-induced myocarditis in HIV-infected patients. Another new method, in situ PCR,[97,98] which combines the sensitivity of PCR with the ability to localize the virus within a cell by the in situ approach (Figure 26-5), is currently under study. If successful, this method will enable the identification of viral genome within the myocytes, allow the investigator to determine the viral load, and detect cell destruction. PCR and antibody analysis of inflammatory mediators could also become useful. The finding that inflammatory mediators are upregulated could be useful as supportive data in a patient with evidence of ventricular dysfunction but little or no inflammatory cell infiltrate in the myocardium. The approach is currently being tested experimentally.

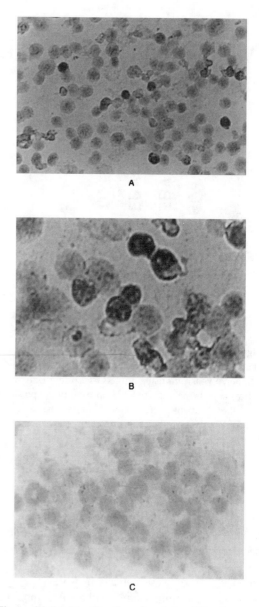

Figure 26-5. Identification of peripheral blood mononuclear cells containing HIV-1 provirus using in situ polymerase chain reaction (PCR). **A**: Peripheral blood mononuclear cells from a patient with HIV-1 infection and persistent generalized lymphadenopathy (stage III). **B**: Peripheral blood mononuclear cells from a patient with AIDS (stage IVA). **C**: Peripheral blood mononuclear cells from a patient who is HIV-1-seronegative (negative control). Note the darkly stained cells in panels A and B, consistent with HIV-1 infection; the negative control (panel C) is devoid of dark stained cells. (From Ref. 98, with permission.)

References

1. Lieberman EB, Herskowitz A, Rose NR, et al. A clinicopathologic description of myocarditis. *Clin Immunol Immunopathol* 1993;68:191–196.

2. Billingham ME. The diagnostic criteria of myocarditis by endomyocardial biopsy. *Heart Vessels* 1985; 1(Suppl):133–137.

3. Waller BF, Slack JD, Orr CD, et al. Flaming, smoldering and burned out: the fireside saga of myocarditis. *J Am Coll Cardiol* 1991;18:1627–1630.

4. Wynne J, Braunwald E. The cardiomyopathies and myocarditis. In: *Heart Disease. A Textbook of Cardiovascular Medicine*, 3rd Ed. Philadelphia: WB Saunders, 1988:1440–1454.

5. Woodruff JF. Viral myocarditis: a review. *Am J Pathol* 1980;101:427–484.

6. Cherry JD. Adenoviral infections. In: Feigin RD, Cherry JD (eds). *Textbook of Pediatric Infectious Diseases*. Philadelphia: WB Saunders, 1992:1670–1687.

7. Martin AM, Webber S, Fricker FJ, et al. Acute myocarditis: rapid diagnosis by PCR in children. *Circulation* 1994;90:330–339.

8. Griffin LD, Kearney D, Ni J, et al. Analysis of formalin-fixed and frozen myocardial autopsy samples for viral genome in childhood myocarditis and dilated cardiomyopathy with endocardial fibroelastosis using polymerase chain reaction (PCR). *Cardiovasc Pathol* 1995;4:3–11.

9. Anderson DW, Virmani R, Reilly JM, et al. Prevalent myocarditis at necropsy in the acquired immunodeficiency syndrome. *J Am Coll Cardiol* 1988; 11:792–799.

10. Anderson DW, Virmani R. Emerging patterns of heart disease in human immunodeficiency virus infection. *Hum Pathol* 1990;21:253–259.

11. Baroldi G, Corallo S, Moroni M, et al. Focal lymphocytic myocarditis in acquired immunodeficiency syndrome (AIDS): a correlative morphologic and clinical study in 26 consecutive fatal cases. *J Am Coll Cardiol* 1988;12:463–469.

12. Beschorner WE, Baughman K, Turnicky RP, et al. HIV-associated myocarditis: pathology and immunopathology. *Am J Pathol* 1990;137:1365–1371.

13. Levy WS, Varghese PJ, Anderson DW, et al. Myocarditis diagnosed by endomyocardial biopsy in human immunodeficiency virus infection with cardiac dysfunction. *Am J Cardiol* 1988;62:658–659.

14. Herskowitz A, Wu FC, Willoughby SB, et al. Myocarditis and cardiotropic viral infection associated with severe left ventricular dysfunction in late-stage infection with human immunodeficiency virus. *J Am Coll Cardiol* 1994;24:1025–1032.

15. Leslie K, Blay R, Haisch C, et al. Clinical and experimental aspects of viral myocarditis. *Clin Microbiol Rev* 1989;2:191–203.

16. Gear JH, Measroch V. *S Afr Inst Med Res Ann Rep* 1953:38–39.

17. Bowles NE, Richardson PJ, Olsen EGJ, Archard LC. Detection of coxsackie B virus-specific RNA sequences in myocardial biopsy samples from patients with myocarditis and dilated cardiomyopathy. *Lancet* 1986;1:1120–1123.

18. Jin O, Sole M, Butany J, et al. Detection of enterovirus RNA in myocardial biopsies from patients with myocarditis and cardiomyopathy using gene amplification by polymerase chain reaction. *Circulation* 1990;82:8–16.

19. Chapman NM, Tracy S, Gauntt CJ, et al. Molecular detection and identification of enterovirus using enzymatic amplification and nucleic acid hybridization. *J Clin Microbiol* 1990;28:843–850.

20. Weiss LM, Movahed LA, Billingham NE, et al. Detection of coxsackievirus B3 RNA in myocardial tissues by the polymerase chain reaction. *Am J Pathol* 1991;138:497–503.

21. Calabrese LH, Proffitt MR, Yen-Lieberman B, et al. Congestive cardiomyopathy and illness related to the acquired immunodeficiency syndrome (AIDS) associated with isolation of retrovirus from myocardium. *Ann Intern Med* 1987;107:691–692.

22. Kishimoto C, Hiraoka Y. Clinical and experimental studies in myocarditis. *Curr Opin Cardiol* 1994; 9:349–356.

23. Kishimoto C, Kuribayashi K, Masuda T, et al. Immunological behavior of lymphocytes in experimental myocarditis: significance of T lymphocytes in the severity of myocarditis and silent myocarditis in BALB/c nu/nu mice. *Circulation* 1985;71:1247–1254.

24. Reyes MP, Ho KL, Smith F, et al. A mouse model of dilated-type cardiomyopathy due to coxsackievirus B3. *J Infect Dis* 1981;144:232–236.

25. Matsumori A, Kawai C. An animal model of congestive (dilated) cardiomyopathy: dilation and hypertrophy of the heart in the chronic stage of DBA/2 mice with myocarditis caused by encephalomyocarditis virus. *Circulation* 1982;66:355–360.

26. Herskowitz A, Ahmed-Ansari A, Neumann DA, et al. Induction of major histocompatibility complex antigens within the myocardium of patients with active myocarditis: a nonhistologic marker of myocarditis. *J Am Coll Cardiol* 1990;15:624–632.

27. Dec GW Jr, Palacios IF, Fallon JT, et al. Active myocarditis in the spectrum of acute dilated cardiomyopathies: clinical features, histologic correlates, and clinical outcome. *N Engl J Med* 1985;312:885–889.

28. Kawai C. Idiopathic cardiomyopathy: a study on the infectious-immune theory as a cause of the disease. *Jpn Circ J* 1971;35:765–768.

29. MacArthur CGC, Tarin D, Goodwin JF, et al. The relationship of myocarditis to dilated cardiomyopathy. *Eur Heart J* 1984;5:1023–1035.

30. Latham RD, Mulrow JP, Virmani R, et al. Recently diagnosed idiopathic dilated cardiomyopathy: incidence of myocarditis and efficacy of prednisone therapy. *Am Heart J* 1989;117:876–882.

31. Ilback NG, Fohlman J, Friman G. Exercise in coxsackie B3 myocarditis: effects on heart lymphocyte subpopulations and the inflammatory reaction. *Am Heart J* 1989;117:1298–1302.

32. Sakakibara S, Konno S. Endomyocardial biopsy. *Jpn Heart J* 1962;3:537–543.

33. Mason JW. Techniques for right and left ventricular endomyocardial biopsy. *Am J Cardiol* 1978;41:887–892.

34. Mason JW, Billingham ME, Ricci DR. Treatment of acute inflammatory myocarditis assisted by endomyocardial biopsy. *Am J Cardiol* 1980;45:1037–1044.

35. Aretz HT, Billingham ME, Edwards WD, et al. Myocarditis: a histopathologic definition and classification. *Am J Cardiovasc Pathol* 1986;1:3–14.

36. Chow LH, Radio SJ, Sears TD, et al. Insensitivity of right ventricular biopsy in the diagnosis of myocarditis. *J Am Coll Cardiol* 1989;14:915–920.

37. Hauck AJ, Kearney DL, Edwards WD. Evaluation of postmortem endomyocardial biopsy specimens from 38 patients with lymphocytic myocarditis: implications for role of sampling error. *Mayo Clin Proc* 1989;64:1235–1245.

38. Lie JT. Myocarditis and endomyocardial biopsy in unexplained heart failure: a diagnosis in search of a disease. [Editorial]. *Ann Intern Med* 1988;109:525–528.

39. Price RW, Brew B, Sidtis J, et al. The brain in AIDS: central nervous system HIV-1 infection and AIDS dementia complex. *Science* 1988;239:586–592.

40. Churchill DR. Gastrointestinal manifestations of AIDS. *Hosp Update* 1991(July):577–584.

41. Acierno LJ. Cardiac complications in acquired immunodeficiency syndrome (AIDS): a review. *J Am Coll Cardiol* 1989;13:1144–1154.

42. Flomenbaum M, Soeiro R, Udem SA, et al. Proliferative membranopathy and human immunodeficiency virus in AIDS hearts. *J AIDS* 1989;2:129–135.

43. Cohen IS, Anderson DW, Virmani R, et al. Congestive cardiomyopathy in association with the acquired immunodeficiency syndrome. *N Engl J Med* 1986;315:628–630.

44. Cammarosano C, Lewis W. Cardiac lesions in acquired immune deficiency syndrome (AIDS). *J Am Coll Cardiol* 1985;5:703–706.

45. Lewis W. AIDS: cardiac findings from 115 autopsies. *Prog Cardiovasc Dis* 1989;32:207–215.

46. Welch K, Finkbeiner W, Alpers CE, et al. Autopsy findings in the acquired immune deficiency syndrome. *JAMA* 1984;252:1152–1159.

47. Kereiakes DJ, Parmley WW. Myocarditis and cardiomyopathy. *Am Heart J* 1984;108:1318–1326.

48. Why HJ, Archard LC, Richardson PJ. Dilated cardiomyopathy: new insights into the pathogenesis. *Postgrad Med J* 1994;70:S2–7.

49. Blanchard DG, Hagenhoff C, Chow LC, et al. Reversibility of cardiac abnormalities in human immunodeficiency virus (HIV)-infected individuals: a serial echocardiographic study. *J Am Coll Cardiol* 1991;17:1270–1276.

50. Lipshultz SE, Chanock S, Sanders SP, et al. Cardiovascular manifestations of human immunodeficiency virus infection in infants and children. *Am J Cardiol* 1989;63:1489–1497.

51. Corboy JR, Fink L, Miller WT. Congestive cardiomyopathy in association with AIDS. *Radiology* 1987;165:139–141.

52. Reilly JM, Cunnion RE, Anderson DW, et al. Frequency of myocarditis, left ventricular dysfunction and ventricular tachycardia in the acquired immune deficiency syndrome. *Am J Cardiol* 1988;62:789–793.

53. Levy WS, Simon GL, Rios JC, et al. Prevalence of cardiac abnormalities in human immunodeficiency virus infection. *Am J Cardiol* 1989;63:86–89.

54. Steinherz LJ, Brochstein JA, Robins J. Cardiac involvement in congenital acquired immunodefi-

ciency syndrome. *Am J Dis Child* 1986;140:1241–1244.

55. Riffanti SR, Chiaramida AJ, Sen P, et al. Assessment of cardiac function in patients with the acquired immunodeficiency syndrome. *Chest* 1988; 93:592–594.

56. Corallo S, Mutinelli R, Moroni M, et al. Echocardiography detects myocardial damage in AIDS: prospective study in 102 patients. *Eur Heart J* 1988; 9:887–892.

57. Stewart JM, Kaul A, Gromische DS, et al. Symptomatic cardiac dysfunction in children with human immunodeficiency virus infection. *Am Heart J* 1989;117:140–144.

58. Fink L, Reichek N, St John Sutton MG. Cardiac abnormalities in acquired immune deficiency syndrome. *Am J Cardiol* 1984;54:1161–1163.

59. Himelman B, Chung WS, Chernoff DN, et al. Cardiac manifestations of human immunodeficiency virus infection: a two-dimensional echocardiographic study. *J Am Coll Cardiol* 1989;13:1030–1036.

60. Joshi VV, Gadol C, Connor E, et al. Dilated cardiomyopathy in children with acquired immunodeficiency syndrome: a pathologic study of five cases. *Hum Pathol* 1988;19:69–73.

61. Moore J, Blanc DF. Immunological incompetence in AIDS. *AIDS* 1995;455–456.

62. Grody WW, Cheng L, Lewis W. Infection of the heart by the human immunodeficiency virus. *Am J Cardiol* 1990;66:203–206.

63. Lipshultz SE, Fox CH, Perez-Atayde AR, et al. Identification of human immunodeficiency virus-1 RNA and DNA in the heart of a child with cardiovascular abnormalities and congenital acquired immune deficiency syndrome. *Am J Cardiol* 1990; 66:240–250.

64. Dittrich H, Chow L, Denaro F, et al. Human immunodeficiency virus, coxsackievirus, and cardiomyopathy. *Ann Intern Med* 1988;108:308–309.

65. Trujillo JR, Gomez-Lucia E, Lee TH, et al. Retroviral effects on muscle cells. [Abstract]. *Proc Int Conf AIDS* 1991;7:1261.

66. Herskowitz A, Willoughby S, Wu TC, et al. Immunopathogenesis of HIV-1-associated cardiomyopathy. *Clin Immunol Immunopathol* 1993;68: 234–241.

67. Herskowitz A, Willoughby S, Oliveira M, et al. HIV-associated cardiomyopathy: evidence for autoimmunity. [Abstract]. *Proc Int Conf AIDS* 1990; 6:510.

68. Ho DD, Pomerantz RJ, Kaplan JC. Pathogenesis of infection with human immunodeficiency virus. *N Engl J Med* 1987;317:278–286.

69. Lahdevirta J, Maury CPJ, Teppo A-M, et al. Cachectin/tumor necrosis factor in AIDS. *Am J Med* 1988;85:289–291.

70. Kandolf R, Ameis D, Kirschner P, et al. In situ detection of enteroviral genomes in myocardial cells by nucleic acid hybridization: an approach to the diagnosis of viral heart disease. *Proc Natl Acad Sci USA* 1987;84:6272–6276.

71. Archard LC, Bowles NE, Cunningham L, et al. Molecular probes for detection of persisting enterovirus infection of human heart and their prognostic value. *Eur Heart J* 1991;12(Suppl D):56–59.

72. Wu T-C, Pizzorno MC, Hayward GS, et al. In situ detection of human cytomegalovirus immediate-early gene transcripts within cardiac myocytes of patients with HIV-associated cardiomyopathy. *AIDS* 1992;6:777–785.

73. Grasso M, Arbustini E, Silini E, et al. Search for coxsackie virus B3 RNA in idiopathic dilated cardiomyopathy using gene amplification by polymerase chain reaction. *Am J Cardiol* 1992;69:658–664.

74. Factor SM. Acquired immune deficiency syndrome: the heart of the matter. *J Am Coll Cardiol* 1990; 13:1037–1038.

75. Rodriguez ER, Nasim S, Hsia J, et al. Cardiac myocytes and dendritic cells harbor human immunodeficiency virus in infected patients with and without cardiac dysfunction: detection by multiplex, nested, polymerase chain reaction in individually microdissected cells from right ventricular endomyocardial biopsy tissue. *Am J Cardiol* 1991;68:1511–1520.

76. Jones AC, Migliorati CA, Baughman RA. The simultaneous occurrence of oral herpes simplex virus, cytomegalovirus, and histoplasmosis in an HIV-infected patient. *Oral Surg Oral Med Oral Pathol* 1992;74:334–339.

77. Reichert CM, O'Leary TJ, Levens DL, et al. Autopsy pathology in the acquired immunodeficiency syndrome. *Am J Pathol* 1983;112:357–382.

78. Andiman WA, Eastman R, Martin K, et al. Opportunistic lymphoproliferations associated with Epstein-Barr viral DNA in infants and children with AIDS. *Lancet* 1985;2:1390–1393.

79. Knox KK, Pietryga D, Harrington DJ, et al. Progressive immunodeficiency and fetal pneumonitis asso-

ciated with human herpesvirus 6 infection in an infant. *Clin Infect Dis* 1995;20:406–413.

80. Robert Y, Samuel B. Immunology of HIV infection. In: Paul WE (ed). *Fundamental Immunology,* 2nd Ed. New York: Lippincott-Raven, 1989:1059–1079.

81. Nelson JA, Ghazal P, Wiley CA. Role of opportunistic viral infections in AIDS. *AIDS* 1990;4:1–10.

82. Hofman P, Michiels JF, Mainguene C, et al. Cardiac toxoplasmosis in acquired immunodeficiency syndrome (AIDS): a postmortem study in 15 cases. [Abstract]. *Proc Int Conf AIDS* 1991;7:2386.

83. Lafont A, Marche C, Wolff M, et al. Myocarditis in acquired immunodeficiency syndrome (AIDS): etiology and prognosis. *J Am Coll Cardiol* 1988; 11:196A.

84. Vynn Adair O, Randive N, Krasnow N. Isolated toxoplasma myocarditis in acquired immune deficiency syndrome. *Am Heart J* 1989;118:856–857.

85. Roldan EO, Moskowit L, Hensley GT. Pathology of the heart in acquired immunodeficiency syndrome. *Arch Pathol* 1987;111:943–946.

86. Lewis W, Lipsick J, Cammarosano C. Cryptococcal myocarditis in acquired immunodeficiency syndrome. *Am J Cardiol* 1985;55:1240.

87. Cox JN, di Dio F, Pizzolato GP, et al. Aspergillus endocarditis and myocarditis in a patient with the acquired immunodeficiency syndrome (AIDS). *Virchows Arch (A) Pathol Anat* 1990;417:255–259.

88. Henochowicz S, Mustafa M, Lawrinson WE, et al. Cardiac aspergillosis in acquired immune deficiency syndrome. *Am J Cardiol* 1985;55:1239–1240.

89. Editorial. Mycoplasma and AIDS: what connection? *Lancet* 1991;337:20–22.

90. Kaminski HJ, Katzman M, Wiest PM, et al. Cardiomyopathy associated with the acquired immune deficiency syndrome. *J AIDS* 1988;1:105–110.

91. Blanche P, Gombert B, Sicard D. Cytomegalovirus myocardium in an AIDS patient. *Presse Med* 1993; 22:597.

92. Brady MT, Reiner CB, Singley G, et al. Unexpected death in an infant with AIDS: disseminated cytomegalovirus infection with pancarditis. *Pediatr Pathol* 1988;8:205–214.

93. Shibata D, Klatt EC. Analysis of human immunodeficiency virus and cytomegalovirus infection by polymerase chain reaction in the acquired immunodeficiency syndrome: an autopsy study. *Arch Pathol* 1989;113:1239–1244.

94. Lawson CM, Grundy JE, Shellam GR. Delayed-type hypersensitivity responses to murine cytomegalovirus in genetically resistant and susceptible strains of mice. *J Gene Virol* 1987;68:2379–2388.

95. Ansari AA, Wang YC, Danner DJ, et al. Abnormal expression of histocompatibility and mitochondrial antigens by cardiac tissue from patients with myocarditis and dilated cardiomyopathy. *Am J Pathol* 1991;139:337–353.

96. Luginbuhl LM, Orav EJ, McIntosh K, et al. Cardiac morbidity and related mortality in children with HIV infection. *JAMA* 1993;269:2869–2875.

97. Haase AT, Retzel EF, Staskus KA. Amplification and detection of lentiviral DNA inside cells. *Proc Natl Acad Sci USA* 1990;87:4971–4975.

98. Bagasra O, Hauptman SP, Lischner HW, et al. Detection of human immunodeficiency virus type 1 provirus in mononuclear cells by in situ polymerase chain reaction. *N Engl J Med* 1992;326:1385–1391.

27

Nursing, Quality of Life, and Social Issues in HIV-Infected Patients

Rachel Diness, MSW, LCSW, Nina Greenbaum, MPH, CHES, Roxellen Auletto, RN, Sheryl Ross, RN, and Karen Lewis, RN

Complex issues in the care of patients with human immunodeficiency virus (HIV) infection may benefit from a multidisciplinary, organized team approach. This chapter is organized into four sections based on distinct care issues. The first part reviews experience with establishing and participating in such organized teams. In the United States, cooperative groups have been determining the most efficacious therapeutic regimens for HIV-infected patients in a way that individual centers with limited numbers of patients cannot. The first section will review the role of the United States National Institutes AIDS Clinical Trials Group Protocols in the care of HIV-infected patients.

The second section covers social issues in the care of HIV-infected patients, including psychosocial issues such as disclosure, anticipatory grief, and bereavement.

The third section reviews quality of life issues. Included in this section are existing models of quality of life and how they are defined, HIV patients' perspective of quality of life during hospitalization, and management strategies for home and hospice care.

The fourth section reviews issues in the care of older adults with HIV infection. Risk factors, risk reduction strategies, social services for the elderly, and the older adult as caregiver are covered.

The Interdisciplinary Team Approach to HIV Care

Most of the routine care of HIV-infected patients occurs within a traditional medical setting and is almost solely connected to the AIDS Clinical Trials Group (ACTG). The principal roles of the ACTG are to test drugs for their pharmacologic and therapeutic effects, to learn more about the natural history of the disease, and to study trends in AIDS-related illnesses.[1] The personnel involved in clinical trials are physicians, nurses, social workers, psychologists and psychiatrists, ethicists, nutritionists and other medical specialists, secretarial support staff, laboratory technicians, data managers, and biostatisticians.

The clinical trial provides access to tested therapies and new therapies, sophisticated diagnostic methods and up-to-date information for patients who might not otherwise have a chance to receive such treatments.

To participate in these studies, a patient must give informed consent.[1] Parents or legal guardians provide consent for children in their care. To encourage participation in and compliance with these studies, various incentives are provided, including social work services, transportation costs, and child care and meal vouchers. Implicit in the agreement to become an experimental subject is the understanding that knowledge regarding treatment is imprecise and incomplete and, despite the best efforts of health care workers, the illness will progress. Many protocols require frequent visits to the clinic and an array of diagnostic and evaluative procedures, some of which are painful and time-consuming. For families in chaos, the death and illness of other family members can make the demands of the protocols seem overwhelming.

The medical care of AIDS patients is complicated by the progressive nature of HIV infection, the psychosocial issues related to the infection, and the incurability of acquired immunodeficiency syndrome (AIDS). Therefore, the skill and knowledge of an interdisciplinary team are crucial. Early management and treatment are critical if there is to be any hope of minimizing the effects of the illness. Currently, state-of-the-art medical care is supportive and consists of antiretroviral therapies and numerous medical interventions. These therapies are rigorous, lifelong, and demand close attention to detail. Members of the team must have an overall understanding of the medical, social, developmental, and psychological aspects of chronic illness. It is unrealistic to expect all members of the team to be expert in meeting all of the complex needs of the patient with HIV infection. Therefore, team members divide up the work based on knowledge and expertise. Communication is the key component in providing quality care. If there is a breakdown in the cooperative efforts of the interdisciplinary team, duplication of services and manipulation of providers may result.

When a plan of care for a person with AIDS is created, the complete spectrum of the disease must be considered. The range of services needed may include hospital and ambulatory care, counseling, child development, psychological services, parenting classes, home care, hospice care, transportation, housing, food, and social, financial, and legal services. Longer survival creates a demand for health services over an extended period in multiple settings, including long-term care facilities, day-care centers, and schools.[2] The team must become the link between the person with AIDS and all the services that are needed; it must be able to give information about treatment options and support

agencies available, both locally and nationally. Providers must be prepared to educate not only the person with AIDS, but also his or her family, friends, and colleagues. Finally, the team must collaborate and share information about the expected course of the disease, the prognosis, continually changing treatment choices, and supportive interventions.

An important goal for a person with AIDS is to be permitted to control his or her life and medical care as much as possible. The team must form a partnership with the patient and the family. Several partnerships may be formed, as each team member plays a different role in offering comprehensive care. These partnerships must be flexible enough to allow for minimal medical intervention during the "well" periods of the disease, while providing support and resources.[3] Additionally, these partnerships allow for extensive medical intervention and delivery of care when appropriate. This partnership must be flexible, adaptable, and supportive to be successful, rendering communication crucial.

Collaborative and interdisciplinary efforts of the health-care team can provide comprehensive care that supports everyone infected with or affected by HIV.[4] An essential component of this approach is the psychosocial assessment that identifies the strengths, specific needs, and resources of each individual. Once an assessment has been made, the team is able to plan appropriate interventions. The psychosocial or needs assessment is the most effective means of ascertaining what the patient feels are the most salient issues, and it helps the team meet the client's needs on the client's own terms. It is not uncommon for providers to create their own agendas for the client. The needs assessment helps to create a client-centered focus to the care plan. This assessment is usually conducted by a social worker or psychologist. However, each team member provides insight and knowledge based on his or her interactions with the client. Important issues that often need to be addressed include, but are not limited to, food, housing, transportation, financial assistance, facilitating proper medical care, coordination of community resources, and helping mothers place their children in day care, school, or respite care.[4] In addition, providers should assist families with planning for the placement and care of their children should their mothers become too ill to look after them. Assistance in finding legal services to prepare a will and helping the family make funeral arrangements are some other examples of services provided by the health-care team.

Crisis intervention has emerged as the predominant psychotherapeutic modality used to assist persons with AIDS.[4] Such interventions include psychiatric referrals for suicidal patients and emergency shelter for families who have lost their homes. Issues addressed in counseling include bereavement, anticipatory grief, substance abuse, domestic and neighborhood violence, disclosure, and the loss of multiple family members.

It is evident that no single discipline is able to meet all of the complex needs of persons with AIDS. The interdisciplinary team must work together in providing a comprehensive, coherent, and client-centered approach to medical, social, and emotional care. The following section focuses on the social and emotional problems faced by persons with AIDS and their families, expanding upon the issues that the interdisciplinary team must address in providing care.

Social Issues

Pyschosocial Issues in the Care of Children With HIV Infection or AIDS

Most children infected with HIV are infected perinatally. This brings with it unique stressors that must be dealt with as the mother and child and often other family members are infected.

The psychosocial histories of the patient and the family can provide insight into how the family deals with HIV/AIDS. The past psychiatric history can greatly affect how the individual approaches the unique stressors associated with HIV/AIDS.

The stressors and psychosocial issues associated with HIV/AIDS are complex, in that they are apparent in both the infected individual and in other people who are affected. Some of those stressors include, fear of rejection and social isolation; feelings of guilt, shame, and anger; denial; altered roles, both familial and societal; the destruction of one's

expectations, hopes, and dreams for the future; and the physical and emotional devastation caused by an HIV/AIDS diagnosis.[5]

Family members may display the same psychological symptoms as the infected person, including agitation, withdrawal, anxiety, and depression. The need for social support becomes crucial for all those affected by the diagnosis. Studies of social support and emotional well-being have demonstrated that people with AIDS report fewer feelings of depression and helplessness if they are able to talk with family and close friends about emotional and physical issues associated with their illness. Although social support can act as a buffer against stress for people with HIV, caregivers themselves may require support in order to continue offering their services and expertise.[6] Support groups for the affected members of the family, as well as for the infected patient can provide healthy options for coping. Support groups can help resolve conflicts through reassurance and shared experiences among persons with the same concerns and by helping to prevent increased loneliness and isolation.[7] The stressors that the family affected by HIV encounter are often multifaceted. In addition to HIV infection, many families also cope with poverty, substance abuse, discrimination, inadequate housing, and limited access to resources.[8] HIV-infected parents must cope with their own illness while also coping with the child's illness. They must manage health-care appointments for the entire family. Another stressor is the stigma associated with HIV infection and its associated risk behaviors that is not characteristic of other chronic illnesses. Thus, secrecy and the fear of ostracism stem from this stigmatization. Another stressor unique to HIV/AIDS is that most families have experienced or will experience multiple deaths due to AIDS.[9] These stressors are often addressed in support groups. Support groups are also becoming increasingly important for professionals working with this growing population. The multiple infections and deaths in a family make HIV infection different from other chronic illnesses. Often an entire family is infected. There are very few other diseases that affect both parent and child. Even seasoned professionals familiar with other progressive, chronic illnesses may find it harder to work with the overwhelming multiple tragedies associated with HIV/AIDS.[10] The dynamic nature of the disease in conjunction with the many psychosocial issues makes support groups crucial for professional caregivers as well as for family and friends.

Children with HIV/AIDS may have many of the same problems as adults in addition to problems of their own. Children infected with HIV may not be able to experience normal socialization, and thus are in jeopardy of growing up in an uncertain, isolating, and often stigmatizing environment. Children may develop a lowered sense of self-esteem. They may also develop maladaptive defenses to deal with their isolation. They maladaptive defenses can include loss of affect and depression. These can lead to acting-out behaviors and poor performance in school, which can further isolate the child. Children may also interpret pain as punishment and blame themselves for causing the disease. These altered perceptions are often perpetuated by a child's reluctance to vent fears and ask questions.[6] Interaction and communication with others may be affected. Children with HIV/AIDS may stare vacantly ahead, not smile, avert their gaze, and appear to be withdrawn. Motivational behavior may also be altered.[11] The psychosocial problems of the child are intertwined with those of the family. The illness of a family member , especially a child, upsets all aspects of family life, including social roles and family relationships. For the parents of a child with AIDS, separation from the child is a painful consequence of long hospital stays and inadequate social supports. Further complications ensue for the infected mother of a child who is infected, because of her need for social and medical support to help care for herself as well as her children. These mothers may also bear an overwhelming sense of guilt associated with the mode of transmission of the disease directly from mother to child. This guilt may be further complicated by the pain and sorrow associated with watching the child's illness progress.[6] These mothers also become consumed with the care of their children and tend to deny or neglect their own health needs for fear that their children will be taken from them. The psychosocial concerns extend beyond the parent and child with HIV. Parents must also make plans for the care of uninfected children after they die or become too sick to care for

them adequately.[12] This has become an increasingly common problem that must be addressed by the family as well as health-care providers.

Normal life patterns are most often altered when a family is affected by HIV/AIDS. This has great impact on all family members, especially children. Children may die before their parents, leaving their parents not only to grieve their loss but also to care for themselves at a time when they may have anticipated future support from their children. Grandparents may also have to take on the role of parents once again to care for grandchildren orphaned by the disease. In other cases, young adults may come home to be cared for at a stage at which they would normally be attempting to establish themselves away from home.

In summary, the psychosocial implications for families affected by HIV/AIDS are numerous. Among the more obvious are secrecy resulting from shame about high-risk behaviors and resulting isolation, altered familial roles, and feelings of guilt and depression about transmission to a child. Existing stressors such as poverty, substance abuse, violence, and psychiatric history are merely exacerbated by the presence of this devastating illness. This illness, like no other, must be dealt with as a family issue.

Disclosure

Disclosure is perhaps the most salient psychosocial issue of HIV/AIDS, in that revealing the diagnosis often implies revealing a lifestyle or high-risk behavior that may have been kept hidden.[5] The fear of social stigma and loss of relationships resulting from disclosure is a powerful force that may lead to secrets or deception in relationships.

Familial patterns of secrecy can be further exacerbated when faced with an issue as salient and profound as HIV/AIDS. Disclosure between adults is often hindered by past difficulties in communication within the families. Disclosure to partners is often avoided because of fear of breakup or rejection, as well as a profound sense of guilt.[5] Deciding whether or not to disclose HIV status to family members, especially children, is the most difficult choice faced by parents with HIV.[13]

The dynamics of disclosure of HIV/AIDS to

children are complex. Parents must decide if, how, and when to tell their child of his or her HIV status. Often the child is ready to hear before the parents are prepared to tell. Children most often know that something is wrong and may start imagining scenarios. The child who is denied the knowledge about his or her HIV status or that of a parent may avoid social stigma, but at the cost of isolation in his or her own family. Although it may be difficult for the child to imagine anything more tragic than the reality of AIDS, the isolation and guilt associated with secrecy interfere with the child's ability to find support during a crucial time. Open communication can help reassure the child that the illness is not his or her fault.[10] Both children and adults may feel a sense of isolation if they are not informed. The burden of keeping the secret of illness from children and families is often as difficult as the act of disclosure itself. When family members, especially children, receive accurate information about their own illness or that of a family member, it opens the lines of communication. This open communication can help all family members find better ways of coping both as individuals and as an integral part of the family unit.[5]

As previously mentioned, most pediatric HIV cases occur in urban minority families. These families have experienced many stressors, such as poverty, early or violent family deaths, racial discrimination, substance abuse, and unstable family relationships. As a result of these stressors, these families' strategies of coping do not include open communication. Discussing HIV might be a difficult exception to their accustomed closed communication and avoidance of salient issues.[14]

Children in our society are loved and represent hope for the future. To discuss a child's terminal illness is to effectively extinguish that hope. Parents resist disclosure of HIV in part to shield their children, but also to shield themselves from the full impact of the child's illness. For infected parents, discussing the child's illness brings pressure to acknowledge their own infection. Parents often fear the child's questions about the source of the infection as they bring on feelings of shame and guilt about past high-risk behaviors.

Many parents feel their children are not old enough to keep their diagnosis secret or to under-

stand the concept of the disease or their impending death. Behind the fear of telling children something they will not understand is the view that children will in fact grasp the diagnosis as emotionally devastating, but may not be able to grasp it cognitively.[14] Children's cognitive and emotional absorption of emotionally charged information such as HIV disclosure will not be spontaneous. Disclosure must be a slow and repetitive process for children to eventually come to grips with their infection.[15] Children's concepts of illness are processed in accordance with their cognitive and emotional development. They do not understand AIDS or death as an adult would.[14] Explanation of the illness process must be tailored to the individual cognitive development of the child. Preschool-aged children do not have the capacity to understand the continuous nature of the illness. They do not understand that they are still infected even if they are asymptomatic. School-aged children are capable of understanding basic body concepts and processes. They can also understand the concept of continuity of illness during an asymptomatic period. Adolescents face the additional burden of establishing autonomy over their bodies and sexuality. Therefore, it becomes important for adolescents to participate in all aspects of their care. The developmental level of the child dictates his or her understanding of death and dying. Children below the age of six tend to view death as a separation from parents. Children between the ages of 6 and 10 view death primarily as a result of bodily injury and physical pain. However, open expression of anxiety about the concept of death is rarely manifested without the combined efforts of family, friends, and professionals.[14]

The choice not to disclose is a personal one. It can be emotionally exhausting, as it also includes the professionals one works with. All those who participate in the health care of the individual must take part in the secrecy or collusion with family members.[5] Often the professional must struggle with conflicting therapeutic responsibilities toward the child and the parent.[14]

As previously mentioned, parents of children with AIDS face an immense burden of guilt and anger associated with the mode of transmission to the child, which can strain family relations and make disclosure much more difficult. Often denial forces relationships to terminate at a time when support and stability are most needed. Families at the limit of their capabilities before diagnosis may not be able to cope with the added stress of disclosure and will need familial and professional support.[16]

Grief and Bereavement

Grief work and bereavement become an important part of that professional support. Grief counseling should begin not when death becomes imminent, but early on in the diagnosis. For many this begins at the time of disclosure, when the barriers of denial have finally been broken down. Grief counseling is a substantial part of the clinical work done by the social worker with these families. The social worker first assesses and identifies the coping mechanisms and style of the family. Assessment of the level of understanding and acceptance of HIV infection is also crucial at this time. Families still experiencing a great deal of denial or avoidance as a means of protection may not yet be psychologically prepared to participate in grief counseling. The social worker helps the family explore how they anticipate coping with the impending loss of a child or family member. This is the first step in the anticipatory grieving process. It is important to normalize the range of feelings that may be experienced as part of the grief reaction.[17]

The patterns experienced with grief and bereavement differ between children and adults. This chapter focuses primarily on children. The process may also differ depending on whether the child is grieving the impending loss of a parent or the child's own impending death. As children begin to sense that a parent is dying, they need to be secure in the knowledge that they will still be cared for.[18] Many people with HIV infection experience several stages of responses, including denial, anger, depression, and acceptance. Many will never reach the feeling of acceptance. Some have an overwhelming sense of apathy and show very little response. This may be attributed to the already diminished quality of life these people have experienced from poverty, substance abuse, and exposure to violence. Their ability to recognize and express their feelings may be impaired. It becomes important to integrate individual experiences into the process of dealing with grief and impending loss.

Psychic trauma occurs when one is exposed to an overwhelming event like the loss of a parent, child, or sibling to AIDS. This can prolong the process of grief, mourning, and bereavement. Children must be included in the process. Like adults, they may feel guilty because of having survived. In addition, if they are excluded from the grieving process as well as from open discussion, they may rely on their imagination, making their experience of loss worse. Children may need a model during this process. They need to see that when someone is going to die, or a loss has already been experienced, it is healthy to grieve.[19]

It is also important to include the sibling of a child lost to AIDS in the grieving process. Often when a child is sick the healthy children in the family are neglected. It is important to ensure that the siblings are not neglected during the grieving process as well. They should be encouraged to express their feelings of sadness, anger, anxiety, and fear. A bereaved sibling may experience depression, social withdrawal, and physical or somatic symptoms. Open communication in families becomes crucial in facilitating the ability of the sibling to mourn. Often a professional must also become involved.[20]

When the child is beginning to deal with his or her own impending death, it is important to allow the child to talk freely about his or her feelings. Often, the pain experienced by parents is so great that they tend to stifle the communication of the child. Parents wish to protect the child from the harsh realities. In this instance parents must realize that ignorance is not bliss and that children must deal with the process in their own way and need to know that open communication will be accepted.

When children do begin to talk about their illness, they may first seek answers to general questions about medical procedures and medications. They may then begin to ask more probing questions about others who are ill or general questions about their illness. It is rare for children to immediately inquire about their own death before gaining general knowledge about illness and death. Children express their emotions in a variety of ways, such as through words, art, play, and often merely through behavioral changes. It is important that children be given the opportunity to express their feelings and concerns in a manner that feels comfortable for them. They must not feel pressured into doing so. Positive as well as negative feelings should be explored with the child.[21]

When working with a child, adults must be careful not to patronize or underestimate the child's ability to cope. Children may feel afraid and sad when facing their death, but they may also find great courage in the knowledge that they are being allowed to take an active part in the process. In acknowledging their own death, children are free to explore the life they have led. Whenever possible, children should be encouraged to exercise control over how and where they die. Some children may even want to write out final wishes in the form of a will. This can be as important for the bereaved family as for the dying child.[21]

The secrecy that often surrounds the diagnosis of AIDS may contribute to feelings of shame and worthlessness for the dying child. The ease with which others associate with this child can influence self-worth, and acceptance of self and of impending death.

When a child is in a bereaved state from the loss of a parent or sibling, open communication is crucial. Parents and family members often avoid the topic in the hope of protecting the child. Again, role modeling is important. Adults should grieve openly with children. It is when those feelings are suppressed that the child becomes isolated in sadness and worried about the existence of feelings that are seemingly not allowed to be expressed.[22]

A bereaved child, for the most part, will look no different from any other child. The child may not behave differently from other children during the course of the day. What is different is the internal knowledge the child possesses. This knowledge may manifest itself in sadness, depression, anger, denial, and many other behaviors at any time. The child must know that this is normal and must be encouraged to express those feelings. A salient feature of childhood bereavement is that it is not contained within a certain time period. These feelings may re-emerge at each new developmental phase. Mourning may become a lifelong commitment to resolving one's childhood loss.

The bereaved child must feel security, trust, and love. The process of bereavement itself can undermine the notion of security. The child must be made to feel safe. The child must also have someone to trust with his or her feelings of grief and loss. This person may be a family member or friend, a clergy person, or a mental health professional.

The realities of death carry with them personal emotions and ways of coping. Professionals must be wary of imposing those personal issues on the grief and bereavement process of the family. When working with children, the professional must remember that children are not isolated individuals. They live within a social environment largely dominated by the beliefs of the adults who care for them. Therefore, it becomes imperative to deal with the grief and bereavement of a child as a family issue. After all, AIDS is a disease that encompasses all aspects of the family. The following section focuses on the need for balance between psychosocial and medical functioning as well as self-perceptions of quality of life in persons with AIDS.

Quality Of Life

Introduction

Quality of life for persons with HIV infection has increasingly become an area of interest and research.[23] Previous studies conducted on the quality of life of HIV-infected patients indicated that HIV classification had the greatest impact on the patient's perception of quality of life.[23,24] The current system, published by the Centers for Disease Control (CDC) in 1987, classifies people with HIV disease into four groups: group I (acute infection), group II (asymptomatic), group III (persistent generalized lymphadenopathy), and group IV (other disease, indicating end-stage HIV disease or AIDS). The CDC proposed changes to the 1987 classification scheme that were implemented in early 1993, focusing on physical changes that occur over time. Previous research reported that changes in quality of life occurred with disease entities[25,26] and varied as a function of the patient's nearness to death.[27] Various nurse researchers have used quality of life as an outcome variable[28–30] in an effort to develop holistic definitions and indications of prevention and recovery from disease. Since there is no cure and no vaccine for HIV infection,[31] there is a need to improve the quality of life of infected persons during the remaining life span. A review of existing models of quality of life may shed some light on the need to develop a model relevant to patients with HIV infection or AIDS.

Defining Quality of Life

There is no universal agreement on how to measure quality of life. The prevalence of chronic diseases has spawned the concept of quality of life and given rise to research and interventions by health-care workers to help patients live with illness. The shift from crisis intervention to the realization that there is no cure for the illness has led nurses and other health-care workers to design and implement patient-care strategies that empower patients to generate and maintain a semblance of control.

According to deTornay,[32] care should include prevention, management of chronic diseases, and meeting social needs. She identified the need to change the emphasis for care from hospitals to community and home settings. Developing models of long-term care is becoming a priority among nurse researchers who recognize the major advances in technology and realize the impact that prolonged survival time will have on the health-care system. Hence, the focus should be on the efficacy of treatment and on providing a better quality of life. Self-esteem, hope, and belief in the ability for improved physical activity are just a few of the variables included in measurement of quality of life in chronic illness.

A poignant definition of quality of life states, "Quality of life should be viewed as the relative effectiveness of a patient's chosen or ascribed management style in solving the practical problems associated with being 'seriously sick.' "[33] The authors describe management style as a specific strategy that the patient uses to understand and respond to problems caused by the disease. Effectiveness in dealing with personal problems, as perceived by the patient, or how management strategies are used, reflects upon one's self-identity and philosophy of life. The patient becomes the center of the health-care team, responsible for managing a multitude of daily tasks and requests that include responses to invasive procedures, relationships with family members and significant others, and interactions with health-care staff. The processes by which patients organize efforts to manage their experiences of hospitalization and their perspective of quality of life during hospitalization will serve as the basis for redefining quality of life for the HIV/AIDS patient.

Existing Models of Quality of Life

Medical models view quality of life from the traditional perspective of the diagnosis of illness, intervention, and subsequent improvement in patient status. The notion of being able to manipulate a patient's quality of life by medical interventions and outcomes is somewhat contradictory to what the nursing models propose. Rather than viewing quality of life as a dependent variable, nursing suggests viewing quality of life as an accomplishment. In other words, the quality of life that results is due to the integrative efforts of all health-care members throughout the patient's health-care encounter. Nursing models propose that the patient and the health-care team collaborate in an effort to manage the effects the illness has on the patient's everyday life. Although this holistic approach to care is reflective of the goals of nursing, the effectiveness of the collaborative process and the overall effect it has on the patient can only be assessed by the patient.[34]

Until recently, models of quality of life addressed traditional or general manifestations of chronic illnesses, such as cancer[35,36] and cardiac failure.[37] Nokes et al.[38] developed an HIV assessment tool that used a visual analog scale to rate the severity of HIV-related symptoms and general well-being.[38] Although they found the tool to be highly reliable, they stressed the importance of calculating reliability estimates whenever the tool is used for different samples. The HIV Self-Care Inventory and the Healthcare Needs Scale for Patients with HIV/AIDS measure subjective and objective dimensions of HIV illness and should be administered in conjunction with the HIV assessment tool to adequately validate this tool. Since symptoms serve as the focus of intervention for nurses as they care for people with acute and chronic diseases,[39] helping a person cope with the multitude of symptoms that are manifested during the natural history of HIV disease may directly impact on well-being. Subsequent management of symptoms by the patient can affect the quality of life.

The differences between HIV/AIDS and other chronic or terminal illnesses are crucial for understanding why quality of life must be measured and looked differently in HIV/AIDS then in other diseases. AIDS is both a chronic and a terminal disease. The lifestyles of persons with AIDS are different from those of patients with other chronic illnesses, thus making it difficult for nurses to understand the relationship of risk factors such as intravenous drug use and unsafe sexual practices to quality of life. The delivery of health care to patients with HIV infection or AIDS differs from that in other chronic diseases in that access to patient information and access to outsiders is more controlled because of the controversial nature of the disease. Finally, most patients with AIDS are not completely dependent on the health-care system for their care and seek alternative therapies, such as holistic healing and meditation.

Patients with HIV infection or AIDS contribute to quality of life through plans made to manage and deal with all the serious indications of the diagnosis. Alternative therapies may encourage the patients to be more involved in deciding how to manage their care. Information from a disease-specific, systematic assessment can assist the patient and the health-care team to plan interventions and promote the attainment of knowledge necessary to provide self-care. Defining quality of life from the perspective of the patient will serve as a conceptual basis for this exploration into sustaining health and supporting wellness.

Patients' Perspectives of Quality of Life and Strategies Used to Manage HIV Infection and AIDS During Hospitalization

An exploratory study conducted in patients with AIDS illustrated the usefulness of studying quality of life through a patient-centered perspective.[33] The small sample size ($N = 13$) and the hospital setting (dedicated AIDS unit in a for-profit community hospital) were two limitations of the study. Yet, the various styles identified appeared autonomous from treatment and care regimes, suggesting that the execution of these styles should not conflict with the delivery of health care.

According to the authors, management styles are apt to change over time, particularly as the patient's physical condition worsens. Increasing the patient's sense of control over self during hospitalization may improve the patient-care outcome by fostering cooperation. Assessing the effectiveness of the responses of nurses and other health-care workers to patient styles needs to be considered when patients describe the positive or negative effects, acceptance or nonacceptance, and support or nonsupport their management styles had on perceptions of quality of life during hospitalization.

Six management styles emerged during the study as a result of semistructured interviews and naturalistic (observations of interactions, such as conversation among patients and nurses). A brief description of each style, as well as suggestions to nurses and other health-care provides for enhancing the effectiveness of these styles, may provide insight into the patients' perspectives of quality of life while hospitalized. But one must realize that these styles are not generalizable to the overall patient population, and further research is needed to examine the management styles of persons with HIV infection or AIDS in nonprofit or teaching hospitals, with a higher proportion of patients who are female, members of minority groups, or intravenous drug abusers.

The six management styles identified are the: loner, activist, mystic, victim, timekeeper, and medic. The loner is a patient who rejects and avoids social interaction. The activist chooses to seek out interactions and perceives HIV infection or AIDS as a social and political phenomenon. The mystic contrives a spiritual explanation to interpret and explain experiences as they relate to the disease. The victim's management style is one of dependence on others. This patient allows others to define what HIV infection or AIDS means and to control quality of life outcomes. The timekeeper is depicted as the "ideal" type of manager who waits for things to happen. Time is central to the organization of the patient's life, and activities are organized within a time frame. Last, the medic manages life through a staggering dependence on medical terminology, its meaning, and its significance in interpreting the disease.

Members of the health-care team may or may not recognize a distinct style or method used by a patient. Recognition of the individuality of each patient's response to the diagnosis and the subsequent interventions they may have to submit to may enable nurses and other health-care workers to gain a better understanding of their values and feelings, thus enhancing communication. The ultimate goal is to improve the quality of care. This can only be accomplished through observations, conversations, and interactions with patients as we encourage them to share their thoughts about HIV infection or AIDS and the caregiving they have experienced.

Understanding Patient Individuality to Improve Quality of Care

Societal discrimination and lack of respect for fundamental human rights and dignity has impeded the prevention of HIV transmission, the care of those who are infected and ill, and the advancement of the health of all people. The psychosocial problems manifested by such discrimination can result in individual and family problems that interfere with and undermine the prevention and treatment of HIV infection and AIDS.[40] The nurse's understanding of the patient's individual value and views can enhance communication and ultimately improve the quality of care. Nurses can further expand their professional roles through a holistic approach to care that uses management strategies recognized by the caregiver and the care receiver.[33] As AIDS continues to evolve towards a chronic disease, the focus on quality of care will be to enhance home care, thus enabling patients and their families to develop consistencies in their management strategies.[33]

Management Strategies for the HIV-Infected Patient at Home or in the Hospice

Self-care management strategies affect families as well as the HIV-infected patient. Concerns re-

garding the quality of life of the other family members are often overlooked. Dealing with an adult child returning to the home, concern about transmission of the disease to other family members, and living with a chronically ill person will have a negative impact on the life of the family.[41] For some HIV-infected patients, the self-perceived quality of life may dictate management strategies after discharge from the hospital to home or hospice care. Nurses can play an important role in assessing and monitoring the mental status of patients and their families, prompting them to make referrals for mental health services accordingly. Further research is warranted in HIV-infected women and children, as relatively little has been written about their mental health concerns and problems. Increasing numbers of women, children, and members of minority groups are being affected by the epidemic.[42] Nurses who have frequent contact with HIV-infected clients can assume a position of advocacy to ensure that client needs are met and changes are made in public policy, funding, research, and access to health care.

AIDS and Older Adults

Introduction

AIDS prevention efforts and research have mainly been directed toward high-risk populations, such as adolescents, young adults, intravenous drug users, and homosexual males.[43] It has become increasingly clear, however, that older adults are also at high risk for contracting AIDS.[43] According to the CDC, 10% of AIDS cases occur in people over the age of 50, and 4% in people over the age of 70.[44]

Older adults are affected by AIDS in many ways. Many older adults with AIDS share many of the same services and resources with their noninfected counterparts and young adults with AIDS. Older caregivers often have to cope not only with a chronically ill adult child, but with their own infirmities and health problems.

Understanding the Issues

It is a challenge to speak to older adults about AIDS and HIV infection. Many older adults became familiar with HIV infection and AIDS after the actor Rock Hudson disclosed that he had been diagnosed with HIV. The news seemed even more surprising considering the fact that he had admitted he was a homosexual. Many older adults grew up in a time where sexuality was never spoken of publicly (Personal communication, 1994). They may feel that they are not at risk for contracting AIDS because they have been married to the same partner for many years and the partner has remained faithful. Older adults may also feel that only young people get AIDS. Society and some medical professionals also think that older adults are not at risk for AIDS because they are not sexually active and do not usually cheat on their partners. These myths perpetuate the false and dangerous belief that older adults are not at risk for AIDS.

The AIDS epidemic affects individuals both directly and indirectly.[45] People are affected directly when they or their loved ones are HIV-positive or develop the disease.[45] People are affected indirectly when they live near people with AIDS or when the demand for long-term care services for older people and others with AIDS puts a further drain on the health-care system, leading to competition.[45] It has been hypothesized that there are three main groups of older adults at risk for contracting or transmitting HIV infection: recipients of HIV-infected blood transfusions, their sexual partners, and people who have unprotected anal or vaginal intercourse outside a mutually monogamous relationship. These three categories include people of all sexual orientations.[46]

These risk factors debunk the myth that older adults do not engage in sexual activity. In a national probability sample, between 2.5% and 3.0% of older Americans (those persons over 50) reported two or more sexual partners in the previous year.[47] The average frequency of sexual activity in older adults is two to four times per month, an adequate rate for transmission of the virus to occur.[47]

There are other ways in which the elderly population is affected by HIV and AIDS. Older adults with AIDS share many of the same services with the frail elderly and the younger population with AIDS, therefore impacting on the services the health-care system can offer.[45] Many elderly people are caring for a loved one with AIDS.[45] AIDS in the elderly also may be misdiagnosed, since many of the symptoms are similar to those of other illnesses.[48]

Blood Transfusions

People infected by blood transfusions constitute the second largest risk group among older adults (the largest risk group is the homosexual/bisexual male population).[43] Although the proportion of AIDS cases due to blood transfusions is higher in children and young adults, the elderly are more likely to receive blood transfusions thus placing them at risk of being infected.[48] Twenty-five percent of patients receiving blood transfusions are between 51 and 60 years of age, 15% are between 61 and 65, 8% are between 66 and 70, and 5% are over 70.[48]

Between 1978 and April 1985, the nation's blood supply was maximally contaminated with HIV.[43] Since April 1985, efforts have been made to protect the blood supply by screening.[43] Although the risk of contracting AIDS from a blood transfusion has decreased because of improved blood screening methods, blood transfusion is still a risk factor.[43]

Estimates are needed of the number of older people who may have received contaminated blood.[43] This is difficult for many reasons. Current estimates of the total number of HIV infections due to blood transfusions do not include older adults; many transfusion recipients died before the availability of HIV testing; the same person may have received repeated transfusions over time.[43] The chances of being infected by blood transfusion also differ across geographic regions. For example, the proportion of patients with HIV infection who were infected through blood transfusion is higher in San Francisco than in Columbus, Ohio.[43]

In another study, 71 college-educated elderly people between the ages of 65 to 78 completed anonymous questionnaires as part of a university-sponsored Urban Elders program. The questionnaires asked for detailed blood-transfusion histories of the respondents and their sexual partner(s), sexual risk behaviors, antibody testing, and attitudes toward condoms.[46] In this group, 51% of the women and 92% of the men were sexually active; 12% of the sexually active had received transfusions between 1977 and 1985. None of these individuals had used condoms, and none had been tested for HIV. Of this sample, 17% had received transfusions between 1977 and 1985; 58% of these had been advised by a health professional to be tested for HIV antibodies. Only 42% of those who had received transfusions obtained HIV antibody testing.[46]

Older Adults and Sexual Activity

HIV infection from blood transfusion is a problem on a larger scale, since people infected from blood transfusions can also pass HIV on to their sexual partners.[43] The number of older people infected by their partners in this way increased rapidly after 1986, approximately 3 years after the initial burst of AIDS cases attributable to blood transfusions.[49]

One of the few concentrated efforts that has focused on AIDS infection in older adults is the National AIDS Behavioral Surveys.[49] The National AIDS Behavioral Surveys telephone survey of randomly chosen older Americans (50 to 75 years old) was divided into two samples: a national sample of 48 contiguous states that oversampled older respondents (2,673 total, including 1,114 over the age of 50 years, with a 70% cooperation rate) and a sample from 23 major metropolitan areas considered "high-risk cities" (11,429 total, including 2,074 over the age of 50).[49]

Among heterosexuals, the proportion of persons with at least one behavioral risk factor for HIV infection was higher in the high-risk cities sample than in the national sample.[49] The sources of risk were nearly equally divided among having a sexual partner with a known risk factor for HIV infection, having a transfusion between 1977 and 1984, and having multiple sexual partners. In the high-risk cities sample, there were glaring differences for gender, race or ethnicity, and marital status.[49] Men were more likely than women to have at least one risk factor, with African-Americans having the highest prevalence rates of risk, followed by whites, Asians, and Hispanics.[49] People who were separated, divorced, or never married had the highest levels of risk, followed by the married, the widowed, and the cohabitating.[49] There was no difference between the two samples in the very low prevalence of condom use during vaginal or anal sexual

contact among sexually active, at-risk Americans aged 50 years or older.[49]

According to the Urban Elders questionnaire: 40% of the total sample and 32% of the sexually active disagreed that condoms can prevent HIV transmission, 58% of the total sample and 50% of the sexually active agreed that condoms were too physically uncomfortable to use,[46] 4% of the total sample and 3% of the sexually active agreed that using condoms was immoral, and 45% of the total sample and 50% of the sexually active agreed that it was too embarrassing to buy condoms in a store.[46]

Many older adults believe they are not at risk because they have been married for many years or widowed. Although monogamy may be one reason that the AIDS epidemic is limited in this population,[49] widowhood or being married to the same partner does not guarantee monogamy as many older people belong to Golden Swinger clubs or employ prostitutes of both sexes.[43]

The main factor that contributes to the increased susceptibility to contracting HIV in older people is the physiologic changes that take place as one ages.[43] Older people have a decrease in the functioning of the immune system, which may explain why they have a lower median HIV incubation time than younger adults.[43] Declining immune function also makes them more susceptible to sexually transmitted diseases, which often serve as cofactors of HIV transmission.[43] Postmenopausal women also experience thinning of the vaginal wall due to a loss of estrogen and may also experience a decrease in the vaginal mucosa,[50] making them more susceptible to tears in the vaginal wall, which can expedite the spread of the virus.[44]

Homosexual men remain the largest group of older AIDS patients, accounting for 65.8% of all cases among older people in 1987.[43] This group is very difficult to study because of its lack of openness about sexual orientation, as older homosexual men are more likely to be closeted and are less subject to changing sexual standards in the homosexual community.[43] However, research has shown that older homosexual men may be more knowledgeable about AIDS than older heterosexuals.[43] The National AIDS Behavioral Surveys found that in the gay or bisexual community, men past the age of 50 are aware of their risk for HIV infection and use risk reduction methods.[49]

Older Adults and Shared Social Services

Frail or infirm older adults and people with AIDS (young and old) require many of the same services and supports.[45] However, rather than combining efforts, they may compete for resources.[45] It is feared that what is perceived as disproportionate spending for people with AIDS or for older people can result in intergenerational conflict.[45]

The young and the elderly with AIDS may be placed in public housing for elderly people. Older adults with AIDS who cannot continue to live independently or in high-crime areas may be placed in senior public housing.[45] Those who need more medical attention and are unable to remain in the hospital or return home are being placed in personal care homes.[45] Many older residents who live in this type of facility and their families are often fearful of people with AIDS living in the same housing complex.[7] Older people are more likely not to be educated about AIDS and its transmission, and neighbors may be afraid of catching the disease.[7] They equate AIDS with other epidemic diseases, such as typhoid, tuberculosis, and polio.[7] Some older adults believe that, like these diseases, AIDS can be spread by casual contact, airborne germs, physical contact, or eating contaminated food.[7] They may also question the moral character and lifestyles of people with AIDS.[7]

Like the sick elderly, HIV-infected persons require both acute and long-term care.[5] The two groups are often dependent on pharmacologic agents and rehabilitative services.[5] Other similarities in the paradigm of geriatric care and care developed for people with AIDS include the use of multidisciplinary teams in care, the incorporation of family members into the overall picture when evaluating the health of the individual, the incorporation of function and cognitive status into patient evaluation and management, and the use of many tiers of institutional and nonhospital settings for care.[6]

The Older Adult as Caregiver

There is an increasing trend in this country for older adults to become the main caregivers for a grandchild, adult child, spouse, or friend with AIDS.[8] In a random sampling of 200 patients with AIDS (ages 21 to 59) registered with an Atlanta-based community AIDS organization, 30% reported a parent or grandparent as the primary caregiver.[7] Other persons reported as primary caregivers were friends (32%), lovers or spouses (20%), and siblings (8%); 10% reported that they had no primary caregiver.[7] Not only do older caregivers need to deal with issues of grief and the stigma of having AIDS in the family, but they are often plagued by their own chronic health problems.[9] The caregiver–patient relationship also includes the relationship between two elderly adults.[9]

In general, there are three areas of stress for caregivers.[9] Primary caregiver strains arise from the demands of the role itself, such as household and managerial tasks, as well as the care of the patient.[9] The second area consists of the indirect stresses associated with caregiving, such as financial problems and the impact of caregiving on leisure activity.[9] A third area consists of intrapsychic strains such as perceptions of personal vulnerability to the disease, reactions from others, and the anticipated loss of the loved one. Another area of strain may be the lack of value assigned by society to the caregiving role.[9]

"Skip-generation parenting" means the care of a child by a grandparent. According to United States census figures, 12.1% of African-American children live with their grandparents, compared with 5.8% of Hispanic-American children and 3.4% of white children. These numbers are probably underestimated.[8] Many of these caregivers have a strong spiritual background and look to religion to help them cope.[8] For this type of caregiver, AIDS often brings about a double loss, the death or impending death of an adult child coupled with the illness and probable death of a grandchild.[9] Many states will not support skip-generation parents raising children who have lost a parent to AIDS, and ironically, some state child welfare agencies provide less financial support to a child's blood relative than to nonrelated foster parents.[8] Children being cared for by elders need special services such as bereavement counseling, transitional services for youth and their new guardians, and housing support such as rent subsidies.[8]

One-third of adult patients with AIDS are dependent on an older parent.[7] This may cause problems for the parent since the elderly are often on a fixed income.[9] Older adults often have less stamina, reduced mobility, diminished sight, and physical deterioration and may not be physically able to care for a person with many health-care needs.[9] However, it is important to remember that "advanced age alone does not place an individual at a dramatically greater risk of being functionally disabled."[9] There is also a fear of diminishing social contacts and loss of status in the family and community because of the stigma associated with AIDS.[8]

Many adults with AIDS have been rejected by their families because of their lifestyle.[9] For older gay men, telling the family of their homosexuality may have resulted in estrangement, since homosexuality was less accepted in the past.[9] Elderly homosexual men may be more likely to have a poor or nonexistent relationship with their families than younger homosexual men.[9] It is not common practice for the older homosexual man to "come out" as a result of a diagnosis of HIV infection. He may have more to lose than his younger counterpart, since ". . . a lifetime has been built on carefully protecting [the older man's] sexual orientation."[9] A history of drug abuse in an adult child also makes the caregiving role even more of a challenge.[9] Often, an elderly caregiver is fearful of abuse by the patient, who may suffer from dementia and have bouts of anger and violence as a manifestation of AIDS or a reaction to medications.[9] Others may be very close to members of their family.[9]

Diagnosing AIDS in the Elderly

One major barrier to educating older adults about AIDS and its transmission is that primary care clinicians usually do not include sexual and HIV risk assessments during the visits.[10] This is unfortunate, since one survey showed that 11% of persons over the age of 50 reported that they had discussed AIDS with their physician, and a majority indicated a willingness to do so if the physician initiated the conversation.[10]

Older patients with AIDS usually present symptoms similar to those of younger patients, although there are differences.[50] Disease progression is more rapid in the elderly, and the shorter survival time

may result in a delayed AIDS diagnosis.[50] Symptoms of HIV infection, such as fatigue, anorexia, weight loss, and decreased physical and cognitive function, often mimic chronic illnesses that are common as one ages.[50] One researcher has described AIDS as the "great imitator" because of its similarities to Alzheimer's disease, dementia, and other illnesses common in older adults.[48]

In addition, elderly persons known to be HIV-positive may still have diseases common in older people and their presentations may be deceptive and misattributed to HIV.[50]

AIDS Risk-Reduction Model

One of the most frequently used health education models for designing AIDS education and prevention programs is the AIDS risk-reduction model devised by Joseph Catania.[46] This model provides a conceptual framework to understand the processes by which people who are at risk for contracting or transmitting HIV may come to label their behavior as putting themselves or others at risk for HIV infection, make a commitment to reduce risk behaviors and increase safe behaviors, and initiate activities that eventuate in the performance of the desired behavior change. In other words, there are stages an individual must go through, and each change process is hypothesized to require different kinds of knowledge, beliefs, and social skills. A person who acknowledges engaging in high-risk activities such as not wearing a condom will have to make an effort to practice safer sex by wearing a condom. This will lead to the person's purchasing the condoms and continuing to use them correctly and consistently.

Stage one, the labeling process, may require education and basic knowledge of the conditions associated with HIV risk and routes of transmission. The type of intervention that targets those in this stage may be influenced by mass media campaigns focused on older people. The campaign geared toward older adults would discuss HIV transmission and how HIV and AIDS can affect them. At this time, there has not been a mass media campaign focused on the older population.

Stage two would require knowledge of alternative behaviors such as risk-reduction techniques and an understanding of the costs and benefits. This stage deals with questions that are more sexually explicit, such as the benefits of using condoms and how to use them so that they do not interfere with sexual pleasure. The mass media tend to avoid these topics, since they are seen as controversial. The most appropriate settings in which to discuss these issues would be health care-related settings and at social organizations, since there would be more of an opportunity for education or counseling.

Stage three may require more social skill, since more communication is involved, such as negotiating changes in sexual behavior. This stage therefore may require more intensive group or individual counseling or therapy.

Conclusion

In the words of one physician, "Age should not be a barrier to considering AIDS as a diagnosis," since ageism in the health care field may lead to poor health outcomes.[44] The biases of concern are the result of ignorance about geriatric medicine or true prejudices against the old that prevent the health-care provider from making appropriate judgments.[44] Despite beliefs to the contrary, studies show that sexuality is maintained well into late life.[44] Physicians should conduct a thorough sexual and AIDS risk assessment on all their elderly patients and ask specific questions about the gender and number of partners, use of condoms, history of sexually transmitted diseases, blood transfusions, or intravenous drug use.[50] Patient education regarding transmission of HIV should also be a part of the session. An older person with risk factors for AIDS should be given the option of confidential (a name is attached to the test result) or anonymous (a number is attached to the test result) testing.[50] The meaning of a positive or negative result should be explained. The patient should also be informed about the incubation period of the virus, the benefits of knowing the test result, and risk reduction. An informed consent must be signed and an appointment for the follow-up test result should be made.[50] No test results should be given out over the telephone.[50]

Counseling and education about HIV risk and condom use are needed for older people.[46] This should include teaching older adults about sexual communication and problem-solving skills, as these skills may be less developed among older people.[43] According to a survey conducted by Gerbert and Maguire in response to the Surgeon General's brochure on AIDS,[47] the elderly are not unreceptive to learning about AIDS. It was found that 69% of the respondents said they read all or almost all of the brochure; 87% did not feel that the brochure was in any way offensive; and 76% said they were glad to get the brochure.[47] Printed materials need to be written in a language that older adults can understand and relate with their experience.

Services and counseling also must be given to older caregivers of people with AIDS.[45] Caregivers need to be linked up to services such as respite programs, to care for another person effectively since they need to take care of themselves physically and mentally[45] Social workers can assist caregivers in helping them understand the service system and may at times need to perform this case management role themselves.[45] Social workers also need to know about the marital status of the caregiver, the relationship between the caregiver and the patient, the caregiver's knowledge of AIDS, and the caregiver's financial, physical, intellectual, and emotional condition.[45]

Providers also need to be educated about AIDS in the elderly. All members of the helping professions should be informed about safe sex, risk reduction, modes of AIDS transmission, and the progression of the illness. Just as importantly, all professionals need guidance in working through their own concerns about dealing with older people and a disease associated with sexuality, homosexuality, and drug addiction.[45]

Health educators and public health professionals can play a role in developing community-based interventions, as this type of education has been shown to be useful in accessing hard-to-reach groups.[43] This type of intervention should be long-term and should target specific segments of the community. Catania and colleagues[46] suggests that mass communication (press, television, mailings, radio), should focus on debunking myths about AIDS (for example, making it clear that AIDS is not just a disease of young, homosexual, white men but has in fact killed a large number of older people), sources of past and present transmission, and encouraging for those at risk to obtain HIV antibody testing.[46] Specific behavioral changes to reduce sexual transmission can be discussed at the group or institutional level.

Older adults should not be underestimated in their ability to act as educators for younger generations. Educating older adults about the prevention of HIV infection and AIDS could "trickle down" to younger people who might understand that if older adults are at risk, that they too are at risk.[10] The hope is that people of all ages will come to understand AIDS as a deadly disease that does not discriminate by race, gender, or age.

Summary

The care of people with HIV infection or AIDS must take account of the relations between the patient and other people who are affected by the patient's illness.

Unlike any other chronic illness, this disease is associated with risk behaviors and lifestyle. A diagnosis of HIV infection or AIDS carries with it a social stigma that is usually not a factor in other chronic, progressive illnesses, such as cancer.

Another unique aspect of this population is that HIV infection or AIDS is perhaps the only disease that involves infection of both the parent and the child. These multiple infections can lead to altered familial roles. The grandparent may have to revisit the primary caregiver role and often must care for infected adult children, as well as their grandchildren.

To address these sensitive issues, an interdisciplinary approach is crucial in providing care that creates a balance between the chronic medical and social needs of families affected by the disease. It is hoped that collaboration between different disciplines will better the quality of life for these families.

References

1. Andiman W. What do children witness? In: Gebelle S, Gruendel J, Andiman W (eds). *Forgotten Children of the AIDS Epidemic.* New Haven: Yale University Press, 1995:46.

2. Boland MG, Santacroce SJ. Nursing role in care of child and family. In: Pizzo PA and Wilfert CM (eds). *Pediatric AIDS: The Challenge of HIV Infection in Infants, Children, and Adolescents.* Baltimore: Williams & Wilkins, 1995:787.

3. Duggan C, Mitchell F. The role of the nurse. In: Mok J, Newell M (eds). *HIV Infection in Children: A Guide to Practical Management.* Cambridge: Cambridge University Press, 1995:238.

4. Weiner L, Septimus A. Psychosocial support for child and family. In: Pizzo PA and Wilfert CM (eds). *Pediatric AIDS: The Challenge of HIV Infection in Infants, Children, and Adolescents.* Baltimore: Williams & Wilkins, 1995:817.

5. Stulberg I, Buckingham SL. Parallel issues for AIDS patients, families, and others. *J Contemp Soc Work* 1988;69:355–360.

6. Lockhart LL, Wodlerski JS. Facing the unknown: children and adolescents with AIDS. *Soc Work* 1989;34:215–221.

7. Flaskerud JH. AIDS: psychological aspects. *J Psychosoc Nurs* 1987;25:9–17.

8. Lewis SY, Haiken HJ, Hoyt LG. Living beyond the odds: a psychosocial perspective on long-term survivors of pediatric human immunodeficiency virus infection. *J Dev Behav Pediatr* 1994;15: S12-S17.

9. Mellins CA, Ehrhardt AA. Families affected by pediatric acquired immunodeficiency syndrome: sources of stress and coping. *J Dev Behav Pediatr* 1994;15:S54-S60.

10. Stuber ML. Psychotherapy issues in pediatric HIV and AIDS. In: Children and AIDS. Washington, DC: American Psychiatric Press, 1992:213–226.

11. Wiener L, Moss H, Davidson R, Fuir C. Pediatrics: the emerging psychosocial challenges of the AIDS epidemic. *Child Adolesc Soc Work J* 1992;9: 381–407.

12. Sherwen LN, Bolan M. Overview of psychosocial research concerning pediatric human immunodeficiency virus infection. *J Dev Behav Pediatr* 1994;15:S5–S11.

13. Levine C, Stein G. Orphans of the HIV epidemic: unmet needs in six US cities. In: Feiden KL (ed). *The Orphan Project: The HIV Epidemic and New York City's Children.* New York: Clarkwood Corporation, 1994:55–62.

14. Lipson M. What do you say to a child with AIDS? *Hastings Center Report* 1993;23:6–12.

15. Lipson M. Disclosure of diagnosis to children with human immunodeficiency virus or acquired immunodeficiency syndrome. *J Dev Behav Pediatr* 1994;15:S61–S65.

16. Lewert G. Children and AIDS: social casework. *J Contemp Soc Work* 1988;69:348–354.

17. Thurlow TJ. The role of the cardiovascular social worker. *Nurs Clin North Am* 1995;30:211–219.

18. Tiblier KB, Walker G, Rolland JS. Therapeutic issues when working with families of persons with AIDS. In: Macklin ED (ed). *AIDS and Families*. New York: Harrington Park Press, 1989:81–128.

19. Dane BO. Death and bereavement. AIDS and the new orphans. In: Dane MO, Levine C (eds). *AIDS and Families*. Connecticut: Auburn House, 1994: 13–33.

20. Fanos JH, Weinger L. Tomorrow's survivors: siblings of human immunodeficiency virus-infected children. *J Dev Behav Pediatr* 1994;15:S43–S48.

21. Lwin R. Talking with the dying child. In: Mok JY, Newell ML (eds). *HIV Infection in Children: A Guide to Practical Management*. Cambridge, UK: Cambridge University Press, 1995:270–282.

22. Hemmings P. The bereaved child. In: Mok J, Newell ML (eds). *HIV Infection in Children: A Guide to Practical Management*. Cambridge, UK: Cambridge University Press, 1995:283–293.

23. Ragsdale D, Morrow JR. Quality of life as a function of HIV classification. *Nurs Res* 1990;39: 355–359.

24. Kelly JA, St. Lawrence JS. *The AIDS Health Crisis: Psychological and Social Interventions*. New York: Plenum, 1988.

25. Aaronson NK, Beckman J. *The Quality of Life of Cancer Patients*. New York: Lippincott-Raven Press, 1987.

26. Wenger NK, Mattson ME, Furberg CD, Slinson, J. *Assessment of Quality of Life in Clinical Trials of Cardiovascular Therapies*. New York: Le Jacq Publishing, 1984.

27. Morris JN, Suissa S, Serwood S, et al. Last days: a study of the quality of life in terminally ill cancer patients. *J Chron Dis* 1986;39:47–62.

28. American Nurses Association. *A Social Policy Statement*. Kansas City, MO: American Nurses Association, 1980.

29. Ferraris C, Powers M. Qualtiy of life index: development and psychometric properties. *Adv Nurs Sci* 1985;10:15–24.

30. Padilla G, Grant M. Quality of life as a cancer nursing outcome variable. *Adv Nurs Sci* 1985; 10:45–60.

31. Solomon GF, Temoshok L. A psychoneuroimmunologic perspective on AIDS research: questions, preliminary findings and suggestions. *J Appl Psychol* 1987;7:286–308.

32. de Tornyay R. An agenda for action. *J Nurs Educ* 1991;31:4.

33. Ragsdale D, Kotarba JA, Morrow JR. Quality of life of hospitalized persons with AIDS. *IMAGE: J Nurs Scholarship* 1992;24:259–265.

34. Kotarba J. The social control function of holistic health care in bureaucratic settings: the case of space medicine. *J Health Soc Behav* 1983;24: 275–288.

35. Morris JN, Sherwood S. Quality of life of cancer patients at different stages in the disease trajectory. *J Chron Dis* 1987;40:545–553.

36. Tchekmedyian NS, Hickman M, Sian J, et al. Treatment of cancer anorexia with megestrol acetate: impact on quality of life. *Oncology* 1990; 4:185–194.

37. Ott CR, Sivarajan ES, Newton KM, et al. A controlled randomized study of early cardiac rehabilitation: the sickness impact profile as an assessment tool. *Heart Lung* 1983;12:162–170.

38. Nolles KM, Wheeler K, Kendrew J. Development of an HIV assessment tool. *IMAGE: J Nurs Scholarship* 1994;26:133–138.

39. Giardino E, Wolf Z. Symptoms: evidence and experience. *Nurs Pract* 1993;7:1–12.

40. Mann J, Tarantola D. The global AIDS pandemic: toward a new vision of health. *Infect Dis Clin North Am* 1995;9:275–285.

41. Durham JD. The changing HIV/AIDS epidemic: emerging psychosocial challenges for nurses. *Nurs Clin North Am* 1994;29:9–18.

42. Kneisl CR. Psychosocial and economic concerns of women affected by HIV infection. In: Durham JD (ed). *Women, Children and HIV/AIDS*. New York: Springer-Verlag, 1993:241–250.

43. Catania JA, Turner H, Kegeles SM, et al. Older Americans and AIDS: transmission risks and primary prevention research needs. *Gerontologist* 1989;29:373–381.

44. Rosenzweig R, Fillit H. Probable heterosexual transmission of AIDS in an aged woman. *J Am Geriatr Soc* 1992;40:1261–1264.

45. Gutheil IA, Chichin ER. AIDS, older people, and social work. *Health Soc Work* 1991;16:227–244.

46. Catania JA, Stall R, Coates TJ, et al. Issues in AIDS primary prevention for late-middle-aged and elderly Americans. *Generations* 1989;13: 50–54.

47. Hinkle KL. A literature review: HIV seropositivitiy in the elderly. *J Gerontol Nurs* 1991;17: 12–17.

48. Weiler PG, Mungas D,Pomerantz S. AIDS as a cuase of dementia in the elderly. *J Am Geriatr Soc* 1988;36:139–141.

49. Stall R, Catania J. AIDS risk behaviors among late middle aged and elderly Americans: the National AIDS Behavioral Surveys. *Arch Intern Med* 1994; 154:57–63.

50. Wallace JI, Paauw DS, Spach DH. HIV infection in older patients: when to suspect the unexpected. *Geriatrics* 1993;48:61–70.

28

Infection Control Considerations in the Care of HIV-Infected Patients With Cardiac Disease

Judith Epstein, M.D., Quentin Eichbaum, Ph.D.,
and Edward O'Rourke, M.D.

The risk of transmission of human immunodeficiency virus (HIV) from infected patients to health-care workers can be minimized and virtually eliminated by careful attention to appropriate infection control principles and practices. Evaluation and treatment of cardiovascular disease in the patient infected with HIV may involve a number of specific procedures, including phlebotomy, catheterization, pericardiocentesis, and endomyocardial biopsy. Occupational exposure to HIV includes any contact of blood or other potentially infectious substances with the mucous membranes, eyes, or nonintact skin, or by parenteral injection. Exposure to the blood and other body fluids of the HIV-infected patient may occur in numerous settings, including nonsurgical (outpatient and inpatient wards, intensive care units) and surgical settings (catheterization and operating rooms).

As of December 1995 the Centers for Disease Control and Prevention (CDC) were aware of 49 health-care workers in the United States who had documented seroconversion to HIV following occupational exposures[1]; 22 of these people have developed acquired immunodeficiency syndrome (AIDS). Of those health-care workers who sero-converted, there were 18 laboratory workers (15 of whom were clinical laboratory workers), 19 nurses, 6 physicians, 2 surgical technicians, 1 dialysis technician, 1 respiratory therapist, 1 health aide, and 1 housekeeper/maintenance worker. Of these exposures, 42 were percutaneous (puncture or cut injury), 5 were mucocutaneous (mucous membrane and/or skin), 1 was both percutaneous and mucocutaneous, and 1 was an exposure by an unknown route. HIV-infected blood was implicated in 44 exposures, concentrated virus in a laboratory in 3 exposures, visibly bloody fluid in 1 exposure, and an unspecified fluid in 1 exposure. The CDC are also aware of 102 other cases of HIV infection or AIDS among health-care workers who report a history of occupational exposure but for whom there is no documentation of seroconversion post-exposure.[1]

Other bloodborne infections account for significant morbidity and mortality in health-care workers, with hepatitis B virus remaining the most prevalent occupational infection in the hospital setting. In a recent 10-year study, the incidence of hepatitis B virus infection in health-care workers was 55 times greater than that of HIV.[2] The CDC have

455

estimated that occupationally acquired hepatitis B virus infection developed in 5,100 health-care workers reporting frequent blood contacts in 1991 in the United States.[3] Of these cases, it was estimated that 225 would require hospitalization, 5 would die of fulminant hepatic failure, and 107 would eventually die of cirrhosis or hepatocelluar carcinoma. The cumulative hepatitis B virus-associated morbidity and mortality constitutes a more significant burden for health-care workers than HIV. Although the focus of this chapter is HIV, many of the points discussed below are applicable to all bloodborne pathogens, including hepatitis B virus.

Our goals in the this chapter are (1) to define risk factors for and prevention of HIV transmission in the hospital setting, (2) to define risk factors for and prevention of occupational exposure to coinfection with pathogens such as *Mycobacterium tuberculosis*, and (3) to discuss the postexposure management of HIV.

The HIV-Infected Patient

Historical: HIV and Nosocomial Infection Control

Health-care workers have always been at risk of acquiring serious infections from patients. Tuberculosis and hepatitis B have been recognized as occupational hazards in the health-care environment for many years. However, in recent times the most dramatic concern in occupational health in the health-care setting has been the furor raised over the risks of acquiring HIV or HIV-associated infection from patients. A parallel concern has been the possibility of transmitting HIV from health-care workers to patients or from one patient to another.

The CDC have published guidelines for preventing the spread of infection from patient to patient and from patient to health-care worker. The initial manual used the "category-specific" system of isolation precautions, which assigned to each organism a type of precaution isolation (e.g., contact isolation, respiratory isolation) depending on the known or presumed mechanism of spread.[4] Although fundamentally sound, this strategy was unable to reli-

ably protect health-care staff against exposure to patients with undiagnosed bloodborne pathogens, such as hepatitis B virus, hepatitis C virus, or HIV. Recognizing this problem, the CDC updated their recommendations in 1985 by adding Universal Precautions as a system to prevent exposure to blood and blood-contaminated body fluids from all patients, regardless of their infectious disease status.[5] The combination of universal and category-specific precautions was admittedly complex. In an attempt to simplify isolation precautions, another system was proposed. The Body Substance Isolation system, which simply required barrier protection (gloves and sometimes face or eye protection) when potentially contacting any patient body substance, was adopted in varying forms by a number of hospitals.[6] However, the Body Substance Isolation system, although simple, did not provide optimal protection against some airborne pathogens, such as *M. tuberculosis*, and thus remained a topic of controversy rather than supplanting the CDC system. In 1994, the CDC proposed a new system that attempted to incorporate the most important elements of Universal Precautions and Body Substance Isolation into one set of precautions called Standard Precautions. This guideline was published in its final form in 1996.[7] Besides the inclusion of the new Standard Precautions, the category-specific precautions were simplified from seven to three categories of Transmission-Based Precautions.[7] The new system, outlined in the following sections, should help to consolidate current recommendations. However, hospital infection control departments will still need to evaluate the options available and adopt a system appropriate to the hospital's circumstances and environment.

Despite the fact that there continues to be confusion regarding the use of precautions systems, it should be clear to the reader that all current and proposed systems emphasize the use of barriers (gloves, mask, eye protection) whenever there is likely to be exposure to any blood or bloody fluids from patients. As HIV has been spread to health-care workers only rarely in the past decade, there is good reason to believe that appropriate use of barriers to prevent contact with blood-contaminated patient material is adequate protection against HIV exposures not involving puncture injuries. Thus, by understanding and following Standard Precautions for all patients, health-care providers can safely provide care for HIV-infected patients without placing themselves at risk. In the following sections, we will discuss the most current recommendations for prevention of exposure to HIV and HIV-associated illnesses, as well as management strategies when suspected exposure to HIV has occurred.

Infection Control Guidelines

Standard Precautions

Standard Precautions are designed to decrease the transmission of bloodborne pathogens and to reduce the spread of pathogens from moist body surfaces. They should be used when the health-care provider may potentially contact any patient body fluid, including blood, mucous membranes, nonintact skin, and all body fluids, secretions, and excretions, regardless of whether or not blood is visible in them. Standard Precautions preserve all the elements of the older Universal Precautions categories and are applied to all patients regardless of their known or suspected infectious disease diagnosis. Thus, Standard Precautions are applied in the care of all patients, including those infected with HIV. These precautions are followed in both surgical and nonsurgical settings, although additional measures to minimize contact with HIV-infected blood may be applied in the intraoperative setting (see the next section).

The utilization of barriers against bloodborne pathogens, as outlined in Standard Precautions, is mandatory under Occupational Safety and Health Administration (OSHA) rules.[7] Other OSHA-mandated initiatives to limit the spread of bloodborne pathogens include immunization with the hepatitis B virus vaccine for any health-care worker who is likely to have contact with blood or blood-contaminated body fluids.[8,9]

Summary of Standard Precautions

See Reference 7 for a full listing of Standard Precautions.

Handwashing. The following handwashing procedure should be applied:

1. Wash hands after touching blood, body fluids, secretions, excretions, or contaminated items, whether or not gloves are worn. Wash hands immediately after gloves are removed between patient contacts, and when otherwise indicated, to avoid transfer of microorganisms to other patients or environments.

2. Use a plain (nonantimicrobial) soap for handwashing, except for specific circumstances (e.g., control of outbreaks), when antimicrobial soaps may be indicated as defined by the infection control program.

Gloves. Wear gloves (clean, nonsterile vinyl or other synthetic gloves are adequate) when touching blood, body fluids, secretions, excretions, or contaminated items; put on clean gloves just before touching mucous membranes or nonintact skin. Remove gloves promptly after use, before touching noncontaminated surfaces, and before going to another patient, and wash hands immediately to avoid transfer of microorganisms to other patients or environments. Although not formally a part of Standard Precautions, many authorities recommend double-gloving during surgery or other procedures when significant and unavoidable contact with an HIV-infected patient's blood is anticipated.[10]

Mask, eye protection, face shield. Wear a mask and eye protection or a face shield to protect mucous membranes of the eyes, nose, and mouth during procedures and patient-care activities that are likely to generate splashes or sprays of blood, body fluids, secretions, or excretions.

Gown. Wear a gown (a clean, nonsterile gown is adequate) to protect skin and prevent soiling of clothing during procedures and patient-care activities that are likely to generate splashes or sprays of blood, body fluids, secretions, or excretions or cause soiling of clothing. Select a gown that is appropriate for the activity and amount of fluid likely to be encountered. Remove a soiled gown as promptly after use as possible and wash hands to avoid transfer of microorganisms to other patients or environments.

Occupational health and bloodborne pathogens. Take care to prevent injuries when using needles, scalpels, and other sharp instruments or devices; when handling sharp instruments after procedures;

when cleaning used instruments; and when disposing of used needles. Never recap used needles or otherwise manipulate them using both hands, or use any other technique that involves directing the point of the needle toward any part of the body; rather, use either a one-handed "scoop" technique or a mechanical device designed for holding the needle sheath. Do not remove used needles from disposable syringes by hand, and do not bend, break, or otherwise manipulate used needles by hand. Place disposable syringes and needles, scalpel blades, and other sharp items in appropriate puncture-resistant containers located as close as practical to the area in which the items were used, and place reusable syringes and needles in a puncture-resistant container for transport to the reprocessing area.

Patient placement. For an HIV-infected patient without any identified coinfections, no special room placement is necessary. However, suspected or documented coinfections, such as *M. tuberculosis*, *Pneumocystis carinii*, and influenza, may mandate special room placement or roommate selection (see the section The HIV-Positive Patient with Known or Suspected Coinfection below). As with any other patient, place a patient who contaminates the environment or who does not (or cannot be expected to) assist in maintaining appropriate hygiene or environmental control in a private room.

Additional Considerations in the Operating Room and Cardiac Catheterization Laboratory

Although Universal Precautions are fundamental to intraoperative infection control, experience has proved that additional guidelines are needed to deal with the unique problems encountered in the surgical setting. Again, the precautions applied in the care of the HIV-infected patient are no different from those applied in the care of any other patient. It is of prime importance that all personnel work with their hospital infection control department in the development and application of specific intraoperative guidelines.

Considerations during surgical procedures should include the following[11]:

1. Layout of the procedure room (visibility, lighting, and spatial locations of team members)
2. Risk of exposure to individual team members
3. Nature of the individual procedure

A hazard-abatement model[11] involves controls in three separate areas: (1) engineering controls, (2) work-practice controls, and (3) personal protective equipment.

Engineering controls. Engineering controls include the use of equipment with inherent safety features, such as the following: blunt suture needles; scalpels with retractable blades; round-ended scalpels; blunt-tipped cautery instruments; tenaculums with blunt edges; redesigned instruments that allow manipulation from a safer distance; magnetic pads to contain metal instruments; improved shielding for lasers and other equipment capable of generating aerosols; devices for removing or containing used blades, suture needles, and other disposable sharps; and plastic substitutes for glass items.

"Needleless" systems for intravenous lines have been marketed and have been shown to be effective in reducing intravenous line-related injuries.[12-15] However, some data suggest that needleless devices may be associated with increased risk of bloodstream infection in certain situations.[16] Appropriate training of personnel in the use of any new safety device is obviously extremely important.[17,18]

Work practice controls. Work practice controls include standard protocols and techniques designed to improve safety:

1. "No-touch techniques" to minimize manipulation: use of instrument to load/unload needles and scalpels, use of instrument to grasp needle.
2. "No-touch" sharps transfers: use of transfer basin, creation of a "neutral zone" (where the instrument is put down and picked up, rather than passed hand to hand), announcement of sharps passage, periodic glove and garment checks.

Personal protective equipment. Protective equipment must be provided, depending on the degree and type of exposures anticipated during a specific procedure.[11,19-22] Factors that have been identified to increase the risk of exposure include major surgical procedures, procedures of greater than 3 hours duration, and blood loss of greater than 300 ml.[21,23,24] In high-risk cases, optimal barrier protection to be considered includes reinforced or impermeable gowns, plastic aprons, double or reinforced sleeves, knee-high foot protection, and face shields or other circumferential eye protection.[11] The use of double gloves (triple gloves in one study[25]) has been associated with a decrease in skin exposures of surgical personnel.[10,20,26–30] For very long procedures, attention should be directed toward the possibility of glove perforations. Perforations are more likely to occur later in a procedure,[28,31,32] and therefore periodic glove examinations or outer-glove changes may prevent contact with patients' blood and tissues.[10,11] Gloves should also be worn by circulating nurses and other persons outside the field who may have contact with contaminated surfaces. Face splashes during surgical procedures are substantially reduced by eyeglasses and are prevented by face shields.[10]

The HIV-Positive Patient With Known or Suspected Coinfection

For the hospitalized patient infected with HIV alone, no additional precautions beyond Standard Precautions are necessary. However, patients with HIV infection are at significant risk for coinfection with other pathogens, and therefore careful consideration of possible coinfection with nosocomially transmissable pathogens must be made on an individual basis. If the patient has secondary infection(s), isolation precautions may be appropriate. Guidelines issued by the CDC form the basis for these recommendations.[7] Transmission-Based Precautions are divided into three areas: Airborne Precautions, Droplet Precautions, and Contact Precautions.

Transmission-based precautions

Isolation precautions, in addition to Standard Precautions, will apply to the patient with HIV infection who has documented or suspected coinfection with one or more of the pathogens included in the categories described below.[7] HIV infection by itself is not a criterion for use of these isolation precautions and would require Standard Precautions alone. See Table 28-1.

Airborne Precautions

Diseases requiring airborne precautions include measles, varicella (including disseminated zoster in the HIV-infected patient), and tuberculosis. In the HIV-infected patient with suspected or confirmed infection with any of these organisms, Airborne Precautions should be applied in addition to Standard Precautions. Consideration of *M. tuberculosis* coinfection in the HIV-infected patient should be a high priority. Airborne Precautions are designed to eliminate transmission of diseases spread by airborne droplet nuclei. These are small-particle residue of evaporated droplets containing viable microorganisms that remain suspended in the air and can be widely dispersed by air currents within a room or over a long distance.

Patient placement.   Place the patient in a private room that has (1) monitored negative air pressure in relation to the surrounding areas, (2) a minimum of six air changes per hour, and (3) appropriate discharge of air outdoors or monitored high-efficiency filtration of room air before the air is circulated to other areas of the hospital. Keep the room door closed and the patient in the room. If a private room is not available, place the patient in a room with another patient who has active infection with the same microorganisms unless otherwise recommended, but with no other infection (cohorting). If a private room is not available and cohorting is not possible, consultation with infection control professionals is necessary before patient placement.

Respiratory protection.   Wear an approved, fitted respirator meeting at least N95 National Institute for Occupational Safety and Health (NIOSH) standard when entering the room of a patient with known or suspected infectious tuberculosis. The hospital infection control department should be notified and will assist in educating staff and providing information on appropriate masking. Individual health-care workers need to be fit-tested to ensure proper function of the mask before entering a pa-

Table 28-1. Coinfection in HIV-Infected Patients: Type and Duration Precautions for Selected Infections

Infection*	Precautions* Type	Duration
Candidiasis, all forms including mucocutaneous	S	
Clostridium difficile	C	DI
Cryptococcosis	S	
Cryptosporidiosis	S[a]	
Hepatitis B virus[b]	S	
Hepatitis C virus	S	
Herpes simplex virus	C	DI
Mucocutaneous, disseminated or primary, severe	S	DI
Mucocutaneous, recurrent (skin, oral, genital)		
Histoplasmosis	S	
Mycobacterium-avium complex (MAC)	S	
Mycobacterium tuberculosis[c]	A	e,f
Extrapulmonary, meningitis[d]		
Pulmonary, confirmed or suspected		
Parainfluenza virus	C	DI
Parvovirus B19	D	g
Pneumocystis carinii	S[h]	
Respiratory syncytial virus	C	DI
Toxoplasmosis	S	
Varicella-zoster virus, localized or disseminated	A, C	i

Adapted from Ref. 7.

*See footnotes *a–i* as applicable.

A, airborne; C, contact; D, droplet; S, standard; DI, duration of illness. When A, C, and D are specified, also use S (see text for full description of transmission-based precautions A, B, C, D)

[a]Use contact precautions for diapered or incontinent children <6 years of age for duration of illness.

[b]Suggested vaccination for employees who may have contact with blood or blood-contaminated body fluids.

[c]Annual skin testing for staff. See Ref. 33.

[d]Patient should be examined for evidence of current (active) pulmonary tuberculosis. If evidence exists, Airborne Precautions are necessary.

[e]Discontinue precautions only when TB patient is on effective therapy, is improving clinically, and has three consecutive negative sputum smears collected on different days, or TB is ruled out. Also see Ref. 33.

[f]Mask required: use approved, fitted respirator meeting at least N95 NIOSH standard.

Adapted from reference 7.

[g]Maintain precautions for duration of hospitalizaation when chronic infection occurs. For patients with transient aplastic crisis or red cell crisis, maintain precautions for 7 days.

Adapted from reference 7.

[hh]Avoid placement in same room with an immunocompromised patient.

Adapted from reference 7.

[h]Maintain precautions until all lesions are crusted. Susceptible persons should stay out of room until all lesions are crusted.

tient's room. If possible, a health-care worker should not enter the room of a patient known or suspected to have measles or varicella if the worker is susceptible to these infections.

Additional precautions for preventing transmission of tuberculosis. Consult Reference 33 for additional prevention strategies.

Droplet Precautions

Pertussis, *Mycoplasma pneumoniae*, *Parvovirus* B19, and influenza are among the diseases for which Droplet Precautions are required. These diseases are transmitted by droplets generated by the patient during sneezing, or talking, or by the performance of procedures such as bronchoscopy. In addition to Standard Precautions, use Droplet Precautions for the HIV-infected patient known or suspected to be infected with these microorganisms.

See Reference 7 for a full listing of organisms requiring Droplet Precautions.

Patient placement. Place the patient in a private room. If a private room is not available, place the patient in a room with another patient(s) who has active infection with the same microorganism, but with no other infection (cohorting). If a private room is not available and cohorting is not possible, maintain spatial separation of at least 3 ft between the infected patient and other patients and visitors.

Mask. In addition to standard precautions, wear a mask when working within 3 ft of the patient.

Contact Precautions

Although some important nosocomial infections are spread by air, most viral, bacterial, and fungal organisms causing nosocomial infections are spread by direct or indirect contact. These microorganisms may be transmitted by skin-to-skin contact that occurs during patient care activities that require touching the patient (direct contact) or by touching environmental surfaces or patient care items that have been contaminated by the patient (indirect contact). Contact Precautions are designed to disrupt this transmission and should be used in addition to Standard Precautions for these microorganisms. Among organisms for which Contact Precautions are required are herpes simplex virus, *Cryptosporidium* (diapered or incontinent patient), respiratory syncytial virus, and varicella-zoster virus. (In HIV-infected patients with varicella-zoster virus, dissemination should be considered a significant risk, and therefore both Airborne and Contact Precautions are required.)

Patient placement. Place the patient in a private room. If a private room is not available, place the patient in a room with a patient(s) who has active infection with the same microorganisms, but with no other infection (cohorting). If a private room is not available and cohorting is not achievable, consider the epidemiology of the microorganism and the patient population when determining pa-

tient placement; consultation with infection control professionals is advised before patient placement.

Gloves and handwashing. In addition to wearing gloves as outlined under Standard Precautions, put on gloves (clean, nonsterile gloves are adequate) upon entering the room if any contact with the patient or possibly contaminated inanimate environment is anticipated. During the course of providing care for a patient, change gloves after having contact with infective material that may contain high concentrations of microorganisms (fecal material and wound drainage). Remove gloves before leaving the patient's room and wash hands immediately with an antimicrobial agent. After glove removal and handwashing, ensure that hands do not touch potentially contaminated environmental surfaces or items in the patient's room to avoid transfer of microorganisms to other patients or environments.

Gown. In addition to wearing a gown as outlined under Standard Precautions, wear a gown (a clean, nonsterile gown is adequate) when entering the room if you anticipate that your clothing will have contact with the patient, environmental surfaces, or items in the patient's room, or if the patient is incontinent or has diarrhea, an ileostomy, a colostomy, or wound drainage not contained by a dressing. Remove the gown before leaving the patient's environment. After removing the gown, ensure that clothing does not contact potentially contaminated environmental surfaces to avoid transfer of microorganisms to other patients or environments.

For a full listing of all pathogens classified according to recommended Transmission-Based Precautions, see Reference 7.

Management of Occupational Exposure to Blood or Blood-Containing Fluids

The following sections will discuss the risk of HIV transmission, postexposure testing, and postexposure prophylaxis. Because of the complexity of addressing issues relating to potential exposure to coinfecting pathogens such as *M. tuberculosis* or hepatitis B virus, the handling of exposures to these other infectious agents will not be discussed here. For these recommendations, consult the hospital infection control department and refer to standard texts.[34,35]

Risk of Transmission of HIV With Occupational Exposure

Percutaneous injury. Analysis of pooled data from 25 prospective studies reveals that the risk associated with percutaneous injury with a blood-contaminated instrument or needle from a known HIV positive-patient is 0.31% (21 infections after 6,498 exposures; 95% confidence interval: 0.18–0.46%).[36] Put another way, about 1 in 300 percutaneous injuries with HIV-contaminated instruments will result in infection with HIV. A recent retrospective case-control study using surveillance data from the United States, France, and United Kingdom analyzed factors that affect this risk.[37] Among the health-care workers in this study, factors associated with HIV transmission included (1) a deep injury, (2) a device visibly contaminated with the patient's blood, (3) procedures involving a needle placed directly in a vein or artery, and (4) terminal illness in the patient. Studies conducted with simulated needle-sticks indicate that the amount of blood transferred during needle-sticks is affected by the type and gauge of needle used, the depth of the needle-stick penetration, and whether or not gloves are used.[38]

Mucocutaneous exposure. The risk of transmission with mucocutaneous exposure has been estimated as 0.053% after pooling data from 15 studies (1 infection per 2,071 mucosal exposures; 95% confidence interval: 0–0.16%).[39] This suggests that the risk of mucocutaneous exposures is lower than that from percutaneous inoculations.[40]

Cutaneous exposure. There has not yet been documented transmission of HIV with cutaneous exposure. In the largest prospective study (2,712 cutaneous exposures of intact skin to HIV), there were no documented cases of transmission.[41]

Body fluids. A number of body fluids have not yet been implicated in occupational transmission but are considered potential sources because they are likely to contain virus or have been implicated in other modes of transmission. These body fluids that are considered *potential sources* include semen, vaginal fluid, cerebrospinal fluid, breast milk, exudates, serosal fluids, amniotic fluid, and saliva (during dental procedures). Body fluids considered unlikely to be a source of transmission of HIV are saliva, urine, and feces unless these fluids are visibly bloody.[40]

Postexposure Testing and Counseling

Each institution should develop a systematic approach to occupational exposure that is consistent with CDC recommendations[42,43] and local regulations. When an occupational exposure has occurred, it should be reported immediately to the hospital employee occupational health service. After informed consent has been obtained, blood should be obtained from the source patient for hepatitis B, hepatitis C, and HIV studies. (Regulations concerning obtaining informed consent may vary from state to state.) Similarly, serologic studies should be done on the exposed health-care worker, and if baseline testing is deferred, a blood sample should be stored in case testing is needed at a later date. Detailed discussions of testing, treatment, and follow-up for hepatitis B and C may be found in detail elsewhere[8,40,44]

The CDC recommends periodic testing for HIV antibody for at least 6 months after occupational exposure (e.g., 6 weeks, 3 months, and 6 months after exposure).[43] During the 6-month period postexposure, the health-care worker should follow the recommendations of the Public Health Service for prevention of human immunodeficiency virus transmission. These recommendations include the following: refrain from blood, tissue, or organ donation; practice abstinence or use measures to prevent the spread of HIV via sexual contact; and in countries such as the United States where safe alternatives to breastfeeding are available, refrain from breastfeeding.[43] Appropriate psychological counseling should be made available at the time of exposure and during follow-up.

Postexposure Chemoprophylaxis

Background

There has been much debate about the use of zidovudine as postexposure prophylaxis. The only prospective controlled clinical trial of the efficacy of zidovudine as postexposure prophylaxis was discontinued because of poor enrollment.[45] The CDC is aware of at least eight instances of failure of zidovudine postexposure prophylaxis after percutaneous injuries to health-care workers.[46] However, there have been encouraging results from a 6-year retrospective case-control study of HIV seroconversion in health-care workers after percutaneous exposure to HIV-infected blood.[37] In this study, zidovudine postexposure prophylaxis was associated with a decrease of approximately 79% in the risk for seroconversion after percutaneous exposure to HIV-infected blood.[37]

Postexposure zidovudine prophylaxis has potentially serious side effects. Zidovudine chemoprophylaxis has been tolerated relatively well in three large studies that evaluated postexposure zidovudine toxicity, although approximately one-third of health-care workers treated with zidovudine after exposure to the virus have had to discontinue therapy due to such subjective toxicities such as nausea, fatigue, insomnia, and headache.[46–48] Although data are limited, there do not appear to be serious adverse side effects for the mother or the infant associated with the use of zidovudine in the second or third trimesters of pregnancy;[49,50] data are even more limited regarding the use of zidovudine in the first trimester.

Recent attention has focused on the use of combination chemotherapy in postexposure prophylaxis. Most of the data about combination chemotherapy comes from studies done with HIV-infected patients. In this population, therapy with zidovudine and lamuvidine resulted in greater antiretroviral activity than treatment with zidovudine alone; with addition of a protease inhibitor, such as idinivir, there was an even greater increase in antiretroviral activity.[51] Gastrointestinal symptoms may be caused by either lamuvidine or idinivir. In rare cases, lamuvidine may cause pancreatitis, while prolonged use of idinivir may lead to mild hyper-bilirubinemia and kidney stones.[51] There are few data on the use of these antiretrovirals during pregnancy.

Recommendations

Based on information that suggests that postexposure zidovudine prophylaxis reduces the risk for HIV seroconversion after occupational exposure to HIV-infected blood,[37] a Public Health Service interagency group has recently published updated provisional Public Health Service recommendations for management of occupational exposure to HIV.[52] It is advised that potential toxicity be carefully considered when prescribing postexposure prophylaxis and that these recommendations be implemented in consultation with persons who have expertise in antiretroviral therapy and HIV transmission. The most recent recommendations are summarized in the remainder of this section. (See Ref. 52 for full text.)

The current Public Health Service recommendation is that chemoprophylaxis should be recommended to health-care workers after occupational exposures associated with the highest risk for HIV transmission. As shown in Table 28-2, the level of risk must be assessed to determine whether postexposure prophylaxis is indicated for other types of exposures. Exposed workers should be informed as follows:

1. Knowledge about the efficacy and toxicity of postexposure prophylaxis is limited.

2. For agents other than zidovudine, data are limited regarding toxicity in persons without HIV infection or who are pregnant.

3. Any or all drugs for postexposure prophyaxis may be declined by the exposed worker.

Because some HIV strains may be resistant to zidovudine, it is strongly recommended that postexposure prophylaxis be coordinated with a specialist in the management of occupational exposures. For HIV strains resistant to both zidovudine and lamuvidine or resistant to a protease inhibitor, or if these drugs are contraindicated or poorly tolerated, the optimal postexposure prophylaxis regimen is uncertain; again, expert consultation is advised.

Table 28-2. Provisional Public Health Service Recommendations for Chemoprophylaxis After Occupational Exposure to HIV, by Type of Exposure and Source Material—1996

Type of Exposure	Source Material*	Antiretroviral Prophylaxis†	Antiretroviral Regimen‡
Percutaneous	Blood§		ZDV + 3TC + IDV
	Highest risk	Recommend	ZDV + 3TC, ± IDV¶
	Increased risk	Recommend	ZDV + 3TC
	No increased risk	Offer	
	Fluid containing visible blood,		ZDV + 3TC
	other potentially infectious	Offer	ZDV + 3TC
	fluid,‖ or tissue	Not offer	
	Other body fluid (e.g., urine)		
Mucous membrane	Blood	Offer	ZDV + 3TC, ± IDV¶
	Fluid containing visible blood,		
	other potentially infectious		ZDV, ± 3TC
	fluid,‖ or tissue	Offer	
	Other body fluid (e.g., urine)	Not offer	
Skin, increased risk#	Blood	Offer	ZDV + 3TC, ± IDV¶
	Fluid containing visible blood,		
	other potentially infectious		ZDV, ± 3TC
	fluid,‖ or tissue	Offer	
	Other body fluid (e.g., urine)	Not offer	

From Ref. 52, with permission.

*Any exposure to concentrated HIV (e.g., in a research laboratory or production facility) is treated as percutaneous exposure to blood with highest risk.

†**Recommend:** Postexposure prophylaxis (PEP) should be recommended to the exposed worker with counseling (see reference 52). **Offer:** PEP should be offered to the exposed worker with counseling (see Ref. 52). **Not offer:** PEP should not be offered because these are not occupational exposures to HIV.

‡Regimens: zidovudine(ZDV), 200 mg three times a day; lamuvidine (3TC), 150 mg two times a day; idinivir (IDV), 800 mg three times a day (if IDV is not available, saquinavir may be used, 600 mg three times a day). Prophylaxis is given for 4 weeks. For full prescribing information, see package inserts.

§**Highest risk:** *Both* larger blood volume (e.g., deep injury with large diameter hollow needle previously in source patient's vein or artery, especially involving an injection of source-patient's blood) *and* blood containing a high titer of HIV (e.g., source with acute retroviral illness or end-stage AIDS; viral load measurement may be considered, but its use in relation to PEP has not yet been evaluated). **Increased risk:** *Either* exposure to larger blood volume *or* blood with a high titer of HIV. **No increased risk:** *Neither* exposure to larger blood volume *nor* blood with a high titer of HIV (e.g., solid suture needle injury from source patient with asymptomatic HIV infection).

¶Possible toxicity of additional drug may not be warranted (see Ref. 52).

‖Includes semen, vaginal secretions, cerebrospinal, synovial, pleural, peritoneal, pericardial, and amniotic fluids.

#For skin, risk is increased for exposures involving a high titer of HIV, prolonged contact, an extensive area, or an area in which skin integrity is visibly compromised. For skin exposures without increased risk, the risk for drug toxicity outweighs the benefit of PEP.

Postexposure prophylaxis should be initiated promptly, preferably 1–2 hours after exposure. Although animal studies suggest that postexposure prophylaxis probably is not effective when started later than 24–36 hours postexposure,[40,53] the interval after which there is no benefit from postexposure prophylaxis is undefined.

If the source patient's HIV status is unknown, initiating postexposure prophylaxis should be decided on a case-by-case basis, based on the exposure risk and the likelihood of HIV infection in known or possible source patients.

If postexposure prophylaxis is used, drug-toxicity monitoring should include a complete blood count and renal and hepatic chemical function tests at baseline and 2 weeks after starting postexposure prophylaxis. If subjective or objective toxicity is noted, dose reduction or drug substitution should be considered with expert consultation and further diagnostic studies may be indicated.

The following sources may provide additional current information regarding management of occupational exposure:

- The CDC National AIDS Hotline: 1-800-342-AIDS (telephone)

- HIV/AIDS Treatment Information Service: 1-800-448-0440 (telephone)

- CDC National AIDS Clearinghouse
  P.O. Box 6003
  Rockville, MD 20849-6003
  1-800-458-5231 (telephone)
  301-738-6616 (fax)

- Internet CDC web site: http://www.cdc.gov

References

1. Centers for Disease Control and Prevention. HIV/AIDS Surveillance Report 1995;7(no 2):21.

2. Gerberding JL. Incidence and prevalence of human immunodeficiency virus, hepatitis B virus, hepatitis C virus, and cytomegalovirus among health care personnel at risk for blood exposure: final report on a longitudinal study. *J Infect Dis* 1994;170:1410–1417.

3. Short LJ, Bell DM. Risk of occupational infection with blood-borne pathogens in operating room and delivery room settings. *Am J Infect Control* 1993;21:343–350.

4. Centers for Disease Control and Prevention. *Isolation Techniques for Use in Hospitals,* 2nd Ed. Washington, DC: U.S. Government Printing Office, 1975. HHS Publ. No. (CDC) 80–8314.

5. Centers for Disease Control and Prevention. Recommendations for preventing transmission of infection with human T-lymphotropic virus type III/lymphadenopathy-associated virus in the workplace. *MMWR* 1985;34:681–686,691–695.

6. Lynch P, Jackson MM, Cummings MJ, et al. Rethinking the role of isolation practices in the prevention of nosocomial infections. *Ann Intern Med* 1987;107:243–246.

7. Garner JS, and the Hospital Infection Control Practices Advisory Committee. Guideline for isolation precautions in hospitals. *Infect Control Hosp Epidemiol* 1996;17:53–80, and *Am J Infect Control* 1996; 24:24–52.

8. Final Standard for Occupational Exposure to Bloodborne Pathogens. 29 CFR 1910. 1991:1030.

9. Centers for Disease Control and Prevention. Protection against viral hepatitis: recommendations of the Immunization Practices Advisory Committee (ACIP). *MMWR* 1990;39(RR2):1–25.

10. Tokars JI, Culver DH, Mendelson MH, et al. Skin and mucous membrane contacts with blood during surgical procedures: risk and prevention. *Infect Control Hosp Epidemiol* 1995;16:703–712.

11. Gerberding JL. Procedure-specific infection control for preventing intraoperative blood exposures. *Am J Infect Control* 1993;21:364–367.

12. Yassi A, McGill ML, Khokhar JB. Efficacy and cost-effectiveness of a needleless intravenous access system. *Am J Infect Control* 1995;23:57–64.

13. Gartner K. Impact of a needleless intravenous system in a university hospital. *Am J Infect Control* 1993;20:75–79.

14. Ippolito G, De Carli G, Puro V, et al. Device-specific risk of needlestick injury in Italian health care workers. *JAMA* 1994;272:607–610.

15. Skolnick R, LaRocca J, Barba D, et al. Evaluation and implementation of a needleless intravenous system: making needlesticks a needless problem. *Am J Infect Control* 1993;21:39–41.

16. Danzig LE, Short LJ, Collins K, et al. Bloodstream infections associated with a needleless intravenous infusion system in patients receiving home infusion therapy. *JAMA* 1995;273:1862–1864.

17. Robert LM, Bell DM. HIV transmission in the health-care setting. *Infect Dis Clin North Am* 1994; 8:319–329.

18. Simpkins SM, Haiduven DJ, Stevens DA. Safety product evaluation: six years of experience. *Am J Infect Control* 1995;23:317–323.

19. Schiff SJ. A surgeon's risk of AIDS. *J Neurosurg* 1990;73:651–660.

20. Gerberding JL, Schecter WP. Surgery and AIDS: reducing the risk. *JAMA* 1991;265:1572–1573.

21. Panlilio AL, Foy DR, Edwards JR, et al. Blood contacts during surgical procedures. *JAMA* 1991; 265:1533–1537.

22. Schecter WP. HIV transmission to surgeons: assessment of risk, infection control precautions, and standards of conduct. In: Becker CE (ed). *Occupational HIV Infection: Risks and Risk Reduction.* Philadelphia: Hanley & Belfus, 1989:65–69.

23. Tokars JI, Bell DM, Culver DH, et al. Percutaneous injuries during surgical procedures. *JAMA* 1992; 267:2899–2904.

24. Quebbeman EJ, Telford GL, Hubbard S, et al. Risk of blood contamination and injury to operating room personnel. *Ann Surg* 1991;214:614–20.

25. Hester RA, Nelson CL, Harrison S. Control of contamination of the operative team in total joint arthroplasty. *J Arthroplasty* 1992;7:267–269.

26. Hester RA, Nelson CL. Methods to reduce intraoperative transmission of blood-borne disease. *J Bone Joint Surg [Am]* 1991;73:1108–1111.

27. Upton LG, Barber HD. Double-gloving and the incidence of perforations during specific oral and maxillofacial surgical precedures. *J Oral Maxillofac Surg* 1993;51:261–263.

28. Quebbemann EJ, Telford GL, Wadsworth K, et al. Double gloving: protecting surgeons from blood contamination in the operating room. *Arch Surg* 1992;127:213–216.

29. Matta H, Thompson AM, Rainey JB. Does wearing two pairs of gloves protect operating theatre staff from skin contamination? *BMJ* 1988;297:597–598.

30. Gani JS, Anseline PF, Bisset RL. Efficacy of double versus single gloving in protecting the operating team. *Aust N Z J Surg* 1990;60:171–175.

31. Cole RP, Gault DT. Glove perforations during plastic surgery. *Br J Plast Surg* 1989;42:481–483.

32. Rose DA, Ramiro NZ, Perlman JL, et al. Two gloves or not two gloves?: intraoperative glove utilization at San Francisco General Hospital. *Infect Control Hosp Epidemiol* 1994;15(Suppl 4):37.

33. Centers for Disease Control and Prevention. Guidelines for preventing the transmission of *Mycobacterium tuberculosis* in health-care facilities, 1994. *MMWR* 43(RR-13):1–132 and *Fed Regist* 1994: 59:54242–54303.

34. Mayhall CG. *Hospital Epidemiology and Infection Control.* Baltimore: Williams & Wilkins, 1996.

35. Wenzel RP. *Prevention and Control of Nosocomial Infections.* Baltimore: Williams & Wilkins, 1993.

36. Gerberding JL. Prophylaxis for Occupational Exposure to HIV. *Ann Intern Med* 1996;125:497–501.

37. Centers for Disease Control and Prevention. Case-control study of HIV seroconversion in health-care workers after percutaneous exposure to HIV-infected blood- France, United Kingdom, and United States, January 1988–August 1994. *MMWR* 1995; 44:929–933.

38. Mast ST, Woolwine JD, Gerberding JS. Efficacy of gloves in reducing blood volumes transferred during simulated needlestick injury. *J Infect Dis* 1993;168:1589–1592.

39. Henderson DK. HIV-1 in the health care setting. In: Mandel GL, Bennett JE, Dolan R (eds). *Principles*

and Practice of Infectious Diseases,* 4th Ed. New York: Churchill Livingstone, 1995:2632–2656.

40. Gerberding JL. Drug Therapy: Management of Occupational Exposures to Blood-Borne Viruses. *N Engl J Med* 1995:332:444–451.

41. Henderson DK, Fahey BJ, Willy M, et al. Risk for occupational transmission of human immunodeficiency virus type 1 (HIV-1) associated with clinical exposures: a prospective evaluation. *Ann Intern Med* 1990;113:740–746.

42. Centers for Disease Control and Prevention. Recommendations for prevention of HIV in health-care settings. *MMWR* 1987;36(Suppl 2S):1S–18S.

43. Centers for Disease Control and Prevention. Public Health Service statement on management of occupational exposure to HIV including considerations regarding zidovudine postexposure use. *MMWR* 1990;39(RR1):1–14.

44. Alter MJ. Occupational exposure to hepatitis C virus: a dilemma. *Infect Control Hosp Epidemiol* 1994;15:742–744.

45. LaFon SW, Mooney BD, McMullen JP, et al. A double-blind, placebo-controlled study of the safety and efficacy of Retrovir (zidovudine, ZDV) as a chemoprophylactic agent in health care workers. *Proc Intersci Conf Antimicrob Agents Chemother,* 1990;30:167.

46. Tokars JI, Marcus R, Culver DH, et al. Surveillance of HIV infection and zidovudine use among health care workers after occupational exposure to HIV-infected blood; the CDC Cooperative Needlestick Surveillance Group. *Ann Intern Med* 1993;118: 913–919.

47. Fahrner R, Beekman SE, Koziol DE, et al. Safety of zidovudine (AZT) administered as post-exposure chemoprophylaxis to healthcare workers (HCW) sustaining occupational exposures (OE) to HIV [Abstract]. *Proc Intersci Conf Antimicrob Agents Chemother* 1994;34:133.

48. Puro V, Ippolito G, Guzzanti E, et al. Zidovudine prophylaxis after accidental exposure to HIV: the Italian experience: the Italian Study Group on Occupational Risk of HIV Infection. *AIDS* 1992; 6:963–969.

49. Connor EM, Sperling DE, Coombs R, et al. Reduction of maternal-infant transmission of human immunodeficiency virus type 1 with zidovudine treatment. *N Engl J Med* 1994;331:1173–1180.

50. Connor E, Sperling R, Shapiro D, et al. Long term side effect of zidovudine exposure among unin-

fected infants born to HIV-infected mothers in pediatric AIDS Clinical Trial Group protocol 076. [Abstracts]. *Proc Intersci Conf Antimicrob Agents Chemother* 1995;35:205.

51. Anonymous. New drugs for HIV infection. *Med Lett Drug Ther*. 1996;38:35–37.

52. Center for Drug Evaluation and Research. Update: provisional public health service recommendations

for chemoprophylaxis after occupational exposure to HIV. *MMWR* 1996;45:468–472.

53. Niu MT, Stein DS, Schnittmann SM. Primary human immunodeficiency virus type 1 infection: review of pathogenesis and early treatment interventions in humans and animal retrovirus infections. *J Infect Dis* 1993;168:1490–501.

Part 5
Conclusion

29

The Global Burden
of Acquired Pediatric
Cardiovascular Disease

Samuel Kaplan, M.D.

There is a marked geographic variation in the incidence of acquired heart disease in children. Until the 1980s, acute rheumatic fever and chronic rheumatic heart disease, as well as Kawasaki disease, were considered to be the common causes of acquired pediatric cardiovascular diseases. Other, less frequent, conditions, some of which can be devastating, include infective endocarditis, dilated and hypertrophic cardiomyopathy, pericardial disease, and cardiovascular manifestations of genetic, metabolic, and nutritional diseases.

Longitudinal follow-up of children infected with the human immunodeficiency virus (HIV) reveals that the cardiovascular system is frequently involved.[1-3] This involvement may be occult because the clinical picture is frequently dominated by intercurrent infections, interstitial lung disease, hepatosplenomegaly, anemia, malnutrition, and wasting. As HIV-infected children are living longer,[4] cardiovascular involvement is being recognized more frequently, with left ventricular dysfunction emerging as the most common cardiac abnormality.[1] Unrecognized left ventricular dysfunction can progress to dilated cardiomyopathy, congestive cardiac failure, and death. (See Chapter 9.) Therefore cardiovascular complications of HIV disease have become major contributing factors in pediatric heart disease.

The purpose of this chapter is to describe the worldwide incidence of these diseases and their socioeconomic impact, with particular reference to HIV disease, rheumatic fever and rheumatic heart disease, and Kawasaki disease.

Rheumatic Fever and Rheumatic Heart Disease

Rheumatic fever and rheumatic heart disease remain important problems in many countries, where these diseases have been the major factors responsible for cardiovascular disease in children. The incidence of rheumatic fever and residual rheumatic heart disease has been attributed to poor economic and social conditions and inadequate delivery of primary health care. Some believe that the incidence of rheumatic fever will be significantly decreased with the improvement of social and economic conditions. There is disagreement with the notion that in industrialized countries the incidence has decreased because of the use of penicillin and other antibiotics.[5]

Trends in Industrialized Countries

In North America and Western Europe, the incidence of rheumatic heart disease began to decrease before the introduction of antibiotics.[6] Thirty to forty years ago, the incidence of rheumatic fever in many parts of the United States ranged from 20 to 50 cases per 100,000 children per year or higher. By the late 1970s, the disease was rare, with an incidence of less than 1/100,000.[7-9] The precise reasons for the decline remain unexplained.[10] The spectacular decline of acute rheumatic fever in the United States and other Western countries is puzzling because of the continued high prevalence of streptococcal (group A) pharyngitis in school children.[11]

In the mid-1980s, localized outbreaks of acute rheumatic fever began to appear in the United States.[12-20] The epidemiology and clinical features of these outbreaks were different from those of previous outbreaks, in that the affected children were from middle-class families living in suburbia or in rural areas with ready access to medical care. The clinical features were also intriguing, in that the preceding pharyngitis was mild and the incidence of documented carditis exceeded 90% in one series.[12] These recent outbreaks have occurred with the appearance of previously uncommon serotypes of group A streptococci,[21,22] namely, mucoid strains, from throat cultures in patients with pharyngitis. It is reasonable to attribute the resurgence of rheumatic fever to the appearance of more virulent group A strains.[6] These scattered outbreaks of acute rheumatic fever in the mid- and late 1980s were not associated with an increased national incidence.[23] The hospital diagnosis of acute rheumatic fever continued to decline gradually from 1984 through 1990.[23]

Trends in Developing Countries

At present, rheumatic fever and rheumatic heart disease cause 25% to 40% of all cardiovascular disease in developing countries,[24] including the tropics, where five or more decades ago rheumatic fever and heart disease were considered rare.[25] In developing countries, with the expansion of urbanization and industrialization, the concomitant increase in the incidence of rheumatic fever is comparable to that reported in the United States 70 to 80 years ago.[26] In 1984 the World Health Organization reported that in Third World countries rheumatic heart disease was the most common cause of cardiac death.[27] The prevalence of rheumatic heart disease in schoolchildren is about 0.1 case per 1,000 children in developed countries and 1–22 cases per 1,000 children in developing countries. These figures suggest that there may be 1.5 million children with rheumatic heart disease in industrialized countries and 30 million in developing countries.[28] The regional prevalence of rheumatic fever and rheumatic heart disease from 1986 to 1990 was 2.2 cases per 1,000 children (range: 0.7–4.7 cases).[29] The prevalence was 4.7 cases per 1,000 children (range: 3.4–12.6 cases) in Africa, 1.5/1,000 (range: 0.1–7.9) in the Americas, 4.4/1,000 (range: 0.9–10.2) in the Eastern Mediterranean, 0.12/1,000 (range: 0.1–1.3) in Southeast Asia, and 0.7/1,000 (range: 0.6–1.4) in the Western Pacific.[29] The World Health Organization Cardiovascular Program for Rheumatic Heart Disease surveyed the incidence of rheumatic heart disease in 16 developing countries from 1986 to 1990.[29] According to this report, the prevalence in screened schoolchildren in Egypt was 5.1 cases per 1,000 children, and the estimated global mean prevalence was 2.2/1,000.

While rheumatic fever was becoming rare in the United States, the incidence was increasing significantly in American and French Polynesia in populations not underfed or poverty-stricken.[26] In New Zealand the incidence of rheumatic fever and chronic rheumatic heart disease is higher in Maoris than in the white population.[30,31] Echocardiographic examination of schoolchildren in Ethiopia showed that chronic rheumatic heart disease was twice as frequent as congenital heart disease.[32] In Egypt acute rheumatic fever has been described as "malignant," with a high incidence of cardiac complications in the initial attack and the early and frequent development of mitral stenosis.[33-35]

There are many socioeconomic factors that have been considered to explain the high incidence of rheumatic fever in developing countries. These include uncontrolled urbanization, with the development of slums, a rapid increase in the number of city-dwelling children, and crowding in schools and public transportation. These factors result in the exposure of new city dwellers to unfamiliar streptococcal serotypes in areas with inadequate facilities for treatment of acute streptococcal pharyngitis. An outbreak of rheumatic fever in New Zealand in 1983 associated with type M-5 streptococcal disease supports the idea that the persistence of rheumatic fever can be related to rheumatogenic strains in affected populations.[36,37] These strains, which spread in Europe and North America during the Industrial Revolution, may have been introduced into developing countries during World War II. This scenario may have occurred in the South African black population in the cities of Johannesburg, Durban, and Cape Town.[38] In 1982, the annual reported incidence of acute rheumatic fever in Soweto (Johannesburg) was greater than 200 cases per 100,000 children, which greatly exceeds the 61 cases per 100,000 children calculated for New York City school children between 1963 and 1965.[26]

Kawasaki Disease

Kawasaki disease, an acute febrile illness of unknown etiology, is characterized by mucosal inflammation, skin rash, and cervical lymphadenopathy. The major cardiovascular complication is vasculitis, especially involving the coronary arteries, with resultant coronary arterial dilatation and aneurysms.

Kawasaki Disease in Japan

The incidence and epidemiologic features of Kawasaki disease were reported from nationwide surveys in Japan from 1970 to 1990.[39] The total number of cases was 116,848 and the number of affected children increased year by year. There were outbreaks in 1979, 1982, and 1986. The fatality rate decreased from 1% in 1974 to 0.04% in 1992. A 2-year survey from January 1991 through December 1992 indicated that in Japan 11,221 cases were reported, with a yearly incidence rate of 90 cases per 100,000 children.[40] The incidence of Kawasaki disease in Japan is 10 times higher than that in Western countries.

In a long-term Japanese study, 594 children with acute Kawasaki disease were followed for 10 to 21 years.[41] The diagnosis was made between 1973 and 1983 before the use of high-dose intravenous gamma globulin. The results of cardiac evaluation were normal in 448 children and remained normal on follow-up. Coronary angiography demonstrated coronary aneurysms in 146 (24.6%) just after the acute phase. Repeat coronary angiography one to two years later revealed that 72 (49.3%) of these patients had regression of the aneurysms. At 10 to 21 years after the onset of the disease, stenosis in the area of the aneurysm developed in 28 patients. Stenotic lesions developed in 12 of 26 patients with giant coronary aneurysm. Myocardial infarction complicated the late course of the disease in 11 patients. Systemic arterial aneurysm occurred in 2.2% and valvular heart disease in 1.2%.[41] The prevalence of coronary artery disease has been reduced significantly with high-dose intravenous gamma globulin therapy and with aspirin given early in the course of the disease.[42,43] Compared with aspirin therapy alone, intravenous gamma globulin with aspirin reduces coronary artery abnormalities by about threefold at 2 weeks and by fivefold at 7 weeks after initiation of therapy.[44]

Kawasaki Disease in Developed Countries Other Than Japan

In the United States, there was a trend toward increasing numbers of patients with Kawasaki disease after 1986, perhaps related to increased physician awareness of clinical features of the disease.[23]

In Sweden, the annual incidence rate was calculated to be 2.9 cases per 100,000 children younger than 16 years and 6.2 cases per 100,000 children younger than 5 years.[45] Epidemiologic data on Kawasaki disease from Finland in patients studied from April 1982 to March 1992 were reported by Salo.[46] The annual attack rate varied from 3.1 to 7.2 cases per 100,000 children under the age of 5 years. Coronary artery lesions were found in 28 of 229 patients, 2 of whom died of myocardial infarction. Race-specific incidence rates of Kawasaki disease were reported from three counties in the state of Washington from 1985 to 1989.[47] Rates were highest among Asian Americans (33.3 cases per 100,000 children younger than 5 years) but were less than in Japan, followed by blacks and whites (23.4 and 12.7/100,000 children under 5, respectively).

A report of the incidence of Kawasaki disease

in Northern Ireland covered the period from 1985 to 1991.[48] The number of cases increased until 1988, when the incidence was 19 cases per 1,000,000 under age 16 years, the highest from any region in the United Kingdom. There was a high incidence of cardiovascular complications in the affected children in Northern Ireland, with proximal coronary artery dilatation or aneurysm in 40%. Pericardial effusion was detected by two-dimensional echocardiography in 17.7%. One year after the onset of the disease, 53% of the children initially affected by coronary disease had persistent coronary artery disease without myocardial infarction or death. In South Australia the epidemiologic data for Kawasaki disease were similar to those from other Australian and New Zealand centers as well as those from North America.[49]

Human Immunodeficiency Virus Infection

The worldwide pandemic due to infection with HIV has become a major public health problem, which is taking a tremendous toll in personal suffering and economic devastation. Heterosexual acquisition has resulted in an increasing number of HIV-infected women of childbearing age. Since vertical transmission (mother to child) is the most frequent mode of infection in children, there is a parallel increase in HIV-infected children. It is estimated that by the year 2000, 10 million children will be infected with HIV, especially in Africa, South and Southeast Asia, and South America.[50,51] A high risk of transmission from contaminated blood and blood products remains in countries where donated blood is not tested for the presence of HIV. This mode of transmission has been highlighted by the large number of infected children in Romania.[52]

Globally, 21 million people are living with various subtypes of the virus; more than 1 million have clinical AIDS, and 8,500 join the ranks daily[53,54]; 90% of HIV-infected people live in the developing world. In some countries in Asia and Africa, one of three urban young and middle-aged adults may be infected, resulting in illness and death from AIDS, which can threaten economies, health systems, and national stability.[53] Since the HIV infection crosses all borders—geographic, social,

cultural, and economic—the current scale of international travel can result in the spread of the epidemic from heavily affected countries.

The global AIDS epidemic has been volatile and ever-expanding. The impact of the epidemic on women who may transmit the virus to their offspring has increased dramatically.

The number of HIV-infected children worldwide is 3,198,000, distributed in the following geographic areas: 672,000 in sub-Saharan Africa, 380,000 in Southeast Asia, 79,000 in Latin America, 36,000 in the Caribbean, 18,000 in North America, 9,000 in Western Europe and from 2,000 to less than 1,000 in each of Northeast Asia, Oceania, Eastern Europe, and Southeast Mediterranean.[54] As of January 1, 1996, 2,289,000 children had died of AIDS, with the largest numbers in the following geographic areas: 1,999,000 in sub-Saharan Africa, 194,000 in Southeast Asia, 27,000 in the Caribbean, 6,000 in North America, and 2,000 in Western Europe.[54]

Worldwide, an estimated 124.1 cases per 100,000 children are estimated to be HIV-infected but have not yet developed AIDS, with the largest concentrations in sub-Saharan Africa (562.5/100,000), the Caribbean (218.5/100,000), Southeast Asia (86.4/100,000), North America (52.4/100,000) and Western Europe (26.2/100,000).[54] As of January 1, 1996, the worldwide prevalence of AIDS in children was 9.0 cases per 100,000, with the largest concentration in sub-Saharan Africa (42.0/100,000).[54]

HIV Infection in Asia

An explosive increase in HIV infection has occurred in certain Asian countries, including Thailand, Myanmar (Burma), and India.[55,56] A sequence of infection is passage of the virus from female sex workers to their male clients, who in turn infect their wives and subsequently their children. Significant numbers of Asian men have sex with relatively small numbers of sex workers, and most women are abstinent before marriage and monogamous afterward.[50]

Recent events are encouraging. In Thailand there has been a reduction in the incidence and prevalence of HIV infection in young men attributed to prevention efforts focused on safer sexual and drug-related behavior.[53] A gratifying decrease in the rate of HIV infection has occurred in northern Thailand. Nelson et al.[57] studied 4,311 men conscripted into the army. The prevalence of HIV infection fell from about 13% to 6.7% during the four-year study period which the authors attributed to the fact that brothel owners and sex workers insisted that their clients use condoms. However, other public health programs could have influenced sexual behavior in Thailand, such as programs to educate people about HIV infection by broadcast media and school curricula, as well as in workplaces and health centers.[50] At the same time, illness and death from AIDS became more prevalent, so that knowledge of the ravages of HIV infection was personalized by men and women having relatives or acquaintances who were sick or had died from AIDS.

In other Asian countries, such as Indonesia, the Philippines, and Bangladesh, the predicted rapid spread of HIV infection has not occurred, even though the virus has been there for many years and commercial sex is common. It has been suggested that a contributing factor is that many men in these Muslim and Catholic societies are circumcised, which apparently reduces the rate of female-to-male transmission.[58] The practice of circumcision is uncommon in most Asian countries, where there is rapid sexual spread of HIV.[50] Few data are available about HIV infection in China, where it is said to be limited to intravenous drug users, sex workers, and their partners in the rural border regions of Yunnan province.[50]

Worldwide Data

As of mid-1993, over 13 million adolescents and adults had become infected with HIV, the majority through heterosexual intercourse, and about 1 million children had become infected perinatally.[59] Conservative worldwide estimates indicate that by the year 2000, 30 to 110 million people will be infected with HIV. In comparison, the "Black Death" killed about 25 million in the fourteenth century.[60]

HIV Infection in Russia and the Former Soviet Republics

At present the spread of HIV infection in Russia, Ukraine, and Belarus is a part of the epidemic of intravenous drug abuse. As in other countries, the spread of the virus is expected to be explosive because of the potential collapse of the health-care system, a growing female sex worker industry, drug abuse, and migration. In the Ukraine, a country of 51 million, 8449 HIV-positive cases have been reported since 1987, of which 8,256 were reported in 1995 and early 1996.[61] In Russia 387 HIV-positive cases were identified in the first part of 1996, which is double the 1995 rate. In the city of Svetlahorsk, Belarus, with 72,000 residents, intravenous drug abuse has resulted in at least 514 HIV-infected people from June to September 1996, and it is estimated that half the 7,000 drug abusers are infected.[61] The epidemic in Belarus could eventually cause more devastation than the nuclear accident in Chernobyl.[61]

United States

The actual number of people infected with HIV in the United States is difficult to estimate, because only cases of AIDS (not HIV infection) are reportable.[62] In the United States as of October 31, 1995, 501,310 persons with AIDS had been reported to the Centers for Disease Control and Prevention (CDC).[63] The percentage of those who were women increased from 8% in 1981–1987 to 18% from 1993 to October 1995.[63] The AIDS epidemic is increasing rapidly among injection-drug users and heterosexual partners of HIV-infected people.[64,65] The epidemic continues to affect blacks and Hispanics disproportionately. Initially the AIDS epidemic was recognized in the Northeast and West,[66] and rates remain highest in the Northeast. The greatest proportionate increases of HIV infection have occurred in the South and Midwest, areas with the largest proportion of the total US population.[63]

Between 1978 and 1993, about 14,920 HIV-infected infants were born in the United States.[67] An estimated 12,240 of these children were living at the beginning of 1994, of whom 26% were under 2 years of age, 35% were aged 2 to 4 years, and 39% were aged 5 years or older. In 1993 about 6,530 HIV-infected women gave birth. Assuming a 25% mother-to-child transmission rate, an estimated 1,630 HIV-infected infants were born in the United States in 1993.[68]

A longitudinal natural history study of more than

2,000 children who had vertically transmitted HIV infection indicated that before the diagnosis of AIDS was established in these children, moderate symptoms developed in the second year of life.[69] These children remained with moderate symptoms for more than half of their expected lives. Since cardiovascular disease remains clinically silent in the majority of patients, the need for careful follow-up of cardiovascular abnormalities is underscored.

HIV Infection in Women

The age of onset of HIV infection in childbearing women has declined substantially.[68] The median age of women at the time of HIV infection was 34 years in 1978 and 26 years in 1990. This decline continues, so that in the mid-1990s HIV infection is frequently acquired by teenaged girls.

As the prevalence of HIV-positive women increases in the United States, the number of newborns infected by vertical transmission increases.[70,71] Annually about 7,000 HIV-positive women become pregnant in the United States, and 1,000 to 2,000 of their newborns become HIV-infected.[71] The ideal way to reduce vertical transmission of the virus is through prevention in women.[72] To date educational efforts for prevention of HIV infection have not been successful. The AIDS Clinical Trials Group (ACTG Protocol 076) showed that offering zidovudine treatment to pregnant HIV-positive women and to their newborns reduced the perinatal transmission rate from 25.5% to 8.3%.[73] The treatment costs for 100 HIV-positive pregnant women and their newborns are estimated to be $104,502. This cost is offset by the reduction of $1,701,333 from the decreased number of HIV-infected newborns, with a net savings of $1,596,831. This strategy would also be successful in sub-Saharan African developing countries, but health-care resources in these countries are limited.[74] Nevertheless, shortened courses of zidovudine therapy are planned or under way in developing African countries, including Burkina Faso, the Ivory Coast, South Africa, Tanzania, and Uganda.[75]

Among pregnant women in São Paulo, Brazil, the rate of HIV infection increased six-fold in the 3 years from 1987 to 1990.[76] In Mexico the ratio of HIV-infected men to HIV-infected women decreased from 25:1 in 1984 to 4:1 in 1990.[76]

In cities in Uganda, where the prevalence of infection is among the highest in the world, the number of HIV-infected pregnant women is lower now than 5 years ago.[53] HIV prevalence in pregnant women is below 1% in North America, Western Europe and many Latin American countries.[77–79] High levels of HIV infection have been found in pregnant women in urban areas of Rwanda (33%), Uganda (29%), Malawi (23%), and Zambia (33.6%).[80]

Orphans and the HIV Epidemic

The number of children whose parents have died of AIDS exceeds 4 million and is steadily rising.[54] In the United States, as in other countries, the number of women infected with HIV is growing exponentially. Women are usually the primary caregivers and decision-makers for the children, with the majority of children being uninfected. Many of these women are low-income single parents living in poor housing.[81] When mothers die of AIDS, their children are at high risk for economic deprivation as well as behavioral and developmental problems.[82]

In the United States, by the turn of the century, the mothers of 72,000 to 125,000 children and adolescents will have died from AIDS.[83] Between 80% and 90% of these orphans will be from economically poor African-American or Latino families. After the death of the parent, usually the mother, children live with guardians, usually grandmothers or aunts. Their understanding of the meaning of death is associated with the child's developmental stage.[84] A major problem faced by guardians of these orphans is that financial benefits and services available to parents while they are alive are no longer available to their orphans, especially the HIV-uninfected child. These financial benefits include support for housing including rent subsides to help keep families together and to develop new stable family units.[82]

The Economic Cost of Pediatric Acquired Heart Disease

Although there is significant information on the epidemiology of rheumatic heart disease and Kawasaki disease, the data on their economic impact are sparse. The detrimental psychosocial effects of chronic rheumatic heart disease have been reported, but their economic costs are generally not clear. However, there is a growing literature on estimates of the economic costs of HIV infection.[54,60,85] By the turn of the century, the cost to the global economy of the HIV pandemic could reach $514 billion, and in the worst-case scenario, could amount to 1.4% of the world gross domestic product, equivalent to the economy of Australia or India.[60,86] Productivity in areas where the incidence of HIV infection is rising exponentially will continue to be affected negatively, because AIDS causes severe illness and death in young adults (aged 25–44 years) during their most productive years.

Personal suffering, family disruption, and the impact on the community have been horrific.[59] The impact of the HIV pandemic continues to worsen. As of January 1, 1996, 20 million people worldwide were living with HIV infection and over 1 million had clinical AIDS.[54] The estimated global cost for medical care has reached $11.6 billion of which 94% is spent for therapy in industrialized countries.[54] The financial resources for medical and preventive care are limited in developing countries, especially Asia and Africa, where most HIV-infected people live.

Economic Costs in the United States

By mid-1995 $75 billion had been spent on HIV infection and AIDS in the United States, with $3 to $6 billion spent annually on the management of new cases.[86] It is estimated that by the year 2000, $81 to $107 billion will have been siphoned off from the economy of the United States.[54,85,86] Since 1986, life and health insurance claims for HIV infection and AIDS have risen 400% to an estimated total of $9.4 billion.[86] In 1994, the cost of HIV infection to the insurance industry was nearly $1.6 billion.[86] These costs do not include losses from decreased productivity and earnings of the HIV-infected person whose disease is progressing to AIDS. The lifetime costs of medical management of a patient with HIV infection or AIDS is $119,000.[86] The enormous costs of social services

and medical care of orphans whose parents have died of AIDS is difficult to estimate.

Economic Costs in Sub-Saharan African Countries

The AIDS epidemic is devastating the economies of these African countries.[54,60,85,86] In 1993, the United Nations Development Program estimated that the HIV/AIDS epidemic had cost sub-Saharan African countries about $30 billion.[86] World Bank officials estimate that there will be an average drop in the growth of per capita income of 0.6% per year, as a result of the epidemic. The United Nations estimates that by the year 2010, illness and death from AIDS will reduce the overall African labor force by 25%. Foreign businesses in Africa have experienced increased worker absenteeism because of sickness due to AIDS or attendance at funerals of relatives and friends. In Kampala, Uganda, some companies are training two workers for each position because of absenteeism, hoping that one worker will be able to continue to work. The government of Uganda estimates that the 5% decline in two years in coffee production is due to in part to AIDS-related illness and death in workers.[86] In the Zambian copper belt, one of five miners is HIV-infected, and there is great concern that the spread of the disease will endanger the copper industry, which provides 95% of the country's foreign earnings.[86]

Cost of Care for HIV Infection and AIDS

With the explosive progression of the HIV pandemic, a new burden is imposed on already stressed health and social service systems.[87] HIV-infected people are now living longer, with increased costs in medical care. In the United States, the life expectancy of a patient with AIDS has nearly doubled since 1986 from 13 to 22 months.[88] HIV infection is now considered to be a chronic disease, and in many instances there is slow progression from HIV infection to AIDS to death. This adds significantly to the cost of medical care and social services.[87]

HIV-infected infants, children and women have special medical, psychosocial, and welfare needs, which are different from those of the adult male population.[54] In the United States, women generally have less access to medical care than men, and they have difficulties with transportation and arranging for child care.

Summary

Acquired heart disease in children continues to exact an awesome toll in personal suffering and economic deprivation. The more common causes of these acquired diseases are rheumatic fever and rheumatic heart disease, Kawasaki disease, and complications from human immunodeficiency viral (HIV) infection. Acute rheumatic fever and chronic rheumatic heart disease are common in developing countries. In industrialized countries these diseases have become rare and the incidence continues to decline except for scattered, localized outbreaks due to the appearance of uncommon serotypes of group A streptococci. The major cardiovascular complication of Kawasaki disease is vasculitis, especially involving the coronary arteries. The disease continues to be frequent in Japan. Longitudinal studies in children infected with HIV have shown that the cardiovascular system is frequently involved with left ventricular dysfunction emerging as the common abnormality. The worldwide increase in the number of HIV-infected children has the potential of greatly increasing the incidence of acquired pediatric heart disease as a complication of HIV infection.

References

1. Lipshultz SE. Cardiovascular problems. In: Pizzo PA, Wilfert CM (eds). *Pediatric AIDS*. Baltimore: Williams &Wilkins, 1994:483–511.

2. Lipshultz SE, Chanock S, Sanders SP, et al. Cardiovascular manifestations of human immunodeficiency infection in infants and children. *Am J Cardiol* 1989;63:1489–1497.

3. Kaplan S, Lipshultz SE. Cardiovascular complications of HIV infection in children. *Cardiol Rev* 1995;32:99–105.

4. Tovo PA, de Martino M, Gabiano C, et al. Prognostic factors and survival in children with perinatal HIV-1 infection. *Lancet* 1992;339:1249–1253.

5. Arguedas A, Mohs E. Prevention of rheumatic fever in Costa Rica. *J Pediatr* 1992;121:569–572.

6. Kaplan EL. Global assessment of rheumatic fever and rheumatic heart disease at the close of the century. [T. Duckett Jones Memorial Lecture]. *Circulation* 1993;88:1961–1972.

7. Fleming DS, Hirschboeck FJ, Cosgriff JA. Minnesota rheumatic fever survey, 1955. *Minn Med* 1956; 39:208–213.

8. Gordis L. The virtual disappearance of rheumatic fever in the United States: lessons in the rise and fall of disease. [T. Duckett Jones Memorial Lecture]. *Circulation* 1985;72:1155–1162.

9. Land MA, Bisno AL. Acute rheumatic fever: a vanishing disease in suburbia. *JAMA* 1983;249: 895–898.

10. Kaplan EL, Markowitz M. The fall and rise of rheumatic fever in the United States: a commentary. *Int J Cardiol* 1988;21:3–10.

11. Holmberg SD, Faich FA. Streptococcal pharyngitis and acute rheumatic fever in Rhode Island. *JAMA* 1983;250:2307–2312.

12. Veasy LG, Wiedmeier SE, Orsmond GS, et al. Resurgence of acute rheumatic fever in the Intermountain Area of the United States. *N Engl J Med* 1987;316:421–427.

13. Hosier DM, Craenen J, Teske DW, et al. Resurgence of rheumatic fever. *Am J Dis Child* 1987; 111:730–733.

14. Congeni B, Rizzo C, Congeni J, et al. Outbreak of acute rheumatic fever in Northeast Ohio. *J Pediatr* 1987;111:176–179.

15. Wald ER, Dashefsky B, Feidt C, et al. Acute rheumatic fever in western Pennsylvania and the tristate area. *Pediatrics* 1987;80:371–374.

16. Westlake RM, Graham TP, Edwards KM. An outbreak of acute rheumatic fever in Tennessee. *Pediatr Infect Dis J* 1990;9:97–100.

17. Griffiths SP, Gersony WM. Acute rheumatic fever in New York City (1969–1988): a comparative study of two decades. *J Pediatr* 1990;116:882–887.

18. Wallace MR, Garst PD, Papadimos TJ, et al. The return of acute rheumatic fever in young adults. *JAMA* 1989;262:2557–2561.

19. Centers for Disease Control. Acute rheumatic fever at a Navy training center: San Diego, California. *MMWR* 1988;37:101–104.

20. Centers for Disease Control. Acute rheumatic fever among army trainees: Fort Leonard Wood, Missouri. 1987–1988. *MMWR* 1988;37:519–522.

21. Kaplan EL, Johnson DR, Cleary PP. Group A streptococcal serotypes isolated from patients and sibling contacts during the resurgence of rheumatic fever in the United States in the mid 1980's. *J Infect Dis* 1989;159:101–103.

22. Johnson DR, Stevens DL, Kaplan EL. Epidemiologic analysis of group A streptococcal serotypes associated with severe systemic infections, rheumatic fever, or uncomplicated pharyngitis. *J Infect Dis* 1992;166:374–382.

23. Taubert KA, Rowley AH, Shulman ST. Seven-year national survey of Kawasaki disease and acute rheumatic fever. *Pediatr Infect Dis J* 1994;13:704–708.

24. Agarwal BL. Rheumatic heart disease unabated in developing countries. *Lancet* 1981;2:910–911.

25. Markowitz M. Observations on the epidemiology and preventability of rheumatic fever in developing countries. *Clin Ther* 1981;4:240–251.

26. Stollerman GH. Rheumatogenic group A streptococci and the return of rheumatic fever. *Adv Intern Med* 1990;35:1–26.

27. World Health Organization. Community prevention and control of cardiovascular diseases: report of a WHO expert committee. *WHO Tech Rep Ser* 1986; 732:1–62.

28. Rotta J, Tikhomirov E. Streptococcal diseases worldwide: present status and prospects. *Bull WHO* 1987;65:769–777.

29. World Health Organization and Principal Investigators. WHO programme for the prevention of rheumatic fever/rheumatic heart disease in 16 developing countries: a report from phase I (1986–1990). *Bull WHO* 1992;70:213–218.

30. Martin DR, Meeking FG, Finch LA. Streptococci: are they different in New Zealand? *NZ Med J* 1983;96:298–301.

31. Neutze JM. The third international conference on rheumatic fever and rheumatic heart disease. *NZ Med J* 1988;101:387–393.

32. Abegaz B. Diagnostic utility of echocardiography in Ethiopia. *Ethiop Med J* 1989;27:129–134.

33. Kassem AS, Zaher SR. An international comparison of the prevalence of streptococcal infections and rheumatic fever in children. *Pediatr Annu* 1992; 21:835–842.

34. Kassem AS, Badr Eldin MD, Abdel Moneim MA, Al Azzouni OF. The pattern of rheumatic fever in Alexandria with 10 years follow up of the valvular lesions. *Gaz Egypt Pediatr Assoc* 1982;30:69–78.

35. El Sharif A. The epidemiological features of rheumatic fever and rheumatic heart disease in Egypt. *Bull Egypt Soc Cardiol* 1975;14:65–70.

36. Barry DMJ, Eastcott RC, Reed PJP, et al. Rheumatic fever outbreak in a school associated with M type 5 streptococci. *NZ Med J* 1983;96:14–15.

37. Martin DR. Rheumatogenic streptococci reconsidered. *NZ Med J* 1988;101:394–396.

38. McLaren MJ, Hawkins DM, Koornhof HS, et al. Epidemiology of rheumatic heart disease in black school children of Soweto, Johannesburg. *BMJ* 1975;3:474–478.

39. Yanagawa H, Yashiro M, Nakamura Y, et al. Results of 12 nationwide epidemiological incidence surveys of Kawasaki disease in Japan. *Arch Pediatr Adolesc Med* 1995;149:779–783.

40. Yanagawa H, Yashiro M, Nakamura Y, et al. Epidemiologic pictures of Kawasaki disease in Japan: from the nationwide incidence survey in 1991 and 1992. *Pediatrics* 1995;95:475–479.

41. Kato H, Sugimura T, Akagi T, et al. Long-term consequences of Kawasaki Disease: a 10- to 21-year follow-up study of 594 patients. *Circulation* 1996;94:1379–1385.

42. Newberger JW, Takahashi M, Burns JC, et al. The treatment of Kawasaki syndrome with intravenous gamma globulin. *N Engl J Med* 1986;315:341–347.

43. Rowley AH, Duffy CE, Shulman ST. Prevention of giant coronary aneurysms in Kawasaki disease by intravenous gamma globulin therapy. *J Pediatr* 1988;113:290–294.

44. Newberger JW. Kawasaki syndrome. In: Fyler DC (ed). *Nadas' Pediatric Cardiology.* Philadelphia: Hanley and Belfus, 1992:319–327.

45. Schiller B, Fasth A, Bjorkhem G, et al. Kawasaki disease in Sweden: incidence and clinical features. *Acta Paediatr* 1995;84:769–774.

46. Salo E. Kawasaki disease in Finland in 1982–1992. *Scand J Infect Dis* 1993;25:497–502.

47. Davis RL, Waller PL, Mueller BA, et al. Kawasaki syndrome in Washington State: race-specific incidence rates and residential proximity to water. *Arch Pediatr Adolesc Med* 1995;149:66–69.

48. Casey F, Craig B, Shanks D, et al. Kawasaki disease: the Northern Ireland experience. *Irish J Med Sci* 1993;162:397–400.

49. Smith PK, Goldwater PN. Kawasaki disease in Adelaide: a review. *J Paediatr Child Health* 1993; 29:126–131.

50. Weniger BC, Brown T. The march of AIDS through Asia. *N Engl J Med* 1996;335:343–344.

51. Chin J. Epidemiology: current and future dimensions of the HIV/AIDS pandemic in women and children. *Lancet* 1990;336:221–224.

52. World Health Organization/EC Collaborating Centre on AIDS 1993. AIDS Surveillance in Europe. Paris: *WHO Q Rep* 1993;39.

53. Piot P. AIDS: a global response. *Science* 1996; 272:1855.

54. Mann J, Tarantola DJM. *AIDS in the World II*. New York: Oxford University Press, 1996.

55. Weniger BC, Limpakarnjanarat K, Ungchusak K, et al. The epidemiology of HIV infection and AIDS in Thailand. *AIDS* 1991;5:S71–S85.

56. Brown T, Xenos P. AIDS in Asia: the gathering storm. *Asia Pac Iss Anal East-West Cent.* 1994; 16:1–15.

57. Nelson KE, Celentano DD, Eiumtrakol S, et al. Changes in sexual behavior and a decline in HIV infection among young men in Thailand. *N Engl J Med* 1996;335:297–303.

58. Moses S, Plummer FA, Bradley JE, et al. The association between lack of male circumcision and risk for HIV infection: a review of the epidemiological data. *Sex Transm Dis* 1994;21:201–210.

59. Merson MH. Slowing the spread of HIV: agenda for the 1990's. *Science* 1993;260:1266–1268.

60. Pertersen JL. *The Road to 2015: Profiles of the Future*. Corte Madera, CA: Waite Group Press, 1994.

61. Boudreaux R. HIV now haunts streets of former Soviet model city. *Los Angeles Times* 1996;29 Sep: A1, A14.

62. Karon JM, Rosenberg PS, McQuillan G, et al. Prevalence of HIV infection in the United States, 1984 to 1992. *JAMA* 1996;276:126–131.

63. Centers for Disease Control. First 500,000 AIDS cases: United States, 1995. *MMWR* 1995;44: 849–853.

64. Centers for Disease Control. Update: trends in AIDS among men who have sex with men—United States, 1989–1994. *MMWR* 1995;44:401–444.

65. Centers for Disease Control. Update: trends in AIDS diagnosis and reporting under the expanded surveillance definition for adolescents and adults—United States, 1993. *MMWR* 1994;43:826–831.

66. Centers for Disease Control. Follow-up on Kaposi's sarcoma and Pneumocystis pneumonia. *MMWR* 1981;30:409–410.

67. Davis SF, Byers RH, Lindegren ML, et al. Prevalence and incidence of vertically acquired HIV infection in the United States. *JAMA* 1995;247: 952–955.

68. Rosenberg PS, Biggar RJ, Goedert JJ, et al. Declining age at HIV infection in the United States. [Letter]. *N Engl J Med* 1994;330:789.

69. Barnhart HX, Caldwell B, Thomas P, et al. Natural history of human immunodeficiency virus disease in perinatally infected children: an analysis from the Pediatric Spectrum of Disease Project. *Pediatrics* 1996;97:710–716.

70. Mauskopf JA, Paul JE, Wichman DS, et al. Economic impact of treatment of HIV-positive pregnant women and their newborns with zidovudine. *JAMA* 1996;276:132–138.

71. Centers for Disease Control. *National HIV Serosurveillance Summary: Results Through 1992*. Atlanta, GA: US Department of Health and Human Services, Public Health Service, 1994:vol 3.

72. Stein Z. HIV prevention: an update on the status of methods women can use. *Am J Public Health* 1993;83:1379–1382.

73. Connor EM, Sperling RS, Gelber R, et al. for the Pediatric AIDS Clinical Trials Group Protocol 076 Study Group. Reduction of maternal-infant transmission of human immunodeficiency virus type I with zidovudine treatment. *N Engl J Med* 1994; 331:1173–1180.

74. Mansergh G, Haddix AC, Steketee RW, et al. Cost-effectiveness of short-course zidovudine to prevent perinatal HIV type 1 infection in a sub-Saharan African developing country setting. *JAMA* 1996; 276:139–145.

75. Cohen J. Bringing AZT to poor countries. *Science* 1995;269:624–626.

76. Mann J, Tarantola DJM, Netter TW. *AIDS in the World*. Cambridge, MA: Harvard University Press, 1992.

77. Wasser SC, Gwinn M, Fleming P. Urban-nonurban distribution of HIV infection in childbearing women in the United States. *J Acquir Immune Defic Syndr* 1993;6:1035–1042.

78. Brossard Y, Larsen M, Meyer L, et al. HIV epidemiological trends (1987–1991) among pregnant women in the Paris area. [Abstract]. *Proc Int Conf AIDS* 1993;9:WS-CO4-I.

79. Chrystie IL, Palmer SJ, Kenny A, et al. HIV seroprevalence among women attending antenatal clin-

ics in London. [Abstract]. *Proc Int Conf AIDS* 1992;8:PoC 4360.

80. Vuylsteke B, Sunkutu R, Laga M. Epidemiology of HIV and sexually transmitted infections in women. In: Mann J, Tarantola DJM (eds). *AIDS in the World II*. New York: Oxford University Press, 1996:97–109.

81. Mok JQY. *HIV Infection In Children*. Cambridge, UK: Cambridge University Press, 1995.

82. Levine C. In whose care and custody?: orphans of the HIV epidemic. *AIDS Clin Care* 1995;7:66–70.

83. Michaels D, Levine C. Estimates of the number of motherless children orphaned by AIDS in the United States. *JAMA* 1992;268:3456–3461.

84. Lewis M. The special case of the uninfected child in the HIV-affected family: normal developmental tasks and the child's concern about illness and death. In: Geballe S, Gruendel J, Andiman W, et al. (eds). *Forgotten Children of the AIDS Epidemic.* New Haven, CT: Yale University Press, 1995: 50–63.

85. Garrett L. *The Coming Plague*. New York: Penguin Books, 1994.

86. Oldham J. The economic cost of AIDS. *Los Angeles Times* 1995;13 Oct.

87. Martin AL. The cost of HIV/AIDS Care. In: Mann J, Tarantola DJM (eds). *AIDS in the World II,* Vol 2. New York: Oxford University Press, 1996: 390–413.

88. Hellinger FJ. Lifetime cost of treating a person with HIV. *JAMA* 1993;270:474–478.

30

Mending A Broken Heart: A Mother's Perspective

Ms. Barrie Wing and Nancy Karthas, R.N.

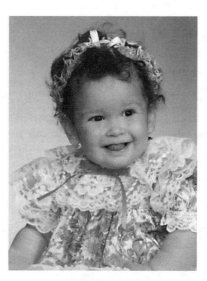

I want to start by telling you about my goals and dreams. I was married in 1980 to my high-school sweetheart and we had a daughter, Heather Ann. The marriage didn't last long. We were both young and we got divorced. I went back to nursing school and started working at a local hospital, a job that I loved.

In 1988, I went to Edgehill, which is a treatment center for drug addiction, for 28 days for my habit of smoking cocaine. After discharge from Edgehill, I continued to work at the hospital. I met "Bear," my present husband, at Narcotics Anonymous meetings. We got married in 1991. We both wanted a new family with at least two more children and a house, the great American Dream!

We tried for a couple of months to get pregnant and finally it happened! This would be Bear's first child. We had put money in the bank and both had good jobs so the house would be next. Heather was also excited about having a new baby brother or sister.

This pregnancy wasn't as easy as my first. I chalked that up to being 10 years older. I developed a rash everywhere and started with diarrhea. Toward the end of my pregnancy, I was retaining fluid and was told to stay in bed as much as possible. That was not easy. I was still working and had Heather to care for and the house to maintain. However, it didn't matter what problems I was having, I was still excited about the pending arrival of my new baby. We had decorated the baby's room completely in Winnie-the-Pooh style. At this point in my life, I was able financially to give our new baby everything I hadn't been able to give Heather, not to mention that I was more stable and more mature.

The joyous and long awaited night *and* day arrived. I was in labor for 15 hours. Bear and my mother stayed with me the whole time. During Alicia's delivery, my platelet count dropped to 22,000. They were considering transfusing me but didn't. On January 26, 1992, Alicia Marie Wing was born! I immediately breastfed my beautiful, healthy, 7 lb 14 oz baby girl. Alicia was a little jaundiced at birth and went under the bili-lights.

My gynecologist said we would just watch my

platelets. My platelets did not rise, so I was referred to a hematologist and told to be careful not to cut myself. He took a brief history. Because of Bear's past history of IV drug use, I asked the hematologist if this could be a symptom of HIV. I was told "no." He stated that he had seen only two cases that turned out to be HIV-related. I had more blood work done and an abdominal CT scan to rule out an enlarged spleen. He ordered a bone marrow and his diagnosis was ITP [idiopathic thrombocytopenic purpura]. His suggestion was to have my spleen removed. At the time I had just gone back to work and couldn't afford to take any more time off. I also could not, and would not, take this time away from my new baby. It would also mean Bear would have to take time off work to help with Heather. My alternative was high doses of prednisone, which meant I had to stop breastfeeding. I felt like a failure and missed that special bond I had with Alicia at feeding time. It seemed that every week we would visit the pediatrician's office. Alicia developed thrush, and the suggested treatment was to wipe her tongue with the rough side of her face cloth. That did not work. We tried nystatin swabs and then gentian violet. Nothing seemed to resolve it completely. I thought I wasn't sterilizing her bottles enough; again, I thought I had failed her just as I had with the breastfeeding.

Alicia started spiking temperatures. Back and forth to the doctor's again. She had chest x-rays and blood work done. The doctor thought she might have some kind of viral pneumonia because her white blood cell count was low and she hadn't responded to the multitude of antibiotics they had prescribed.

What could be wrong with my baby? She was going through so much poking, prodding, and blood work. She was a "little chub chub" and most of her milestones were on time. Despite these problems, she remained cheerful. When I prepared supper I would sing to her and tell her how to cook things. That was "our time" together.

In August 1992 I came home from work and noticed Alicia's eyes were a little yellow and she had another fever. That was it. I took her to the doctor's office again. The pediatrician who was there this time was also an immunologist. I described to him the problems that she had been hav-

ing, and when I finished, he asked my other daughter Heather to leave the room. I was so scared my heart was pounding a mile a minute. He told me he thought Alicia should be tested for HIV! My heart sank to my feet, and I just looked at him as he started explaining why he thought it might be wise. Alicia was admitted that night. Heather and I were crying, and I called Bear at work to come to the hospital.

Bear kept trying to reassure me that she couldn't be HIV-positive. I continuously prayed, "Please God, don't let my baby have AIDS—please." We had to wait a full week for the results while she stayed in the hospital. I stayed with her constantly and Bear would come when he wasn't working. I did take a break here and there to be with Heather. Needless to say, we didn't tell any family or friends what was being questioned.

Then came that fateful morning. The doctor did his rounds on the floor and passed our door to save us for last. My heart was racing as he came in with the nurse and closed the door. "Alicia is positive for HIV." "Oh my God, are you sure? There can be no mistake?" How could God do this to my baby and our family! I hated God then. Bear and I had to go downstairs to the outpatient department to get tested. How humiliating! Of course, I knew I had to be positive, but did I get it from Bear? I was thinking that would have been easier for me to take because then I could blame him. But I thank God *now* he is negative. I carried all the guilt, shame, and remorse.

The very day she was diagnosed, she was sent to Children's Hospital in Boston by ambulance. That day had to be one of the longest days of my life. There was a constant stream of doctors, residents, fellows, medical students, nurses, and social workers all asking questions about Alicia's first seven months of life. It was all a blur. I don't know how I answered all the questions because I kept repeating, "This can't be happening." My baby was poked and prodded by all the medical staff. I remember her looking at me as if asking "Why are you letting them do this to me, Mommy?" It broke my heart.

This was to be Alicia's longest admission, two and a half months. During this stay, she had cytomegalovirus, hepatitis, cytomegalovirus pneumonitis, cytomegalovirus retinitis, and *Pneumocystis carinii* pneumonia. She also had a couple of bronchoscopies. They were unable to extubate her after one of them. Alicia spent two weeks in intensive care on a ventilator. That was very hard and heartbreaking to watch. I just wanted to hold her and make everything all right.

During the hospitalization, I stayed with Alicia Sunday night through Friday evening, and Bear would stay the weekends. We did not want her to ever wake up without one of us there. On the weekends I would go home to try and spend some quality time with Heather. My mother was suffering from bone cancer and was in and out of the hospital. I tried to be with my mother and help her when I could. Heather was being shuffled around a lot and she was not happy about all this so, she began acting out. I was also trying to come up with lies or untruths about what was wrong with Alicia. I had a hard time keeping track of what I told to who.

During the admission Bear and I made a decision to put Alicia on protocol 152, which was comparing zidovudine versus dideoxyinosine versus both zidovudine and dideoxyinosine. We made this decision knowing she would be watched more closely. We also enrolled her in the heart/lung study, which ended up helping her by performing echocardiograms, pulmonary function tests, and lung scans at regular intervals.

After being taken off the ventilator, Alicia had trouble eating so she had a nasogastric tube inserted. It was during this time that the doctors discovered Alicia had cytomegalovirus retinitis. She had to have a central line placed for her daily IV infusions. All during this nightmare, my baby was still able to laugh, smile, and definitely touch some hearts.

Finally her day of discharge, October 30, 1992, arrived. I must say I was scared but very happy. Alicia was to have 16 hours of nursing every day, weekly physical therapy, and weekly occupational therapy. Our home had a revolving door. Not much time or space for privacy, but my baby was home! Heather had a hard time with the privacy issue, and continued to be acting out in all the wrong ways. We also had a miniature schnauzer, Ashley, and a black cat, Shadow. Because of all I had read about pets and HIV, I felt we had to get rid of Ashley and Shadow. That was a hard thing for all of us,

but we knew it was the best thing to do for Alicia as well as my own health. It didn't take long for Bear and me to split up under all the stress. We were at each other's throats, so he moved out in December 1992.

In December I finally told my family about our diagnosis, and I told Heather in January. Heather was devastated, to say the least. She began running away, doing drugs, drinking, and doing poorly in school, and even stole my car (she was 12 years old) and got arrested. I tried all kinds of punishments and counseling, but even to this day nothing and no one has been able to reach her.

We all tried to get Alicia back to eating by mouth, but nothing worked. So she again was admitted to Children's Hospital for a G-tube placement. During that procedure, they discovered she had esophageal candidiasis, which meant a longer hospital stay.

Despite the difficulty in living with this diagnosis, I am very grateful that we enrolled Alicia in the heart/lung study, because they found she had a right lower lobe collapse. Chest physical therapy was initiated and the lobe did reinflate sporadically. Another potential problem was averted because of her participating in the heart/lung study. After a routine echocardiogram, it was determined that Alicia had developed cardiomyopathy. She had a cardiac catheterization with a biopsy to determine if she had any infection, such as cytomegalovirus, causing her cardiomyopathy. Because of the special nature of the procedure, she was admitted to a whole new floor. No one knew Alicia or that much about AIDS. After the biopsy, Alicia was treated with IV Lasix, IV digitalis, and enalapril until we were sure her stomach was absorbing the medications. Alicia received multiple blood transfusions when her heart rate was up and her hematocrit was down. We had to keep a close eye on that so her poor little heart was not under any undue strain. The next echocardiogram did show improvement, and we went back home again.

When she was at home, she went to school (Early Intervention) once a week for two hours with other toddlers. Boy, did she enjoy that! She was unable to walk but would kick her legs when she was excited, and we had special chairs to help her sit alone. She could speak a few words. In fact, her first word was "Heather." She used some sign language of her own to get her point across. It was such a joy seeing her interact with so-called normal kids.

My mother passed away on September 16, 1993, and shortly after that Alicia was admitted again, this time for pancreatitis. My poor baby was in such pain and in intensive care. We tried everything to make her comfortable. The only thing that helped was pain control medications and gut rest. We were told that this was the beginning of the end. This was another long admission, because we were trying to regulate her parenteral nutrition. She was hospitalized for Halloween, so I dressed her up like the angel she was. We went around to different floors saying, "Trick or treat, I can't eat." I decorated her room with all kinds of Halloween lights, she enjoyed that!

We finally went home, and now she had 24 hours of nursing a day. We needed it with all the medications being given IV, the total parenteral nutrition, and daily fingersticks to check her blood sugar.

Her last Thanksgiving came, and we went to my in-laws' house. She was very happy feeding her daddy and being around everyone. Christmas came and I hadn't bought anything in advance. We lived day by day, not knowing what was going to happen next. On Christmas Eve I decided it would be all right to go downstairs for a party. I figured I would still be close and the nurse could get me if there were any emergencies. Alicia had been spilling sugar in her urine. When I came home, her blood sugar was over seven hundred! She was miserable. Christmas was postponed for Alicia because she was feeling so lousy. We did go to my father's house but couldn't stay long. I vowed never to leave her again.

Alicia continued to have intermittent problems with pancreatitis, and we were using IV morphine to control the pain. She was still able to enjoy watching Barney and to play with all her new toys.

Her second birthday was coming up on January 26, so I planned a big "Barney Bash". We all knew this would be her last birthday, and I just prayed she would make it. I invited lots of kids and Barney too. Her pain seemed to worsen, and the morphine was increased. Her party was to be on a Sunday.

The Friday before her party, my Alicia stopped breathing in my arms from the morphine. I kept screaming "Not yet! Not yet!" and I tried to do cardiopulmonary resuscitation on her. Thank God the nurse was there. She took her from me and got her back with cardiopulmonary resuscitation. Alicia was rushed to Boston by ambulance.

I kept telling her doctor she had to get home for her party. Thanks to his perseverence, she was set up with a PCA pump, and sent home Saturday night. I still hadn't bought any food or gifts, so I ran around like a nut that night.

We had her party and it was a huge success! Alicia was afraid of Barney but got a kick out of watching the other kids with him. Her infectious disease nurse even came down from Boston. Alicia wasn't quite herself, but she was at home and with her family and friends.

Alicia's last admission lasted about three weeks. All that time was spent in intensive care due to respiratory syncytial virus, except for her last two days of life. This was a difficult time for her; she had to have ribavirin treatments three times a day and needed 100% oxygen. It was very difficult for me to hold her without her oxygen sats dropping. The subject of her code status came up quite often. That had to be the most difficult decision I ever had to make in my life. Finally, after three weeks of ribavirin and no change, Alicia got transferred to "her" floor in a private room. Bear stayed up with her most of her final night. She would ask to suck on her wet face cloth, and I tried to get some sleep.

After lying there for awhile, I just had this gut feeling that this was it. I got up around 6:00 A.M. and asked her nurse to help get her out of bed so I could rock her and hold her. She wasn't responding. I told my baby it was okay to go. I told her I loved her and would miss her, but she had gone through enough. Her heart rate and sats started dropping. Bear held her one last time. Her monitor was turned off. My baby, Alicia Marie, died in my arms at 8:15 a.m., March 16, 1994. Most of her nurses and doctors came to say their good-byes. I washed and dressed my baby for the last time.

I am thankful that one month before she died I went back to church and forgave God. He, and the belief that I will see her again, have been the biggest part of my healing. Initially, I tried to keep very busy. I did speaking for Pediatric AIDS and volunteered for committees and boards. I even went to Washington, D.C. a couple of times lobbying for pediatric AIDS. I also attended support groups and counseling. I found working on Alicia's quilt very healing. I can definitely say it hasn't been easy. I have tried to commit suicide a couple of times. I wanted to hurry up and be with my baby again. Now I realize that she was in my life for a reason, and she has taught me many lessons. I believe she has helped some doctors and nurses to see things a little differently as well.

Bear and I got back together. This has helped to mend my broken heart. We have that special bond and can share Alicia's memories. We also have a two-year-old German shepherd "Alicia's Rocky," and he has a very calming effect on me. It has been over two years since Alicia passed away, but not a day goes by that I don't think about her and miss her.

With this disease, you lose control of things a little at a time. It's hard enough fighting for your daughter's life without having to deal with people trying to control aspects of her treatment without involving you. I certainly learned the other side, going from nurse to mother of the patient.

I think one of the most important lessons to be learned is that doctors and nurses must listen to the child's mother. No one knows her child better than a mother. The other important message I hope to be learned is compassion—try putting yourself in my shoes and see if you just might have more compassion.

Index

ISBN 0-412-08861-4